WITHDRAWN

Clinical
Companion
for
PEDIATRIC
NURSING

3/11/10

Clinical
Companion
for
PEDIATRIC
NURSING

BONITA E. BROYLES, RN, BSN, MA, PhD
AUTHOR AND NURSING EDUCATION CONSULTANT
INSTRUCTOR
ADN PROGRAM
PIEDMONT COMMUNITY COLLEGE
PIEDMONT, NORTH CAROLINA

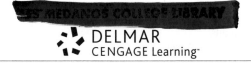

DELMAR
CENGAGE Learning™

Australia • Brazil • Japan • Korea • Mexico • Singapore • Spain • United Kingdom • United States

DELMAR
CENGAGE Learning™

Clinical Companion for Pediatric Nursing
Bonita E. Broyles

Vice President, Career and Professional Editorial: Dave Garza

Director of Learning Solutions: Matthew Kane

Senior Acquisitions Editor: Maureen Rosener

Managing Editor: Marah Bellegarde

Senior Product Manager: Elisabeth F. Williams

Editorial Assistant: Meaghan O'Brien

Vice President, Career and Professional Marketing: Jennifer McAvey

Senior Marketing Manager: Michele McTighe

Marketing Coordinator: Scott Chrysler

Director of Production: Carolyn Miller

Senior Content Project Manager: Stacey Lamodi

Senior Art Director: Jack Pendleton

Library of Congress Control Number: 2007938958

ISBN-13: 978-1-4283-0537-3

ISBN-10: 1-4283-0537-8

Delmar Cengage Learning
5 Maxwell Drive
Clifton Park, NY 12065-2919
USA

Cengage Learning products are represented in Canada by Nelson Education, Ltd.

For your lifelong learning solutions, visit **delmar.cengage.com**

Visit our corporate website at **www.cengage.com**

Notice to the Reader

Publisher does not warrant or guarantee any of the products described herein or perform any independent analysis in connection with any of the product information contained herein. Publisher does not assume, and expressly disclaims, any obligation to obtain and include information other than that provided to it by the manufacturer. The reader is expressly warned to consider and adopt all safety precautions that might be indicated by the activities described herein and to avoid all potential hazards. By following the instructions contained herein, the reader willingly assumes all risks in connection with such instructions. The publisher makes no representations or warranties of any kind, including but not limited to, the warranties of fitness for particular purpose or merchantability, nor are any such representations implied with respect to the material set forth herein, and the publisher takes no responsibility with respect to such material. The publisher shall not be liable for any special, consequential, or exemplary damages resulting, in whole or part, from the readers' use of, or reliance upon, this material.

Printed in Canada
1 2 3 4 5 XX 11 10 09 08

Contents

Appendices

PREFACE

The landscape of pediatric nursing is ever-changing. Caring for children and their families can be a challenging and rewarding endeavor. Technological advances, health care reform, length of hospital stays, increased acuity levels, and care delivered outside the acute setting all contribute to the fabric of the pediatric health care scene. Nurses must be prepared for these realities and strive to bring competency and knowledge to their practice. They must know how to think critically, in a problem-solving manner, while mastering knowledge about pediatric health alterations—all while working within the confines of demanding lives and schedules.

The reader's need for quick access to important information was the driving force in the creation of the user-friendly style and easy-to-follow presentation found in *Clinical Companion for Pediatric Nursing*. This clinical reference will serve both nursing students and practicing professional nurses. Students will appreciate its handy size and versatility as a quick reference for pediatric content in the clinical setting; for practicing nurses, it serves as an invaluable reference to help sharpen critical-thinking skills as well as to augment knowledge.

Clinical Companion for Pediatric Nursing is specifically designed to help readers learn to approach client care in a critical-thinking manner while gaining knowledge about pediatric health conditions. Each chapter focuses on a single health alteration, presenting material in a logical and consistent format:

Definition: A description of the disorder and its effects, including a brief review of anatomy and physiology specific to the topic.

Pathophysiology: A logical, easy-to-follow presentation of the pathophysiologic changes that result in the health alteration.

Complications: A listing of the most commonly encountered problems associated with the health alteration if treatment is not sought or is ineffective.

Incidence: The most current statistical data of occurrence, giving insight into how often the nurse may encounter the condition.

Etiology: A discussion of the identified causes of the condition or factors that place certain children at increased risk for the disorder.

Clinical Manifestations: A thorough explanation of the signs and symptoms the child exhibits as a result of the pathological process.

Diagnostic Tests: A presentation of diagnostic and laboratory tests used to diagnose the condition so the nurse can anticipate what family teaching may be required and what treatments may be prescribed.

Medical Management: A discussion of the medical and surgical standards of care in treating children with the condition.

Nursing Management: A presentation in the nursing process format. **Assessment** focuses on the data the nurse must collect and analyze in order to determine client needs. **Nursing Diagnoses** are drawn from the current NANDA listing and offer a starting point from which readers can customize care for a specific client. The nursing diagnoses are followed by associated **Planning/Goals**, written as realistic, measurable, and observable outcome criteria; accepted terminology from the *Nursing Outcomes Classification (NOC)* nomenclature is included with each condition. The **Implementation** section focuses on nursing interventions, including pertinent assessments the nurse should make while addressing identified client needs, as well as actions related to collaborative care; *Nursing Interventions Classification (NIC)* terminology supports these actions. Included as a part of the Implementation section for each entry is coverage of discharge teaching and home care. An **Evaluation** section rounds out each nursing management discussion.

References are included at the end of each chapter. The reference lists include extensive scholarly Internet resources for acquiring further information about each condition. These resources will help the reader in pursuing evidence-based practice, as many of these sites provide information about research, changes in health practices, and current clinical trials.

Nine appendices provide information on diagnostic tests, laboratory values, physical assessment, vital signs, growth and development, play, immunizations, common conversions, and abbreviations.

ABOUT THE AUTHOR

Dr. Broyles began her nursing career in obstetrics in 1968, when she began work as a student nursing assistant. She remained in this area through her graduation from The Ohio State University in 1970, with her BSN. She combined staff nursing and teaching in maternal-child for the next 11 years in Columbus, Ohio. In 1981, she changed her nursing focus to medical-surgical nursing, where she has been staffing and teaching since. In 1984, she and her husband relocated to North Carolina, where she continued her combined career in staff nursing and teaching.

In 1986, Dr. Broyles began teaching at Piedmont Community College in Roxboro, North Carolina, at which time she added another content focus—pediatrics. She has taught pediatric nursing for 21 years, as well as pharmacology and medical-surgical nursing. Her teaching career includes experience in Practical Nursing, Diploma, and Associate Degree Nursing education. The bedside nursing focus of ADN education is her career love.

Dr. Broyles received her Master of Arts degree from North Carolina Central University in 1988 and her Doctorate of Education from LaSalle University in 1996. In 2004 she completed her PhD in Education from St. Regis University. She has written a number of nursing texts including *Clinical Companion for Nursing of Children: Principles and Practice* (1997), *Pharmacological Aspects of Nursing Care* (6th and 7th editions, 2002 and 2007), *Dosage Calculation Practice for Nurses* (2003), *Medical-Surgical Nursing Clinical Companion* (2005), and *Case Studies in Pediatrics* (2006).

Dr. Broyles and her husband Roger reside in Creedmoor, North Carolina, and between them have five grown children and ten grandchildren.

ACKNOWLEDGMENTS

This text is dedicated to my husband, whose support and encouragement allowed this project to remain a work of heart from its conception to the finished product. This text also is dedicated to the nursing students (past, present, and future) at Piedmont Community College, who serve to inspire my writing.

A special thanks to the reviewers of this text for their expertise and passion for nursing care of children.

A special thanks also to Beth Williams at Delmar Cengage Learning for believing in this project. Thank you for the countless e-mails and phone calls and for your gentle support.

REVIEWERS

ABUSE

Definition

According to the Child Abuse Prevention and Treatment Act (CAPTA) amendments of 1996 (42 U.S.C.A. § 5106g), child abuse and neglect are defined as follows: "Any recent act or failure to act on the part of a parent or caretaker which results in death, serious physical or emotional harm, sexual abuse or exploitation; or an act or failure to act which presents an imminent risk of serious harm" (Child Welfare Information Gateway, 2006a, p. 1).

Pathophysiology

Most states in the United States recognize four major types of child abuse, including (1) neglect, (2) physical maltreatment, (3) sexual abuse, and (4) emotional abuse. Although any of the forms of abuse may occur separately, they often are found in combination. Some states' definitions are less rigid (but must maintain the minimum standards as defined in the federal law), and some states have more stringent definitions.

Neglect is defined as "failure to provide for a child's basic needs." Examples include physical neglect, such as failure to provide necessary food or shelter, or lack of appropriate supervision that could result in harm to the child; medical neglect, such as failure to provide for the necessary medical or mental health treatment of the child; educational neglect, or failure to provide education for a child or attend to the child's special education needs; and emotional neglect including not paying attention to a child's emotional needs, failing to provide psychological care, or permitting the child to use alcohol or other drugs. These situations do not always mean a child is neglected. "Sometimes cultural values, the standards of care in the community, and poverty may be contributing factors, indicating the family is in need of information or assistance. When a family fails to use information and resources, and the child's health or safety is at risk, then child welfare intervention may be required" (Child Welfare Information Gateway, 2006a, p. 1).

Physical abuse includes beating, kicking, shaking (as with shaken-baby syndrome), throwing, biting, stabbing, choking, burning, or hitting (with a hand or another object) that results in physical injury to the child. The injuries can range from minor bruises to severe fractures or death and are considered to be abuse regardless of whether the parent or caretaker intended to hurt the child (Child Welfare Information Gateway, 2006a).

Sexual abuse is defined by CAPTA as "the employment, use, persuasion, inducement, enticement, or coercion of any child to engage in, or assist any other person to engage in, any sexually explicit conduct or simulation of such conduct for the purpose of producing a visual depiction of such conduct; or the rape, and in cases of caretaker or interfamilial relationships, statutory rape, molestation, prostitution, or other form of sexual exploitation of children, or incest with children" (Child Welfare Information Gateway, 2006a, p. 1). Activities that also are included in this definition are the fondling of a child's genitals by a parent or caretaker, penetration, sodomy, and indecent exposure.

Emotional abuse involves behavior on the part of the parent or caretaker that impairs a child's emotional development or sense of self-worth. This may include constant criticism, threats, or rejection, as well as withholding of love, support, or guidance. The greatest difficulty is in proving that emotional abuse is occurring; but if it is suspected, other forms of abuse are likely present and may provide more solid manifestations that can be proven.

Complications

Physical wounds

Psychosocial wounds

Death

Incidence

According to the Administration for Children & Families of the U.S. Department of Health & Human Services, "An estimated 3.6 million children in the 50 States, the District of Columbia, and Puerto Rico received investigations by CPS (Child Protective Services) agencies" (Administration for Children & Families of the U.S. Department of Health & Human Services, 2007a, p. 1). Of those investigations, however, 60% were unsubstantiated. Further, the report states, "more than three-quarters (76.6%) of children who were killed (as a result of child maltreatment) were younger than 4 years of age, 13.4 percent were 4–7 years of age, 4.0 percent were 8–11 years of age, and 6.1 percent were 12–17 years of age. The youngest children experienced the highest rates of fatalities. Infant boys (younger than 1 year) had a fatality rate of 17.3 deaths per 100,000 boys of the same age. Infant girls (younger than 1 year) had a fatality rate of 14.5 deaths per 100,000 girls of the same age. In general, fatality rates for both boys and girls decreased as the children get older" (Administration for Children & Families of the U.S. Department of Health & Human Services, 2007b, p. 1).

Etiology

Child abuse and neglect cross all racial and socioeconomic groups. The etiologies of child abuse and neglect can be categorized according to (1) characteristics of the abused child, (2) characteristics of the abusive parent or caretaker, and (3) characteristics of the environment in which the abuse occurs. Characteristics of the child include (1) infants separated at birth from their parents because of prematurity, (2) infants who are chronically ill, (3) infants with fussy temperaments, (4) infants with developmental delays, (5) female children, who are 3 times as likely to experience sexual abuse, (6) male children, who are more likely to experience physical abuse or neglect, (7) children born into a large family unit with limited resources, and/or (8) children of the same sex as the abusing parent (Anbarghalami, Yang, Van Sell, & Miller-Anderson, 2007). Characteristics of the abusive parent or caregiver include (1) having a history of being abused as a child, (2) abusing alcohol or other substances, (3) having low self-esteem, (4) being a single parent (77% higher incidence of physical abuse), (5) having an annual income usually less than $15,000, (6) lacking knowledge about growth and development, (7) being in mid-20s to mid-30s, (8) lacking a high school education, and/or (9) lacking social supports (Potts & Mandleco, 2007). Environmental characteristics include (1) ethnic and racial prejudices, (2) poverty-level living conditions, (3) lack of family support, (4) lack of community resources, (5) poor access to health care, and/or (6) ineffective child protection laws and agencies.

Clinical Manifestations

GENERAL MANIFESTATIONS

THE CHILD

Exhibits sudden changes in behavior or school performance.

Has not received help for physical or medical problems brought to the parents' attention.

Exhibits learning problems (or difficulty concentrating) that cannot be attributed to specific physical or psychological causes.

Is always anxious.

Lacks adult supervision.

Is overly compliant, passive, or withdrawn.

Comes to school or other activities early, stays late, and does not want to go home.

THE PARENT OR OTHER ADULT CAREGIVER

Exhibits little concern for the child.

Denies the existence of—or blames the child for—the child's problems in school or at home.

Requests that teachers or other caretakers use harsh physical discipline if the child misbehaves.

Views the child as entirely bad, worthless, or burdensome.

Demands a level of physical or academic performance the child cannot achieve.

Views the child primarily as a source of care, attention, and satisfaction of their emotional needs.

THE PARENT AND CHILD

Seldom touch or make eye contact.

View their relationship as entirely negative.

Verbalize that they do not like each other.

MANIFESTATIONS OF PHYSICAL ABUSE

THE CHILD

Has unexplained burns.

Has burn marks that fit a particular pattern, such as a cigar or cigarette.

Has bruises or welts in the shape of a belt buckle or a hand.

Has teeth bite marks.

Has multiple fractures in varying stages of healing.

Shows bruising under the upper arm.

Shows bruising on the face and/or abdomen.

Has retinal hemorrhages (indicative of shaken-baby syndrome).

Has fading bruises or other marks noticeable after an absence from school.

Visits emergency department frequently for injuries.

Appears frightened of the parents and protests or cries when it is time to go home.

Is anxious when approached by adults.

Reports injury by a parent or another adult caregiver.

THE PARENT OR OTHER ADULT CAREGIVER

Offers a conflicting or unconvincing explanation or no explanation for the child's injury.

Does not maintain eye contact when asked about child's injuries.

Describes the child in a very negative way, such as "evil."

Uses harsh physical discipline with the child.

Has a history of being abused as a child.

Is usually a young adult in mid-20s to mid-30s.

Lacks a high school education.

MANIFESTATIONS OF EMOTIONAL ABUSE

THE CHILD

Exhibits extremes in behavior, such as overly compliant or demanding behavior, extreme passivity, or aggression.

Exhibits behaviors that are inappropriate for child's level of growth and development (parenting other children or frequently rocking or banging the head).

Exhibits physical or developmental delays.

Has suicidal ideation or has attempted suicide.

Reports a lack of attachment to the parent.

THE PARENT OR OTHER ADULT CAREGIVER

Constantly blames, belittles, or berates the child.

Appears unconcerned about the child.

Refuses to consider offers of help for the child's problems.

Is in obvious rejection of the child.

MANIFESTATIONS OF NEGLECT

THE CHILD

Exhibits frequent school absences.

Begs or steals food or money.

Lacks needed medical or dental care, immunizations, or glasses.

Exhibits consistently dirty appearance and has severe body odor.

Is inappropriately dressed for the weather.

Abuses alcohol or other drugs.

Denies the presence of anyone at home to provide care.

THE PARENT OR OTHER ADULT CAREGIVER

Shows indifference to the child.

Seems apathetic or depressed.

Exhibits irrational or bizarre behavior.

Abuses alcohol or other drugs.

MANIFESTATIONS OF SEXUAL ABUSE

THE CHILD

Exhibits difficulty walking or sitting.

Suddenly refuses to change for gym or to participate in physical activities.

Reports nightmares or enuresis.

Experiences a sudden change in appetite.

Exhibits bizarre, sophisticated, or unusual sexual knowledge or behavior.

Becomes pregnant or contracts a venereal disease, particularly when under 14 years of age.

Runs away from home.

Reports sexual abuse by a parent or another adult caregiver.

THE PARENT OR OTHER ADULT CAREGIVER

Is unduly protective of the child or severely limits the child's contact with other children, especially of the opposite sex.

Exhibits secretive and isolated behaviors.

Is jealous or controlling with family members.

(Adapted from Child Welfare Information Gateway, 2006b)

Diagnostic Tests

Radiography

Developmental testing

Ultrasonography

Magnetic resonance imaging (MRI)

Computed tomography

Head circumference

Abdominal circumference

Height and weight percentiles

Pregnancy screening

Screening for sexually transmitted disease

Cerebrospinal fluid analysis

Interview with child

Interview with child's teacher

Interview with parent or caretaker

Medical Management

The goals of treatment are to (1) manage the child's present condition and (2) activate resources to prevent further abuse or neglect. When a child is brought to the health care provider's office, health department, health clinic, or emergency department, treating the child's present physical condition is the priority of health care professionals. All of the injuries should be carefully documented with color photographs and recorded as specifically as possible. Once the child's condition has been stabilized, the suspicions of child abuse must be reported to the local child protective agency mandated by law. A referral to the facility's social services also should be completed. Many acute health care facilities that treat children have protocols regarding child abuse that include not allowing the parent to visit the child alone while in the facility. Data that should be assessed and documented include (1) location, color, size, and shape of any injury, (2) specific characteristics of bruise, including an outline and the depth of injury, (3) pain or tenderness associated with the injury, (4) complete assessment of all body systems, (5) general level of hygiene, (6) exact date, time, and place of event, (7) chronological account of injury, (8) witnesses present at time of injury, and (9) exact quotations by child and caregiver of how the injury occurred (Potts & Mandleco, 2007).

Nursing Management

ASSESSMENT

1. Obtain history, if possible
2. Assess for evidence of abuse or neglect
3. Obtain vital signs
4. Perform pediatric physical assessment
5. Assess interactions (verbal and nonverbal) between child and parent/caregiver

NURSING DIAGNOSES (INCLUDING BUT NOT LIMITED TO)

1. Risk for injury R/T evidence of abuse or neglect
2. Acute pain R/T injuries sustained as a result of abuse or neglect
3. Fear R/T abusive actions of parent/caregiver
4. Delayed growth and development R/T abuse and neglect
5. Impaired parenting R/T presence of characteristics that increase risk of abuse
6. Deficient knowledge R/T child's needs, growth and development, effective coping strategies, and community support services

PLANNING/GOALS

1. Client will be identified as having the potential for abuse or neglect before further injury occurs.
2. Client will demonstrate effective pain control through verbal and nonverbal behavior.
3. Client will verbalize feelings, fears, and concerns.
4. Client will achieve developmental milestones and highest level of wellness.
5. Family will identify and use effective coping strategies to prevent further abuse.
6. Family will demonstrate understanding of child's needs, growth and development, effective coping strategies, and community support services.

NOC

1. Risk Control
2. Pain Control
3. Fear Level: Child
4. Child Development
5. Family Coping
6. Knowledge: Parenting, Health Promotion

IMPLEMENTATION

1. Risk for injury
   a. Resuscitate and stabilize as needed
   b. Protect from further injury
   c. Assist with diagnosis of abuse
   d. Provide supportive care
   e. Report suspected abuse
   f. Facilitate referral to social worker
   g. Document assessment of child's physical finding and parent/child interactions
   h. Discuss and role-model behaviors to foster child/family positive interactions
   i. Assess stress level of child and parent
   j. Discuss normal growth and development
   k. Discuss alternative methods of discipline
   l. Discuss need for community resources
2. Acute pain
   a. Assess pain level hourly or more often as indicated by child's condition
   b. Treat pain proactively, avoiding intramuscular pain medications
   c. Assess wounds
   d. Position for comfort
   e. Provide emotional support for child
   f. Provide for diversionary age-appropriate activities
3. Fear
   a. Encourage verbalization of fears
   b. Facilitate referral to recreation therapy
   c. Participate in therapeutic and dramatic play
   d. Assess stress level of child and parent

4. Growth and development
   a. Assess child's present level of growth and development
   b. Document presence of developmental milestones
   c. Discuss normal growth and development
   d. Discuss alternative methods of discipline
   e. Discuss need for community resources
   f. Role-model appropriate interactions with child
   g. Facilitate positive interactions between child and family
5. Family coping
   a. Assess for indications of ineffective coping
   b. Encourage verbalization of feelings and concerns
   c. Discuss need and ways to activate community resources
   d. Assist family to identify positive coping strategies
   e. Document interactions between child and family
6. Family teaching
   a. Assess family's current level of understanding
   b. Provide verbal and written information regarding:
      1) Growth and development and ways to assist child in meeting developmental milestones
      2) Alternative methods of discipline
      3) Community resources including Parents Anonymous
      4) Referral information as indicated
      5) Positive coping strategies
      6) Behaviors to encourage parent-child attachment
      7) Positive parenting skills
      8) Importance of follow-up with health care provider
      9) Contact numbers for health care provider and community resources
   c. Provide adequate time for teaching
   d. Document teaching, referrals, and family response

NIC

1. Risk Identification, Surveillance: Safety
2. Pain Management
3. Security Enhancement
4. Risk Identification: Developmental Enhancement
5. Coping Enhancement
6. Teaching: Child Rearing, Child Safety, Growth and Development, Health Education, Health Resources

EVALUATION

1. Client is identified as having the potential for abuse or neglect before further injury occurs.
2. Client demonstrates effective pain control through verbal and non-verbal behavior.
3. Client verbalizes feelings, fears, and concerns.
4. Client achieves developmental milestones and highest level of wellness.
5. Family identifies and uses effective coping strategies to prevent further abuse.
6. Family demonstrates understanding of child's needs, growth and development, effective coping strategies, and community support services.

References

Administration for Children & Families of the U.S. Department of Health & Human Services. (2007a). *Child maltreatment 2005*—Summary. Retrieved May 10, 2007, from http://www.acf .dhhs.gov/programs/cb/pubs/cm05/summary.htm

Administration for Children & Families of the U.S. Department of Health & Human Services. (2007b). *Child maltreatment 2005*—Chapter 4: Fatalities. Retrieved May 10, 2007, from http://www.acf.dhhs.gov/programs/cb/pubs/cm05/chapterfour.htm#child

Anbarghalami, R., Yang, L., Van Sell, S. L., & Miller-Anderson, M. (2007). When to suspect child abuse. *RN. 70*(4).

Child Welfare Information Gateway. (2006a). *What is child abuse and neglect?* Retrieved February 15, 2007, from http://www.childwelfare.gov/pubs/factsheets/whatiscan.cfm

Child Welfare Information Gateway. (2006b). *Recognizing signs of child abuse and neglect*. Retrieved February 15, 2007, from http://www.childwelfare.gov/can/identifying/recog_signs.cfm

Potts, N. L., & Mandleco, B. L. (2007). *Pediatric nursing: Caring for children and their families* (2nd ed.). Clifton Park, NY: Delmar Cengage Learning.

ACID-BASE IMBALANCES

Definition

Acid-base imbalances are alterations in the serum pH level as a result of increases or decreases in the concentration of hydrogen ions. These changes alter three things: function at the cellular level, enzyme activity, and integrity of the neuromuscular membrane. An increase in the hydrogen ion concentration results in a decrease in the serum pH below 7.35, causing acidosis. A decrease in the hydrogen ion concentration leads to an increase in the serum pH above 7.45, resulting in alkalosis. There are four types of acid-base imbalances: (1) respiratory acidosis, (2) respiratory alkalosis, (3) metabolic acidosis, and (4) metabolic alkalosis.

Pathophysiology

The body's pH is maintained within a narrow normal range of 7.35 to 7.45 by buffer systems to regulate the functioning of all body systems. When this delicate balance is altered, cellular function and integrity are compromised. Because acid is produced as a by-product of metabolism, the chemical and cellular buffer systems work continuously to ensure no buildup of acid. In addition to neutralizing excess acids, these buffer systems also control bases to maintain a slightly alkaline body environment, optimal for cellular function. The four types of acid-base imbalances reflect either altered respiratory function or altered metabolic function and depend on whether the health alteration that causes the imbalance is in the respiratory system or in other systems in the body (Broyles, 2005).

When changes in the acid-base balance exceed what the buffer systems can regulate, compensatory mechanisms are activated in both the respiratory and renal systems. Regardless of the cause (respiratory or metabolic) of the acid-base imbalance, the respiratory system responds immediately in an attempt to correct it. The respiratory system responds first by removing carbon dioxide from the blood through increased rate and depth of respirations (hyperventilation) to reduce the level of carbonic acid and increase the serum pH in the presence of acidosis; conversely, the respiratory system conserves carbon dioxide in the blood by slowing the rate and depth of respiration to increase the serum level of carbonic acid and lower the pH in the presence of alkalosis. The respiratory system activates quickly to compensate for pH imbalances; however, because of the body's need for oxygen, this system is only 80% effective in returning the pH to normal values.

The renal system regulates levels of bicarbonate (base) and hydrogen ions. In the presence of pH imbalances that the respiratory system is unable to rectify, the renal system is activated in 24 hours. In the presence of acidosis, the kidneys remove excess hydrogen ions from the blood and conserve bicarbonate ions, thus increasing the serum pH. In alkalosis, the kidneys conserve hydrogen ions, lowering the blood pH. Renal compensation functions more slowly than respiratory compensation, but its potential for effectiveness is higher. When the compensatory mechanisms are not adequate, acid-base imbalances result in changes in cellular function that can become pathological and potentially life-threatening.

The compensatory mechanisms (buffers) also can result in an acid-base imbalance in the event that the mechanism is forced to act beyond the compensatory status (Broyles, 2005). This occurs when the underlying pathophysiology of the causative condition is not resolved. An example of this is in the presence of asthma (reactive airway disease) exacerbation. The acute phase of asthma causes constriction of the bronchi, resulting in the trapping of carbon dioxide in the lungs, which leads to respiratory acidosis. This activates the respiratory buffer system to increase the respiratory rate to exhale the excess carbon dioxide. At the same time, the amount of oxygen reaching the lungs decreases because of the bronchoconstriction activating the respiratory system to further increase the respiratory rate in an effort to increase oxygen intake. This results in hyperventilation and the development of respiratory alkalosis.

Complications

Cellular dysfunction

Altered neuromuscular membrane integrity

Altered enzyme activity

Cellular, tissue, and organ damage

Cardiac dysrhythmias ("Supraventricular arrhythmias are increased in the presence of a severe respiratory acidosis, but these problems are most likely caused by concomitant hypoxemia, electrolyte shifts, and increased catecholamines rather than a direct hypercapnia-induced cardiac irritability" [Priestley, 2006, p. 1]).

Electrolyte imbalances

Seizures

Shock

Coma

Death resulting from multiple organ failure if not corrected rapidly

Incidence

The incidence of acid-base imbalances is reflected in the occurrence of the pathophysiologic conditions that lead to each imbalance. Consequently, the exact incidence of acid-base imbalances is difficult to calculate.

Etiology

Each type of acid-base imbalance has its own group of causes as follows:

RESPIRATORY ACIDOSIS (HAYES, 2005A)

Respiratory conditions including asthma (reactive airway disease), airway obstruction, foreign body aspiration, respiratory distress syndrome, severe pneumonia, bronchopulmonary dysplasia (BPD), bronchiolitis, cystic fibrosis, croup, epiglottitis

Sleep apnea

Neonatal resuscitation

Trauma to the central nervous system (CNS), such as head injuries and spinal cord injuries

Muscular dystrophy

Chest trauma

Near drowning

Extensive burns that result in elevated CO_2 levels

Pharmacologic agents including CNS depressants

Chronic metabolic alkalosis with respiratory compensation

RESPIRATORY ALKALOSIS (HAYES, 2005B; MANCINI, 2006)

Respiratory conditions resulting in decreased lung compliance and hypoxemia, including pneumonia, reactive airway disease, interstitial lung disease

Hyperventilation from CNS stimulation, fear, anxiety, compensation for
   respiratory acidosis or metabolic acidosis

Salicylate poisoning

Pregnancy

Gram-negative sepsis

Meningitis

Encephalitis

CNS tumor

Hyperthyroidism

Heat exhaustion

Hepatic failure

METABOLIC ACIDOSIS

Ketoacidosis associated with uncontrolled diabetes (Stavile, 2005)

Conditions that increase the body's metabolic rate, including fever,
   shock, burns, seizures, respiratory distress syndrome

Acute or chronic renal failure

Conditions that result in a loss of bicarbonate, including diarrhea, excess
   ostomy drainage

Hyperkalemia (Thomas & Hamawi, 2005)

METABOLIC ALKALOSIS (YASEEN & THOMAS, 2006)

Conditions resulting in body fluid depletion, including vomiting and
   excess gastric drainage

Potassium loss secondary to diuretic therapy

Decreased renal perfusion

Hypochloremia

Cystic fibrosis

Clinical Manifestations

Refer to Table 2-1.

Table 2-1 | Manifestations According to Each Acid-Base Imbalance

Imbalance	Manifestations
Respiratory Acidosis	pH < 7.35
	$pCO_2 > 45$ mm Hg
	Tachypnea, hyperventilation
	Increased use of accessory muscles for breathing
	Tachycardia
	Hypertension
	Potential atrial and ventricular dysrhythmias
	Headache
	CNS changes such as restlessness, apprehension, drowsiness, increased intracranial pressure (ICP)
	Presence of underlying causative pathology

(*continues*)

Table 2-1 | Manifestations According to Each Acid-Base Imbalance (continued)

Imbalance	Manifestations
Respiratory Alkalosis	pH > 7.45 pCO_2 < 35 mm Hg CNS changes including dizziness, tinnitus, decreasing level of consciousness (LOC) Diaphoresis Dysrhythmias including changes in ST segment and T wave Neuromuscular changes such as muscle twitching, prolonged muscle spasms, facial and extremity paralysis Presence of underlying causative pathology
Metabolic Acidosis	pH < 7.35 Cold, clammy skin with mild to moderate acidosis Dry, warm skin with severe acidosis Tachycardia Tachypnea Kussmaul respirations Increased use of accessory muscles for breathing Visual disturbances including diplopia, blurred vision Headache Decreasing LOC Muscle spasms Nausea and vomiting Diarrhea Presence of underlying causative pathology
Metabolic Alkalosis	Potassium loss resulting in cardiac dysrhythmias Tachycardia Changes in LOC including lethargy and confusion Muscle weakness Presence of underlying causative pathology

Diagnostic Tests

Presence of clinical manifestations
Arterial blood gases
Serum chemistries
Pulmonary function tests
Chest radiography
Computed tomography

Medical Management

Medical management is directed at resolving the acid-base imbalance. For management of respiratory acid-base imbalances, the goal is to reestablish effective gas exchange. Therapy for metabolic acid-base imbalances focuses on correcting the underlying causative pathology (Broyles, 2005). Refer to Table 2-2.

Table 2-2 | Treatment Standards for Each Acid-Base Imbalance

Acid-base imbalance	Treatment
Respiratory Acidosis	Treatment of underlying cause Use of oxygen, intubation, and mechanical ventilation Administration of sodium bicarbonate ($NaHCO_3$) intravenously Use of sympathomimetic bronchodilators (albuterol, epinephrine, isoproterenol, metaproterenol), xanthine bronchodilators (theophylline, aminophylline), and anticholinergic bronchodilator (ipratropium) Use of naloxone if respiratory acidosis resulted from use of CNS depressants

Respiratory Alkalosis	Treatment focused primarily on management of underlying cause
	If hyperventilation-related:
	  oxygen
	  rebreathing mask
	  psychological reassurance
	  if severe, mechanical ventilation
	Use of anxiolytic agents such as benzodiazepines (those with pediatric safety and efficacy shown) such as lorazepam

Metabolic Acidosis	Treatment of underlying cause Intravenous administration of $NaHCO_3$ with caution Intravenous insulin if cause is ketoacidosis
Metabolic Alkalosis	Treatment of underlying cause Use of fluid resuscitation including replacement of electrolytes Intravenous hydrogen chloride

Nursing Management

ASSESSMENT

1. Obtain client history
2. Perform respiratory assessment
3. Perform neurologic assessment
4. Assess for presence of clinical manifestations
5. Assess results of diagnostic tests

NURSING DIAGNOSES (INCLUDING BUT NOT LIMITED TO)

1. Impaired gas exchange R/T altered breathing pattern
2. Risk for injury R/T impaired cerebral tissue perfusion and altered thought processes
3. Decreased cardiac output R/T altered neurotransmitter levels

4. Imbalanced fluid volume R/T fluid deficit or excess
5. Injury R/T adverse effects of pharmacologic agents and therapy
6. Anxiety (child and parents) R/T difficulty breathing, medical therapies such as mechanical ventilation, and treatment in the critical care environment
7. Deficient knowledge R/T health alterations that cause acid-base imbalances, medical and nursing management, and home care

PLANNING/GOALS

1. Client will experience restoration of effective gas exchange as evidenced by arterial blood gases within defined limits (WDL), pulse oximetry readings of oxygen saturation WDL (> 94%), and no adventitious breath sounds.
2. Client will not experience injuries secondary to impaired cerebral perfusion.
3. Client will not experience decreased cardiac output as evidenced by vital signs WDL for age and individual client, no adventitious heart sounds, and serum electrolyte levels WDL.
4. Client will not experience injury and will regain fluid and electrolyte balance.
5. Client will not experience injury from adverse effects of pharmacologic agents or medical and nursing management.
6. Client/parents will demonstrate decreased anxiety as evidenced by verbalization of decreasing fear and anxiety, relaxed posture, ability to rest, and ability to control breathing pattern.
7. Client/parents will demonstrate understanding of condition, medical and nursing management, and home care.

NOC

1. Respiratory Status: Gas Exchange
2. Risk Control, Neurological Status
3. Cardiac Pump Effectiveness
4. Electrolyte and Acid/Base Balance
5. Risk Control
6. Anxiety Level
7. Knowledge: Disease Process, Illness Care, Medication, Treatment Regimen

IMPLEMENTATION

1. Gas exchange
   a. Assess respiratory status every 2–4 hours and as needed
   b. Maintain patent airway
   c. Initiate and maintain patency of intravenous access, monitoring hourly
   d. Monitor arterial blood gases
   e. Monitor continuous pulse oximetry
   f. Administer oxygen and titrate to maintain oxygen saturation > 94%
   g. Instruct client (if possible) on therapeutic breathing techniques
   h. Position head of bed to facilitate breathing effort
   i. Administer medications as prescribed following seven rights of medication administration

    j.   Explain all procedures, equipment, and therapies to client/parents

    k.   Follow appropriate facility protocols and health care provider prescriptions if mechanical ventilation is required

2. Neurologic status

    a.   Assess neurologic status every 2–4 hours and as needed

    b.   Monitor central venous pressure as indicated

    c.   Maintain side rails in raised position and bed level in lowest position

    d.   Maintain patency of intravenous access, monitoring hourly

    e.   Administer osmotic diuretics as prescribed for increased ICP

    f.   Monitor continuous urine output as measure of effectiveness of diuretic therapy

    g.   Explain all procedures, equipment, and therapies to client/parents

    h.   Administer sodium bicarbonate, anticonvulsants, and potassium chloride as appropriate and prescribed

    i.   Administer titrate oxygen to maintain oxygen saturation > 94%

3. Cardiac output

    a.   Monitor cardiac status continuously in the critical care environment

    b.   Monitor cardiac output to maintain at 200 mL/kg/minute in infants and 100 mL/kg/minute in adolescents

    c.   Assess skin and peripheral circulation status

    d.   Administer oxygen to maintain pulse oximetry readings > 94% or as prescribed

    e.   Maintain mechanical ventilation as prescribed

    f.   Monitor electrolyte and cardiac enzyme levels

    g.   Maintain patency of intravenous access, monitoring hourly

    h.   Administer cardiac pharmacologic agents as prescribed

    i.   Monitor intake and output

    j.   Respond to changes in cardiac status according to facility protocol

    k.   Ensure that defibrillator is present and in working order

4. Fluid balance

    a.   Monitor intake and output at intervals appropriate for client condition

    b.   Monitor serum electrolyte levels

    c.   Maintain patency of intravenous access, monitoring hourly

    d.   Administer intravenous fluids as prescribed

    e.   Monitor for manifestations of electrolyte imbalances

    f.   Administer electrolytes as prescribed

5. Injury related to pharmacologic therapy

    a.   Maintain the seven rights of medications administration

        1) Right client

        2) Right medication

        3) Right dose

        4) Right time

        5) Right route

      6) Right documentation

      7) Right to refuse

  b. Monitor for manifestations of adverse effects of therapy

  c. Report any abnormal findings to health care provider

6. Anxiety

  a. Monitor for verbal and nonverbal indicators of fear and anxiety in client/parents

  b. Provide explanations for all equipment and procedures

  c. Listen actively to concerns

  d. Answer questions honestly

  e. Collaborate with health care provider for appropriate referrals as needed

  f. Maintain calm affect

  g. Monitor sleep pattern

  h. Administer anxiolytics to client as prescribed and indicated

7. Parent/child teaching

  a. Assess client's/parents' current level of knowledge

  b. Provide verbal and written information concerning:

      1) Predisposing factors for acid-base imbalances

      2) Manifestations of fluid and electrolyte imbalances

      3) Manifestations of acid-base imbalances

      4) Importance of obtaining medical care in the event the manifestations occur

      5) Contact information for health care providers as needed

      6) Importance of follow-up care with child's health care provider

  c. Provide sufficient time for teaching and client/parent questions

  d. Refer questions as needed to health care provider or appropriate health care team member

  e. Document teaching and client/parent response.

NIC

1. Acid-Base Management, Oxygen Therapy, Ventilation Assistance

2. Risk Identification, Surveillance: Safety, Cerebral Perfusion Promotion, Neurologic Monitoring

3. Cardiac Care, Hemodynamic Monitoring

4. Acid-Base Management, Fluid/Electrolyte Management

5. Risk Identification, Surveillance: Safety

6. Anxiety Reduction, Fear Reduction, Calming Technique

7. Teaching: Disease Process, Illness Care, Medication, Treatment Regimen

EVALUATION

1. Client experiences restoration of effective gas exchange as evidenced by arterial blood gases WDL, pulse oximetry readings of oxygen saturation WDL (> 94%), and no adventitious breath sounds.

2. Client does not experience injuries secondary to impaired cerebral perfusion.

3. Client does not experience altered cardiac output as evidenced by vital signs WDL for age and individual client, no adventitious heart sounds, and serum electrolyte levels WDL.

4. Client does not experience injury and will regain fluid and electrolyte balance.

5. Client does not experience injury from adverse effects of pharmacologic agents or medical and nursing management.

6. Client/parents demonstrate decreased anxiety as evidenced by verbalization of decreasing fear and anxiety, relaxed posture, ability to
rest, and ability to control breathing pattern.

7. Client/parents demonstrate understanding of condition, medical
and nursing management, and home care.

References

Broyles, B. E. (2005). *Medical-surgical nursing clinical companion*. Durham, NC: Carolina
Academic Press.

Hayes, J. A. (2005a). *Respiratory acidosis*. Retrieved December 9, 2006, from http://www
.emedicine.com/med/topic2008.htm

Hayes, J. A. (2005b). *Respiratory alkalosis*. Retrieved December 9, 2006, from http://www
.emedicine.com/med/topic2009.htm

Mancini, M. C. (2006). *Alkalosis, respiratory*. Retrieved December 9, 2006, from http://www
.emedicine.com/ped/topic70.htm

Priestley, M. A. (2006). *Acidosis, respiratory*. Retrieved December 9, 2006, from http://www
.emedicine.com/ped/topic16.htm

Stavile, K. L. (2005). *Metabolic acidosis*. Retrieved December 9, 2006, from http://www
.emedicine.com/emerg/topic312.htm

Thomas, C., & Hamawi, K. (2005). *Metabolic acidosis*. Retrieved December 9, 2006, from
http://www.emedicine.com/med/topic1458.htm

Yaseen, S., & Thomas, C. (2006). *Metabolic alkalosis*. Retrieved December 9, 2006, from
http://www.emedicine.com/MED/topic1459.htm

ACQUIRED IMMUNODEFICIENCY SYNDROME (AIDS)

Definition

Acquired immunodeficiency syndrome (AIDS) is a chronic, life-threatening immunosuppressive condition caused by the human immunodeficiency virus (HIV) (Broyles, 2005). The presence of the virus and the infection it causes are termed *HIV infection*. The later stages of the HIV infection constitute AIDS.

Pathophysiology

HIV is an RNA virus belonging to the lentivirus family of retroviruses and known to have two strains—HIV-1 and HIV-2. HIV-1 is very mutant and has a number of sub-types. It causes persistent viremia and is associated with long periods of clinical latency and asymptomatic infection. The virus can be found in blood and almost any body tissue including saliva, vaginal secretions, semen, tears, urine, and tracheal secretions (Broyles, 2005).

HIV is comprised of two envelopes (inner and outer) of glycoproteins, gp120 and gp41, as well as a viral core. The outer glycoproteins are needed to bind HIV-1 to CD4+ lymphocytes. These lymphocytes, also called helper T cells, are the white blood cells necessary for humoral and cell-mediated immunity and coordinate the function of the entire immune system. The viral core capsule consists of the core proteins p24, p7, and p9. The viral core has two single strands of viral RNA and essential viral enzymes for replication, reverse transcriptase, RNAse, polymerase, integrase, and protease (aids.org, 2007b).

When the body is infected by HIV-1, the HIV-1 attaches to the host CD4+ cell binding of the gp120 and the CD4+ receptor site. The gp41 assists the fusion of the envelope with the CD4+ cell membrane. The virus then penetrates the cell wall into the host cell. The HIV-1 virus releases two strands of viral RNA into the cytoplasm of the host cell and copies the DNA using the reverse transcriptase enzyme. The RNAse, polymerase, integrase, and protease then separate the RNA and DNA, combine with two DNA strands, and move into the DNA of the host cell nucleus. This forms the HIV-1 provirus. This provirus remains dormant until activation of the CD4+ cell causes it to replicate. Once the CD4+ cell is activated, it transcribes the DNA of the provirus into messenger RNA. This moves out of the cell nucleus and facilitates the production of more HIV envelopes and cores (Potts & Mandleco, 2007).

The initial replication occurs in the lymph nodes and plasma membrane. It then gradually produces cellular death. The decrease in CD4 lymphocytes reduces the body's immune defenses, resulting in decreased ability of the body to prevent infections caused by bacteria, viruses, and fungi. The normal range of CD4 cells is 500–1500 cells/mm^3. When the number of these cells falls below 200 cells/mm^3, the individual becomes susceptible to opportunistic infections as well as certain types of cancers including Kaposi's sarcoma and non-Hodgkin's lymphoma. The nature of the infections may be life-threatening. In addition, HIV results in progressive wasting disorders (including neurodegeneration) that also can be life-threatening.

At the time of the initial infection, the body activates an anti-HIV immune response that acts to neutralize free HIV and eliminate HIV-infected cells. During the acute infection, these anti-HIV antibodies inhibit the infectivity of the HIV. Anti-HIV CD4+ cells and cytotoxic T lymphocytes and macrophages manage to remove large numbers of circulating HIV-infected cells. This may explain why people are asymptomatic during the acute phase of HIV infection. However, the HIV's ability to use CD4 molecules as receptor sites as well as its ability to mutate and replicate makes the body's natural defenses ineffective for controlling the long-term HIV infection. The average incubation period for HIV to the development of AIDS remains approximately ten years. However, the length of this period depends on how the HIV infection was contracted. For instance, most AIDS in children (91% of the cases) occurs as a result of prenatal transmission of the virus from an infected mother to her fetus (Potts & Mandleco, 2007), resulting in a shorter incubation period (15–20% of these infants will die by age 1 year if not treated), whereas contamination resulting from a single sexual contact with an infected person may result in a much longer latency period. Perinatal transmission can occur through the placental membrane during pregnancy or during delivery. Transmission from tainted blood used in transfusions dropped to less than 3% following the testing of all blood in the United States beginning in April 1985 (aids.org, 2007b).

As the HIV infection progresses to late symptomatic AIDS disease (CD4 T-cell count below 200 cells/mm^3), the infected child develops the AIDS-related complex. The respiratory system is the first to display opportunistic infections associated with this complex, with the most distinguishing characteristic medical condition being *Pneumocystis carinii* pneumonia (PCP). Another common associated condition is *Mycobacterium avium-intracellulare* complex (MAC), a complex bacterial infection that affects the respiratory and gastrointestinal (GI) systems. The GI tract is susceptible to numerous pathogenic bacterial microorganisms including *Salmonella, Shigella, Giardia lamblia, Entamocha, Candida albicans, Histoplasmosis capsulatum,* and cytomegalovirus (CMV). The diarrhea associated with these infections becomes so severe that the person experiences dehydration and electrolyte imbalances. Eventually, this progresses to the protein wasting syndrome. CMV can infect other body systems in addition to the respiratory and GI systems, including the eyes and the central nervous system. Other common infections including herpes simplex, which affects the mucous membranes of the oral, genital, and perianal areas, and varicella-zoster virus, which causes painful shingles, are common during this period. Peripheral neuropathies, central nervous system lymphomas, and AIDS-related dementia (non-focal encephalopathy) represent neurologic manifestations of the AIDS-related complex. Another complication of AIDS is Kaposi's sarcoma, which results in lesions occurring anywhere in or on the body from the skin to internal organs, including the lungs. The pressure that visceral and lymphatic tumors create on nerves can result in moderate to severe pain. As a result of newer pharmacologic treatment (highly active antiretroviral therapy—HAART), this condition has decreased in incidence during recent years. AIDS-related myopathy also causes moderate to severe pain in these children; however, the most common cause of death is opportunistic infections resulting in organ failure.

According to the Centers for Disease Control and Prevention (CDC), in 1986, the second type of HIV, called HIV-2, was identified in AIDS clients in West Africa. It may have been present decades earlier. Although studies of the natural history of HIV-2 are limited, at this point, differences and similarities have been noted when comparing HIV-1 and HIV-2. Both HIV-1 and HIV-2 are transmitted the same way and are associated with similar opportunistic infections and AIDS. In those individuals infected with HIV-2, immunodeficiency seems to develop slower, is milder in form, and is less infectious early in the course of infection. As the disease advances, HIV-2 infectiousness seems to increase. However, when compared with HIV-1, the duration of this increase in infectiousness is shorter. The two types differ in geographic patterns of infection. The United States has few reported cases of HIV-2 (Centers for Disease Control and Prevention, 2006b).

Complications

Life-threatening infections
Protein wasting syndrome
Kaposi's sarcoma
Peripheral and CNS lymphomas
Myopathy
Non-focal encephalopathy
Death

Incidence

HIV-1 is present worldwide, while HIV-2 exists primarily in West Africa (aids.org, 2007a). The subtypes of HIV-1 vary depending on their location throughout the world. In its statistics through 2004, the CDC provides estimates of AIDS cases according to the person's age at diagnosis. According to these estimates, 9,443 cases are in children under the age of 13 years, 959 cases are in teens 13–14 years of age, and 4,936 cases occur during the remaining adolescent years (15–19 years). The CDC further estimates that 1 million to 1.2 million U.S. residents are living with HIV infection, about one-quarter being unaware of their infection. Each year there are about 40,000 new infections. Of these, about 70% are among men and 30% are among women. The cumulative estimates of perinatal AIDS cases through 2004 are 8,779. The estimated cases for 2004 include 48 in children under 13 years of age, 60 in children 13 to 14 years, and 326 in the remaining adolescent years (Centers for Disease Control and Prevention, 2006a).

According to the World Health Organization (WHO) HIV/AIDS is an important health issue in children and adolescents. Since the first clinical evidence of AIDS was reported two decades ago, HIV/AIDS has spread to every corner of the world. According to estimates by Uniting the World Against AIDS (UNAIDS) and WHO, more than 4 million children under the age of 15 have been infected with HIV since the epidemic began. More than 90% of them were infants born to HIV-positive mothers; these infants acquired the virus before or during birth or through breastfeeding. Because HIV infection often quickly progresses to AIDS in children, most of the children under 15 who have been infected have developed AIDS; most of these children have died. Another 13 million children have lost their mother or both parents to the disease. An estimated 10.3 million young people aged 15–24 are living with HIV/AIDS, and half of all new infections—over 7,000 daily—are occurring among young people. Young people are vulnerable to HIV because of risky sexual behavior, substance use, and their lack of access to HIV information and prevention services. Many young people do not believe that HIV is a threat to them, and many others do not know how to protect themselves from HIV (World Health Organization, 2007).

According to information from the CDC, in 2004, an estimated 15,798 (including 15,737 adults and adolescents and 61 children under age 13) died from AIDS and AIDS-related illnesses. The cumulative data estimates that 529,113 individuals (including 523,598 adults and adolescents and 5,515 children under age 13) succumbed to AIDS through 2004. From 2000 through 2004, the estimated number of AIDS cases in the United States decreased 61% among children less than 13 years of age (Centers for Disease Control and Prevention, 2006b).

According to the organization Save the Children, of the more than 39.4 million people throughout the world with HIV/AIDS, 2.2 million are children under the age of 15. Sub-Saharan Africa is the home of almost 70% of these children (Save the Children, 2008).

Etiology

HIV is transmitted through contact with the blood or body secretions of an infected person. Ninety percent of HIV infections in children occur as a result of fetuses being infected through the placental blood supply of HIV-infected women, contact with the infected blood during delivery, or through breastfeeding after birth. HIV infections in adolescents result from having sexual contact with an infected person or sharing needles with infected intravenous drug users. According to the CDC, there is no scientific evidence to support the contracting of HIV/AIDS through casual contact, such as hand-shaking (Centers for Disease Control and Prevention, 2006a).

Clinical Manifestations

The onset of clinical manifestations of AIDS depends on the mode of transmission. Because of immature immune systems and developing organs of fetuses and neonates, 15–20% of those who contract HIV prenatally will die by the age of 1 year if not treated. In the other 80–85%, the disease progresses more slowly; and although this group may experience laboratory indications (leukopenia), the onset of AIDS-defining symptoms often does not appear until after the age of 4 years.

In 1994, the CDC revised the Pediatric Classification System for AIDS, outlining the four clinical categories based on how the disease is manifested in children. Table 3-1 contains the latest revision available.

Table 3-1 | CDC's Pediatric Classification System for AIDS

Category	Manifestations
N	Non-symptomatic
A	Symptomatic: Lymphadenopathy (0.5 cm at more than two sites) Hepatomegaly Splenomegaly Dermatitis Recurrent or persistent upper respiratory infections including otitis media and sinusitis
B	Moderately Symptomatic: Anemia (hemoglobin less than 8 grams/dL) Neutropenia (less than 1000 cells/mm³) Thrombocytopenia (less than 100,000 cells/mm³) Bacterial meningitis Pneumonia Sepsis Candidiasis (persisting for more than two months in children older than 6 months) Cardiomyopathy Cytomegalovirus infection in children less than 1 month of age Recurrent or chronic diarrhea Hepatitis Herpes simplex viral stomatitis (recurrent, more than two episodes within one year) Herpes simplex viral pneumonitis, bronchitis, or esophagitis with onset at less than 1 month of age Herpes zoster involving at least two episodes Leiomyosarcoma Lymphoid interstitial pneumonia or pulmonary interstitial hyperplasia complex

(continues)

Table 3-1 | CDC's Pediatric Classification System for AIDS (continued)

Category	Manifestations
	Nephropathy
	Nocardiosis
	Persistent fever lasting more than one month
	Toxoplasmosis (onset prior to 1 month of age)
	Complicated varicella
C	Severely Symptomatic:
	Serious bacterial infection, multiple or recurrent
	Pneumocystis carinii pneumonia (PCP)
	Esophageal or pulmonary candidiasis
	Disseminated coccidioidomycosis
	Extrapulmonary cryptococcosis
	Cryptosporidiosis or isosporiasis with persistent diarrhea
	Cytomegaloviral disease
	Encephalopathy
	Herpes simplex viral infection causing a mucocutaneous ulcer persisting for more than one month
	Disseminated histoplasmosis at site other than lungs, cervix, or hilar lymph nodes
	Kaposi's sarcoma
	Primary brain lymphoma
	Burkitt's or large B-cell lymphoma
	Wasting syndrome

Adapted from Centers for Disease Control and Prevention: Revised Pediatric Classification Systems (AIDS): Clinical Categories (Centers for Disease Control and Prevention, 2006c)

Diagnostic Tests

ELISA (enzyme-linked immunosorbent assay) HIV antibody test (children older than 15–18 months of age)—most commonly known (Broyles, 2005)

Western blot test

For children from birth to 15 months of age:

HIV DNA polymerase chain reaction (PCR) test (most common)

Plasma HIV RNA assay (most expensive)

HIV whole cell viral culture

CD4+T lymphocyte counts and percentages

Medical Management

There remains no known cure for HIV/AIDS, so management is a coordinated multidisciplinary team approach with a medical manage focusing on pharmacologic agents that inhibit or block HIV replication and the aggressive treatment of infections. Because the treatment of opportunistic infections is specific to the causative pathogenic microorganisms, this discussion is limited to agents used to inhibit HIV replication and immune enhancement therapy. The development of HAART (combination of three or four antiretroviral drugs) has improved the quality of life in children infected with HIV/AIDS. There are two main classifications of antiretroviral agents used for HIV: non-nucleoside reverse transcriptase inhibitors (NNRTIs) and protease inhibitors (PIs). NNRTIs bind directly to reverse transcriptase and prevent the conversion of RNA and DNA. PIs prevent the pooling and release of HIV-1 and HIV-2 from the infected CD4 cells by inhibiting the proteases, rendering them ineffective and leading to the production of immature noninfectious HIV particles (Broyles, Reiss, & Evans, 2007). The NNRTIs approved for use in children include zidovudine, didanosine, lamivudine, stavudine, zalcitabine, saquinavir, indinavir, and efavirenz. The PIs include nelfinavir and ritonavir. The initial treatment usually includes one or two NNRTIs, one nucleoside reverse transcriptase inhibitor (NRTI), and one PI. Long-term use in the adult population of PIs suggests that they may cause lipodystrophy; however, long-term effects of all antiretrovirals in children are not known at this time.

In July 2006, a new combination agent was approved by the Food and Drug Administration (FDA), called efavirenz 600 mg/emtricitabine 200 mg/tenofovir disoproxil fumarate 300 mg (ATRIPLA). However, this agent has not been studied sufficiently for use in children under the age of 18 years but is approved for those 18 years and older.

Agents used for prophylaxis for *Pneumocystis carinii* are trimethoprim-sulfamethoxazole, dapsone, and intravenous or aerosol pentamidine. Prophylaxis for Mycobacterium avium-intracellulare infections include clarithromycin, azithromycin, and rifabutin; and for candidiasis prevention, nystatin, clotrimazole, and fluconazole are the agents of choice.

Well-child care is an important component in the treatment of children with HIV/AIDS. This includes following the immunization schedule recommended by the American Academy of Pediatrics (Appendix G) with the exception of using only the inactivated formulation of IPV, receiving an annual influenza vaccine, and considering only the use of varicella vaccines for children in the N or A pediatric categories.

Psychosocial and developmental monitoring remains a critical facet in the care of these children. Due to the cost of the pharmacologic management required, a social service referral should be initiated shortly after the diagnosis of HIV/AIDS is confirmed.

Nursing Management

ASSESSMENT

1. Assess vital signs, breath sounds, heart sounds, and bowel sounds
2. Assess for history of the presence of conditions noted in the Pediatric Classifications System (Refer to Clinical Manifestations section)
3. Assess for history of fever, diarrhea, ear pulling, and changes in appetite, sleep patterns, and behavior
4. Assess hydration status, respiratory status, and presence of mouth lesions, skin lesions, blisters, or dryness
5. Perform pain assessment using developmentally-appropriate pain rating scale
6. Assess the family's understanding about the child's condition
7. Assess the child's level of growth and development
8. Perform psychosocial assessment of both parent(s) and child

NURSING DIAGNOSES (INCLUDING BUT NOT LIMITED TO)

1. Ineffective protection R/T cell-mediated immunodeficiency
2. Impaired gas exchange R/T inadequate immune system function and opportunistic infections
3. Imbalanced nutrition: Less than body requirements R/T increased metabolic needs, recurrent infections, diarrheal losses, and inadequate caloric intake
4. Acute pain R/T effects of disease on nerve endings
5. Risk for impaired skin integrity R/T potential skin lesions associated with HIV/AIDS
6. Delayed growth and development R/T effects of chronic and potentially terminal illness

7. Risk for caregiver role strain R/T insufficient finances, support, and knowledge of community resources

8. Grieving R/T child's prognosis

9. Deficient knowledge (parental) R/T child's condition, medical management, and home care

PLANNING/GOALS

1. Client will remain free of opportunistic infections and will maintain an up-to-date immunization record.

2. Client will maintain clear breath sounds, pulse oximetry within defined limits (WDL) of greater than 94%, pulse and respiratory rates WDL for age, and lack of dyspnea on minimal exertion.

3. Client will maintain optimal weight for height and age, consume adequate calories to meet metabolic and growth needs, and have formed stools every one to two days.

4. Client will verbalize a pain level of 0–1 on an age-appropriate pain assessment tool.

5. Client's skin will remain intact.

6. Client's motor, cognitive, and psychosocial development will be WDL.

7. Parents' care of child at home will promote wellness and utilize community and support resources.

8. Parents will verbalize feelings about expected loss and plans for treatment as disease progresses.

9. Parents will demonstrate understanding of disease, the way transmission occurs, medical management, and management of acute illness and chronic symptoms.

NOC

1. Immune Status, Infection Status, Knowledge: Infection Control, Risk Detection

2. Respiratory Status: Gas Exchange

3. Nutritional Status: Nutrient Intake

4. Comfort Level, Pain Control, Pain Level

5. Tissue Integrity: Skin, Risk Control

6. Child Development, Knowledge: Parenting

7. Caregiver Emotional Health

8. Family Coping

9. Knowledge: Treatment Regimen

IMPLEMENTATION

1. Infection
   a. Maintain an infection-free environment
   b. Use Standard Precautions and teach child and family
   c. Teach family need for follow-up with health care provider
   d. Instruct family about recommended immunization schedule and alterations for their child
   e. Administer antipyretics as needed for fever
   f. Reinforce infection control, classification manifestations, prophylaxis, and medication administration
   g. During hospitalization:
      1) Monitor temperature every 4 hours and as needed
      2) Assess breath sounds and oxygen saturation at least once per shift depending on child's diagnosis on admission

        3) Assess for diarrhea

        4) Monitor intake and output

        5) Monitor CD4 T-lymphocyte counts

        6) Administer antimicrobials, antivirals, and immune enhancement as prescribed

        7) Monitor for effectiveness of drug therapy

        8) Monitor for adverse effects of drug therapy

2. Gas exchange

  a. Maintain patent airway

  b. Monitor vital signs and pulse oximetry every 4 hours and as needed

  c. Assess breath sounds each shift and as needed

  d. Administer supplemental oxygen as prescribed

  e. Administer medications as prescribed

  f. Monitor for effectiveness and for adverse effects of medications

  g. Monitor intake and output

  h. Maintain adequate fluid intake to maintain urine output > 2 mL/kg/hour

  i. Position for maximum ventilatory efficiency

  j. Provide parent teaching regarding prophylaxis for PCP

3. Nutrition

  a. Assess child's likes and dislikes

  b. Offer foods high in protein and calories

  c. Administer vitamin and mineral supplements as prescribed

  d. Monitor intake and output

  e. Offer milk, juice, and water after meals so child does not fill up on fluids before meals

  f. Provide age-appropriate foods and avoid spicy foods

  g. Avoid procedures prior to and immediately following meals

  h. Offer six small meals per day

  i. Monitor child's weight daily

  j. Initiate enteral or parenteral feedings as prescribed

  k. Assess bowel movements for frequency, consistency, and blood

4. Pain

  a. Assess for pain hourly using age-appropriate pain assessment tool

  b. Be proactive in pain management

  c. Offer acetaminophen and non-steroidal anti-inflammatory drugs (NSAIDs) for mild pain, oxycodone or acetaminophen with codeine for moderate pain, and morphine sulfate for severe pain as prescribed

  d. Cluster activities and provide rest periods

  e. Use palms when lifting and provide padding, floatation, and soft linens

  f. Turn every 2 hours

  g. Assist with activities of daily living

  h. Maintain calm environment

  i. Assess for mucous membrane and skin lesions

5. Skin integrity

  a. Assess skin for lesions

  b. Turn every 2 hours

   c. Provide pressure-relieving mattresses

   d. Use mild soap for bathing

   e. Offer liquids throughout the day

   f. Avoid tight ponytails and braids

   g. Cleanse open lesions with warm water and apply antiviral agents as prescribed

   h. Clean child's teeth with soft-bristled toothbrush; clean infant's mouth with swabs and plain water

   i. Leave diaper area open to air as much as possible if diaper rash or lesions occur

   j. Reinforce meticulous skin and mouth care and hand washing

6. Growth and development

   a. Encourage family to visit and play with child as much as possible within limitations of child's condition

   b. Provide age-appropriate activities within limitations of child's condition

   c. Administer HAART as prescribed

   d. Interact with child according to child's level of development

7. Caregiver strain

   a. Assess for indications of caregiver strain

   b. Encourage caregiver to express feelings and concerns

   c. Listen actively

   d. Provide information about community resources and support groups

   e. Involve caregiver in child's care during hospitalization and consider needs of caregiver and child

   f. Involve caregiver in decision making concerning child's care

   g. Assist caregiver in problem solving regarding delegation of child's care to other family members

   h. Document caregiver interactions with child

8. Grieving

   a. Encourage expression of feelings and concerns

   b. Help family identify support sources

   c. Encourage family to be honest with child

   d. Use therapeutic communication and support techniques

   e. Explain all procedures and equipment

   f. Encourage family to seek help from health care professionals if process becomes too difficult to manage within support systems

   g. Collaborate with health care provider for needed referrals

9. Parent/child teaching (if age-appropriate)

   a. Assess child's/family's level of understanding of child's condition

   b. Provide verbal and written instructions regarding:

      1) Signs and symptoms of infection

      2) Skin care and mouth care

      3) Medication administration and importance of compliance

      4) Adverse effects of medications to report to health care provider

      5) Changes in child's condition to report to health care provider

      6) Nutritional counseling

       7) Names and phone numbers of referral contact persons

       8) Importance of follow-up care with health care provider

  c. Provide sufficient time for client/family questions, providing honest answers

  d. Document teaching and client/family response

NIC

1. Infection Control, Health Screening, Infection Protection
2. Oxygen Therapy, Calming Technique
3. Nutrition Management, Weight Gain Assistance
4. Medication Management, Pain Management
5. Skin Surveillance, Health Education
6. Developmental Enhancement: Child
7. Caregiver Support
8. Grief Work Facilitation, Family Support
9. Health Education, Risk Identification, Teaching

EVALUATION

1. Client remains free of opportunistic infections and maintains an up-to-date immunization record.
2. Client maintains clear breath sounds, pulse oximetry WDL of greater than 94%, pulse and respiratory rates WDL for age, and lack of dyspnea on minimal exertion.
3. Client maintains optimal weight for height and age, consumes adequate calories to meet metabolic and growth needs, and has formed stools every one to two days.
4. Client verbalizes a pain level of 0–1 on an age-appropriate pain assessment tool.
5. Client's skin remains intact.
6. Client's motor, cognitive, and psychosocial development remains WDL.
7. Parents care of child at home promotes wellness and community and support resources are utilized.
8. Parents verbalize feelings about expected loss and plans for treatment as disease progresses.
9. Parents demonstrate understanding of disease, the way transmission occurs, medical management, and management of acute illness and chronic symptoms.

References

aids.org. (2007a). *Children and HIV*. Retrieved April 21, 2007, from http://www.aids.org/factSheets/index

aids.org (2007b). *What is AIDS?* Retrieved April 21, 2007, from http://www.aids.org/FactSheets/101-what-is-aids.htm

Broyles, B. E. (2005). *Medical-surgical nursing clinical companion*. Durham, NC: Carolina Academic Press.

Broyles, B. E., Reiss, B. S., & Evans, M. E. (2007). *Pharmacological aspects of nursing care* (7th ed.). Clifton Park, NY: Delmar Cengage Learning.

Centers for Disease Control and Prevention. (2006a). *AIDS/HIV*. Retrieved December 10, 2006, from http://www.cdc.gov/hiv/topics/basicindex.html

Centers for Disease Control and Prevention. (2006b). *HIV-2*. Retrieved December 10, 2006, from http://www.cdc.gov/hiv/resources/factsheets/hiv2.html

Centers for Disease Control and Prevention. (2006c). *Revised pediatric classification systems (AIDS): Clinical categories*. Retrieved December 10, 2006, from http://www.wonder.cdc.gov/wonder/help/AIDS/MMWR-09–30–1994.html

Potts, N. L., & Mandleco, B. L. (2007). *Pediatric nursing: Caring for children and their families* (2nd ed.). Clifton Park, NY: Delmar Cengage Learning.

Save the Children. (2008). Retrieved March 12, 2008, from http://www.savethechildren.org/technical/health/aids.pdf

World Health Organization. (2007). *WHO/HIV surveillance*. Retrieved April 21, 2007, from http://www.who.int/hiv/topics/me/en/index.html

4

AIRWAY OBSTRUCTION

Definition

Airway obstruction occurs when edema, a foreign body, or the tongue blocks the larynx, trachea, or bronchi, disrupting the inflow of air into the lungs. The obstruction may be partial or complete (Potts & Mandleco, 2007).

Pathophysiology

Foreign bodies can be any solid object (food, toys, balloons, hard candy, popcorn, nuts, pencil erasers, coins, buttons, or hot dogs) inhaled through the mouth that becomes lodged in the larynx, trachea, or bronchi as it attempts to move through any of these smaller structures. The trachea is a common place for the obstruction to occur; however, most often obstruction occurs in the cricopharyngeal area. The object becomes lodged there because the propulsive pharyngeal muscles carry it to this anatomical point. If the object is smaller than the trachea, it may pass into the bronchial tree. The trachea ends in the bifurcation that divides into the right and left bronchi. The orifice of the right main bronchus is slightly wider than the left bronchus; and because of the angle of this bifurcation, foreign bodies usually enter the right main bronchus. Obstruction interferes with the intake of air into the lungs, resulting in atelectasis. Hyperinflation or air trapping may result when air is inhaled; but because of the obstruction, it is unable to be completely exhaled. This leads to respiratory acidosis. When the obstruction is not cleared, hypoxia followed by hypoxemia occurs; lack of oxygen to the brain for more than 4 minutes can result in brain damage or death. Larger objects may obstruct the glottic inlet and lead to respiratory arrest.

Complications

Hypoxia
Atelectasis
Hypoxemia
Respiratory acidosis
Asphyxiation
Brain injury
Respiratory arrest

Incidence

Airway obstruction is the leading cause of accidental injury-related death among children under 1 year of age. Infants and children under age 4 are at high risk for choking or aspirating food or small objects because their upper airways are smaller, they are less experienced in chewing food properly, and their oral fixation leads them to explore items with their mouths. Current statistics indicate that 88% of children who died from airway obstruction injuries were ages 4 and under. In 2003, 18,000 children were treated in emergency rooms for airway obstruction (Lucille Packard's Children's Hospital at Stanford, 2007). The incidence of foreign body aspiration in children under 5 years of age occurs more frequently in boys and often occurs when running or falling (Broyles, 2005).

Etiology

Foreign body aspiration and subsequent airway obstruction usually occur as a result of the (1) oral needs of children, (2) natural curiosity of children, and (3) lack of parental supervision of young children. Peanuts and other nuts account for approximately half of aspirated foreign bodies. Other foods easily aspirated include raisins, vegetable pieces, seeds, and hot dogs.

Clinical Manifestations

IMMEDIATE MANIFESTATIONS

Sudden and violent coughing, gagging, or choking
Wheezing
Vomiting
Dyspnea
Cyanosis

LARYNGEAL AND TRACHEAL OBSTRUCTION

Hoarseness
Croupy cough
Stridor
Sternal and intercostal retractions
Severe dyspnea
Inability to speak
Decreasing level of consciousness
Respiratory arrest

BRONCHIAL OBSTRUCTION

Hemoptysis
Cough
Unilateral decreased breath sounds
Atelectasis
Excessive mucous production
Wheezing
Hoarseness
Inspiratory stridor
Ineffective ventilation
Decreasing level of consciousness

Diagnostic Tests

Chest radiography
Laryngoscopy
Bronchoscopy
Fluoroscopy
Xeroradiography
Pulse oximetry

Medical Management

Emergency treatment using the Heimlich maneuver is necessary when the child cannot speak and is unable to exchange gases. In the infant, back blows and chest thrusts are the emergency actions to take. Both bronchoscopy and laryngoscopy provide a method of diagnosing airway obstruction, identifying the object, and removing the object to prevent complications. Following either of these procedures, the child must remain in the health care facility until the gag reflex returns and no signs of laryngeal edema or respiratory distress are present.

Inhaled bronchodilators may be prescribed for bronchospasms or laryngospasms, as well as short-term corticosteroids to decrease airway edema. Systemic antibiotics are usually prescribed prophylactically to prevent respiratory infection resulting from the object itself or from the possibility of remaining fragments.

In the event that attempts to remove the object are unsuccessful, emergency medical personnel or the health care provider in the emergency department may need to perform a cricothyroidotomy or tracheostomy to administer oxygen below the level of the obstruction to maintain gas exchange and tissue perfusion. Mechanical ventilation usually is required in this situation.

Nursing Management

ASSESSMENT

1. Assess airway, breathing, and circulation (ABCs)
2. Obtain history if possible
3. Assess degree of obstruction as evidenced by clinical manifestations

NURSING DIAGNOSES (INCLUDING BUT NOT LIMITED TO)

1. Ineffective airway clearance/Impaired gas exchange R/T airway obstruction
2. Anxiety R/T difficulty exchanging gases and fight-or-flight response
3. Deficient knowledge R/T child safety

PLANNING/GOALS

1. The patency of the child's airway will be restored and maintained, and adequate gas exchange will be evidenced by pulse oximetry > 94%.
2. The child's/family's anxiety will be reduced as evidenced by relaxing body posture and decreasing distress.
3. The age-dependent child/family will demonstrate understanding of the risk factors for airway obstruction and ways to avoid them, emergency treatment, and home care.

NOC

1. Respiratory Status: Airway Patency, Gas Exchange
2. Anxiety Control, Coping
3. Knowledge: Risk Identification, Safety

IMPLEMENTATION

1. Airway patency/gas exchange
   a. Assess respiratory status as indicated by presence of symptoms
   b. Place on continuous pulse oximetry
   c. Administer blow-by oxygen while trying to resuscitate child
   d. Perform back blows and chest thrusts when client is an infant or a toddler (depending on size) and continue until object is expelled or infant becomes unconscious; then convert to care of unconscious choking infant, remembering to do mouth sweep only when the object can be seen
   e. Perform Heimlich maneuver to older child until object is expelled or child becomes unconscious; then convert to care of unconscious choking client
   f. Prepare child for procedures (bronchoscopy)
   g. Following procedure, monitor respiratory status continuously
   h. Withhold fluids until gag reflex returns
   i. Administer oxygen to maintain pulse oximetry > 94%

    j. Administer systemic antimicrobials as prescribed

    k. After child recovers, stress importance of avoiding risk factors

2. Anxiety

    a. Provide respiratory support prior to and after object is removed

    b. Explain all procedures and equipment to child and parents

    c. Project a relaxed, calm affect

    d. Encourage parents to express feelings and concerns

    e. Encourage parents to remain with child

    f. Use play therapy as child's condition allows

3. Client teaching

    a. Assess child's (if possible) and parents' current level of understanding

    b. Provider verbal and written information regarding:

        1) Adverse effects, importance of fluid intake during antibiotic course, and importance of completing entire prescription if child is placed on antibiotic therapy

        2) Normal growth and development activities

        3) Risk factors for foreign body aspiration and airway obstruction

        4) Removal of toys with small parts from environment of infants, toddlers, and preschoolers

        5) Age-appropriate foods and dangers of small children eating nuts and popcorn

        6) Importance of child chewing foods well and not running while eating

        7) Manifestations of airway obstruction that should be reported to health care provider

        8) Importance of follow-up with health care provider

    c. Allow sufficient time for child/family questions, providing honest answers

    d. Document teaching and child/family responses

NIC

1. Airway Management

2. Anxiety Reduction, Coping Enhancement

3. Teaching: Child Safety

EVALUATION

1. Patency of the child's airway is restored and maintained, and adequate gas exchange is evidenced by pulse oximetry > 94%.

2. Child's/family's anxiety is reduced as evidenced by relaxing body posture and decreasing distress.

3. Child/family demonstrate understanding of what the risk factors are for airway obstruction and how to avoid them, emergency treatment, and home care.

References

Broyles, B. E. (2005). *Medical-surgical nursing clinical companion.* Durham, NC: Carolina Academic Press.

Lucille Packard's Children's Hospital at Stanford. (2007). *Safety and injury prevention: Airway obstruction—Injury statistics and incidence rates.* Retrieved April 21, 2007, from http://www.lpch.org/DiseaseHeathInfo/healthlibrary/safety/airstats.html

Potts, N. L., & Mandleco, B. L. (2007). *Pediatric nursing: Caring for children and their families* (2nd ed.). Clifton Park, NY: Delmar Cengage Learning.

5

ANOREXIA NERVOSA

Definition

Anorexia nervosa is a potentially life-threatening condition characterized by severe weight loss and deliberate lack of sufficient nutritional intake to sustain metabolic functions.

Pathophysiology

The underlying pathophysiology of anorexia nervosa is the child's distorted body image and an attempt to use food and weight to deal with emotional issues. According to the National Alliance on Mental Illness, anorexia nervosa is "defined by a refusal to maintain minimal body weight within 15 percent of an individual's normal weight" (National Alliance on Mental Illness, 2007, p. 1). Regardless of how thin a child is, the child feels overweight. In addition, the child may focus on the size and shape of particular body parts. Even in the most severe cases, the child continues to deny the seriousness of the weight loss. The child is obsessed with being thin and is terrified of gaining weight.

There are two types of anorexia nervosa. In the restrictive type, the person severely limits food intake and compulsively exercises. The binge eating and purging type involves limiting dietary intake used in combination with intermittent episodes of binge eating followed by purging. The purging commonly is accomplished by self-induced vomiting and the use of laxatives, diuretics, and enemas. Both are characterized by the excessive use of appetite suppressants.

The starvation and purging can lead to electrolyte imbalances including hypokalemia, hyponatremia, and hypochloremia that can result in metabolic alkalosis and cardiac dysfunction. Further, there are changes in growth hormone levels, decreased secretion of sex hormones, altered bone marrow tissue development, structural abnormalities in the brain, and gastrointestinal health alterations. A specific dysfunction associated with anorexia in the adolescent is the risk for growth retardation, delay in menarche, amenorrhea, blood dyscrasias, and reduction in bone mass. Because of loss of muscle mass, cold intolerance is common. Without sufficient glucose to provide energy for neurological functioning, difficulty concentrating occurs as well as the mental preoccupation with food. Over 87% of young people affected by anorexia develop cardiac dysfunction. Anyone with anorexia may be at risk for death resulting from starvation or cardiac arrest (National Association of Anorexia Nervosa and Associated Disorders, 2006).

Complications

Amenorrhea and anovulation in females

Decreased gonadotropin levels and hypogonadism in males

Growth retardation and other endocrine dysfunction (hypercortisolemia, thyroid function suppression, delayed puberty, low estrogen states, increased growth hormone, decreased antidiuretic hormone, hypercarotenemia, and hypothermia)

Gastrointestinal dysfunction (constipation, delayed gastric emptying, and gastric dilation and rupture)

Anemia, leukopenia, and thrombocytopenia

Electrolyte imbalances including hypokalemia, hyponatremia, and hypochloremia

Renal dysfunction (decreased glomerular filtration rate (GFR), elevated blood urea nitrogen (BUN), edema, metabolic acidosis with dehydration, hypokalemia, hypochloremic metabolic alkalosis with vomiting, and hyperaldosteronism)

Neurological changes

Cardiac dysfunction (mitral valve prolapse, supraventricular and ventricular dysrhythmias, bradycardia, orthostatic hypotension, shock due to heart failure, and cardiac arrest)

Death

(Broyles, 2005)

Incidence

Anorexia nervosa usually occurs in adolescent girls and young adult women; but it also can occur in adolescent boys and adult women and men. Although most frequently found in the Caucasian population of most developed countries, anorexia nervosa is found in all races and cultural backgrounds. Conservative estimates suggest that 1/2–1% of females in the United States develop anorexia nervosa. According to the National Association of Anorexia Nervosa and Associated Disorders (ANAD), approximately 7 million women and 1 million men experience anorexia nervosa. Over 90% of those who are affected are adolescent and young women; as a result, the disorder has been characterized as primarily a woman's illness. However, anorexia nervosa has been diagnosed in children as young as 7 years old and in women between the ages of 50 and 80 years (National Association for Anorexia Nervosa and Associated Disorders, 2006).

The following shows the results of a ten-year study by ANAD:

Age at onset of illness
86% report onset of illness by the age of 20
10% report onset at 10 years or younger
33% report onset between ages of 11–15
43% report onset between ages of 16–20

Duration of illness/mortality
77% report duration from 1–15 years
30% report duration from 1–5 years
31% report duration from 6–10 years
16% report duration from 11–15 years
It is estimated that 6% of serious cases die
Only 50% report being cured

National Association of Anorexia Nervosa and Associated Disorders, 2006.

Finally, according to Dr. Tracy Farkas, "Anorexia nervosa has one of the highest mortality rates of all psychiatric disorders, with rates reported from 5–18%" (Farkas & Waldrop, 2006, Section 2).

Etiology

The cause of anorexia is the child's poor self-image, the use of food and weight to deal with emotional issues, and the vulnerability of adolescent girls and young women to strive to achieve the "ideal" body form in response to today's societal pressure to be thin.

Anorexia nervosa gives the individual whose emotional life is chaotic and painful a sense of control (over food and weight) (National Association of Anorexia Nervosa and Associated Disorders, 2006).

Clinical Manifestations

Decreased weight (usually less than 85% of ideal body weight)

Deliberate self-starvation with sudden, unexplained weight loss

Emaciated appearance

Fear of gaining weight

Refusal to eat

Caloric intake of less than 1000 kcal/day

Denial of hunger

Obsessive exercising

Greater amounts of hair on the body or the face

Cold sensitivity

Dry skin

Amenorrhea (absence of at least 2 consecutive cycles when they are otherwise expected)

Loss of scalp hair

Lanugo on extremities, back, and face

Chronic constipation or diarrhea

Esophageal erosions (from vomiting)

Depressed affect

Erosion of teeth enamel

Self-perception of being fat when the person is really too thin

Diagnostic Tests

History and physical examination

The following are performed to rule out other potential causes for weight loss as well as to diagnose damage resulting from starvation:

Electrocardiogram

Serum electrolytes including glucose level

Complete blood count

Liver function tests

Thyroid function tests

Bone density

Test for body composition

Psychological evaluation

Medical Management

Medical management of anorexia nervosa is difficult because individuals with this disorder believe that nothing is wrong with them. The goals of management are to provide adequate nutritional intake to meet each client's metabolic needs and to assist each client with resolution of the psychosocial problems that precipitated the anorexia. Clients in the early stages of anorexia (less than six months with the disorder or with minimal weight loss) may be successfully treated without hospitalization. But for successful treatment, clients must want to change and must have the support and assistance of family and friends. The focus of this treatment is teaching the client and family about the importance of nutrition and the assistance of psychological counselors, psychologists, or psychiatrists to help with body image perception and behavior modification.

Clients experiencing more serious anorexia require hospitalization, usually in a unit that specializes in individuals with anorexia nervosa and bulimia. Treatment involves more than changing the person's eating habits. Clients with anorexia nervosa often need counseling for a year or more so that they can work on modifying the feelings responsible for their eating problems. These feelings may be about their weight, family problems, or difficulties with self-esteem. As deemed by the health care provider, antidepressant agents may be prescribed in conjunction with psychological counseling (Broyles, 2005).

Nursing Management

Assessment

1. Measure vital signs
2. Perform physical assessment with anthropometric measurements
3. Obtain nutritional history and assessment
4. Obtain family and psychosocial history including coping skills

Nursing Diagnoses (including but not limited to)

1. Imbalanced nutrition: less than body requirements R/T inadequate nutritional intake or binging or purging
2. Decreased cardiac output R/T inadequate nutritional intake to meet metabolic needs
3. Disturbed body image R/T psychosocial factors
4. Deficient knowledge R/T condition, treatment, and psychosocial needs

Planning/Goals

1. Client will achieve adequate nutrition as evidenced by gradual weight gain to within defined limits (WDL) for age, height, and metabolic needs.
2. Client will not experience a decrease in cardiac output or evidence of cardiac dysfunction associated with anorexia nervosa.
3. Client will be compliant with psychosocial therapy and demonstrate and verbalize positive change in body image.
4. Client and family will demonstrate understanding of client's condition, treatment regimen, and psychosocial needs.

NOC

1. Nutritional Status: Food and Fluid Intake, Nutrient Intake, Weight, Body Mass
2. Cardiac Pump Effectiveness; Tissue Perfusion, Cardiac; Vital Signs
3. Body Image: Child Development, Adolescence: Self-Esteem
4. Knowledge: Diet, Health Behavior, Health Promotion, Treatment Regimen

Implementation

1. Nutrition
   a. Monitor intake and output
   b. Maintain calorie count as prescribed
   c. Assess food likes and dislikes
   d. Collaborate with dietician and health care provider to create nutritional plan
   e. Include family in developing dietary supplementation plan
   f. Organize eating of meals so client does not eat alone
   g. Monitor activity for two hours after eating

    h. Promote trusting relationship and actively listen to client and family

    i. Participate in interdisciplinary team planning of treatment modalities

    j. Promote client sense of responsibility and involvement in treatment and recovery

2. Cardiac output

    a. Obtain client history for clinical manifestations of decreased cardiac output

    b. Monitor vital signs and heart sounds

    c. Assess for activity tolerance

    d. Promote sense of trust

    e. Educate client and family about the cardiac risks of anorexia nervosa

    f. Document teaching and client/family response

    g. Collaborate with interdisciplinary team

    h. Monitor diagnostic findings

3. Body image

    a. Assess client's current body concept

    b. Encourage client to verbalize feelings

    c. Assess for nonverbal cues indicating ineffective coping strategies

    d. Assess client's need/desire for spiritual counseling

    e. Provide information concerning expected body mass distribution

    f. Assist in psychotherapy treatment plan

    g. Provide consistent positive feedback

    h. Support involvement of significant others in treatment plan

4. Client teaching

    a. Assess client's/family's current level of knowledge about condition

    b. Provide verbal and written information regarding:

        1) Nutritional plan and importance of compliance with plan

        2) Follow-up visits with interdisciplinary team members

        3) Referrals to adolescent and family community and support services

        4) Reinforcement of psychotherapy behavioral modification plan

        5) Contact phone numbers for interdisciplinary team involved in treatment plan

    c. Encourage client/family questions and respond honestly

    d. Document teaching and client/family response

NIC

1. Nutritional Monitoring, Fluid Monitoring, Eating Disorders Management, Weight Gain Assistance

2. Hemodynamic Regulation, Vital Signs Monitoring

3. Body Image Enhancement, Developmental Enhancement: Adolescence, Risk Identification, Self-Esteem Enhancement, Parent Education: Adolescence, Self-Esteem Enhancement

4. Health Education, Teaching Individual, Health System Guidance, Teaching: Condition, Treatment

EVALUATION

1. Client achieves adequate nutrition as evidenced by gradual weight gain to WDL for age, height, and metabolic needs.
2. Client does not experience a decrease in cardiac output or evidence of cardiac dysfunction associated with anorexia nervosa.
3. Client is compliant with psychosocial therapy and demonstrates and verbalizes positive change in body image.
4. Client/family demonstrates understanding of client's condition, treatment regimen, and psychosocial needs.

References

Broyles, B. E. (2005). *Medical-surgical nursing clinical companion*. Durham, NC: Carolina Academic Press.

Farkas, T. A., & Waldrop, R. (2006). *Anorexia nervosa*. Retrieved November 23, 2006, from http://www.emedicine.com/emerg/topic34.htm

National Alliance on Mental Illness. (2007). Retrieved April 21, 2007, from http://www.nami.org/Template.cfm?Section=By_Illness&template=/ContentManagement

National Association of Anorexia Nervosa and Associated Disorders. (2006). Retrieved April 21, 2007, from http://www.ANAD.org/site/anadweb/content.php?id=2118

6

AORTIC STENOSIS

Definition

Aortic stenosis is a stenotic congenital heart defect involving the narrowing of the valve (aortic valve) of the main artery exiting the left ventricle of the heart. This valve is located where the blood leaves the left ventricle to enter the aorta to be dispersed into systemic circulation. Refer to Figure 6-1.

Pathophysiology

Aortic stenosis occurs when the valve leaflets are abnormally formed during fetal development, resulting in the obstruction of the left ventricular outflow. A normal valve has three thin and pliable leaflets or cusps, but a stenotic valve may be unicuspid (only one cusp) or bicuspid (two cusps) with cusps that are thick and stiff (American Heart Association, 2008). This leads to a decrease in the amount of blood that can be ejected from the left ventricle and, consequently, reduced systemic blood supply. The heart then increases its rate to compensate, causing increased afterload and increased workload for the left ventricle with resulting decreasing left ventricular efficiency as the

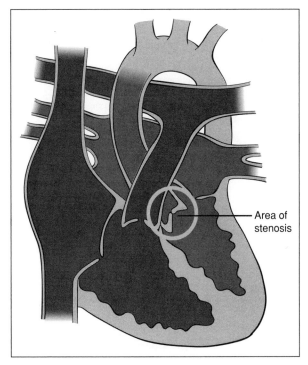

Area of stenosis

Figure 6-1: Aortic Stenosis.

heart muscle works harder against the obstructive stenosis. This leads to left ventricular hypertrophy and furthers the heart's inefficiency in meeting body demands (Potts & Mandleco, 2007).

This lesion can vary in degrees of obstruction and, consequently, differing severity of symptoms from asymptomatic to moderate to severe dyspnea (shortness of breath) on exertion. There are three types of aortic stenosis: subvalvular, valvular, and supravalvular. Subvalvular involves the narrowing below the aortic valve, valvular is obstruction at the valve itself, and supravalvular is aortic narrowing immediately above the valve.

Complications
Decreased cardiac output
Left ventricular hypertrophy
Growth retardation
Failure to thrive
Cardiac failure

Incidence
One percent of the world's population has congenital heart disease (International Children's Heart Foundation, 2006). Congenital heart defects are the most frequent birth defects, with 25,000 babies born with these defects annually. This is an incidence of approximately 1 in 115 to 150 births (Congenital Heart Defects.com, 2006). Of these, the incidence of aortic stenosis is "approximately 3–6% of individuals with CHD (congenital heart defect) with a 4:1 ratio of males to females" (Potts & Mandleco, 2007, p. 785). "The most common abnormality occurs when the aortic valve has only two . . . leaflets: a bicuspid aortic valve" (Cincinnati Children's Hospital Medical Center, 2006, p. 1).

Etiology
Congenital aortic stenosis is caused by a defect in the development of the aortic valve during the first eight weeks of fetal development. According to Children's Hospital of Philadelphia, congenital aortic stenosis can be caused by a number of factors, although most of the time this heart defect occurs sporadically with no apparent reason for its development (Children's Hospital of Philadelphia, 2006).

Clinical Manifestations
Mild stenosis (usually asymptomatic in the infant)
Murmur
Dyspnea on exertion
Syncope on exertion
Hypertension

Diagnostic Tests
Auscultation of a heart murmur
Echocardiography
Chest X-ray
Cardiac catheterization—may be used for diagnostics but usually is used
    as a method of treatment (refer to next section)

Medical Management
The goals of medical management are to provide adequate cardiac output for optimal tissue perfusion and prevent the irreversible congestive heart failure. Outpatient management is used for children with mild symptoms. Medications may be prescribed to

increase cardiac output, decrease pulmonary edema, and manage the hypertension associated with aortic stenosis. These medications usually include the cardiac glycoside digoxin, the loop diuretic furosemide, the beta-blocking agent propranolol, and an angiotensin-converting enzyme inhibitor.

For infants with moderate to severe aortic stenosis, the treatment of choice is balloon valvuloplasty performed during cardiac catheterization. In the neonate, this can be performed through the umbilical artery. This method is preferred in the neonate to spare potential damage to the femoral arteries. The procedure involves dilation of the aortic valve with use of a balloon. In most facilities, this procedure has replaced the more invasive commissurotomy to open the fused cusps, which requires open heart surgery. The primary complication of the balloon valvuloplasty is aortic regurgitation. "If this becomes severe, the aortic valve may need to be surgically repaired or replaced" (Potts & Mandleco, 2007, p. 786). If an artificial valve is used to replace the damaged valve, the child must be on anticoagulant therapy (warfarin) for life to prevent clots from forming as blood passes through the artificial valve.

Nursing Management

Refer to Chapter 26: Congenital Heart Disease/Open Heart Sugery.

ASSESSMENT

1. Assess for dyspnea on exertion or activity intolerance
2. Obtain history for evidence of difficulty with feedings (fatigue)
3. Auscultate heart sounds for presence of murmur
4. Assess for manifestations of left-sided heart failure

NURSING DIAGNOSES (INCLUDING BUT NOT LIMITED TO)

1. Activity intolerance R/T decreased cardiac output
2. Parental anxiety R/T child's diagnosis of heart defect
3. Ineffective cerebral tissue perfusion R/T decreased cardiac output
4. Decreased cardiac output R/T overworked left ventricle
5. Excess fluid volume R/T decreased cardiac output
6. Delayed growth and development R/T inadequate tissue perfusion
7. Deficient knowledge R/T condition, treatment, and home care

PLANNING/GOALS

1. Client will participate in age-appropriate activities without experiencing dyspnea on exertion or unexpected fatigue.
2. Parents will verbalize feelings and concerns, participate in child's care, and demonstrate decreased anxiety.
3. Client will not exhibit manifestations of decreased cerebral tissue perfusion (syncope).
4. Client will maintain adequate cardiac output to maintain metabolic functioning as evidenced by absence of tachycardia, diaphoresis, mottling of extremities, and tachypnea.
5. Client will maintain fluid and electrolyte balance as evidenced by urine output of 1–2 mL/kg of body weight/hour.
6. Client will maintain standardized guidelines for growth and development.
7. Client (if age-appropriate) and parents will demonstrate understanding of child's condition, treatment, and home care.

NOC

1. Activity Tolerance
2. Anxiety Level

3. Circulation Status, Neurological Status
4. Cardiac Pump Effectiveness
5. Fluid Balance
6. Child Development (Age-Appropriate)
7. Knowledge: Cardiac Disease Management, Energy Conservation, Treatment Regimen

IMPLEMENTATION

1. Activity tolerance
   a. Assess response to age-appropriate activities
   b. Space activities if fatigue or dyspnea occur
   c. Assess respiratory status
   d. Assess nutritional intake
   e. Plan activities to allow for adequate rest periods
   f. Encourage participation in age-appropriate activities as energy level allows
2. Parental anxiety
   a. Assess for parental behaviors that indicate anxiety
   b. Facilitate parental expression of feelings and concerns
   c. Encourage parents to participate in child's care
   d. Assist parents in decision making concerning child's care
   e. Provide parents with information about aortic stenosis, medication administration, and treatment options discussed with health care provider
3. Tissue perfusion
   a. Keep child as free from stress as possible
   b. Assess for syncope when child moves from lying to sitting or standing position
   c. Monitor oxygen saturation using pulse oximetry
   d. Administer medications as prescribed
   e. Administer oxygen as prescribed, titrating to maintain oxygen saturation at prescribed level
   f. Maintain safe environment for child
   g. Monitor vital signs as appropriate
4. Cardiac output
   a. Assess vital signs as appropriate
   b. Teach parents about medications prescribed
   c. Administer medications as prescribed
   d. Auscultate heart sounds
   e. Monitor intake and output
   f. Administer oxygen as prescribed, titrating to maintain oxygen saturation at prescribed level
5. Fluid volume
   a. Monitor intake and output
   b. Report to health care provider if urine output is less than 1 mL/kg/hour
   c. Obtain daily weight
   d. Change child's position at least every 2 hours to prevent skin breakdown from edema
   e. Provide skin care for child with edema to prevent skin breakdown

6. Growth and development
   a. Assess child's current level of growth and development
   b. Provide parents with information on age-appropriate play activities
   c. Plot weight and height on growth chart, comparing to standardized chart
   d. Encourage child participation in age-appropriate activities as energy level allows
7. Child/parent teaching
   a. Assess parents' current level of knowledge about child's condition
   b. Assess parental readiness to learn
   c. Provide verbal and written information regarding:
      1) Age-appropriate activities and ways to adjust these according to child's energy level
      2) Prescribed medication administration
      3) Importance of follow-up with cardiologist
      4) Manifestations of worsening condition
      5) Contact numbers needed to report adverse effects of medications or worsening of condition
   d. Encourage client/family questions and respond honestly
   e. Document teaching and client/family response

NIC

1. Activity Therapy
2. Anxiety Reduction
3. Cerebral Perfusion Promotion, Neurologic Monitoring, Risk Management
4. Vital Signs Monitoring, Medication Administration
5. Fluid/Electrolyte Monitoring, Fluid/Electrolyte Management
6. Developmental Enhancement: Child
7. Teaching: Disease Process, Prescribed Activities, Treatment

EVALUATION

1. Client participates in age-appropriate activities without experiencing dyspnea on exertion or unexpected fatigue.
2. Parents verbalize feelings and concerns, participate in child's care, and demonstrate decreased anxiety.
3. Client does not exhibit manifestations of decreased cerebral tissue perfusion (syncope).
4. Client maintains adequate cardiac output to maintain metabolic functioning as evidenced by absence of tachycardia, diaphoresis, mottling of extremities, tachypnea.
5. Client maintains fluid and electrolyte balance as evidenced by urine output of 1–2 mL/kg/hour.
6. Client maintains standardized guidelines for growth and development.
7. Client (if age-appropriate) and parents demonstrate understanding of child's condition, treatment, and home care.

References

American Heart Association. (2008). *Congenital heart defects*. Retrieved March 12, 2008, from http://www.americanheart.org/presenter.jhtml?identifier=12012

Children's Hospital of Philadelphia. (2006). *Aortic stenosis*. Retrieved March 12, 2008, from http://www.chop.edu/consumer/your_child/condition_section_index.jsp?id=-9326

Cincinnati Children's Hospital Medical Center. (2006). *Aortic stenosis.* Retrieved April 21, 2007, from http://www.cincinnatichildrens.org/health/heart-encyclopedia/anomalies/avs.htm

Congenital Heart Defects.com. (2006). *Aortic stenosis.* Retrieved April 21, 2007, from http://www.congenitalheartdefects.com/typesofCHD.html#Aortic

International Children's Heart Foundation. (2006). *Children and congenital heart defects.* Retrieved April 21, 2007, from http://www.ichf.org/doc/2354

Potts, N. L., & Mandleco, B. L. (2007). *Pediatric nursing: Caring for children and their families.* (2nd ed.). Clifton Park, NY: Delmar Cengage Learning.

7

APLASTIC ANEMIA/PANCYTOPENIA

Definition

Aplastic anemia, also called aplastic pancytopenia, is a condition of bone marrow suppression (Broyles, 2005) resulting in a severe reduction in the production of erythrocytes (red blood cells), granulocytes (leukocytes or white blood cells), and platelets.

Pathophysiology

The dramatic reduction of hematopoesis by the bone marrow results in peripheral pancytopenia, a triad of (1) severe anemia, (2) leukopenia, and (3) thrombocytopenia resulting from bone marrow hypoplasia. The primary function of erythrocytes is to carry oxygen and carbon dioxide in the blood, which is necessary for adequate tissue perfusion. The normal red blood cell count varies from 4.8–7.1 million/mm^3 in the neonate to 4.5–5.3 million/mm^3 in the adolescent male and 4.1–5.1 million/mm^3 in the adolescent female. The resulting anemia in aplastic anemia causes a decrease in tissue perfusion necessary for cellular function.

Granulocytes are responsible for maintaining the immune system and preventing and fighting infection in the body. The normal leukocyte count ranges from 9,000–30,000 cells/mm^3 in the neonate to 4,500–13,500 cells/mm^3 in 8–13 year olds. Leukocytes are classified according to one of five types and are measured based on the percentage of each in the leukocyte count: neutrophils (57–67%), lymphocytes (25–33%), monocytes (3–7%), eosinophils (1–3%), and basophils (0–0.75%). Because neutrophils account for the largest number of leukocytes, they are most representative of the status of the immune system. Dramatic reductions in granulocytes place the person at high risk for infection, including potentially life-threatening infections.

Platelets play a significant role in blood coagulation. The normal platelet count is 150,000–400,000 cells/mm^3. A reduction in circulating platelets places the individual at risk for thrombocytopenia and bleeding episodes.

Of the three types of cells involved in aplastic anemia, "RBCs (red blood cells) are the last to demonstrate a reduction in numbers because of their relatively long life span" (Potts & Mandleco, 2007, p. 835). Aplastic anemia can vary in severity from mild to severe.

Complications

Infection
Bleeding
Anemia
Tissue and organ failure
Graft-versus-host disease
Bone marrow graft failure
Death (in severe cases)

Incidence

According to one study, "The annual incidence of aplastic anemia in Europe, as detailed in large, formal epidemiologic studies, is similar to that in the United States, with 2 cases per million population. Aplastic anemia is thought to be more common in Asia than in the West. The incidence was accurately determined to be 4 cases per million population in Bangkok, but may be closer to 6 cases per million population in the rural areas of Thailand and as high as 14 cases per million population in Japan. . . . This increased incidence may be related to environmental factors, such as increased exposure to toxic chemicals, rather than to genetic factors because this increase is not observed in people of Asian ancestry who are presently living in the United States" (Bakhshi, Baynes, & Abella, 2006, Section 2). The incidence of aplastic anemia in the United States is approximately 500 new cases annually.

Etiology

Aplastic anemia is classified as hereditary or acquired. The hereditary type is called Fanconi's anemia, a rare autosomal recessive condition that becomes evident early in life and usually is accompanied by multiple congenital anomalies. "The distinction between acquired and inherited disease may present a clinical challenge, but more than 80% of cases are acquired. In acquired aplastic anemia, clinical and laboratory observations suggest that this is an autoimmune disease" (Bakhshi et al., 2006, Section 2).

A number of toxic substances have been identified as causes of aplastic anemia; they include benzene; toluene; insecticides; arsenic; and medications such as chloramphenicol, sulfonamides, gold salts, phenybutazone, phenytoin, mephenytoin, trimethadione, carbamazepine, quinacrine, Pyridium, and tolbutamide.

Clinical Manifestations

Increased bruising (usually the first sign)
Petechiae
Pallor
Fatigue
Tachycardia
Infection
Dyspnea

Diagnostic Tests

Complete blood count
Bone marrow aspiration

Medical Management

If the aplastic anemia is acquired, the first intervention is alleviating the underlying cause, including preventing further exposure to the causative toxin. Treatment then is symptomatic. Red blood cell transfusions are used to elevate erythrocyte counts and improve tissue perfusion. Transfusion of platelets may be performed depending on the criticality of the platelet count. Antimicrobials are employed to treat bacterial infections. To achieve remission in children with acquired aplastic anemia, bone marrow transplantation or immunosuppression with steroids, cyclosporine, antihymocyte globulin, and antilymphocyte globulin may be needed.

Nursing Management

Assessment

1. Obtain history and physical
2. Assess for manifestations of anemia
3. Obtain baseline temperature
4. Assess for ecchymosis, petechiae, and changes in mental status

NURSING DIAGNOSES (INCLUDING BUT NOT LIMITED TO)

1. Ineffective protection R/T decreased production of leukocytes
2. Risk for injury, bleeding R/T decreased production of platelets
3. Ineffective tissue perfusion R/T decreased production of erythrocytes
4. Deficient knowledge R/T condition, treatment regimen, and home care

PLANNING/GOALS

1. Client will remain free of infection; or if infection occurs, client will be effectively treated.
2. Client will not experience episodes of uncontrolled bleeding.
3. Client will maintain adequate tissue perfusion to meet metabolic needs as evidenced by oxygen saturation within defined limits (WDL).
4. Parents/client will demonstrate understanding of condition, treatment, and home care.

NOC

1. Immune Status
2. Risk Control
3. Circulation Status
4. Knowledge: Illness Care, Health Promotion

IMPLEMENTATION

1. Risk for infection
   a. Monitor temperature at least every 4 hours, avoiding rectal temperatures (can damage rectal mucosa causing bleeding)
   b. Place child in private room
   c. Activate compromised host or reverse isolation precautions
   d. Assess wounds for redness, swelling, and purulent drainage
   e. Monitor white blood cell count and differential
   f. Administer antimicrobials as prescribed and appropriate
   g. Assess breath sounds
   h. Activate neutropenic precautions according to facility protocol
2. Risk for bleeding
   a. Monitor skin and mucous membranes carefully for bleeding (if child is receiving oxygen per nasal cannula, be sure to closely monitor nares for epistaxis)
   b. Monitor stools for blood
   c. Monitor platelet count
   d. Activate bleeding precautions according to facility protocol
   e. Avoid all injections
   f. Use soft-bristled toothbrush for oral hygiene
   g. Involve child in age-appropriate quiet (low-impact) activities
   h. Administer contraceptives as prescribed to decrease menstrual flow in adolescent girls
   i. Administer stool softeners as prescribed
   j. Administer intravenous platelets as prescribed
3. Tissue perfusion
   a. Monitor continuous pulse oximetry
   b. Administer oxygen to maintain oxygen saturation at prescribed levels

    c. Monitor erythrocyte count

    d. Monitor cardiopulmonary status every 4 hours

    e. Monitor vital signs

    f. Administer packed red blood cells as prescribed following facility protocol, monitoring closely for transfusion reactions and fluid overload

    g. Administer medications as prescribed to stimulate production of red blood cells

    h. Administer medications to achieve remission as prescribed

4. Parent/client teaching

    a. Assess current level of knowledge

    b. Provide parents and child (if age-appropriate) verbal and written information regarding:

        1) The way aplastic anemia is acquired or hereditary aplastic anemia occurs

        2) All procedures and medications used to treat child

        3) Infection prevention

        4) Accident and injury prevention (age-appropriate)

        5) Medication administration as needed

        6) Importance of follow-up care

        7) Contact information to report worsening of condition or adverse effects of medications

    c. Provide adequate time for teaching and parental questions

    d. Document teaching and parent/client response

NIC

1. Laboratory Data Interpretation, Infection Protection, Medication Administration

2. Risk Identification, Bleeding Precautions

3. Fluid Management, Oxygen Therapy, Laboratory Data Interpretation, Medication Administration

4. Teaching: Disease Process, Treatment, Health Education

EVALUATION

1. Client did contract opportunistic infection; however, it was promptly treated.

2. Client does not experience episodes of uncontrolled bleeding.

3. Client maintains adequate tissue perfusion to meet metabolic needs as evidenced by oxygen saturation WDL.

4. Parents/client demonstrate understanding of condition, treatment, and home care.

References

Bakhshi, S., Baynes, M. B., & Abella, E. (2006). *Aplastic anemia*. Retrieved January 3, 2007, from http://www.emedicine.com/med/topic162.htm.

Broyles, B. E. (2005). *Medical-surgical nursing clinical companion*. Durham, NC: Carolina Academic Press.

Potts, N. L., & Mandleco, B. L. (2007). *Pediatric nursing: Caring for children and their families*. (2nd ed.). Clifton Park, NY: Delmar Cengage Learning.

8

APPENDICITIS AND APPENDECTOMY

Definition

Appendicitis is defined as "the inflammation and infection of the vermiform appendix, a small lymphoid, tubular blind sac at the [proximal] end of the cecum of the large intestines (below the ileocecal valve). Appendectomy is the surgical removal of the appendix" (Broyles, 2005, p. 71).

Pathophysiology

The appendix is a wormlike projection with the diameter of a lead pencil. Early in life the appendix is theorized to have immune qualities that decrease early in childhood. As food passes from the small intestine into the large intestine, the appendix fills and empties with the rhythm of peristalsis. "In 70% of cases (appendicitis), the lumen between the appendix and the cecum becomes obstructed with agents such as a fecalith, fecal matter that becomes petrified and stone-like, calculi, tumors, parasites, and foreign bodies" (Potts & Mandleco, 2007, p. 681). As normal mucous secretions accumulate around these particles, capillary and venous engorgement occurs, resulting in intra-lumenal pressure. This causes inflammation, leading to further engorgement of the appendix followed by infection from invasion by bacteria and/or viruses. The infection creates the classic manifestations of temperature elevations, umbilical pain radiating to the right lower abdominal quadrant, and nausea and vomiting secondary to intestinal obstruction from the enlarged appendix. If left untreated, the appendix may rupture, spilling the infectious contents into the peritoneal cavity, resulting in peritonitis. This may progress to life-threatening septicemia.

Complications

Appendix rupture
Appendix perforation
Abscess formation
Peritonitis
Septicemia

Incidence

"Appendicitis is the most common condition requiring abdominal surgery in child-hood, occurring at a rate of 4 per 1,000 children younger than 14 years of age" (Potts & Mandleco, 2007, p. 681). The peak incidence of appendicitis is between the ages of 20 and 30 years.

Etiology

According to the National Institute of Diabetes and Digestive and Kidney Diseases (NIDDK) of the National Institutes of Health, most commonly, fecal material blocks the inside of the appendix. Also, bacterial or viral infections in the digestive tract can result in swelling of lymph nodes (lymphoid hyperplasia) that squeezes the appendix and causes obstruction. Traumatic injury to the abdomen may lead to appendicitis in a small number of individuals. Genetics may be a factor in other cases; for instance, appendicitis that runs in families may result from a genetic variant that predisposes a person to obstruction of the appendiceal lumen (National Institute of Diabetes and Digestive and Kidney Diseases, 2007).

Clinical Manifestations

Umbilical abdominal pain radiating to the lower right quadrant

Anorexia

Nausea and vomiting

Constipation

Diarrhea

Fever

Abdominal distention

Diagnostic Tests

Complete blood count

Serum electrolyte levels

Abdominal ultrasound

Abdominal computed tomography

Medical Management

The goals of treatment for acute appendicitis are the surgical removal of the appendix (appendectomy) and treatment of any infection present. An intravenous access is established, and the child is not permitted to consume anything by mouth until after surgery. The appendectomy may be performed through a standard small incision into the right lower quadrant of the abdomen or through laparoscopy, which requires three or four smaller incisions. The laparoscopic appendectomy is preferred because the skin incision is smaller, postoperative pain is less, and recovery time is shorter. If an abscess has formed at the appendix site, after the appendix is removed, a drain is placed to ensure complete drainage of the area.

If the appendix ruptures prior to or during surgery, antimicrobials are prescribed. Those most frequently used are cephalosporins, which are administered intravenously during hospitalization and then continued orally following discharge.

Nursing Management

ASSESSMENT

1. Obtain history and physical
2. Assess for manifestations of appendicitis
3. Obtain baseline vital signs
4. Assess for signs of rupture (sudden relief of pain), perforation, or abscess formation
5. Interpret laboratory and diagnostic tests
6. Perform psychosocial assessment of child and parents for anxiety, fear of the unknown, presence of emergency situation, and unplanned surgery

NURSING DIAGNOSES (INCLUDING BUT NOT LIMITED TO)

1. Acute pain R/T appendix inflammation and postoperative incision
2. Risk for deficient fluid volume R/T inadequate intake and fluid loss from vomiting
3. Risk for infection R/T possible rupture or perforation of appendix and surgical incision
4. Deficient knowledge R/T condition, medical management, and home care

PLANNING/GOALS

1. Client will demonstrate adequate pain management as evidenced by pain level of 2 on a scale of 0–10, with 10 being the most severe pain. *NOTE:* The numerical pain scale indicates the client's pain level by a continuum from 0 (meaning no pain) to 10 (indicating the worst pain the client has ever felt).
2. Client will maintain fluid and electrolyte balance as evidenced by urine output >1 mL/kg/hour.
3. Client will not experience appendix rupture and will remain free of infection.
4. Parents/client will demonstrate understanding of condition, medical management, and home care.

NOC

1. Comfort Level, Pain Control, Pain, Disruptive Effects, Pain Level
2. Fluid Balance, Hydration
3. Immune Status, Infection Status, Wound Healing, Primary Intention
4. Knowledge: Illness Care, Health Promotion

IMPLEMENTATION

1. Pain
   a. Assess pain preoperatively and administer analgesics as prescribed
   b. Assess pain hourly using developmentally-appropriate pain scale
   c. Assess for behavioral cues of discomfort
   d. Position for comfort
   e. Encourage to request medication before pain becomes too intense (Rocca, 2007)
   f. Avoid applying heat to abdomen preoperatively as this can trigger perforation or rupture
   g. Initiate patient-controlled analgesia (PCA) postoperatively as prescribed, monitoring for effectiveness
   h. Use age-appropriate activities as child indicates desire to play
   i. Encourage early ambulation to decrease stiffness and soreness from being in bed
2. Fluid volume
   a. Administer intravenous fluids as prescribed
   b. Maintain strict intake and output
   c. Monitor wound drainage
   d. Monitor output of nasogastric tube and replace with intravenous volume as prescribed if tube has been placed
   e. Encourage fluids postoperatively as soon as bowel sounds return and as prescribed
3. Infection
   a. Do not apply moist heat to abdomen prior to surgery as this increases risk of rupture
   b. Monitor vital signs
   c. Report abnormal findings
   d. Administer antipyretics and antimicrobials as prescribed
   e. Monitor wound and provide wound care as indicated

4. Parent/child teaching
   a. Assess current level of knowledge
   b. Provide parents and child (if age-appropriate) verbal and written information regarding:
      1) All procedures and medications used to treat child
      2) Infection prevention
      3) Postoperative guidelines including no lifting or strenuous activity until cleared by health care provider
      4) Medication administration as needed, stressing importance of completing antimicrobial prescriptions
      5) Importance of follow-up care
      6) Contact information to report worsening of condition or adverse effects of medications
   c. Provide adequate time for parental questions
   d. Document teaching and parent/client response

NIC

1. Analgesic Administration, Medication Management, Pain Management, PCA Assistance
2. Fluid Management, Fluid Monitoring, Hypovolemia Management, Intravenous (IV) Therapy
3. Infection Control, Infection Protection, Incision Site Care
4. Teaching: Disease Process, Treatment, Health Education

EVALUATION

1. Client demonstrates adequate pain management as evidenced by pain level of 1–2 on a scale of 1–10, with 10 being the most severe pain.
2. Client maintains fluid and electrolyte balance as evidenced by urine output >1 mL/kg/hour.
3. Client does not experience appendix rupture and remains free of infection.
4. Parents/client demonstrate understanding of condition, medical management, and home care.

References

Broyles, B. E. (2005). *Medical-surgical nursing clinical companion*. Durham, NC: Carolina Academic Press.

National Institute of Diabetes and Digestive and Kidney. (2007). *Appendicitis*. Retrieved April 21, 2007, from http://digestive.niddk.nih.gov/ddiseases/pubs/appendicitis/index.htm

Potts, N. L. & Mandleco, B. L. (2007). *Pediatric nursing: Caring for children and their families*. (2nd ed.). Clifton Park, NY: Delmar Cengage Learning.

Rocca, J. D. (2007). Hospital nursing: Minimizing the perils of appendicitis. *Nursing 2007, 37*(1), 64hn2.

9

Asthma/Reactive Airway Disease

Definition

Asthma, or reactive airway disease (RAD), is a hypersensitivity obstructive airway disease characterized by chronic inflammation, bronchoconstriction, and increased airway reaction to a variety of stimulants (Broyles, 2005). Once thought to be a reversible response, now it is believed to result in chronic damage to the airways as a result of chronic inflammation (Potts & Mandleco, 2007). Formerly called asthma, it was renamed reactive airway disease as a more accurately descriptive term for the condition.

Pathophysiology

The airways, especially the bronchi, of individuals with RAD constrict and narrow in response to exposure to irritants (allergens) and other stimuli that normally would not elicit a response. When the person is exposed to irritants, the inflammatory response is initiated, the smooth muscle of the bronchi spasm, and additional events cascade. Antibodies such as immunoglobulin E (IgE) are formed against the allergens as well as the increase in mast cells and macrophages. In response, histamine, basophils, eosinophils, neutrophils, T lymphocytes, prostaglandins, and platelets are released resulting in bronchoconstriction from contracted hypertrophied muscle, mucosal edema, and an increased production of mucus from enlarged mucous glands (Potts & Mandleco, 2007). Refer to Figure 9-1.

This cascade of events causes the lumen of bronchi to narrow, resulting in airway obstruction, dyspnea, orthopnea, and hypoxia. Because the airways are normally larger during inspiration than expiration, the child can inhale but has difficulty exhaling. This is reflected in the characteristic expiratory wheeze. The inability to completely exhale leads to hyperinflation of the alveoli from the trapped air and resultant decrease in gas exchange and respiratory acidosis.

The body's drive for oxygen, the anxiety response to the inability to breathe effectively, and the respiratory buffer to acid-base imbalances stimulate tachypnea.

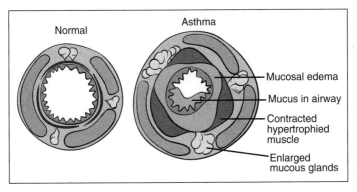

Figure 9-1: Pathophysiology of Asthma.

This hyperventilation lowers carbon dioxide levels in the blood (hypocapnea), which can lead to compensatory respiratory alkalosis. As the child tires from the tachypnea and in response to the compensatory respiratory alkalosis, hypoventilation occurs, causing further retention of carbon dioxide, recurrent respiratory acidosis, and eventually respiratory failure. A reactive airway response that is not effectively reversed results in status asthmaticus, which can lead to death due to respiratory failure and exhaustion.

Complications

Ineffective gas exchange
Respiratory acidosis
Compensatory respiratory alkalosis
Hypoxia
Recurrent respiratory acidosis
Status asthmaticus
Respiratory failure
Death

Incidence

"Asthma is the most common pediatric chronic illness" (Potts & Mandleco, 2007, p. 724). According to the National Heart Lung and Blood Institute of the National Institutes of Health, in the United States, approximately 20 million people are diagnosed with asthma and almost 9 million of them are children. Although asthma affects individuals of all ages, it most commonly starts in childhood. Boys are affected more than girls; however, during adulthood, it affects more women than men. African Americans are more likely than Caucasians to be hospitalized for asthma attacks and to die from asthma. African-American children are three times as likely to die from asthma as Caucasian children (National Heart Lung and Blood Institute, 2007a).

Etiology

Reactive airway disease is caused by an individual's hypersensitivity to irritants in the environment. Exercise, allergens, irritants, and viral infections have been identified as risk factors for stimulating an "attack." Animal dander, dust mites, tree and grass pollen, mold, and even cockroaches are among the allergens. Cigarette smoke, air pollution, cold air, strong odors from cooking or painting, and scented products are irritants that have been responsible for asthmatic episodes. Other factors include pharmacological agents such as aspirin and beta-adrenergic blockers, sulfites in foods and beverages (wine), gastroesophageal reflux disease, infections, and chemicals that the child may be exposed to at school or play (National Heart Lung and Blood Institute, 2007b).

Clinical Manifestations

Coughing, especially worse at night
Dyspnea
Orthopnea
Tachypnea
Wheeze (expiratory)
Chest tightness
Irritability
Restlessness

Diaphoresis

Use of accessory muscles to breathe

Increased anteroposterior diameter of the chest (barrel chest)

Nasal flaring

Diagnostic Tests

White blood cell count differential

Allergy testing

Spirometry

Pulmonary function test (PFT)

Pulse oximetry

Peak expiratory flow rate (PEFR)

Chest radiography

Arterial blood gases if child presents with manifestations of acid-base imbalance

Medical Management

The goals of management are to restore effective gas exchange and minimize chronic damage to the airways. Although there are a number of guidelines for consistency in the treatment of asthma, according to Kavuru, Lang, and Erzurum of the Cleveland Clinic in their 2005 report, the guidelines developed by the National Asthma Education and Prevention Program (NAEPP) are the most practiced. The authors caution, however, that "specific treatment regimens must be tailored to individual patient needs. Also, since asthma research is a rapidly evolving area and new therapeutics are anticipated, these guidelines will be revised periodically" (Kavuru, Lang, & Erzurum, 2005a, p. 1).

The NAEPP guidelines are based on asthma severity and provide a stepwise approach to the treatment of infants and children 5 years of age and younger and a separate approach for adults and children 5 years of age and older. The approaches are based on a four-step classification of asthma: Step 1: Mild Intermittent (least severe), Step 2: Mild Persistent, Step 3: Moderate Persistent, and Step 4: Severe Persistent. The guidelines identify medications required to maintain long-term control (Potts & Mandleco, 2007; Kavuru, Lang, & Erzurum, 2005b).

The major difference in the approaches is the dosing of the medications. The classifications remain consistent. These classifications are as follows:

Step 1	No daily medications
Step 2	Low-dose corticosteroids (inhalation) or cromolyn or leukotriene receptor antagonist; in adults and children over 5 years of age, an alternative of the use of sustained release theophylline to achieve a serum concentration of 5–15 ug/mL
Step 3	Low- to medium-dose inhaled corticosteroids and long-acting beta-agonists or medium-dose corticosteroids and either leukotriene modifier or theophylline
Step 4	High-dose inhaled corticosteroids and long-acting beta-agonist and, if needed, oral corticosteroids

Adapted from National Asthma Education and Prevention Program. (2003). Expert panel report: Guidelines for the diagnosis and management of asthma: Update on selected topics 2002 by Karuru, M. S., Lang, D. M., & Erzurum, S. C. 2005b.

Systemic corticosteroids used in the treatment of RAD include methylprednisolone, prednisolone, and prednisone. Inhaled corticosteroids used are beclomethasone, budesonide DPI, flunisolide, fluticasone, and triameinolone acetonide. Long-acting inhaled beta$_2$-agonists include salmeterol and formoterol and combined fluticasone/salmeterol. Leukotriene modifiers or leukotriene receptor antagonists (Broyles, Reiss, & Evans, 2007) used include montelukast, zafirlukast, and zileuton. Theophylline remains the xanthine derivative or methylxanthine of choice. A number of short-acting inhaled beta$_2$-agonists are employed in the treatment of asthmatic episodes, including albuterol, albuterol HFA, pirbuterol, albuterol rotahaler, levalbuterol, and albuterol and bitolterol nebulizer solutions.

Nursing Management

ASSESSMENT

1. Obtain history and physical
2. Assess vital signs
3. Obtain focused assessment of respiratory system
4. Assess parent's/child's knowledge of asthma/RAD
5. Obtain pulse oximetry reading

NURSING DIAGNOSES (INCLUDING BUT NOT LIMITED TO)

1. Ineffective airway clearance R/T bronchial inflammation, bronchospasms, mucosal edema, and increased mucus production
2. Impaired gas exchange R/T bronchoconstriction and bronchial edema
3. Anxiety R/T difficulty breathing and hospitalization
4. Risk for deficient fluid volume R/T increased respiratory rate (insensible fluid loss) and decreased oral intake
5. Deficient knowledge R/T condition, medication treatment, preventative measures, and home care

PLANNING/GOALS

1. Client will exhibit improved airway clearance as evidenced by a respiratory rate less than 24 per minute and absence of dyspnea, orthopnea, use of accessory muscles, or nasal flaring.
2. Client will experience sufficient oxygen for body demands, acid-base balance, and oxygen saturation within defined limits (WDL).
3. Client/parents will exhibit decreased anxiety as evidenced by verbal and nonverbal indicators.
4. Client will maintain adequate fluid balance as evidenced by urine specific gravity of 1.005–1.012 and urine output greater than 1 mL/kg/hour.
5. Client (if appropriate) and parents will verbalize understanding of disease process and treatment and will be compliant with prescribed treatment regimen.

NOC

1. Respiratory Status: Airway Patency
2. Respiratory Status: Gas Exchange
3. Anxiety Level

4. Fluid Balance

5. Asthma Self-Management

IMPLEMENTATION

1. Airway

   a. Assess respiratory status every 2–4 hours and as needed (prn)

   b. Monitor vital signs according to client's condition

   c. Collaborate with health care provider regarding changes in client's condition

   d. Administer fast-acting beta$_2$-agonist (e.g., albuterol) nebulizers as prescribed

   e. Maintain intravenous access, monitoring hourly

   f. Administer inhaled or intravenous corticosteroids as prescribed

   g. Assist client to position to facilitate breathing

   h. Monitor arterial blood gases if client's condition warrants these measurements

   i. Place on cardiopulmonary monitor at bedside

2. Gas exchange

   a. Monitor pulse oximetry

   b. Administer oxygen to maintain oxygen saturation within prescribed parameters

   c. Assess respiratory status every 2–4 hours and prn

   d. Collaborate with health care provider regarding changes in client's condition

   e. Administer medications as prescribed, monitoring theophylline levels

   f. Maintain intravenous access, monitoring hourly

   g. Assist child into position to facilitate respiratory effort

3. Anxiety

   a. Assess for verbal and nonverbal manifestations of anxiety

   b. Encourage client and parents to express feelings and concerns

   c. Explain all procedures and medications

   d. Provide age-appropriate explanations

   e. Encourage age-appropriate nontaxing play

4. Fluid balance

   a. Maintain intravenous access, monitoring hourly

   b. Monitor strict intake and output

   c. Assess skin, mucous membranes, and urine specific gravity

   d. Administer intravenous fluids and medications as prescribed

   e. Encourage oral intake of 1 ounce per hour for children 6 years and younger as condition allows, monitoring closely for choking

   f. Provide humidification to environment

   g. Collaborate with health care provider if client's urine output falls below 1 mL/kg/hour

5. Client/parent teaching

   a. Assess current level of knowledge

   b. Provide parents and child (if age-appropriate) verbal and written information regarding:

      1) Asthma triggers or precipitating factors

      2) All procedures and medications used to treat child

3) Role of emotions and stress on asthma exacerbations

4) Age-appropriate activities

5) Medication administration including use of inhalers and adverse effects of medications

6) Importance of compliance with medication regimen

7) Importance of breathing exercises as prescribed

8) Importance of follow-up care and monitoring of therapeutic blood levels of medications

9) Contact information to report worsening of condition and adverse effects of medications

c. Provide adequate time for parental questions

d. Document teaching and parent/client response

NIC

1. Airway Management

2. Asthma Management, Respiratory Monitoring, Acid-Base Management, Anxiety Reduction

3. Anxiety Reduction

4. Fluid Management

5. Asthma Management

EVALUATION

1. Client exhibits improved airway clearance as evidenced by a respiratory rate less than 24 per minute and absence of dyspnea, orthopnea, use of accessory muscles, or nasal flaring.

2. Client experiences sufficient oxygen for body demands, acid-base balance, and oxygen saturation WDL.

3. Client and parents exhibit decreased anxiety as evidenced by verbal and nonverbal indicators.

4. Client maintains adequate fluid balance as evidenced by urine specific gravity of 1.005–1.012 and urine output greater than 1 mL/kg/hour.

5. Client (if appropriate) and parents verbalize understanding of disease process and treatment and are compliant with prescribed treatment regimen.

References

Broyles, B. E. (2005). *Medical-surgical nursing clinical companion*. Durham, NC: Carolina Academic Press.

Broyles, B. E., Reiss, B. S., & Evans, M. E. (2007). *Pharmacological aspects of nursing care*. (7th ed.). Clifton Park, NY: Delmar Cengage Learning.

Kavuru, M. S., Lang, D. M., & Erzurum, S. C. (2005a). *Asthma: Asthma management algorithms*. Retrieved January 4, 2007, from http://www.clevelandclinicmeded.com/diseasemanagement/pulmonary/asthma/asthma2.htm#algorithms

Karuru, M. S., Lang, D. M., & Erzurum, S. C. (2005b). *Asthma: Asthma management algorithms. Table 1*. Retrieved January 4, 2007, from http://www.clevelandclinicmeded.com/diseasemanagement/pulmonary/asthma/asthmatable1b.htm

National Asthma Education and Prevention Program. (2003). *Expert panel report: Guidelines for the diagnosis and management of asthma: Update on selected topics 2002*. Retrieved January 4, 2007, from http://www.clevelandclinicmeded.com/diseasemanagement/pulmonary/asthma/asthmatable1b.htm

National Heart Lung and Blood Institute. (2007a). *Who is at risk?* Retrieved April 21, 2007, from http://www.nhlbi.nih.gov/health/dci/Diseases/Asthma/Asthma_WhoIsAtRisk.html

National Heart Lung and Blood Institute. (2007b). *Causes.* Retrieved April 21, 2007, from http://www.nhlbi.nih.gov/health/dci/Diseases/Asthma/Asthma_Causes.html

Potts, N. L., & Mandleco, B. L. (2007). *Pediatric nursing: Caring for children and their families.* (2nd ed.). Clifton Park, NY: Delmar Cengage Learning.

10

ATRIAL SEPTAL DEFECT (ASD)

Definition

An atrial septal defect (ASD) is an abnormal connection between the two upper chambers of the heart that occurs during fetal development, arising from the foramen ovale (American Heart Association, 2007). Refer to Figure 10-1.

Pathophysiology

The ASD can vary in size from as small as a hole that is 1 mm in diameter to as large as the complete absence of the septum. Small defects usually produce no symptoms beyond a vague murmur, whereas larger defects can produce symptoms of decreased cardiac output requiring open-heart surgery to close the connection between the two atria. There are three different types of ASDs. The most common type is the secundum defect that usually occurs as an isolated defect. The primum ASD is associated with a cleft in the mitral valve that may cause the valve to leak. The third type is the sinus venosus defect, located in the superior portion of the atrial septum. This is typically associated with abnormal drainage of the right upper pulmonary vein (Congenital Heart Defects.com,

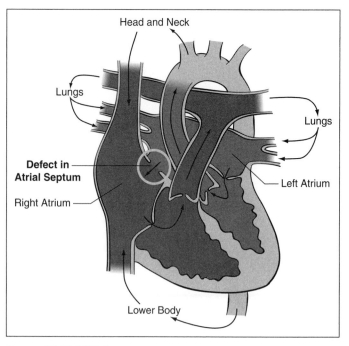

Figure 10-1: Atrial Septal Defect.

2006). Most infants/children with ASD are asymptomatic, requiring neither medical nor surgical intervention.

Normally, the pressure is greater on the left side of the heart so that in the presence of an ASD, blood flows from the left to the right across the defect (Potts & Mandleco, 2007). This left-to-right shunting of blood leads to increased volume on the right side of the heart, resulting in an increased size of the right heart chambers. There is a mixing of oxygenated blood from the left atria and deoxygenated blood entering the right atria from systemic circulation. The increased blood volume results in a greater workload in the right side of the heart and can eventually lead to right ventricular hypertrophy, decreased right-sided efficiency, and decreased cardiac output. Further, this process has the potential to result in chronic increased pulmonary blood flow, pulmonary hypertension, and ineffective gas exchange.

Complications

Right ventricular hypertrophy
Decreased cardiac output
Pulmonary hypertension
Altered gas exchange

Incidence

ASDs occur in "approximately 6–10% of all congenital heart defects" (Potts & Mandleco, 2007, p. 772). ASD is twice as common in girls as in boys (Congenital Heart Defects.com, 2006).

Etiology

According to the American Heart Association, in most cases, the etiology of congenital heart defects is unknown. The reason defects occur is presumed to be genetic; however, only a few genes have been discovered that are linked to the presence of heart defects. Only occasionally, the ingestion of certain drugs and the occurrence of certain infections during pregnancy can result in congenital heart defects (American Heart Association, 2007).

Clinical Manifestations

Most ASD produces no symptoms except a murmur. Severe defects can produce:

Murmur
Dyspnea on exertion
Growth retardation
Failure to thrive
Diaphoresis
Right ventricular hypertrophy
Right-sided heart failure

Diagnostic Tests

Auscultation of a murmur
Pulse oximetry
Electrocardiogram
Holter monitor
Chest radiography
Echocardiogram
Cardiac catheterization

Medical Management

Most infants/children with ASD are asymptomatic and require no medical intervention. However, since it is a possibility, complex ASD medical/surgical management is discussed in Chapter 26: Congenital Heart Disease/Open Heart Surgery.

Nursing Management

Refer to Chapter 26: Congenital Heart Disease/Open Heart Surgery.

References

American Heart Association. (2007). *Atrial septal defect*. Retrieved April 21, 2007, from http://www.americanheart.org/presenter.jhtml?identifier=11065

Congenital Heart Defects.com. (2006). *Atrial septal defect*. Retrieved April 21, 2007, from http://www.congenitalheartdefects.com/typesofCHD.html#Atrial

Potts, N. L., & Mandleco, B. L. (2007). *Pediatric nursing: Caring for children and their families* (2nd ed.). Clifton Park, NY: Delmar Cengage Learning.

11

ATTENTION-DEFICIT HYPERACTIVITY DISORDER (ADHD)

Definition
Attention-deficit hyperactivity disorder is a neurobehavioral disorder characterized by inattention, hyperkinetic activity, and impulsive behavior.

Pathophysiology
ADHD frequently is associated with other neurobehavioral dysfunction and has three specific characteristics: (1) inattention, (2) hyperactivity, and (3) impulsivity. According to the National Institute of Mental Health (NIMH) of the National Institutes of Health, the most recent version of the *Diagnostic and Statistical Manual of Mental Disorders* (DSM-IV-TR) divides ADHD into three patterns of behavior. Children and adults with ADHD may show several signs of being consistently inattentive. They may have a pattern of being hyperactive and impulsive far more than others of their age, or they may show all three types of behavior. As a result, professionals recognize three subtypes of ADHD. These are the (1) predominantly hyperactive-impulsive type (behavior that does not show significant inattention), (2) predominantly inattentive type (behavior that does not show significant hyperactive-impulsive behavior), and (3) combined type (behavior that displays both inattentive and hyperactive-impulsive symptoms) (DSMIV-TR workgroup, 2000). At one time, the predominantly inattentive type of ADHD was termed attention-deficit disorder; however, this is an outdated term (National Institute of Mental Health, 2007).

ADHD has been linked to a deficiency in the neurotransmitter dopamine. Dopamine is responsible for initiating purposeful movement and increasing and maintaining alertness and motivation. Dopamine also decreases appetite and causes insomnia (Potts & Mandleco, 2007). There appears to be a strong genetic association.

Complications
Difficulty with establishing and maintaining social relationships
Negative impact on school performance
Developmental delays

Incidence
According to the NIMH, an estimated 3–5% of children have ADHD, accounting for approximately 2 million children in the United States. Boys are 3 to 6 times more likely to experience ADHD than girls (National Institute of Mental Health, 2007).

Etiology
The exact cause(s) of ADHD is not known; however, genetic, environmental, neurophysiological, and dietary factors have been identified as potential causes. The genetic connection is evident in statistics showing a 10–15% higher incidence in children of parents with a history of ADHD than in the general pediatric population. In addition, in identical twins, there is a high probability that if one twin has ADHD, the other twin also will be affected (Potts & Mandleco, 2007). This probability does not appear to be as high in fraternal twins. A deficiency of dopamine also has been implicated in children and adults with ADHD. Environmental factors include perinatal insult, head trauma, lead poisoning, and maternal prenatal use of alcohol or tobacco. Food allergies or sensitivities, food additives, and excess intake of sugar have been associated with ADHD.

In 2002, researchers at the NIMH completed a long-term study of children with ADHD and found that "as a group, the ADHD children showed 3–4 percent smaller brain volumes in all regions—the frontal lobes, temporal gray matter, caudate nucleus, and cerebellum" (National Institute of Mental Health, 2007, p. 4). Other disorders that sometimes accompany ADHD include learning disabilities, Tourette's syndrome, oppositional defiant disorder (ODD), conduct disorder, anxiety, depression, and bipolar disorder.

Clinical Manifestations

HYPERACTIVITY-IMPULSIVITY

Is constantly in motion
Cannot think before acting
Cannot curb immediate responses
Feels restless
Cannot remain seated or is constantly squirming when seated
Fidgets with hands and feet
Blurts out answers to questions before the entire question has been asked
Has difficulty taking turns

INATTENTION

Is easily distracted
Cannot pay attention to details
Cannot follow directions for task
Loses or forgets things
Moves from one activity to another before completing the first activity
Has difficulty maintaining social relationships because of lack of
    attention span

Diagnostic Tests

Interviews with past and present teachers
Interview with parents
Behavior rating scale
Intelligence testing
Learning achievement testing
Functional magnetic resonance imaging (fMRI)
Positive emission tomography
Single photon emission computed tomography (SPECT)

Medical Management

The goals of treatment for ADHD are to modify the dysfunctional behaviors and facilitate normal growth and development. This can be achieved using a multimodal approach (Children and Adults with Attention Deficit/Hyperactivity Disorder (CHADD) that includes pharmacotherapeutics, psychotherapy, social skills training, behavior management, educational interventions, and family education (CHADD, 2006). Of importance is the fact that pharmacotherapy alone does not provide the same management outcomes as the multimodal approach. The provision for the educational needs of these children is addressed in Public Law 94-142, the Education for All Handicapped Children Act, revised and presently called the Individuals with Disabilities Education Act (IDEA), which states that children between the ages of 3 and 21 years must receive free public education in the least restrictive learning environment (The ARC, 1999). Children with ADHD are included in this act.

Pharmacological agents currently used to treat ADHD include methylphenidate (Ritalin), long-acting methylphenidate (Concerta), a mixture of amphetamine salts (Adderall), dextroamphetamine (Dexedrine), pemoline (Cylert), and dexmethylphenidate

(Focalin) to help increase the availability of dopamine and norepinephrine in the neural synapses to increase concentration and attention. Because of the seriousness of the adverse effects associated with the use of pemoline, it is not considered a first-line drug therapy for ADHD. In 2006, the Food and Drug Administration (FDA) approved the label revision for methylphenidate to include a warning of the risk of serious cardiovascular events including sudden death in children and adults using stimulant therapy for ADHD. In 2002, the FDA approved atomoxetine HCl (Straterra) specifically for the treatment of ADHD in children 6 years of age and older as well as adults (Broyles, Reiss, & Evans, 2007). Unlike the stimulant medications used to treat ADHD, atomoxetine controls the neurotransmitter norepinephrine, whereas the stimulants work primarily on dopamine. Although more studies to contrast atomoxetine with the other medication already in use need to be done, current evidence indicates that over 70% of children with ADHD given atomoxetine manifest significant improvement in their symptoms (National Institute of Mental Health, 2007).

Currently, a study entitled the Preschool ADHD Treatment Study (PATS) is under way to determine the best treatment options for preschool-age children affected by ADHD. Because many children in the preschool years are diagnosed with ADHD and are given medication, it is important to know the safety and efficacy of such treatment. The NIMH-sponsored multisite PATS initiative is the first major effort to examine the safety and efficacy of a stimulant, methylphenidate, for ADHD in this age group. "The PATS study uses a randomized, placebo-controlled, double-blind design. Children ages 3 to 5 who have severe and persistent symptoms of ADHD that impair their functioning are eligible for this study. To avoid using medications at such an early age, all children who enter the study are first treated with behavioral therapy. Only children who do not show sufficient improvement with behavior therapy are considered for the medication arm of the study. This study is being conducted at New York State Psychiatric Institute, Duke University, Johns Hopkins University, New York University, the University of California at Los Angeles, and the University of California at Irvine. Enrollment in the study will total 165 children" (National Institute of Mental Health, 2007, p. 10).

Nursing Management

ASSESSMENT

1. Perform neurological assessment
2. Perform psychosocial assessment of child and parents
3. Gather other input information from child's school
4. Assess for manifestations of ADHD

NURSING DIAGNOSES (INCLUDING BUT NOT LIMITED TO)

1. Impaired social interaction R/T poor impulse control, short attention span, and hyperactivity
2. Risk for injury R/T impulsive behavior, inability to perceive danger, and adverse effects of prescribed medications for ADHD
3. Chronic low self-esteem R/T lack of satisfactory peer relationships and positive feedback; academic underachievement
4. Ineffective family coping R/T child's disruptive behavior, hyperactivity, inability to follow directions, and academic underachievement
5. Deficient knowledge (parents) R/T understanding of ADHD, multifocal treatment modalities, and home care

PLANNING/GOALS

1. The client will demonstrate acceptable and safe social skills and improved ability to interact with others.
2. The client will not experience injury or unnecessary risk behaviors.
3. The client will verbalize increased feelings of self-worth.

4. The family will identify and use coping strategies for managing child's disruptive behaviors.
5. Parents will demonstrate understanding of ADHD, multifocal treatment modalities, and home care.

NOC

1. Social Interaction Skills
2. Risk Control
3. Self-Esteem
4. Coping, Impulse Self-Control
5. Knowledge: Illness Care, Treatment

IMPLEMENTATION

1. Social interaction
   a. Assess level of growth and development
   b. Assess social interactions with family and peers
   c. Encourage compliance with treatment modalities
   d. Assess effectiveness of treatment modalities
   e. Provide for consistency in health care professionals working with child and family
   f. Encourage child/family to verbalize feelings and concerns
   g. Collaborate with health care provider for appropriate referrals to assist child and family
   h. Coordinate information sharing with child's school
2. Risk for injury
   a. Assess for risk-taking behavior
   b. Assess effectiveness of treatment modalities
   c. Assist parents in identifying modifications in environment to provide for child safety
   d. Assess for presence of adverse effects of medications
   e. Encourage compliance with treatment modalities
3. Self-esteem
   a. Assess for indications of low self-esteem
   b. Assist family/child to identify positive traits
   c. Encourage family interactions according to family dynamics
   d. Maintain nonjudgmental and caring affect
   e. Encourage child/family to verbalize feelings and concerns
4. Family coping
   a. Encourage family to verbalize feelings and concerns
   b. Assist family in identifying positive coping strategies
   c. Provide emotional support
   d. Provide for spiritual support
   e. Assist family in identifying and using support systems
5. Family teaching
   a. Assess family's current level of understanding
   b. Provide verbal and written information regarding:
      1) Prescribed medications, schedule of administration, and adverse effects and reassurance that use of stimulant medications for ADHD does not lead to substance abuse problems, rather that it decreases the incidence of substance abuse issues (Potts & Mandleco, 2007)

    2) Behavior modification guidelines

    3) Educational guidelines and topics to discuss with child's school

    4) Community support services and referral information

    5) Psychotherapy information

    6) Social skills enhancement

    7) Importance of compliance with child's multimodal treatment regimen

    8) Referral information

    9) Information to report to health care provider

  c. Provide adequate time for teaching, encouraging verbalization of feelings and concerns

  d. Document teaching and family response

NIC

1. Behavior Modification: Social Skills
2. Safety Surveillance
3. Self-Esteem Enhancement
4. Coping Enhancement
5. Teaching: Illness Care, Treatment

EVALUATION

1. Client demonstrates acceptable and safe social skills and improved ability to interact with others.

2. Client does not experience injury or unnecessary risk behaviors.

3. Client verbalizes increased feelings of self-worth.

4. Family identifies and uses coping strategies for managing child's disruptive behaviors.

5. Parents demonstrate understanding of ADHD, multifocal treatment modalities, and home care.

References

Broyles, B. E., Reiss, B. S., & Evans, M. E. (2007). *Pharmacological aspects of nursing care.* (7th ed.). Clifton Park, NY: Delmar Cengage Learning.

Children and Adults with Attention Deficit/Hyperactivity Disorder (CHADD). (2006). Retrieved February 13, 2007, from http://www.chadd.org/Content/CHADD/Understanding/TermstoKnow/default.htm

DSM-IV-TR workgroup. (2000). *The diagnostic and statistical manual of mental disorders* (4th ed.). Washington, DC: American Psychiatric Association.

National Institute of Mental Health. (2007). *Attention-deficit hyperactivity disorder.* Retrieved May 10, 2007, from http://www.ninds.nih.gov/disorders/adhd/adhd.htm

Potts, N. L., & Mandleco, B. L. (2007). *Pediatric nursing: Caring for children and their families* (2nd ed.). Clifton Park, NY: Delmar Cengage Learning.

The ARC. (1999). *The Individuals with Disabilities Education Act (IDEA): Eligibility, IEPs and placement.* Retrieved February 13, 2007, from http://www.thearc.org/faqs/qa-idea.html

12

AUTISM

Definition

According to the Autism Society of America, "Autism is a complex developmental disability that typically appears during the first three years of life and is the result of a neurological disorder that affects the normal functioning of the brain, impacting development in the areas of social interaction and communication skills" (Autism Society of America, 2007, p. 1). It is one of five disorders that is classified according to the Society as Pervasive Developmental Disorders (PDD).

Pathophysiology

The pathophysiology of autism can best be explained by examining the causes currently under investigation and the clinical manifestations. However, although a list of common manifestations is presented here, the exact behaviors in a child with autism are as unique as each autistic child. Brain scans show differences in the shape and structure of the brains of autistic versus non-autistic children. Heredity, genetics, and predisposition in the presence of coexisting congenital abnormalities are considered the most likely etiologies. Regardless of the cause, the brain of the child with autism does not process or communicate information in the same way as that of a "normal" child. The neurological alterations are reflected in the child's difficulty to synthesize environmental stimuli and to reach developmental milestones and in the child's tendency to exhibit repetitive and often disruptive behaviors that interfere with the child's ability to develop self-care skills. This creates anxiety in both the child and the family, disruption of family processes, the need for education alternatives, and life-long adjustments.

Complications

> Interference with development
> Family anxiety
> Disruption of family processes and roles
> Life-long adjustments to developmental challenges

Incidence

According to the Autism Society of America, autism occurs in 1 of every 166 births and between 1 million and 1.5 million Americans have autism. It is considered the fastest-growing developmental disability. According to the National Institute of Neurological Disorders and Stroke (NINDS) of the National Institutes of Health, an estimated 3 to 6 children out of every 1,000 will have autism and males are 4 times more likely to have autism than females. Identical twins demonstrate a congruence of 36–91% if one has autism (National Institute of Neurologic Disorders and Stroke, 2007).

Etiology

No single cause is known for autism, but the consensus among researchers is that children with autism are born with it or are born with the potential to develop the disorder. According to the Autism Society of America, heredity, genetics, and the coexistence of certain medical disorders are considered the most likely causes of autism. Research is considering other possible causative factors, such as clusters of unstable genes interfering with fetal brain development, abnormalities during pregnancy, metabolic imbalances, viral infections, and environmental factors. Research has identified that autism occurs more frequently in children with certain health alterations including Fragile X syndrome, tuberous sclerosis, congenital rubella syndrome, and untreated phenylketonuria (Autism Society of America, 2007). According to NINDS, studies of people with autism have found irregularities in several areas of the brain while other studies suggest abnormal levels of serotonin or other neurotransmitters in the brain that may cause autism. Either of these abnormalities could be caused by the disruption of normal brain development early in fetal development resulting from defects in genes that control brain growth and that regulate how neurons communicate with each other (National Institute of Neurologic Disorders and Stroke, 2007).

Clinical Manifestations

Talking at others instead of to or with them
Giving manic monologues
Being very resistant to change
Having obsessive attachments to objects
Displaying ritualistic behavior
Having difficulty in expressing needs
Using gestures or pointing instead of using words
Using repetitious speech
Exhibiting emotional lability
Preferring to being alone
Throwing tantrums
Having difficulty communicating or socializing with others
Being unresponsive to normal teaching methods and to verbal cues
Not wanting affection or not wanting to be hugged or cuddled
Using little or no eye contact
Being consistently hyperkinetic or underactive
Showing developmental delays in gross/fine motor skills

Diagnostic Tests

There is no one medical test for autism.
National Institute of Child Health & Human Development identified
    behaviors that warrant further evaluation (National Institute of Child
    Health & Human Development, 2006)
Developmental testing
Childhood Autism Rating Scale (CARS)
Checklist for Autism in Toddlers (CHAT)
Autism Screening Questionnaire

Medical Management

There is no cure for autism, so the goal of care is to allow the child the highest level of independence within the constraints of the disorder through treatment and education to decrease some of the daily challenges the child with autism experiences and to lessen disruptive behaviors. As the Autism Society notes, "Just as there is no one symptom or behavior that identifies autistic children, there is no single treatment. Children can learn to function within the confines of their disability, but treatment must be tailored to the child's individual behaviors and needs" (Autism Society of America, 2007, p. 1). Any child under the age of 3 years is eligible for "early intervention" assistance available from The National Information Center for Children and Youth with Disabilities, which is available in every state in the United States. Children ages 3–21 years are guaranteed by the federal Individuals with Disabilities Education Act (IDEA) to a free appropriate public education supplied by the child's local education agency.

Nursing Management

ASSESSMENT

1. Obtain history and physical
2. Identify child's routines, rituals, likes, and dislikes
3. Assess child's abilities regarding self-care
4. Assess child's communication skills and presence of specific autistic behaviors
5. Obtain information from parents (caregivers) regarding medication administration or other anticipated procedures

NURSING DIAGNOSES (INCLUDING BUT NOT LIMITED TO)

1. Risk for injury R/T potential for sensory deficits or self-destructive behaviors
2. Impaired verbal communication R/T limited language skills
3. Impaired social interaction R/T inability to develop and sustain relationships appropriate for child's developmental level
4. Delayed growth and development R/T altered neurological brain activity
5. Deficient knowledge (caregiver, parent, and child) R/T condition, treatment modalities, home care, and respite care

PLANNING/GOALS

1. Client will not sustain injury.
2. Client will develop a means of communicating needs to others.
3. Client will demonstrate awareness of others in the environment and attempt to interact with them.
4. Client will demonstrate ability to master average academic tasks consistent with level of growth and development.
5. Parents/caregivers will demonstrate understanding of condition, treatment modalities, home care, and use of respite care.

NOC

1. Personal Safety Behavior
2. Communication
3. Social Involvement
4. Child Development: Knowledge: Parenting
5. Knowledge: Child Physical Safety, Health Promotion, Health Resources

IMPLEMENTATION

1. Risk for injury
   a. Assess child's personal behavior that could result in injury
   b. Incorporate the caregivers in child's care
   c. Listen actively to both child and caregivers
   d. Identify ritualistic behavior
   e. Encourage 24-hour visitation by caregivers when child is hospitalized
   f. Assess caregivers for caregiver strain
   g. Assess caregivers' understanding of autism
   h. Provide information to fill caregivers' gaps in knowledge

2. Communication
   a. Assess child's form of communication
   b. Listen actively
   c. Incorporate caregivers to provide information concerning how child communicates at home and how they communicate with child
   d. Collaborate with other members of the multidisciplinary team to discuss potential for improving communication with child

3. Socialization
   a. Collaborate with health care provider for referral to recreation or play therapy
   b. Assess child's interactions with other children of same level of growth and development
   c. Ask caregivers to provide information concerning child's social skills at home and in school
   d. Collaborate with other members of multidisciplinary team to enhance child's social skills
   e. Remind child to use the "golden words" (*please* and *thank-you*)
   f. Encourage caregivers to spend time in the child's classroom, especially during the first days of school
   g. Provide caregivers with information concerning community and governmental services for child
   h. Encourage caregivers to volunteer at school and to participate in school activities

4. Growth and development
   a. Assess child's level of growth and development
   b. Identify milestones child has and has not reached
   c. Encourage caregivers to participate in teacher conferences at school at least twice monthly
   d. Encourage caregivers to collaborate with teachers to provide at-home materials that duplicate or resemble schoolwork
   e. Provide caregivers information about tutors and summer school programs (Potts & Mandleco, 2007)
   f. Teach caregivers to expect child to succeed

5. Caregiver/parent/child teaching
   a. Assess client's/family's current level of knowledge about condition
   b. Provide verbal and written information regarding:
      1) Delicacy of the child's condition
      2) Importance of collaborating with school nurse and teachers
      3) Importance of involvement in child's education and school activities
      4) Referrals to support groups, community, and government services
      5) Reinforcement of multidisciplinary team recommendations
      6) Importance of follow-up care with health care provider
      7) Contact phone numbers for interdisciplinary team involved in treatment plan
   c. Encourage client/family questions and respond honestly
   d. Document teaching and client/family response

NIC

1. Impulse Control Training, Environmental Management: Safety
2. Communication Enhancement, Active Listening
3. Socialization Enhancement, Teaching: Individual
4. Developmental Enhancement: Child, Learning Readiness Enhancement, Learning Facilitation
5. Behavior Modification, Health System Guidance, Learning Readiness Enhancement, Learning Facilitation

EVALUATION

1. Client does not sustain injury.
2. Client develops an effective means of communicating needs to others.
3. Client demonstrates awareness of others in the environment and, with practice, attempts to interact with them.
4. Client demonstrates ability to master average academic tasks consistent with level of growth and development.
5. Parents/caregivers demonstrate understanding of condition, treatment modalities, home care, and use of respite care.

References

Autism Society of America. (2007). *Defining autism.* Retrieved April 21, 2007, from http://www.autism-society.org/site/PageServer?pagename=about_whatis_home

National Institute of Child Health & Human Development. (2006). *Autism spectrum disorders (ASDs).* Retrieved April 21, 2007, from http://www.nichd.nih.gov/health/topics/asd.cfm

National Institute of Neurological Disorders and Stroke. (2007). *Autism fact sheet.* Retrieved April 21, 2007, from http://www.ninds.nih.gov/disorders/autism/detail_autism.htm

Potts, N. L., & Mandleco, B. L. (2007). *Pediatric nursing: Caring for children and their families* (2nd ed.). Clifton Park, NY: Delmar Cengage Learning.

13

BETA-THALASSEMIA MAJOR

Definition

Beta-thalassemia major (β-thalassemia), also referred to as Cooley's anemia, is the most severe form of a group of hematological autosomal recessive hereditary conditions characterized by the inadequate production of the β-chain necessary for the synthesis of hemoglobin. β-thalassemia "occurs in four forms: two heterozygous forms: thalassemia minor, an asymptomatic silent carrier, and thalassemia trait which produces a mild microcytic anemia; thalassemia intermedia, which is manifested as splenomegaly and moderate to severe anemia; and a homozygous form, thalassemia major . . ." (Hockenberry, 2005, pp. 949–950).

Pathophysiology

Each normal hemoglobin molecule is comprised of four globin components or polypeptide chains—two α-polypeptide chains and two β-polypeptide chains. These four chains combine with four heme components, the oxygen-carrying portion, to form one hemoglobin compound. In β-thalassemia, there is impairment of the synthesis of the beta chains (or β-chains), resulting in erythrocytes with less hemoglobin (or oxygen-carrying capacity) than normal hemoglobin. In addition, because the alpha chains (or α-chains) are not bound, they are less stable and precipitate easily, causing the destruction of a number of erythrocytes in the bone marrow. As a result, anemia develops from the decreased number of circulating red blood cells (Potts & Mandleco, 2007).

The severe anemia stimulates the release of erythropoietin from the kidneys to stimulate the bone marrow to produce more red blood cells that cannot match the numbers of red blood cells being destroyed. These destroyed red blood cells then are stored in the liver and spleen, causing hepatosplenomegaly. The additional stimulation of the bone marrow causes it to become hyperplastic, leading to an increase in bone size to accommodate the proliferation of red blood cells produced. As the bones enlarge, they thin and become more fragile, increasing the incidence of pathological fractures. Without transfusion support, cardiac failure and death in early childhood result.

Complications

Bone thinning and fragility leading to pathological fractures
Hepatosplenomegaly
Iron toxicity from transfusion therapy
Cardiac failure
Death

Incidence

According to the National Institutes of Health Genetics Home Reference, "Worldwide, beta-thalassemia is considered a fairly common blood disorder, affecting thousands of infants each year. Beta-thalassemia occurs most frequently in Mediterranean countries, North Africa, the Middle East, India, and southeast Asia. In North America, the disorder is less common; an estimated 750–1000 people have beta-thalassemia" (Genetics Home Reference, 2007, p. 1).

These children also are found in the Arabian peninsula, Iran, and southern China. It is estimated that in excess of 2 million people in the United States carry the genetic β-thalassemia trait (Genetics Home Reference, 2007).

Etiology

As previously noted, β-thalassemia is the most severe form of a group of hematological autosomal recessive hereditary conditions caused by the genetic absence of hemoglobin β-chains.

Clinical Manifestations

Pallor
Unexplained fever
Poor feeding
Hepatosplenomegaly
Headache
Bone pain
Dyspnea on exertion
Anorexia
Small stature
Delayed sexual maturation
Enlarged head with prominent frontal and parietal bosses
    (Refer to Figure 13-1.)

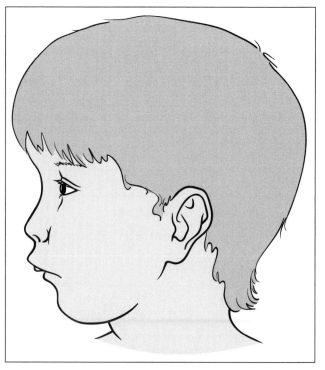

Figure 13-1: Face of a Child with β-Thalassemia.

Flat or depressed nasal bridge
Enlarged maxilla
Protrusion of the lip and central incisors
Microlytic, hypochromic red blood cells

Diagnostic Tests

Complete blood count
Peripheral smear
Serum iron
Serum ferritin
Total iron binding capacity
Bone marrow aspiration

Medical Management

There is no cure for β-thalassemia, but medical interventions are necessary to support and prolong life for children with the disease. Chronic transfusions, which for many children mean transfusions every two to three weeks, remain the treatment of choice with the goal of maintaining hemoglobin levels between 9 and 10 g/dL. In addition to the transfusions, a splenectomy often is performed to eliminate the site of hemolysis, which can decrease the child's need for frequent transfusions. However, a splenectomy places the child at risk for infection requiring prophylactic antibiotics for life. To eliminate the need for lifelong transfusions, bone marrow transplants and cord blood transplants are being attempted in the United States and in other countries. One of the most difficult hurdles with bone marrow transplantation is finding a suitable donor.

The major adverse effect of chronic transfusions is hemosiderosis, or iron overload. This requires chelation therapy to prevent organ damage. Deferoxamine is the chelation agent of choice to prevent or reduce the toxic effects of elevated serum iron levels or to accelerate the excretion of iron from the body. Deferoxamine is administered parenterally (intravenous or intramuscular) five to seven times a week, requiring infusions of up to 12 hours per dose. Adverse effects of deferoxamine include potential allergic reactions, hypotension, and neurotoxicity following long-term treatment (Potts & Mandleco, 2007).

Nursing Management

ASSESSMENT

1. Obtain family history
2. Perform physical examination with focus on clinical manifestations of β-thalassemia
3. Obtain baseline vital signs
4. Obtain weight and height and compare findings with standardized normal values
5. Assess for psychosocial impact of disease on family members and child

NURSING DIAGNOSES (INCLUDING BUT NOT LIMITED TO)

1. Ineffective tissue perfusion R/T defective oxygen-carrying capacity of hemoglobin
2. Risk for injury and iron toxicity R/T chronic transfusions
3. Ineffective coping R/T chronicity of disease
4. Deficient knowledge R/T condition, treatment modalities, and home care

PLANNING/GOALS

1. Client will demonstrate improved tissue perfusion as evidenced by oxygen saturation within prescribed parameters, hemoglobin levels within prescribed parameters, age-appropriate activity tolerance, and vital signs within defined limits (WDL).
2. Client will be effectively treated for elevated serum iron levels through chelation therapy.
3. Client/family will verbalize feelings and concerns and actively participate in child's care and activities of daily living.
4. Client/family will demonstrate understanding of condition, medical treatment, and home care.

NOC

1. Circulation Status
2. Risk Identification
3. Acceptance Health Status
4. Knowledge: Disease Process, Infection Control, Treatment Regimen

IMPLEMENTATION

1. Tissue perfusion
   a. Monitor vital signs every 4 hours during hospitalization
   b. Maintain intravenous access, monitoring hourly
   c. Administer intravenous fluids as prescribed
   d. Administer red blood cell transfusions as prescribed following facility protocol
   e. Monitor closely for transfusion reaction
   f. Stop transfusion immediately, maintain patency of intravenous access, and notify health care provider if transfusion reaction occurs
   g. Monitor hemoglobin levels pre- and post-transfusion
   h. Monitor oxygen saturation via pulse oximetry
   i. Administer oxygen to maintain oxygen saturations within prescribed parameters
2. Risk for injury
   a. Monitor serum iron levels pre- and post-chelation therapy
   b. Administer deferoxamine as prescribed
   c. Monitor vital signs
   d. Monitor for adverse effects of chelation therapy
3. Coping
   a. Assess family/child for manifestations of anxiety and coping interferences
   b. Encourage verbalization of feelings and concerns
   c. Collaborate with members of multidisciplinary team
   d. Refer to chaplain or contact family spiritual leader if requested
   e. Provide information about condition, treatments, and home care
   f. Maintain calm, therapeutic environment
   g. Provide age-appropriate activities for child
   h. Encourage family to participate in child's care
   i. Provide information concerning family support services

4. Family/client teaching
   a. Assess parents'/family's/child's current level of understanding of child's hospital and home care
   b. Provide verbal and written information regarding:
      1) Prevention of infection (family/client can provide a return demonstration of hand washing prior to child's discharge)
      2) Clinical manifestations of worsening of condition
      3) Clinical manifestations of iron toxicity
      4) Importance of monitoring child's temperature and prescribed parameters for notifying health care provider
      5) Importance of follow-up care and schedule for next appointment
      6) Discussion of manifestations to report to health care provider
      7) Contact numbers
   c. Provide adequate time for teaching and parental questions
   d. Document teaching and parental response

NIC

1. Oxygen Therapy, Vital Signs Monitoring, Intravenous Therapy
2. Risk Control
3. Coping Enhancement, Emotional Support
4. Teaching: Disease Process, Infection Control, Treatment Regimen

EVALUATION

1. Client demonstrates improved tissue perfusion as evidenced by oxygen saturation within prescribed parameters, hemoglobin levels within prescribed parameters, age-appropriate activity tolerance, and vital signs WDL.
2. Client is effectively treated for elevated serum iron levels through chelation therapy.
3. Client/family verbalize feelings and concerns and actively participate in child's care and activities of daily living.
4. Client/family demonstrate understanding of condition, medical treatment, and home care.

References

Genetics Home Reference. (2007). *Beta thalassemia*. Retrieved April 21, 2007, from http://ghr.nlm.nih.gov/condition=betathalassemia

Hockenberry, M. J. (2005). *Wong's essentials of pediatric nursing* (7th ed.). St. Louis, MO: Mosby Elsevier.

Potts, N. L., & Mandleco, B. L. (2007). *Pediatric nursing: Caring for children and their families* (2nd ed.). Clifton Park, NY: Delmar Cengage Learning.

BILIARY ATRESIA/LIVER TRANSPLANTATION

Definition

Biliary atresia is the congenital lack of or obstruction of the bile ducts outside and sometimes inside the liver.

Pathophysiology

With biliary atresia, the obstruction of the bile ducts prevents the flow of bile from the liver to the small intestines. This results in a backup of bile in the liver. Because food intake stimulates the release of bile and subsequent production of more bile, the bile becomes "trapped in the liver, quickly causing damage and scarring of the liver cells (cirrhosis, and finally liver failure)" (Cincinnati Children's Hospital Medical Center, 2006, p. 1).

Liver cirrhosis and eventual liver failure are characterized by deterioration of the normal functions of the liver with pathophysiology presented in Table 14-1.

Table 14-1 | Pathophysiology of Liver Failure

Normal function	Presence of cirrhosis/liver failure
Synthesis of prothrombin and fibrinogen	Altered clotting factors and increased bleeding
Manufacture of heparin	Altered clotting factors
Metabolism and detoxification of chemicals	Inability to detoxify substances including drugs
Synthesis of almost all plasma proteins	Decreased serum albumin, altered serum osmolarity, edema, skin breakdown, and ascites
Hemolysis	Anemia, hepatosplenomegaly, jaundice —› pruritis
Manufacture and release of bile for digestion	Malabsorption
Storage of large amounts of vitamins (A, B$_{12}$, D, E)	Vitamin deficiencies
Metabolism of carbohydrates and proteins	Hyperglycemia from inability to convert glucose to glycogen and store glycogen
Regulation of blood sugar by converting glycogen to glucose	Hypoglycemia
Synthesis of protein and formation of ammonia	Elevated ammonia levels —› hepatic encephalopathy
Major producer of body heat secondary to multiple metabolic functions	Hypothermia and cold intolerance
	Changes terminate in death

Adapted from Broyles, 2005

Complications

Cirrhosis

Portal hypertension

Liver failure

Incidence

"Biliary atresia is a serious but rare disease of the liver that affects newborn infants. It occurs in about one in 10,000 children and is more common in girls than in boys and in Asian and African-American newborns than in Caucasian newborns" (National Institutes of Diabetes and Digestive and Kidney Diseases, 2006, p. 1). "Within the same family, it is common for only one child in a pair of twins or only one child within the same family to have it" (Cincinnati Children's Hospital Medical Center, 2006, p. 1). Between 10 and 15% of infants with biliary atresia are born with other anomalies including cardiac anomalies, polysplenia, inferior vena caval abnormalities, preduodenal portal vein anomalies, malrotation of the intestines, or situs inversus.

Etiology

Although the exact causes of biliary atresia are not completely understood, congenital biliary atresia is believed to occur due to the bile ducts not forming during fetal development. Biliary atresia also can be acquired, and this type is believed to be the result of damage to the bile ducts secondary to an autoimmune response to a viral infection acquired after birth (National Institutes of Diabetes and Digestive and Kidney Disorders, 2006; American Liver Foundation, 2007).

Clinical Manifestations

Jaundice

Dark urine

Clay-colored stools

Irritability

Weight loss

Diagnostic Tests

Complete blood count

Liver function tests

Abdominal ultrasound

Abdominal computed tomography

HIDA nuclear scan (determine bile flow)

Operative cholangiogram

Coagulation studies

Liver biopsy

Medical Management

There is no known cure for biliary atresia, and it cannot be treated with medication. A surgical procedure called a hepatoportoenterostomy, or Kasai procedure, can be performed, which creates an open duct (with a piece of the infant's own intestine) that drains the bile from the liver. Although not a cure, it does allow some infants to grow and experience good health for several years. When performed by surgeons familiar with the procedure, the success rate is 60–85% (National Institutes of Diabetes and Digestive and Kidney Diseases, 2006).

When the Kasai procedure is unsuccessful, the reason usually is because both the intrahepatic and extrahepatic bile ducts are obstructed. Liver transplantation is the only treatment to correct this. Nearly 50% of infants who have experienced the Kasai procedure require transplantation before they are 5 years of age.

Unlike liver transplants in adults that use cadaver livers, live liver transplants with the mother of the infant as the donor have become the most frequent option in children and have been increasingly successful in effectively treating this condition (eMedicine Health, 2007). "International 1-year success rates for pediatric liver transplantation now exceed 90%, and 5- to 10-year survival rates are 80%" (Carter & Kilic, 2006, p. 2). This procedure is most effective when performed on infants less than 2 to 3 months of age. Prior to the transplant, an alternative method for feeding the infant is established (enteral feedings) to meet caloric needs and to conserve energy.

An important part of the transplantation process is the method of determining which client is in most critical need of a transplant. The United Network for Organ Sharing has established criteria for adults and children. The pediatric criteria are used for clients younger than 18 years and are outlined in the Pediatric End-Stage Liver Disease (PELD) scoring system. The priority factor on which this system is based is the risk or probability of death within three months if the child does not receive a transplanted liver. The PELD score is calculated by assessing laboratory data (albumin level, bilirubin level, and INR (or International Normalized Ratio) for determining blood clotting capability) and growth parameters. Infants/children with severe biliary atresia (determined not to be manageable by the Kasai procedure) are considered high-status candidates. However, with live donor transplantation and a suitable donor, these children avoid the usual period of waiting for a donor liver (eMedicine Health, 2007). In addition, within six to eight weeks following transplantation, both the donated segments of liver and the remaining part in the donor grow to normal size (eMedicine Health, 2007).

Liver transplantation involves harvesting the donor liver portion (approximately 50% of the recipient infant's current liver size), which is then flushed with cold Lactated Ringers solution to remove potassium and air bubbles. Due "to the proximity of the diaphragm to the liver, atelectasis and the subsequent placement of chest tubes must be accomplished. The failed organ is removed and the lengthiest and perhaps the most difficult part of the procedure (progresses). . . . Biliary reconstruction and end-to-end anastomosis of the donor and recipient common bile ducts is [*sic*] performed as well as end-to-end anastomosis of the blood vessels and bile ducts from the recipient to the donor liver. A T-tube is placed for external drainage" (Broyles, 2005, p. 502). Following the transplant, the infant/child is transferred to the Pediatric Intensive Care Unit (PICU).

To prevent organ rejection, lifelong immunosuppressant therapy is necessary following liver transplantation. Among the agents used are cyclosporine, azathioprine, OKT3, tacrolimus, mycophenolate mofetil HCl, daclizumab, and corticosteroids such as prednisone. Careful monitoring of these medications must be maintained to determine their effectiveness and to provide early recognition of adverse effects of these agents. Just as critical a problem as organ rejection is risk of life-threatening infections occurring secondary to the immunosuppression. Infection is the leading cause of death following liver transplantation.

Nursing Management

ASSESSMENT

PRETRANSPLANTATION

1. Obtain history and baseline vital signs
2. Perform physical assessment
3. Assess parents/family for psychosocial impact of diagnosis and prospect of transplantation
4. Monitor laboratory values

POSTTRANSPLANTATION

5. Assess for infection (temperature elevation is primary manifestation)
6. Monitor respiratory function (most common site of opportunistic infections)
7. Monitor for manifestations of rejection (tachycardia, fever, flank pain, right upper quadrant pain, increased jaundice)
8. Monitor laboratory values

NURSING DIAGNOSES (INCLUDING BUT NOT LIMITED TO)

PRETRANSPLANTATION

1. High risk for injury, bleeding R/T altered clotting mechanisms
2. Ineffective breathing pattern R/T ascites
3. Risk for impaired skin integrity R/T edema, ascites, and pruritis
4. Excess fluid volume R/T decreased serum osmotic pressure, edema
5. Imbalanced nutrition: less than body requirements R/T fatigue, vitamin deficiencies, loss of appetite, and abdominal distention
6. Disturbed sleep pattern R/T pruritis, hospital environment, and parental anxiety
7. Deficient knowledge (parental) R/T condition, treatment modalities, and home care

POSTTRANSPLANTATION

8. High risk for infection R/T immunosuppressant therapy and surgical recovery
9. Risk for injury, organ failure R/T body's immune response to attack foreign bodies
10. Impaired gas exchange R/T loss of lung inflation due to surgical approach
11. Risk for injury, complications secondary to liver transplantation R/T cardiovascular, renal, neurologic, and metabolic functioning
12. Acute pain R/T surgical incision and chest tubes
13. Risk for delayed growth and development R/T criticality of child's condition and long-term care and parental lack of knowledge of growth and development needs
14. Deficient knowledge R/T posttransplant therapy and home care

PLANNING/GOALS

PRETRANSPLANTATION

1. Client will not experience bleeding injuries.
2. Client will demonstrate improved breathing pattern as evidenced by vitals signs and oxygen saturation within defined limits (WDL).
3. Client will maintain skin integrity.
4. Client will regain and maintain fluid balance as evidenced by decrease in edema and urine output > 1 mL/kg/hr.
5. Client will regain and maintain adequate nutritional intake to meet metabolic needs.
6. Client will experience undisturbed periods (1–2 hours) of sleep between feedings.
7. Family will demonstrate understanding of condition, medical treatment, and home care.

POSTTRANSPLANTATION

8. Client will not experience infection; but if it does occur, manifestations will be recognized and antimicrobial therapy will be initiated in a timely manner.
9. Client will not experience rejection of transplanted organ as evidenced by liver function tests WDL and absence of manifestations of organ rejection.
10. Client will regain and maintain effective gas exchange as evidenced by hemodynamic stability and oxygen saturation within prescribed parameters.

11. Client will not experience complications secondary to liver transplant as evidenced by cardiovascular, renal, neurologic, and metabolic functioning WDL.
12. Client will demonstrate adequate pain management as evidenced by a level of 1 on a 5-point scale with 5 indicating severe pain based on infant behaviors.
13. Client will participate in age-appropriate activities within the constraints of immunosuppressive therapy and will achieve highest level of growth and development.
14. Family/parents will demonstrate understanding of posttransplantation therapy and home care.

NOC

PRETRANSPLANTATION

1. Risk Control
2. Vital Signs, Respiratory Status
3. Risk Control
4. Fluid Overload Severity
5. Nutritional Status: Food and Fluid Intake
6. Sleep
7. Knowledge: Condition, Treatment, Health Promotion

POSTTRANSPLANTATION

8. Risk Control
9. Risk Control
10. Respiratory Status: Gas Exchange
11. Risk Control
12. Comfort Level
13. Risk Control, Knowledge: Condition, Health Promotion
14. Knowledge: Condition, Infection Control, Medication

IMPLEMENTATION

PRETRANSPLANTATION

1. Risk for bleeding
   a. Assess for bleeding, including mucous membranes
   b. Closely monitor infants receiving oxygen per nasal prongs for epistaxis
   c. Monitor laboratory values
   d. Assist with liver biopsy if it is performed
   e. Use soft toothbrush (for older children) or toothettes for oral hygiene
   f. Avoid injections
2. Breathing pattern
   a. Place infant on continuous cardiorespiratory monitor and pulse oximetry
   b. Position infant with head of bed elevated to facilitate breathing
   c. Administer oxygen to maintain oxygen saturation at prescribed levels
   d. Monitor vital signs
   e. Report any abnormal changes immediately to health care provider
   f. Administer diuretics as prescribed

3. Skin integrity
   a. Assess skin for redness and breaks in the skin
   b. Keep fingernails trimmed
   c. Apply mittens to hands to prevent scratching secondary to pruritis
   d. Reposition every 1–2 hours
   e. Provide frequent skin care (bathing reduces bilirubin on the skin)
4. Excess fluid volume
   a. Monitor strict intake and output
   b. Weigh daily
   c. Obtain daily abdominal girths
   d. Maintain patency of intravenous access, monitoring hourly
   e. Administer diuretics as prescribed
   f. Administer albumin as prescribed
5. Nutrition
   a. Monitor daily weight
   b. Monitor intake and output
   c. Administer enteral feedings as prescribed
   d. Monitor for residual every 2–4 hours for continuous tube feedings
   e. Collaborate with dietician and health care provider to provide adequate calorie intake
   f. Use pacifier to maintain infant's suck reflex if infant is not receiving oral feedings
   g. Encourage parents/family to participate in child's care
6. Sleep pattern
   a. Monitor sleep pattern, comparing with normal needs of infants
   b. Provide environment conducive for sleep
   c. Encourage parents/family to hold and rock infant
7. Parent teaching
   a. Assess parents' current level of knowledge about child's condition
   b. Provide verbal and written information regarding:
      1) Explanation of all procedures
      2) Skin care
      3) Importance of bonding with infant
      4) Enteral feeding administration
      5) Pretransplantation procedures and testing
      6) Explanation of what parents can expect following liver transplantation
   c. Provide adequate time for teaching and parental questions
   d. Document teaching and parents' response

POSTTRANSPLANTATION

8. High risk for infection
   a. Monitor body temperature continuously with skin probe per critical care protocol
   b. Monitor body temperature every 4 hours following acute postoperative period

   c. Monitor incision, chest tube drainage, and intravenous access sites

   d. Obtain cultures if purulent drainage is noted

   e. Monitor complete blood count with differential

   f. Maintain patency of central venous access device, monitoring hourly

   g. Administer antimicrobials as prescribed

   h. Collaborate with health care provider to remove invasive lines when possible

   i. Perform meticulous hand washing

   j. Change central venous access dressing using sterile technique and following facility protocol

   k. Instruct parents on appropriate hand washing technique

9. Risk for organ failure

   a. Monitor for manifestations of liver failure

   b. Monitor liver function tests

   c. Monitor coagulation studies

   d. Monitor for increasing jaundice and report abnormal findings immediately to health care provider

   e. Administer immunosuppressive therapy as prescribed

   f. Monitor for adverse effects of immunosuppressive therapy

   g. Provide information to parents regarding manifestations of organ failure

10. Gas exchange

   a. Place on continuous cardiorespiratory and pulse oximetry monitoring

   b. Monitor capillary wedge pressure

   c. Monitor serial arterial blood gases from arterial line

   d. Maintain closed chest drainage system

   e. Have plastic or rubber-tipped hemostats at infant's bedside

   f. Routinely check connections on closed chest drainage system for leaks

   g. Assess breath sounds every 1–2 hours and as needed

11. Risk for complications

   a. Monitor cardiovascular status including central venous pressure, cardiac output, and vital signs

   b. Monitor pulmonary function

   c. Monitor renal function including hourly urine output

   d. Monitor neurologic functioning using Pediatric Glasgow Coma Scale

   e. Monitor metabolic functioning

   f. Report abnormalities immediately to health care provider

12. Acute pain

   a. Assess pain level hourly using age-appropriate pain assessment tool

   b. Medicate proactively to maintain pain control

   c. Maintain patency of intravenous access, monitoring hourly

   d. Monitor cardiorespiratory status continuously

   e. Position for comfort

   f. Explain to parents the need for proactive pain management

13. Coping
    a. Assess parents for manifestations of ineffective coping
    b. Encourage parents to verbalize feelings and concerns
    c. Explain all equipment and procedures to parents
    d. Provide accurate information and answers to parents' questions
    e. Encourage parental visitation and participation in care as client's condition allows
14. Parent/Family posttransplantation teaching
    a. Assess parental level of understanding of posttransplantation care
    b. Provide verbal and written information regarding:
       1) Infant protection from infection
       2) Immunosuppressant medication administration
       3) Importance of monitoring infant's axillary temperature (avoiding rectal temperatures)
       4) Dressing changes as needed
       5) Manifestations of organ failure (increasing jaundice)
       6) Adverse effects of immunosuppressant therapy
       7) Observations to report to health care provider immediately
       8) Referral information if needed
       9) Contact numbers
       10) Importance of follow-up and long-term posttransplant care
    c. Provide sufficient time for parents' return demonstration of needed procedures and their questions
    d. Document teaching and parental response

NIC

Pretransplantation

1. Surveillance: Safety
2. Vital Signs Monitoring, Respiratory Monitoring, Positioning
3. Surveillance: Safety, Skin Integrity
4. Fluid/Electrolyte Management, Medication Administration
5. Nutrition Therapy, Nutrition Management, Enteral Tube Feeding
6. Sleep Enhancement
7. Health Teaching: Condition, Treatment, Health Promotion

Posttransplantation

8. Surveillance: Safety, Vital Signs Monitoring
9. Surveillance: Safety
10. Oxygen Therapy, Positioning: Chest Tube Management
11. Surveillance: Safety, Vital Signs Monitoring
12. Medication Management, Pain Management, Analgesic Administration, Positioning
13. Health Education: Infant Care, Child Development
14. Health Education: Condition, Infection Control, Medication

Evaluation

Pretransplantation

1. Client does not experience bleeding injuries.
2. Client demonstrates improved breathing pattern as evidenced by vitals signs and oxygen saturation WDL.

3. Client maintains skin integrity.

4. Client regains and maintains fluid balance as evidenced by decrease in edema and urine output >1 mL/kg/hr.

5. Client regains and maintains adequate nutritional intake to meet metabolic needs.

6. Client experiences undisturbed periods (1–2 hours) of sleep between feedings.

7. Family/parents demonstrate understanding of condition, medical treatment, and home care.

POSTTRANSPLANTATION

8. Client does not experience infection; but if it does occur, manifestations will be recognized and antimicrobial therapy will be initiated in a timely manner.

9. Client does not experience rejection of transplanted organ as evidenced by liver function tests WDL and absence of manifestations of organ rejection.

10. Client regains and maintains effective gas exchange as evidenced by hemodynamic stability and oxygen saturation within prescribed parameters.

11. Client does not experience complications secondary to liver transplant as evidenced by cardiovascular, renal, neurologic, and metabolic functioning WDL.

12. Client demonstrates adequate pain management as evidenced by a level of 1 on a 5-point scale with 5 indicating severe pain based on infant behaviors.

13. Client participates in age-appropriate activities within the constraints of immunosuppressive therapy and continues to achieve highest level of growth and development.

14. Family/parents demonstrate understanding of posttransplantation therapy and home care.

References

American Liver Foundation. (2007). *Biliary atresia*. Retrieved April 21, 2007, from http://www.liverfoundation.org/education/info/biliaryatresia

Broyles, B. E. (2005). *Medical-surgical nursing clinical companion*. Durham, NC: Carolina Academic Press.

Carter, B. A., & Kilic, M. (2006). *History of pediatric liver transplantation*. Retrieved April 21, 2007, from http://www.emedicine.com/ped/topic2840.htm

Cincinnati Children's Hospital Medical Center. (2006). *Biliary atresia*. Retrieved April 21, 2007, from http://www.cincinnatichildrens.org/svc/alpha/l/liver/diseases/biliary.htm

eMedicine Health. (2007). *Liver transplant*. Retrieved April 21, 2007, from http://www.emedicine-health.com/liver_transplant/article_em.htm

National Institutes of Diabetes and Digestive and Kidney Diseases. (2006). *Biliary atresia*. Retrieved April 21, 2007, from http://digestive.niddk.nih.gov/ddiseases/pubs/atresia/index.htm

15

BITES AND STINGS

Definition

Bites and stings are injuries that occur when children experience impact with animals, insects, and snakes. These injuries can cause minor discomforts or may produce severe trauma, infection, and even life-threatening anaphylaxis.

Pathophysiology

When an animal bites, the bacteria on the animal's teeth enter through the broken skin caused by the bite. Most animal bites involve the face and cause abrasions, lacerations, or tearing of facial tissue. Infection is the leading complication associated with animal bites. However, in the presence of severe bites of the head area, major vessels can be injured, resulting in the risk of massive blood loss, hypovolemia, and shock.

Another significant threat from animals is rabies. Animals such as foxes, bats, skunks, raccoons, opossums, and bats carry the greatest risk of transmitting rabies. However, domestic animals that have not been vaccinated also pose a risk requiring immediate rabies prophylaxis to be initiated with rabies immune globulin (Potts & Mandleco, 2007).

With biting insects, antigens in the insect's saliva initiate reactions in the host. The sensitivity of the child to the antigens determines the extent of the reaction. Although most bites cause only local responses, anaphylaxis can occur. Stings from bumblebees, wasps, hornets, and ants contain antigens, histamine, and mast cell degranulating peptides. Venom is injected from the stinger into the skin. Hypersensitivity responses are the most common reactions and occur as a consequence of the release of endogenous cellular mediators in the child. Toxic reactions can result from the poisonous effects of venom injected by insects such as the black widow spider or the brown recluse spider. Fire ants both bite and sting their victims. They "inject their venom by biting the victim with their mandibles and then inserting an abdominal stinger into the skin repeatedly in an arc around the bite site. The venom contains hemolytic factors that induce the release of histamine and other vasoactive amines" (Nunnelee, 2005, p. 57).

Bites from mosquitoes, fleas, and flies can be painful and pruritic. When the mosquito stings, saliva with digestive enzymes and anticoagulants are injected into the host's skin. The first time a person is bitten, there is no reaction. However, with subsequent bites, young children become sensitized to the foreign proteins and small, itchy red bumps appear about 24 hours later. Following many more bites, in older children and adolescents, the formation of a pale, swollen hive or wheal occurs minutes after a bite. This is followed by the red bump 24 hours later.

Mosquitoes also can act as vectors transmitting blood-borne disorders such as West Nile virus, yellow fever, malaria, dengue fever, and encephalitis. Bites from ticks acting as vectors can result in conditions such as Lyme disease and Rocky Mountain spotted fever. Harvest mites (chiggers) attach to human skin with their claws and produce digestive enzymes that liquefy epidermal tissue of the host, creating pruritic erythematous papules. The larvae of these mites feed from the epidermal and dermal tissues of the host (Potts & Mandleco, 2007).

A bite from a nonvenomous snake can result in infection and even an allergic response in sensitized individuals. Venomous snakebites occur most commonly (90%) on the arms and legs of the victim (Lucile Packard Children's Hospital at Stanford, 2007). The venom can cause responses that range from mild swelling, pain, and erythema to shock and a disseminated intravascular coagulation-like syndrome (Brown, 2005). Snake venoms cause damage either to the blood and other tissues (hemotoxic) or to nerves (neurotoxic). The pit vipers (rattlesnakes, copperheads, and water moccasins), with the exception of some Mojave rattlesnakes, have hemotoxic venom. Coral snakes have neurotoxic venom. The characteristic manifestations of hemotoxic bites are intense pain and swelling. Neurotoxic manifestations include local parenthesia, ptosis, dysphasia, diplopia, diaphoresis, excessive salivation, diminished reflexes, respiratory depression, and paralysis.

Complications

Infection
Intense pain
Hypersensitivity responses
Shock
Death from anaphylaxis
Hemotoxic responses from pit viper bites
Neurotoxic responses from coral snake bites
Lyme disease (deer tick)
Rocky Mountain spotted fever (wood tick)

Incidence and Etiology

Dog and cat bites represent 90% of all animal bites occurring in the United States annually, with dog bites accounting for 80%. As a result, several million individuals receive animal bites each year. Although bites from other mammals including raccoons, squirrels, bats, foxes, and skunks are not as significant in number, the morbidity from these bites cannot be ignored (Potts & Mandleco, 2007).

Stings from insects in the Hymenoptera order, which includes honeybees, bumblebees, hornets, wasps, yellow jackets, and ants, result in 30 to 50 deaths and more than 500,000 emergency department visits annually in the United States. "Yellow jacket stings are the leading cause of allergic reactions to insect stings" (Nunnelee, 2005, p. 50).

More infants and children are bitten by mosquitoes than by any other insect. Of the 20,000 spider species in the United States, only the brown recluse and the black widow pose any danger to humans. "It is estimated that spider bites cause fewer than three deaths per year in the United States" (Nunnelee, 2005, p. 60).

Approximately 45,000 people receive snakebites annually in the United States. Of these, 7,000 to 8,000 are venomous snakebites that result in 9 to 15 deaths per year. More than half of the venomous snakebites involve children, and most occur between April and October. Of the venomous bites in the United States, 55% are from rattlesnakes, 34% are from copperheads, 10% are from water moccasins, and 1% are from coral snakes. Rattlesnakes have the most deadly venom and are responsible for most of the venomous snakebite deaths (North Carolina State University, n.d.).

"Only about 5 percent, or roughly 25 species of snakes in the US are venomous. The most common venomous snakebites are caused by the following snakes: 1) pit vipers—rattlesnakes, copperheads and cottonmouth (water moccasin) snakes and 2) coral snakes. Rattlesnake bites cause most of the venomous bites in the US. Coral snakes cause less than 1 percent of venomous snakebites" (Children's Hospital Central California, n.d., p. 1).

Clinical Manifestations

Animal Bites

Tissue tears
Bleeding from wounds

Abrasions

Lacerations

Avulsion

Pain

Swelling

INSECT STINGS/BITES

Localized pain and pruritis

Brown recluse spider bite:

    Mild stinging 2–3 hours following bite

    Mild erythematous, painful macule

    Fever

    Chills

    Malaise

    Erosion of skin and tissue surrounding bite 2–3 days following bite

Black widow spider bite:

    Manifestations that peak within 24 hours and may continue for 2–5 days

    Immediate pain

    Puncture marks

    Severe muscle cramping and spasm

    Diaphoresis

    Anxiety

    Parenthesia

    Decreased coordination

    Increasing irritability

    Hypertension

    Shock

Hematotoxic snake bites:

    Puncture (fang) marks in the skin

    Severe localized pain, burning, and warmth

    Weakness

    Tachycardia

    Parenthesia

    Tingling sensations

    Ecchymosis

    Bleeding disorders (generalized bleeding or coagulation disorders)

    Vomiting

    Unusual metallic taste

    Confusion

Neurotoxic snake bites:

    Ptosis

    Dysphagia

    Diplopia

    Diaphoresis

    Excessive salivation

    Diminished reflexes

    Respiratory depression

    Paralysis

Diagnostic Tests

Identification of the animal, insect, or snake that created the wound

Wound cultures

Complete blood count

Medical Management

The goals of treatment for children experiencing bites and stings are to effectively manage the symptoms, administer antivenin if appropriate, monitor for infection and anaphylaxis, and prevent further bites and stings. Animal bites should be cultured; then the wound should be irrigated with large amounts of sterile saline under sufficient pressure to debride the wound. The administration of a local anesthetic should be completed before suturing (or stapling) the wound(s). Administration of antibiotics may be prescribed depending on the depth and severity of the wound, the immune status of the child, and the presence of overt signs of infection. Amoxicillin-clavulanate is the oral broad-spectrum antibiotic of choice, and ticarcillin-clavulanate is the intravenous antimicrobial of choice. Rabies prophylaxis is initiated; and if appropriate, a tetanus booster is administered. In the presence of hypovolemia and hypotension, the intravenous administration of volume expanding fluids and vasogenic support should be available (Potts & Mandleco, 2007).

Most insect bites require symptomatic therapy including cleansing the wound, administering diphenhydramine or hydrocortisone topically, and monitoring for the onset of more severe symptoms requiring emergency treatment. When coming to the aid of a child who has been stung by a bee, wasp, or hornet, the rescuer needs to maintain his/her own safety and remove the child from the vicinity of the stinging insects. Maintaining a calm affect will help keep the child calm. The child's airway, breathing, and circulation (ABCs) should be assessed; and if the child is having difficulty breathing, he/she should be positioned upright. If manifestations of shock present, the victim should be placed in a supine position and 911 should be notified. If the child is known to be allergic to bee stings and carries an epinephrine pen, the epinephrine should be administered. If not, the child needs to be taken immediately to the emergency department of the closest acute health care facility for epinephrine administration. If the stinger remains in the wound, it should be removed as quickly as possible. This can be accomplished by scrapping it out with the edge of a credit card, a nail file, a dull knife blade, tweezers, or a needle. Then the wound should be cleaned with soap and water and antiseptic/antibiotic ointment should be applied (Laskowski-Jones, 2006).

With the child who has been bitten by a snake, identifying the type of snake is important to assist with treatment options. However, this should be accomplished without placing the rescuer or the child in further danger. The rescuer must remain calm and reassure the child. The child should be moved to a nearby safe area away from the snake, and emergency assistance should be requested immediately. If it is possible to kill the snake without harming the rescuer or the child further, it is important to do so, remembering that the snake may bite up to one hour after being killed. The snake should be placed in a glass jar or plastic container so it can be positively identified.

Antivenin (an antitoxin specific to the venom of a particular animal or insect) for poisonous snakebites should be given within four hours when possible, so it is important that the rescuer note the time that the bite occurred. Antivenin is not usually effective when given more than 12 hours after the bite. While waiting for emergency assistance, the rescuer should continuously monitor the child's ABCs while having the child lie down, rest, and remain calm, washing the bite with soap and water and loosely immobilizing the bitten area and maintaining it below the level of the heart. If a pump suction device is available, the manufacturer's directions should be used in placing it over the bite to help draw venom out of the wound; but a tourniquet should not be applied as this can cause further damage to the limb where the bite occurred.

Once the child is in the hospital, treatment includes the use of antivenin. Treatment also may include lab work, pain or sedation medications, a tetanus booster, antibiotics, and supportive care. Antivenin is derived from antibodies created in a horse's blood serum when the animal is injected with snake venom. In humans, antivenin is administered through the veins or is injected into muscle; it works by neutralizing snake venom that has entered the body. Because antivenin is obtained from horses, snakebite victims sensitive to horse products must be carefully managed. The danger is that they could develop an adverse reaction or even a potentially fatal allergic condition called anaphylactic shock (Daley & Barbee, 2007). Antivenin is used to treat poisonous spider bites in children (Holcomb, 2006).

Nursing Management

ASSESSMENT

1. Assess child's airway, breathing, and circulation
2. Obtain history of bite/sting, including time of event
3. Assess wound
4. Obtain cultures in the event these are needed
5. Assess vital signs and perform physical assessment

NURSING DIAGNOSES (INCLUDING BUT NOT LIMITED TO)

1. Risk for injury R/T effects of bite/sting
2. Risk for infection R/T break in the skin and injection of microorganisms from bite
3. Deficient knowledge R/T condition, treatment, home care, and prevention of further bites/stings

PLANNING/GOALS

1. Client will not experience serious consequences resulting from the bite/sting; however, if a serious reaction occurs, it will be effectively treated.
2. Client will not experience wound infection.
3. Client/family will demonstrate understanding of condition, treatment, home care, and prevention of further bites/stings.

NOC

1. Risk Control
2. Wound Healing: Primary Intention, Wound Healing: Secondary Intention
3. Knowledge: Illness Care, Treatment, Injury Prevention

IMPLEMENTATION

1. Risk for injury
   a. Monitor airway, breathing, and circulation
   b. Identify animal/insect/snake responsible for bite
   c. Identify time of event
   d. Provide calm reassurance to child/family
   e. Establish and maintain intravenous access if prescribed
   f. Administer medications as prescribed
   g. Provide proactive pain management for hemotoxic bites
   h. Monitor neurologic status for neurotoxic bites
   i. Monitor vital signs
   j. Cleanse wound with soap and water
   k. Irrigate animal bites as prescribed

2. Risk for infection
   a. Assess wound for manifestations of infection
   b. Obtain cultures of wound
   c. Send cultures to lab as prescribed
   d. Wash wound with soap and water
   e. Prepare for wound suturing if health care provider prescribes
   f. Monitor vital signs
   g. Apply antiseptic/antibiotic ointment to wound
3. Client/family teaching
   a. Assess client's/family's current level of knowledge
   b. Provide verbal and written information regarding:
      1) Medication administration and importance of completing prescription
      2) Use of epinephrine pen if child is allergic to bites/stings and importance of wearing medical identification
      3) Clinical manifestations of worsening condition
      4) Importance of follow-up as prescribed by health care provider
      5) Prevention principles for bites/stings
         a) Do not approach wild animals
         b) Do not approach domestic animals that are not familiar
         c) Keep domestic animals properly vaccinated
         d) Have children wear DEET products when they are outside in areas and during seasons in which insects are prevalent (no greater than a 10% solution should be used on young children), make sure children's clothing covers as much of their body as possible, and avoid clothing with bright and flowery prints
         e) Avoid perfumes, colognes, and scented soaps during peak insect seasons
         f) Inform children to leave snakes alone
         g) Inform children to stay out of tall grass unless wearing thick leather boots
         h) Inform children to remain on hiking trails
         i) Inform children to keep their hands and feet out of areas they cannot see
         j) Inform children not to pick up rocks or firewood
         k) Maintain caution when climbing rocks
         l) Maintain a distance of at least 6 feet or walk away when a snake is encountered
   c. Provide adequate time for teaching and questions
   d. Document teaching and client/family response

NIC
1. Risk Identification, Safety Surveillance
2. Infection Control
3. Teaching: Illness Care, Treatment, Injury Prevention

EVALUATION
1. Client does not experience serious consequences resulting from the bite/sting. Serious reactions are effectively treated.
2. Client does not experience wound infection.

3. Client/family demonstrate understanding of condition, treatment, home care, and prevention of further bites/stings.

References

Brown, H. (2005). Venomous snakebite. *Nursing, 35*(5).

Children's Hospital Central California. (n.d.). *Snake bites*. Retrieved April 22, 2007, from http://www.childrenscentralcal.org/printpage.asp?id=1532

Daley, B. J. & Barbee, J. (2007). *Snakebite*. Retrieved March 16, 2008, from http://www.emedicine.com/med/topic2143.htm

Holcomb, S. S. (2006). Black widow spider bite. *Nursing, 36*(5).

Laskowski-Jones, L. (2006). First aid for bee, wasp, and hornet stings. *Nursing, 36*(7).

Lucile Packard Children's Hospital at Stanford. (2007). *Common childhood injuries and poisonings: Snake bites*. Retrieved April 22, 2007, from http://www.lpch.org/DiseaseHealthInfo/HealthLibrary/poison/snake.html

North Carolina State University. (n.d.). *Avoiding snake bites*. Retrieved February 13, 2007, from http://www.ces.ncsu.edu/gaston/Pests/reptiles/avoidsnakebite.htm

Nunnelee, J. D. (2005). Bites & stings. *RN, 68*(4).

Potts, N. L., & Mandleco, B. L. (2007). *Pediatric nursing: Caring for children and their families* (2nd ed.). Clifton Park, NY: Delmar Cengage Learning.

16

BRONCHIOLITIS

Definition

Bronchiolitis is the inflammation and usually the infection of the small airway passages in the lower respiratory track distal to the bronchi.

Pathophysiology

With bronchiolitis, the smaller bronchial passages leading into the bronchioles and the bronchioles themselves become inflamed; the inflammation causes edema in the walls lining these passages, increased mucus production, and cellular infiltrates. The changes lead to varying degrees of obstruction of the bronchioles. This "causes air trapping (distally that) leads to hyperinflation of some alveoli and atelectasis in others" (Potts & Mandleco, 2007, p. 720). The obstructions do not occur in a uniform manner throughout the lungs, but rather in a patchy pattern. Airway resistance increases, which is reflected in decreased tidal volumes, tachypnea, and dyspnea. This condition is especially severe in infants because the lumina of the bronchioles are smaller. The airtrapping can cause hypercapnia, resulting in respiratory acidosis and hypoxia.

Complications

> Atelectasis
> Hypoxia
> Respiratory acidosis

Incidence

The highest incidence of bronchiolitis is in infants and toddlers ages 2 months to 2 years. In the United States, the "annual incidence is 11.4% in children younger than 1 year and 6% in those aged 1–2 years. The illness accounts for 4500 deaths and 90,000 hospital admissions per year" (Louden, 2006, Section 2). The international incidence in developed countries is similar to that in the United States (Louden, 2006).

Etiology

Respiratory syncytial virus (RSV) is the causative organism in 85% of all cases of bronchiolitis. Adenovirus is responsible for approximately 11% of cases; and a few cases are due to *Mycoplasma pneumoniae,* enterovirus, influenza virus, rhinovirus, and *Chlamydia pneumoniae* (Louden, 2006).

Clinical Manifestations

> Symptoms of upper respiratory infection for 1–4 days (rhinorrhea, low-grade fever, and coughing)
> Poor feeding
> Irritability
> Malaise
> Tachypnea
> Nasal flaring
> Sternal retractions

Increased mucus production

Adventitious breath sounds (wheezing, crackles, and prolonged
    expiratory phase)

Intermittent cyanosis

Diagnostic Tests

History of upper respiratory infection—primary diagnostic data

Complete blood count

Chest radiography

Culture of nasopharyngeal secretions

Antigen assay

Medical Management

The goals of medical management are to resolve infection and reestablish gas
exchange. Mild cases (approximately 95% of cases) usually are treated at home with
oral fluid resuscitation, humidification, fever management, and rest. Infants who
manifest respiratory distress or dehydration are treated in the hospital setting with
humidified oxygen, intravenous fluid resuscitation, mechanical ventilation (in severe
cases resulting in respiratory failure), and antimicrobials for secondary bacterial
infections.

Ribavirin is the only antiviral agent currently approved for the treatment of RSV.
It acts by interfering with RNA and DNA synthesis, thus inhibiting viral replication.
Ribavirin is administered in aerosol form. Consequently, because of the risk of terato-
genic effects, it may be hazardous to anyone coming in contact with it. Thus, nurses
or parents who are pregnant or are planning pregnancy should not care for infants on
ribavirin therapy (Broyles, Reiss, & Evans, 2007).

Nursing Management

ASSESSMENT

1. Obtain client history
2. Perform physical examination with special attention to the infant's/
   child's respiratory status
3. Obtain baseline vital signs
4. Obtain length and weight

NURSING DIAGNOSES (INCLUDING BUT NOT LIMITED TO)

1. Impaired gas exchange R/T increased mucus production, airtrapping, and ineffective airway clearance
2. Deficient fluid volume R/T inadequate fluid intake and insensible
   fluid loss secondary to tachypnea
3. Risk for ineffective thermoregulation R/T potential secondary
   bacterial infectious process
4. Anxiety (parental) R/T infant's/child's condition, hospitalization,
   and intensive care environment
5. Deficient knowledge R/T infant's/child's condition, medical
   management, and home care

PLANNING/GOALS

1. Client will regain and maintain effective gas exchange and airway
   clearance as evidenced by respiratory rate return to within defined
   limits (WDL), oxygen saturation WDL, clear breath sounds, and
   absence of manifestations of respiratory distress.

2. Client will regain and maintain adequate hydration as evidenced by moist mucous membranes, fluid intake, and urinary output WDL for age.

3. Client will maintain effective thermoregulation as evidenced by body temperature WDL.

4. Parents will demonstrate a reduction in anxiety level as evidenced by verbal and nonverbal cues.

5. Parents will demonstrate understanding of infant's/child's condition, medical management, and home care.

NOC

1. Respiratory Status: Gas Exchange, Airway Patency
2. Fluid Balance
3. Risk Control
4. Anxiety Level
5. Knowledge: Disease Process, Illness Care, Infection Control, Health Promotion

IMPLEMENTATION

1. Gas exchange
   a. Assess respiratory status continuously in acute care or intensive care environment
   b. Assess vital signs with frequency consistent with infant's/child's condition
   c. Initiate continuous pulse oximetry
   d. Position to maintain airway patency and support respiratory effort
   e. Maintain mechanical ventilation as required and prescribed
   f. Maintain meticulous hand washing to protect infant from nosocomial infections
   g. Administer oxygen, titrating to maintain oxygen saturation within prescribed parameters
   h. Administer nebulizer medication as prescribed
   i. Maintain emergency equipment at bedside
   j. Provide calm, supportive environment
   k. Provide age-appropriate play within constraints of infant's/child's condition
   l. Encourage parents to visit and participate in care within constraints of condition

2. Fluid balance
   a. Assess mucous membranes and skin turgor at least every 4–8 hours
   b. Monitor strict intake and output
   c. Weigh daily
   d. Maintain intravenous access device, monitoring hourly
   e. Administer intravenous fluids as prescribed
   f. Offer oral fluids frequently within constraints of infant's/child's condition
   g. Monitor energy level during oral fluid intake
   h. Monitor serum electrolytes
   i. Monitor urine specific gravity

3. Thermoregulation
   a. Monitor temperature at least every 4 hours
   b. Maintain stable environmental temperature
   c. Administer antipyretics as prescribed
   d. Encourage oral fluid intake within constraints of infant's/child's condition
4. Parental anxiety
   a. Assess parents (caregivers) for manifestations of anxiety
   b. Encourage parents to verbalize fears and concerns
   c. Listen actively
   d. Explain all procedures, equipment, and medications
   e. Encourage parents to visit and stay with their child when possible
   f. Provide calm environment as much as possible
   g. Keep parents informed of child's condition
   h. Involve parents in child's care
5. Parent teaching
   a. Assess parental current level of knowledge
   b. Provide parents with verbal and written information regarding:
      1) Avoidance of infection by restricting exposure to crowds
      2) All procedures and medications used to treat child
      3) Manifestations of worsening condition
      4) Age-appropriate activities
      5) Importance of follow-up care and monitoring
      6) Contact information to report worsening of condition
   c. Provide adequate time for parental questions
   d. Document teaching and parent/client response

NIC

1. Airway Management, Acid-Base Management, Oxygen Therapy, Ventilation Assistance
2. Fluid Resuscitation
3. Risk Identification
4. Anxiety Reduction
5. Teaching: Disease Process, Illness Care, Infection Control, Health Promotion

EVALUATION

1. Client regains and maintains effective gas exchange and airway clearance as evidenced by respiratory rate return to WDL, oxygen saturation WDL, clear breath sounds, and absence of manifestations of respiratory distress.
2. Client regains and maintains adequate hydration as evidenced by moist mucous membranes, fluid intake, and urinary output WDL for age.
3. Client maintains effective thermoregulation as evidenced by body temperature WDL.
4. Parents demonstrate a reduction in anxiety level as evidenced by verbal and nonverbal cues.
5. Parents demonstrate understanding of infant's/child's condition, medical management, and home care.

References

Broyles, B. E., Reiss, B. S., & Evans, M. E. (2007). *Pharmacological aspects of nursing care* (7th ed.). Clifton Park, NY: Delmar Cengage Learning.

Louden, M. (2006). *Pediatrics, bronchiolitis.* Retrieved April 22, 2007, from http://www.emedicine .com/emerg/topic365.htm

Potts, N. L., & Mandleco, B. L. (2007). *Pediatric nursing: Caring for children and their families* (2nd ed.). Clifton Park, NY: Delmar Cengage Learning.

BRONCHOPULMONARY DYSPLASIA (BPD)

Definition

Bronchopulmonary dysplasia (BPD) is a chronic obstructive lung disease that occurs in preterm and full-term infants as a complication of prolonged oxygen therapy and mechanical ventilation to survive during the neonatal period (Hockenberry, 2005).

Pathophysiology

The maturing of the respiratory system begins during the third trimester of gestation (from about 36 weeks' gestation) and continues until the child is approximately 18 months of age. Preterm infants (usually 30 weeks' gestation or less) are born with immature lungs that place them at risk for respiratory distress and failure. Respiratory insufficiency impairs gas exchange and leads to ineffective tissue perfusion to meet the increased metabolic needs of the preterm neonate. To prevent neurologic damage from inadequate oxygenation and death from respiratory failure, high concentration oxygen and mechanical ventilation may be required. In addition, long-term mechanical ventilation may require the placement of a tracheostomy tube.

High concentrations of oxygen can be toxic to the cells and tissues in the respiratory system; and when the oxygen is delivered under increased pressure as seen with mechanical ventilation, this damage is more severe. This creates damage to the bronchial epithelium and alveoli. The damage to the epithelium decreases the airway's resistance to microorganisms, thus increasing the risk of opportunistic respiratory microbial growth. The inflammation that occurs increases airway resistance and mucus production, further providing microorganisms with media for growth. Damage to the alveoli involves thickening of the alveolar walls and fibrosis, or scarring, of these pockets of gas exchange. This decreases the numbers of functional alveoli, resulting in impaired gas exchange and decreased oxygen available in circulation to meet the metabolic needs of the body. Severe BPD can result in pulmonary hypertension and abnormal pulmonary vascular development (Rajiah & Banerjee, 2006).

Unlike the mature immune system of the adult, the immune systems of neonates are normally immature, placing newborns at risk for infection. Preterm infants are at greater risk for infection, especially respiratory infections. Infants with BPD have increased risk of recurrent pneumonia.

According to the National Heart Lung and Blood Institute of the National Institutes of Health, although some of these infants may experience chronic oxygen dependency, "Today, most babies with BPD recover" (National Heart Lung and Blood Institute, 2006, p. 1).

Complications

Atelectasis
Recurrent pneumonia
Pulmonary hypertension
Respiratory failure

Incidence

BPD usually occurs in preterm infants less than 30–36 weeks' gestation. However, it can occur in full-term infants who require high percentage oxygen therapy especially via mechanical ventilation. According to the National Heart Lung and Blood

Institute of the National Institutes of Health, "[M]ost babies with BPD (9 of 10) weigh 1,500 grams (about $3\frac{1}{2}$ pounds), or less, at birth" (National Heart Lung and Blood Institute, 2006, p. 1). It most frequently is seen in infants with respiratory distress syndrome; however, it has been seen in adults with ARDS (adult respiratory distress syndrome) (American Lung Association, 2007). With the routine use of surfactant replacement, the survival rate of preterm infants has dramatically improved. Along with other advances in technology and improved understanding of neonatal physiology, infants with BPD appear to have a less severe disease compared to infants with BPD in years past. Infants with severe BPD remain at high risk for pulmonary morbidity and mortality during the first two years of life (Rajiah & Banerjee, 2006). "About 5,000 to 10,000 babies in the United States develop BPD each year. Because more babies weighing less than 3 pounds live past 4 weeks, more babies develop BPD today than 30 years ago" (National Heart Lung and Blood Institute, 2006, p. 1).

Etiology

Four major factors predispose infants to the development of bronchopulmonary dysplasia: (1) preterm birth, (2) respiratory distress syndrome, (3) exposure to high concentrations of supplemental oxygen, and (4) treatment with mechanical ventilation.

Clinical Manifestations

Tachypnea

Tachycardia

History of preterm birth

History of treatment with high concentration oxygen and/or mechanical ventilation after birth

Dyspnea, sternal retractions, nasal flaring, and use of accessory muscles

Pallor

Feeding intolerance

Weight loss or inadequate weight gain

Restlessness

Irritability

Cyanosis and fatigue

Diagnostic Tests

Chest radiography

Arterial blood gases to determine acid base

Pulse oximetry

Medical Management

The goals of treatment for respiratory distress syndrome (RDS) in neonates are to (1) provide adequate gas exchange until the newborn's lungs can perform this function on their own and (2) prevent the development of BPD. However, once BPD has been diagnosed, supportive therapy to prevent further lung damage is the goal of care. Oxygen therapy may be continued after discharge from the hospital for as long as a year. Positive pressure mechanical ventilation is discontinued as soon as the infant's condition allows, and invasive procedures that may compromise lung tissue are avoided. Antimicrobial agents are used to treat infections. Bronchodilators and corticosteroids may be prescribed to decrease the inflammation and lower airway resistance. These infants require close monitoring of respiratory status to detect any signs of third spacing of fluid in the lungs. Diuretics may be prescribed to treat fluid overload. Infant nutrition is of utmost importance for the child with BPD. Prescribing high-calorie infant formulas and providing additional enteral feedings help the infant grow stronger and healthier.

Providing age-appropriate growth and development activities is critical for the infant/child with BPD to achieve the highest level of wellness.

Nursing Management

ASSESSMENT

1. Obtain history and note whether child experienced preterm birth, oxygen dependency, use of high concentration oxygen, or mechanical ventilation during neonatal period
2. Assess respiratory status including breath sounds and vital signs
3. Monitor chest radiography findings
4. Assess fluid status
5. Assess growth and development
6. Assess psychosocial needs of parents/caregivers

NURSING DIAGNOSES (INCLUDING BUT NOT LIMITED TO)

1. Impaired gas exchange R/T air trapping, ineffective airway clearance
2. Ineffective protection R/T preterm birth, disease process, immature immune system
3. Deficient fluid volume R/T inadequate fluid intake and insensible fluid loss secondary to tachpnea
4. Risk for ineffective thermoregulation R/T potential secondary bacterial infectious process
5. Anxiety (parental) R/T infant's preterm birth or infant's/child's condition, hospitalization, and intensive care environment
6. Deficient knowledge R/T infant's/child's condition, medical management, and home care

PLANNING/GOALS

1. Client will regain and maintain effective gas exchange and airway clearance as evidenced by respiratory rate return to within defined limits (WDL), oxygen saturation WDL, clear breath sounds, and absence of manifestations of respiratory distress.
2. Client's respiratory ineffective protection will be effectively managed, and infections will be promptly and effectively treated.
3. Client will regain and maintain adequate hydration as evidenced by moist mucous membranes, fluid intake, and urinary output WDL for age.
4. Client will maintain effective thermoregulation as evidenced by body temperature WDL.
5. Parents will demonstrate a reduction in anxiety level as evidenced by verbal and nonverbal cues.
6. Parents will demonstrate understanding of infant's/child's condition, medical management, and home care.

NOC

1. Respiratory Status: Gas Exchange, Airway Patency
2. Immune Status
3. Fluid Balance
4. Risk Control
5. Anxiety Level
6. Knowledge: Disease Process, Illness Care, Infection Control, Health Promotion

IMPLEMENTATION

1. Gas exchange
   a. Assess respiratory status continuously in intensive care environment
   b. Assess vital signs with frequency consistent with infant's/child's condition
   c. Initiate continuous pulse oximetry
   d. Position to maintain airway patency and support respiratory effort
   e. Maintain mechanical ventilation as required and prescribed
   f. Maintain meticulous hand washing to protect infant from nosocomial infections
   g. Administer oxygen, titrating to maintain oxygen saturation within prescribed parameters
   h. Administer surfactant therapy as prescribed
   i. Administer nebulizer medication as prescribed
   j. Maintain emergency equipment at bedside
   k. Provide calm, supportive environment
   l. Provide age-appropriate play within constraints of infant's/child's condition
   m. Encourage parents to visit and participate in care within constraints of infant's/child's condition

2. Ineffective protection
   a. Monitor continuous temperature in critical care using a skin probe
   b. Maintain meticulous infection protection
   c. Teach parents/caregivers appropriate hand washing technique
   d. Administer antimicrobials as prescribed
   e. Encourage parents/caregivers to spend time bonding with child in the critical care environment
   f. Explain all equipment and procedures

3. Fluid balance
   a. Assess mucous membranes and skin turgor at least every 4–8 hours
   b. Monitor strict intake and output
   c. Weigh daily
   d. Maintain intravenous access device, monitoring hourly
   e. Administer intravenous fluids as prescribed
   f. Offer oral fluids frequently within constraints of infant's/child's condition
   g. Monitor energy level during oral fluid intake
   h. Monitor serum electrolytes
   i. Monitor urine specific gravity

4. Thermoregulation
   a. Monitor temperature at least every 4 hours
   b. Maintain stable environmental temperature
   c. Administer antipyretics as prescribed
   d. Encourage oral fluid intake within constraints of infant's/child's condition

5. Parental anxiety
   a. Assess parents (caregivers) for manifestations of anxiety
   b. Encourage parents to verbalize fears and concerns
   c. Listen actively
   d. Explain all procedures, equipment, and medications
   e. Encourage parents to visit and stay with child when possible
   f. Provide calm environment as much as possible
   g. Keep parents informed of child's condition
   h. Involve parents in child's care
6. Parent teaching
   a. Assess parental current level of knowledge
   b. Provide parents with verbal and written information regarding:
      1) Avoidance of infection by restricting exposure to crowds
      2) All procedures and medications used to treat child
      3) Tracheostomy care and suctioning if needed
      4) Manifestations of worsening condition
      5) Age-appropriate activities
      6) Referral information including home oxygen therapy
      7) Importance of follow-up care and monitoring
      8) Contact information to report worsening of condition
   c. Provide adequate time for parental questions and return demon-strations of procedures (tracheostomy care, changing, suctioning, and oxygen and medication administration using tracheostomy)
   d. Document teaching and parent/client response

NIC

1. Airway Management, Acid-Base Management, Oxygen Therapy, Ventilation Assistance
2. Infection Protection
3. Fluid Resuscitation
4. Risk Identification
5. Anxiety Reduction
6. Teaching: Disease Process, Illness Care, Infection Control, Health Promotion

EVALUATION

1. Client regains and maintains effective gas exchange and airway clearance as evidenced by respiratory rate return to WDL, oxygen saturation WDL, clear breath sounds, and absence of manifestations of respiratory distress.
2. Client's respiratory ineffective protection is effectively managed, and infections are promptly and effectively treated.
3. Client regains and maintains adequate hydration as evidenced by moist mucous membranes, fluid intake, and urinary output WDL for age.
4. Client maintains effective thermoregulation as evidenced by body temperature WDL.
5. Parents demonstrate a reduction in anxiety level as evidenced by verbal and nonverbal cues.
6. Parents demonstrate understanding of infant's/child's condition, medical management, and home care.

References

American Lung Association. (2007). *Bronchopulmonary dysplasia.* Retrieved April 22, 2007, from http://www.lungusa.org/site/pp.asp?c=dvLUK9O0E&b=35017#whatis

Hockenberry, M. J. (2005). *Wong's essentials of pediatric nursing* (7th ed.). St. Louise, MO: Mosby Elsevier.

National Heart Lung and Blood Institute. (2006). *Bronchopulmonary dysplasia.* Retrieved April 22, 2007, from http://www.nhlbi.nih.gov/health/dci/Diseases/Bpd/Bpd_WhatIs.html

Rajiah, B., & Banerjee, B. (2006). *Bronchopulmonary dysplasia.* Retrieved April 22, 2007, from http://www.emedicine.com/radio/topic120.htm

18

BULIMIA NERVOSA

Definition

Bulimia nervosa is an eating disorder characterized by episodes of consuming large amounts of food with a lack of control (binge eating) followed by various compensatory behaviors to control weight gain (Potts & Mandleco, 2007). These behaviors include vomiting, consuming laxatives, and using enemas.

Pathophysiology

As with most eating disorders, bulimia nervosa is a psychosocial condition. The person is unable to express his/her feelings effectively and has a low self-esteem and feelings of inadequacy especially in controlling impulse behavior. Although the person receives comfort from food, he/she has an intense fear of gaining weight and being perceived as fat. There are two types of bulimia: (1) the purging type and (2) the nonpurging type. Often bulimia occurs in individuals with coexisting psychological problems such as substance abuse, self-mutilation, obsessive-compulsive disorder, bipolar disorder, and dissociative identity disorder (Broyles, 2005).

Binge eating usually occurs in private and involves the consumption of large quantities of food, usually high-calorie, high-fat, high-carbohydrate, and sweet and with a texture that allows for quick consumption. Characteristics of purging behavior include self-induced vomiting and abuse of diuretics, laxatives, and/or enemas. Nonpurging behaviors include fasting and excessive exercise activities (Foster & Smith-Coggins, 2007).

The binge and purge behaviors can result in gastrointestinal irritability, pancreatitis (from overstimulation of the pancreas from binge foods), peptic ulcer disease, and life-threatening electrolyte imbalances (hypokalemia and hyponatremia) that may lead to cardiac muscle dysfunction, dysrhythmias, and cardiac failure. Hyponatremia and hypochloremia (from vomiting and loss of gastric secretions) can cause fluid and acid-base imbalances. Frequent vomiting can result in esophageal erosions, increased dental caries, erosion of dental enamel, and parotid gland enlargement (Potts & Mandleco, 2007).

Complications

Electrolyte imbalances
Dehydration
Esophageal erosion
Peptic ulcer disease and gastric rupture
Pancreatitis
Erosion of tooth enamel
Increased dental caries
Life-threatening cardiac dysrhythmias
Death from cardiac failure

Incidence

The lifetime prevalence of bulimia is approximately 3%. It "affects about 6% of adolescent girls and 5% of college women. More than 5 million individuals are believed to experience an eating disorder (BN or anorexia nervosa) in this country alone. Symptoms of bulimia, such as isolated episodes of binge eating and purging, have been reported in up to 40% of college women" (Foster & Smith-Coggins, 2007,

Section 2). The majority (90–95%) of individuals with bulimia nervosa are female; women are 10 to 20 times more likely to develop the eating disorder than men (Foster & Smith-Coggins, 2007).

Etiology

Although the exact cause of bulimia nervosa is not known, neurochemical, psychosocial, and cultural factors are believed to contribute to the development of this condition. One theory identifies a lack of the neurotransmitter serotonin as a potential cause, and ongoing research seems to be supporting this theory. The frequent coexisting psychiatric disorders may have an impact on the development of this and other eating disorders. Depression is a frequent manifestation of bulimia and may be a part of its cause. However, the usual factors identified as leading to bulimia are pressures, conflicts, familial obesity, sexual abuse within the family unit, and society's current obsession with thinness (Foster & Smith-Coggins, 2007).

Clinical Manifestations

Constant concern about food and weight

Secretive eating

Purging behaviors

Scarring of knuckles

Manifestations of dehydration and electrolyte imbalances

Compulsive exercising

Diagnostic Tests

Serum electrolyte levels

Serum albumin level

Complete blood count

Physical examination revealing enlarged parotid glands, knuckle scarring, and dental erosion

Medical Management

The primary treatment for bulimia involves individual, family, and/or group psychotherapy. Most individuals with bulimia can be treated through individual outpatient therapy because they are not in danger of starving themselves as are people with anorexia nervosa. However, if the bulimia is out of control, admission to an eating disorders treatment program may assist the individual in identifying why the behaviors exist and how to resolve the bulimia nervosa.

Group therapy has been found to be especially effective for college-aged and young adult women because of the growth and development characteristics of this group. These individuals are very peer-focused and find talking with peers about similar experiences to be very comforting. Communication with peers, especially in light of their communication difficulties, is more likely than with other people with whom the individuals with bulimia do not believe they can identify.

Cognitive-behavioral therapy, either in a group setting or individual therapy session, has been beneficial to many people with bulimia. This type of therapy is based on self-monitoring eating and purging behaviors as well as changing the distorted thinking patterns associated with the disorder (MedlinePlus Medical Encyclopedia, 2006).

The use of selective serotonin uptake inhibitor antidepressants such as fluoxetine hydrochloride (Prozac), sertraline hydrochloride (Zoloft), and paroxetine hydrochloride (Paxil) and monoamine oxidase inhibitors such as isocarboxazide (Marplan), phenelzine sulfate (Nardil), and tranylcypromine sulfate (Parnate) to control binge behavior have been successful in treating bulimia when used in conjunction with psychotherapy.

The combined therapies have proven to be more successful than either modality when used as monotherapy (Broyles, 2005).

Nursing Management

ASSESSMENT

1. Obtain history of client's eating patterns
2. Obtain height and weight
3. Assess vital signs
4. Assess for manifestations of dehydration and electrolyte imbalances

NURSING DIAGNOSES (INCLUDING BUT NOT LIMITED TO)

1. Imbalanced nutrition: less than body requirements R/T purging and inadequate nutrition intake
2. Disturbed body image R/T distorted perception of body size and shape
3. Compromised family coping R/T issues of control and dysfunctional dynamics
4. Deficient knowledge R/T condition, treatment regimen, and home care

PLANNING/GOALS

1. Client will regain and maintain adequate nutritional intake to meet metabolic needs as evidenced by weight within normal range for height and age, maintenance of a pattern of consuming nutritionally adequate foods, reduction of energy expenditure, and verbalization of understanding of individual needs.
2. Client will demonstrate realistic attitudes and perceptions of body size and shape and the development of a positive self-image.
3. Family members will demonstrate understanding of dysfunctional family dynamics, establish clearly defined boundaries within the family, and use effective communication patterns.
4. Client/family will demonstrate understanding of condition, treatment regimen, and home care.

NOC

1. Nutritional Status: Food and Fluid Intake
2. Body Image
3. Family Coping
4. Knowledge: Health Behavior, Health Promotion

IMPLEMENTATION

1. Nutrition
   a. Assess weight and compare height and age according to standardized chart
   b. Explain this comparison with client
   c. Assess client's food preferences
   d. Collaborate with dietician to provide prescribed nutritionally balanced diet incorporating client preferences when possible
   e. Involve client in selection of balanced diet with gradual increase in caloric intake
   f. Provide supervision during and after meals
   g. Supervise selection and performance of activity plan

2. Body image
   a. Assess for individual manifestations of disturbed body image
   b. Discuss client's misconceptions about his/her body image
   c. Develop trusting relationship conducive for communication
   d. Encourage client to identify and express feelings and concerns
   e. Provide positive support and encouragement
   f. Assist in identification of strengths and ways to enhance them
3. Family coping
   a. Assess family for specific behaviors that identify dysfunctional family dynamics
   b. Assess family's current level of understanding of client's condition and impact of family dynamics on client
   c. Provide information about healthy boundaries within the family and normal separation and individuation of family members
   d. Discuss controlling behaviors exhibited by family or perceived by client
   e. Collaborate with health care provider for appropriate referrals
4. Family/client teaching
   a. Assess client's/family's current level of knowledge about condition
   b. Provide verbal and written information regarding:
      1) Nutritional plan and importance of compliance with plan
      2) Medication administration and importance of compliance with medication regimen
      3) Potential adverse effects of medications
      4) Importance of reporting adverse effects of medications to health care provider
      5) Follow-up visits with interdisciplinary team members
      6) Referrals to adolescent and family community and support services
      7) Reinforcement of psychotherapy behavioral modification plan
      8) Contact phone numbers for interdisciplinary team involved in treatment plan
   c. Encourage client/family questions and respond honestly
   d. Document teaching and client/family response

NIC

1. Nutritional Monitoring, Eating Disorder Management
2. Body Image Enhancement
3. Family Integrity Promotion: Family Therapy
4. Health Education, Teaching: Individual, Family

EVALUATION

1. Client regains and maintains adequate nutritional intake to meet metabolic needs as evidenced by weight within normal range for height and age, maintenance of a pattern of consuming nutritionally adequate foods, reduction of energy expenditure, and verbalization of understanding of individual needs.
2. Client demonstrates realistic attitudes and perceptions of body size and shape and the development of a positive self-image.

3. Family members demonstrate understanding of dysfunctional family dynamics, establish clearly defined boundaries within the family, and use effective communication patterns.
4. Client/family demonstrates understanding of condition, treatment regimen, and home care.

References

Broyles, B. E. (2005). *Medical-surgical nursing clinical companion.* Durham, NC: Carolina Academic Press.

Foster, T., & Smith-Coggins, R. (2007). *Bulimia.* Retrieved April 22, 2007, from http://www.emedicine.com/emerg/topic810.htm

MedlinePlus Medical Encyclopedia. (2006). *Bulimia.* Retrieved April 22, 2007, from http://www.nlm.nih.gov/medlineplus/ency/article/000341.htm

Potts, N. L., & Mandleco, B. L. (2007). *Pediatric nursing: Caring for children and their families* (2nd ed.). Clifton Park, NY: Delmar Cengage Learning.

19

BURNS

Definition

Burns are thermal injuries that occur to tissues from contact with thermal, chemical, electrical, or radiation sources.

Pathophysiology

The pathophysiologic changes that occur with burns are based on alteration of structure and function of the skin and the tissues beneath the skin and can impact other major body systems as well. The severity of the burn and the extent of physiologic changes depend on the depth of the tissue injury and the percentage of total body surface area (TBSA) involved.

Burns are classified according to depth of the burn to the skin and corresponding tissues and are further graded as minor, moderate, or major in severity. Superficial-thickness burns (first-degree burns) involve the destruction of the epidermis although physiologic functions remain intact. Partial-thickness burns (second-degree burns) destroy the epidermis and some (superficial) or all (deep) of the dermis. Refer to Figure 19-1.

The severity grading system adopted by the American Burn Association further grades partial-thickness burns as minor (if > 10% of TBSA), moderate (if > 10–20% of TBSA), or major (if > 20% of TBSA). Full-thickness burns are divided into third- and fourth-degree burns. Third-degree burns involve damage of the epidermis and dermis down to and including part of the subcutaneous tissue. Fourth-degree burns encompass all other depths discussed and include muscle tissue and may extend as far as the bone. Full-thickness burns also are further graded based on care requirements, with minor full-thickness burns "usually requiring outpatient care; may require 1- to 2-day admission, [moderate full-thickness burns needing] admission to hospital, preferably a hospital with expertise in burn care, [and major full-thickness burns requiring] admission to a burn center" (Hockenberry, 2005, p. 1131).

First-degree burns are very painful and are characterized by erythema. These burns heal spontaneously in approximately five to ten days without leaving scar tissue. Second-degree burns result in painful, reddened, moist skin that commonly forms

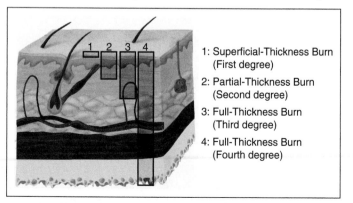

1: Superficial-Thickness Burn (First degree)

2: Partial-Thickness Burn (Second degree)

3: Full-Thickness Burn (Third degree)

4: Full-Thickness Burn (Fourth degree)

Figure 19-1: Depths of Burns. Courtesy of Dr. Robert Arensman, Chief Pediatric Surgery, Children's Memorial Medical Center, Chicago.

blisters that require two to three weeks to heal and may result in scarring depending on the depth of the dermal layer destroyed. Third-degree burns are not as painful as first- and second-degree burns because of cauterization of the nerves within the subcutaneous tissue. Eschar generally forms with this level of burn. Healing may require weeks to months and usually involves some level of skin grafting. Fourth-degree burns appear whitish, leathery, and dry with further reduction in sensation. Healing of these burns requires skin grafting that usually occurs in stages (Potts & Mandleco, 2007).

Full-thickness burns are considered major burns and result in systemic changes that may be life-threatening depending on the TBSA involved. Refer to Figure 19-2. Tissue injury stimulates the inflammatory response resulting in increased fluids being sent to the injury site. This increases the fluid loss because of the destruction to protective skin and tissue that usually control the external loss. The fluid loss leads to hypovolemia, the most cause of death during the first 24 hours following a major burn. In addition, the fluids being lost contain large volumes of plasma proteins that normally maintain vascular and interstitial osmotic pressure to maintain homeostasis in the fluid compartments. A cascade of systemic changes result.

Cardiovascular changes occurring in the first 24 to 48 hours following the burn event include increased capillary permeability and vasodilation resulting in hypovolemia and decreased cardiac output. This causes the cells to convert from aerobic to anaerobic

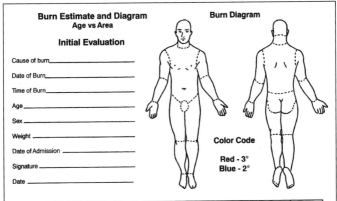

Burn Estimate and Diagram
Age vs Area

Initial Evaluation

Cause of burn_____

Date of Burn_____

Time of Burn_____

Age _____

Sex _____

Weight _____

Date of Admission _____

Signature _____

Date _____

Burn Diagram

Color Code

Red - 3°
Blue - 2°

Area	Birth 1 yr.	1-4 yrs.	5-9 yrs.	10-14 yrs.	15 yrs.	Adult	2°	3°	Total	Donor Areas
Head	19	17	13	11	9	7				
Neck	2	2	2	2	2	2				
Ant. Trunk	13	13	13	13	13	13				
Post. Trunk	13	13	13	13	13	13				
R. Buttock	2 1/2	2 1/2	2 1/2	2 1/2	2 1/2	2 1/2				
L. Buttock	2 1/2	2 1/2	2 1/2	2 1/2	2 1/2	2 1/2				
Genitalia	1	1	1	1	1	1				
R.U. Arm	4	4	4	4	4	4				
L.U. Arm	4	4	4	4	4	4				
R.L. Arm	3	3	3	3	3	3				
L.L. Arm	3	3	3	3	3	3				
R. Hand	2 1/2	2 1/2	2 1/2	2 1/2	2 1/2	2 1/2				
L. Hand	2 1/2	2 1/2	2 1/2	2 1/2	2 1/2	2 1/2				
R. Thigh	5 1/2	6 1/2	8	8 1/2	9	9 1/2				
L. Thigh	5 1/2	6 1/2	8	8 1/2	9	9 1/2				
R. Leg	5	5	5 1/2	6	6 1/2	7				
L. Leg	5	5	5 1/2	6	6 1/2	7				
R. Foot	3 1/2	3 1/2	3 1/2	3 1/2	3 1/2	3 1/2				
L. Foot	3 1/2	3 1/2	3 1/2	3 1/2	3 1/2	3 1/2				
						Total				

Figure 19-2: Estimation of TBSA Extent of Burns in Children. Courtesy of The Shriners Burn Hospital: Cincinnati, Ohio.

metabolism, which is not as efficient and produces increased levels of lactic acid leading to metabolic acidosis. The hypovolemia occurs because of fluid and blood loss causing the body's compensatory mechanisms to shift vascular volume away from the periphery, gastrointestinal system and the kidneys to increase the blood supply to the vital organs, the brain, heart, and lungs. As renal blood flow is shifted, urine output decreases and the risk of acute renal failure increases. The fluid shift away from the gastrointestinal tract leads to decreased peristalsis that presents the risk of paralytic ileus and the development of Curling's ulcers. The shift of blood supply from the integument results in the characteristic cool, clammy skin of the client experiencing shock. As the heart's workload increases to meet tissue perfusion needs, cardiac efficiency decreases resulting in risk of cardiac dysrhythmias and heart failure.

In addition to the cellular changes in metabolism that occur from burns, the metabolic rate of the client dramatically increases causing increased blood glucose levels (and losses) due to insulin resistance and the breakdown of glycogen as well as rapid protein breakdown and muscle wasting. Although the body temperature usually rises with increased metabolism, heat losses from the damaged skin are so great that hypothermia occurs.

With the loss of skin, the body's primary protection from infection, burn clients are at high risk for developing life-threatening infections and septicemia. Infection is the most common cause of death in burn victims after the first 48 hours following a major burn. Burn-related encephalopathy results from hypoxemia, hypovolemia, and septicemia.

Respiratory changes occurring in major burns include upper airway edema from inhalation of heated gases. This results in lower airway obstruction and pneumonia. Carbon monoxide poisoning and hypoxia from inhalation injuries cause edema and erythema of the mucous membranes. Restrictions of chest excursion from edema and eschar formation decrease lung vital capacity and gas exchange. The lungs' compensatory response to acid-base imbalances places increased demands on the respiratory system and leads to acute respiratory failure.

Complications

Hypovolemic or burn shock
Hypermetabolism
Metabolic acidosis
Fluid and electrolyte losses
Hyperglycemia
Life-threatening infections
Acute respiratory distress
Inhalation injuries
Multiple organ failure

Incidence

According to the data from the National Institute of General Medical Sciences of the National Institutes of Health, "[E]ach year in the United States, 1.1 million burn injuries require medical attention. Approximately 45,000 of these require hospitalization, and roughly half of those burn patients are admitted to a specialized burn unit. Each year, approximately 4,500 of these people die. Up to 10,000 people in the United States die every year of burn-related infections; pneumonia is the most common infectious complication among hospitalized burn patients" (National Institute of General Medical Sciences, 2006, p. 1). According to Sidor, Benson, Swartz, Desposito, and Lucchesi, children younger than 4 years of age account for 50% of all pediatric burn clients. Deaths from fires and burns are the second leading cause of death in children under 15 years of age (Sidor, Benson, Swartz, Desposito, & Lucchesi, 2006, Section 2). According to the American Burn Association, "Over one-third of admissions (38%) exceeded 10% TBSA, and 10% exceeded 30% TBSA. Most included severe burns of such vital body areas as the face, hands and feet" (American Burn Association, 2007, p. 1). Seventy percent of burn victims are male; 30% are female. Caucasians accounted for 62% of burn victims admitted to an acute care facility for treatment, 18% are African-American, and 12% are Hispanic (American Burn Association, 2007).

Etiology

Scalding injuries in children account for 85% of all burn injuries. These occur most commonly in toddlers. Flame burns are most prevalent in older children and adolescents, accounting for 13%. Chemical, electrical, and radiation burns compose the rest. Child abuse accounts for 16% of burns. (Potts & Mandleco, 2007). According to the American Burn Association, statistics related to burn causes indicate that 46% are due to contact with fire/flame, 32% due to scald injuries, 8% involve hot object contact, 4% are electrical burns, 3% are chemical burns, and 6% are classified as "other." Forty-three percent of burn injuries occur in the home (American Burn Association, 2007).

Clinical Manifestations

Dependent on the severity of the burn

SUPERFICIAL (FIRST-DEGREE)

Erythema

Hypersensitivity (pain)

PARTIAL-THICKNESS (SECOND-DEGREE)

Superficial—moist, weepy pink or red blisters; blanching;
  hypersensitivity

Deep-pale, decreased moistness, prolonged and absent blanching;
  decreased sensation

FULL-THICKNESS (THIRD-DEGREE)

Pale, mottled, brown

Dry, leathery appearance

Visible thrombosed vessels

No sensation

Eschar

FULL-THICKNESS (FOURTH-DEGREE)

Dry and charred

Mottled brown, red, or white

Impaired movement of extremity or digit

No sensation

Diagnostic Tests

Primary mode of diagnosis is visual assessment of wounds.

Carboxyhemoglobin level

Arterial blood gases

Pulse oximetry

Serial chest radiography

Culture and sensitivity studies of wound

Urinalysis and culture and sensitivity

Complete blood count

Serum electrolyte levels

Laryngoscopy

Bronchoscopy

(Broyles, 2005)

Medical Management

The goals of medical management are to regain and maintain homeostasis by sustaining a patent airway, adequate gas exchange, hemodynamics, and acid-base and fluid and electrolyte balance. The American Burn Association recommends that all victims of third- (and fourth-) degree burns; electrical burns; chemical burns; inhalation injuries; burns on the face, hands, feet, genitalia, or major joints; burned children being treated in hospitals without qualified personnel or equipment specific to pediatric care; burn injury clients that require long-term rehabilitative care; and those with second-degree burns covering more than 10% TBSA be transported to a burn center or a hospital with a burn unit (American Burn Association, 2007).

The ABC (airway, breathing, and circulation) needs are addressed first. In major burns, this usually requires a minimum of oxygen therapy and possibly intubation and mechanical ventilation as well as rapid fluid resuscitation. Establishment of an intravenous access may be a special challenge in the victim of major burns because of the lack of peripheral vessels. A central venous access device is preferred because of the multiple uses this vascular access will serve including fluid resuscitation, medication administration, and parenteral nutrition. In the event of carbon monoxide inhalation, 100% oxygen is administered. Any burned clothing still present on the victim must be removed to prevent further tissue damage from the heat retained in the clothing. Also, a part of the initial treatment of a major burn victim is covering him/her with sterile sheets to reduce further fluid loss through evaporation.

Intravenous fluids are administered to restore and maintain urine output of 1–2 mL/kg/hour. Lactated Ringer's solution is the volume expander of choice not only because it rapidly replaces fluids but also because the lactate ions convert to bicarbonate to help treat the metabolic acidosis. An arterial line is placed to monitor acid-base balance by assessing arterial blood gases. The Parkland formula for fluid resuscitation is a standard used with children and describes the first 24-hour fluid resuscitation. This formula is applied as follows: 4 mL Lactated Ringer's solution multiplied by kilogram of body weight multiplied by the percentage of TBSA burned. One-half of the total volume is administered in the first 8 hours following the burn (not from the time of admission to the health care facility, but from the time of the injury); one-fourth of the total is administered in the second 8 hours postburn; and one-fourth of the total is administered during the third 8 hours postburn (Broyles, 2005).

Central venous pressure monitoring is necessary as well as other forms of hemodynamic monitoring. Continuous cardiorespiratory monitoring and pulse oximetry are needed as well as assessment of breath and heart sounds. Respiratory management may further include an incision into the eschar (escharotomy) to "restore peripheral blood circulation . . . and release chest constriction" (Potts & Mandleco, 2007, p. 609).

After initial fluid resuscitation is performed, blood product replacement may be needed. Children must be closely monitored for both transfusion reactions and fluid overload during the transfusion process. Frequently, acetaminophen and diphenhydramine are used as premedications for transfusions in children.

Monitoring bowel sounds, assessing liver enzymes, and placing a nasogastric tube for gastric decompression and assessment of gastric juices for blood provide means of assessing and treating loss of gastric motility and the possible development of Curling's ulcers. In addition, proton pump inhibitors and histamine (H_2) antagonists are used to maintain gastric pH and help prevent Curling's ulcers.

Because of the state of hypermetabolism, the burn client requires 2–3 times the normal calorie intake. This usually is achieved through administration of total parenteral nutrition via a central venous access device. Close monitoring for manifestations of infection is critical not only because the burn injuries pose this risk but also because the major complication of central venous accesses and the use of total parenteral nutrition is infection.

Pain management is critical for the burn victim. The victim already is experiencing a hypermetabolic state, and pain increases metabolism and energy demands. Further, pain increases intracranial pressure. Continuous intravenous infusion of morphine sulfate is the standard of care for pain management.

Wound care is initiated by covering the victim with a sterile sheet. Maintaining strict asepsis in wound care is critical. Eschar is incised or removed to provide circulation to the wound. As healing progresses, regular debridement is performed through surgery or hydrotherapy or is performed pharmacologically. Debriding drugs "promote the removal of dead skin at the site of skin damage . . . [and are] of particular importance in the treatment of second- and third-degree burns . . ." (Broyles, Reiss, & Evans, 2007, p. 1020). Silver sulfadiazine is applied to all open wounds to help prevent infection. "As blood supply to the burned area may be impaired, topical anti-infective [agents] may represent the only possible source of therapy to prevent infection at the burn site" (Broyles et al., 2007, p. 1022). Intravenous antimicrobial agents are used prophylactically and are used for the treatment of any diagnosed infection.

The recovery process involves skin grafting and physical therapy. Skin grafting is performed in stages and usually is a long-term process. Physical therapy is needed to prevent muscle atrophy as well as to restore and maintain joint mobility. It also serves to facilitate graft healing.

Rehabilitation following major burns is a long, tedious, and painful process for the victim as well as the parents or caregivers of the child. This process may take months and years, and emotional as well as physical scars usually remain. In situations where burn injuries occurred as a result of a house fire or an automobile accident, the child may have lost one or both parents in addition to enduring the burn injuries and prolonged physical recovery process.

Nursing Management

ASSESSMENT

1. Assess airway immediately
2. Assess breathing and circulation
3. Obtain baseline hemodynamic data
4. Assess wounds and the presence of eschar
5. Perform psychosocial assessment of child and parents/caregivers

NURSING DIAGNOSES (INCLUDING BUT NOT LIMITED TO)

1. Ineffective airway clearance and impaired gas exchange R/T upper airway edema, pulmonary injury secondary to inhalation, carbon dioxide poisoning, and hypoxia
2. Altered tissue perfusion R/T hypovolemic state
3. Deficient fluid volume R/T fluid loss
4. Risk for infection R/T impaired skin and tissue integrity and prolonged use of invasive therapies
5. Acute pain R/T tissue injury and related treatment procedures
6. Imbalanced nutrition: less than body requirements R/T hypermetabolic state, inability to consume oral nutrition, and increased demands for healing
7. Disturbed body image R/T disfigurement from burns and skin grafting
8. Ineffective individual/family coping R/T child's injuries and long-term rehabilitation
9. Delayed growth and development R/T burn injuries, long-term rehabilitation, and alterations in family processes

10. Deficient knowledge R/T child's condition, medical regimen, growth and development needs, long-term rehabilitation needs, and home care

PLANNING/GOALS

1. Client will experience patent airway within 1–5 minutes following burn injury. Client will regain adequate gas exchange within 30 minutes following initiation of therapy as evidenced by spontaneous respirations, clear breath sounds, arterial blood gases within defined limits (WDL), and oxygen saturation within prescribed parameters.

2. Client will regain and maintain adequate tissue perfusion as evidenced by urine output of 1–2 mL/kg/hr within 24 hours following burn injury, return of bowel sounds with 48–72 hours postburn, maintenance of mean arterial pressure within prescribed parameters, vital signs WDL, and neurologic status WDL.

3. Client will regain and maintain adequate fluid volume as evidenced by urine output of 1–2 mL/kg/hr.

4. Client will experience burn wound healing without manifestations of infection; however, if infection occurs, it will be promptly identified and effectively treated.

5. Client will demonstrate pain level of 1–2 on an age-appropriate pain scale, vital signs WDL, and by absence of nonverbal pain indicators.

6. Client will regain and maintain adequate nutritional intake as evidenced by stable weight, balanced nitrogen state, serum albumin WDL, and evidence of wound healing within reasonable timeframe considering extent of burn injury.

7. Client/parents will demonstrate recovery of positive body image.

8. Client/parents will demonstrate effective coping strategies as evidenced by decrease in manifestations of anxiety and guilt and through participation in child's care.

9. Client will regain and maintain highest level of growth and development within the constraints of burn injuries.

10. Parents will demonstrate understanding of child's ongoing condition, medical regimen, long-term rehabilitation needs, growth and development needs, and home care.

NOC

1. Respiratory Status: Gas Exchange/Airway Patency
2. Tissue Perfusion: Cardiopulmonary, Tissue Perfusion: Peripheral
3. Fluid Balance
4. Risk Control
5. Pain Control
6. Nutritional Status
7. Body Image
8. Coping
9. Child Development
10. Knowledge: Illness Care, Health Promotion, Infection Control, Treatment Regimen

IMPLEMENTATION

1. Airway/Gas exchange
   a. Monitor respiratory status continuously during critical period
   b. Assess breath sounds hourly

    c.   Monitor arterial blood gases, pulse oximetry, and carboxyhemoglobin levels

    d.   Place on hemodynamic monitoring

    e.   Assist with intubation and maintain mechanical ventilation as prescribed

    f.   Administer humidified oxygen to maintain oxygen saturation within prescribed parameters

    g.   Elevate head of bed

    h.   Perform endotracheal, tracheal, and nasopharyngeal suctioning as needed

    i.   Administer chest physiotherapy within constraints of client's wounds

    j.   Encourage turning, coughing, and deep breathing when not receiving mechanical ventilation assistance

    k.   Administer medications as prescribed

2. Tissue perfusion

    a.   Place on continuous hemodynamic monitoring

    b.   Maintain patency of intravenous access device, monitoring hourly

    c.   Administer intravenous fluid resuscitation as prescribed

    d.   Maintain strict intake and output

    e.   Weigh daily

    f.   Monitor urine specific gravity

    g.   Monitor complete blood count results

    h.   Monitor for electrolyte imbalances

    i.   Monitor neurologic status hourly

    j.   Premedicate as prescribed prior to transfusion of blood products

    k.   Administer blood products as prescribed according to facility protocol

    l.   Monitor peripheral pulses hourly

    m. Monitor skin temperature and hydration

3. Fluid volume

    a.   Maintain continuous hemodynamic monitoring

    b.   Maintain patency of intravenous access device, monitoring at least hourly

    c.   Administer fluid therapy as prescribed

    d.   Monitor hourly urine output

    e.   Monitor central venous pressure as prescribed

    f.   Weigh daily

    g.   Monitor hemoglobin, hematocrit, and serum electrolytes

    h.   Monitor for manifestations of electrolyte imbalances

    i.   Monitor breath sounds for signs of fluid overload

    j.   Monitor neurologic status

    k.   If fluid volume excess occurs in the form of increased intracranial pressure, health care provided should be consulted concerning initiation of mannitol.

4. Risk for infection

    a.   Monitor vital signs

    b.   Place skin probe for continuous temperature monitoring

    c.   Shave hair within 5 cm of burn margins

    d. Assess wound drainage with each dressing change

    e. Culture if purulent or malodorous drainage is noted

    f. Document use of antimicrobials when sending cultures to be analyzed

    g. Perform meticulous hand washing and maintain compromised host precautions

    h. Maintain asepsis during dressing changes

    i. Apply topical antimicrobials

    j. Maintain patency of intravenous access device, monitoring at least hourly

    k. Administer intravenous antimicrobials as prescribed

    l. Identify indications for discontinuing use of invasive lines and procedures

    m. Turn, cough, and deep-breathe client every 2 hours

    n. Assess appearance of skin graft site

    o. Monitor graft donor site for signs of infection

    p. Assess for clinical manifestations of sepsis

    q. Administer antipyretics as prescribed

5. Acute pain

    a. Assess pain level hourly using age-appropriate pain assessment scale

    b. Maintain patency of intravenous access device, monitoring at least hourly

    c. Maintain continuous infusion of opioid analgesics

    d. Administer prescribed analgesics for break-through pain

    e. Explain all procedures and equipment to child and parents

    f. Encourage parents to visit child and assist in child's care (if they are comfortable with this)

    g. Minimize time of wound exposure and manipulation

    h. Premedicate prior to hydrotherapy or application of debriding agents

    i. Perform passive range-of-motion exercises two or three times per day

    j. Administer anxiolytics as prescribed and indicated

    k. Provide for uninterrupted sleep when possible

6. Nutrition

    a. Monitor intake and output

    b. Weigh daily

    c. Monitor serum albumin, blood urea nitrogen, thyroxine-binding prealbumin, and retinal-binding protein

    d. Maintain hemodynamic monitoring

    e. Monitor for manifestations of protein deficiency

    f. Provide high-calorie, high-carbohydrate, high-protein diet as prescribed

    g. Maintain patency of central venous access device, monitoring hourly

    h. Administer total parenteral nutrition as prescribed and as facility protocol dictates

    i. Schedule procedures so they do not occur immediately before or after meals

    j. Assess for constipation and diarrhea
    k. Administer medications as prescribed
    l. Encourage parents to visit during mealtimes when possible
    m. Administer supplemental tube feedings as prescribed as recovery progresses
7. Body image
    a. Encourage child (if age-appropriate) and parents to verbalize feelings
    b. Answer questions honestly within scope of practice
    c. Refer questions as appropriate to health care provider
    d. Explain all equipment and procedures
    e. Assist in expressing spiritual needs and make referrals consistent with family's expressed needs
    f. Participate in multidisciplinary team planning for client care
    g. Provide information regarding use of cosmetics and clothing to conceal burn areas
    h. Provide information about support groups for child and family
    i. Provide information concerning American Burn Association, National Headquarters Office, 625 N. Michigan Avenue, Suite 1530, Chicago, IL 60611
    j. Provide encouragement for use of compression netting to skin graft and burn sites
8. Coping
    a. Encourage child (if age-appropriate) and family to express concerns and feelings
    b. Provide support for family as members move through grief and guilt process
    c. Discuss with family the coping strategies previously used in times of stress
    d. Discuss use of relaxation techniques
    e. Coordinate multidisciplinary team approach to care
    f. Provide information concerning support services available
    g. Provide for family spiritual needs
    h. Discuss use of diversion and guided imagery techniques
9. Growth and development
    a. Assess child's current level of growth and development
    b. Address child consistent with growth and development communication level
    c. Be aware of child's overwhelming fear of mutilation if child is a preschooler
    d. Provide play activities within constraints of child's condition that foster growth and development
    e. Provide growth and development information to family, discussing the importance of meeting these needs for their child
    f. Serve as role model for family when caring for child
    g. Provide child contact with other children with similar growth and development needs if possible
10. Client/parent teaching
    a. Assess family's level of understanding in preparation for child's discharge

   b. Provide verbal and written information regarding:

     1) Care of burn wounds

     2) Medication administration as appropriate

     3) Use and importance of burn garments

     4) Infection protection

     5) Community and national support services including respite care

     6) Importance of follow-up care with health care provider

     7) Contact information for health care provider and referral support providers

   c. Provide adequate time for teaching and needed return demonstrations of skills necessary to care for child

   d. Document teaching and family members' responses

NIC

1. Airway Management, Respiratory Monitoring, Acid-Base Management, Oxygen Therapy, Ventilation Assistance
2. Acid-Base Management, Hemodynamic Regulation, Shock Management
3. Fluid/Electrolyte Management
4. Infection Protection
5. Pain Management
6. Nutrition Management, Fluid/Electrolyte Management
7. Body Image Enhancement
8. Coping Enhancement
9. Developmental Enhancement: Child
10. Teaching: Treatment, Illness Care, Infection Control, Health Promotion

EVALUATION

1. Client experiences patent airway within 1–5 minutes following burn injury. Client regains adequate gas exchange within 30 minutes following initiation of therapy as evidenced by spontaneous respirations, clear breath sounds, arterial blood gases WDL, and oxygen saturation within prescribed parameters.
2. Client regains and maintains adequate tissue perfusion as evidenced by urine output of 1–2 mL/kg/hr within 24 hours following burn injury, return of bowel sounds with 48–72 hours postburn, maintenance of mean arterial pressure within prescribed parameters, vital signs WDL, and neurologic status WDL.
3. Client regains and maintains adequate fluid volume as evidenced by urine output of 1–2 mL/kg/hr.
4. Client experiences burn wound healing without manifestations of infection; however, if infection occurs, it will be promptly identified and effectively treated.
5. Client demonstrates pain level of 1–2 on an age-appropriate pain scale, vital signs WDL, and by absence of nonverbal pain indicators.
6. Client regains and maintains adequate nutritional intake as evidenced by stable weight, balanced nitrogen state, serum albumin WDL, and evidence of wound healing within reasonable timeframe considering extent of burn injury.

7. Client/parents demonstrate recovery of positive body image.

8. Client/parents demonstrate effective coping strategies as evidenced by decrease in manifestations of anxiety and guilt and through participation in child's care.

9. Client regains and maintains highest level of growth and development within the constraints of burn injuries.

10. Parents demonstrate understanding of child's ongoing condition, medical regimen, long-term rehabilitation needs, growth and development needs, and home care.

References

American Burn Association. (2007). *Burn incidence and treatment in the US: 2007 fact sheet.* Retrieved April 23, 2007, from http://www.ameriburn.org/resources_factsheet.php

Broyles, B. E. (2005). *Medical-surgical nursing clinical companion.* Durham, NC: Carolina Academic Press.

Broyles, B. E., Reiss, B. S., & Evans, M. E. (2007). *Pharmacological aspects of nursing care* (7th ed.). Clifton Park, NY: Delmar Cengage Learning.

Hockenberry, M. J. (2005). *Wong's essentials of pediatric nursing* (7th ed.). St. Louis, MO: Mosby Elsevier.

National Institute of General Medical Sciences. (2006). *Fact sheet: Trauma, shock, burn, and injury: Facts and figures.* Retrieved April 23, 2007, from http://www.nigms.nih.gov/Publications/trauma_burn_facts.htm

Potts, N. L., & Mandleco, B. L. (2007). *Pediatric nursing: Caring for children and their families* (2nd ed.). Clifton Park, NY: Delmar Cengage Learning.

Sidor, M. I., Benson, B. E., Swartz, R. A., Desposito, F., & Lucchesi, M. (2006). *Thermal burns.* Retrieved April 23, 2007, from http://www.emedicine.com/ped/topic301.htm

20

CELIAC DISEASE

Definition

Celiac disease, also called gluten-sensitive enteropathy is a lifelong autoimmune genetic gastrointestinal malabsorption disorder. It is believed to result from an autoimmune response triggered by a permanent intolerance to gluten, a component of the breakdown of the protein portion of wheat, barley, rye, triticale, and oats.

Pathophysiology

Gluten is comprised of two protein components, glutenin and gliadin. In celiac disease, the gastrointestinal tract is unable to digest gliadin and the gliadin acts as an antigen causing an immune response that leads to inflammation of and damage to the fingerlike projections in the small intestines (Potts & Mandleco, 2007). These fingerlike projections called villa function to move digestive products along the small intestines and absorb nutrients through the intestinal wall. The inflammatory response in celiac disease causes the villa to flatten out and atrophy, leading to a decrease in the absorptive surface of the intestines. Because the chemical digestion of fats begins in the duodenum, fats are the first nutrients affected by this malabsorption, followed by fat-soluble vitamins and proteins. Carbohydrates are the last macronutrient to be malabsorbed because carbohydrates have experienced chemical digestion in the mouth and in the stomach; as a result, their nutrient components are more easily absorbed even on a limited surface area. Eventually, the absorption of all macronutrients is impaired. When not absorbed, the nutrients pass quickly through the digestive tract resulting in diarrhea, dehydration, anemia, and metabolic acidosis from loss of electrolytes. "Celiac disease is second only to cystic fibrosis as a cause of malabsorption in children" (Hockenberry, 2005, p. 885) and is a leading cause of organic or physiological failure to thrive.

Complications

Diarrhea
Electrolyte imbalances
Dehydration
Anemia
Metabolic acidosis
Failure to thrive

> NOTE: The Celiac Disease Foundation has identified additional long-term conditions that can result from untreated celiac disease. These conditions include osteoporosis, vitamin deficiencies, iron deficiency anemia, central and peripheral nerve disorders, pancreatic insufficiency, intestinal lymphomas and other gastrointestinal cancers, and lactose intolerance (Celiac Disease Foundation, 2007).

Incidence

According to the National Institute on Diabetes and Digestive and Kidney Disorders of the National Institutes of Health, the data concerning the incidence of celiac disease is "spotty"; however, the disease appears to affect European populations (in Italy, about

1 in 250 people and in Ireland about 1 in 300 people) more than populations in the United States (0.1 in 1,000 births). The incidence is believed to coincide with the introduction of gluten-containing foods (National Institute of Diabetes and Digestive and Kidney Diseases, 2007).

Etiology

Celiac disease is a genetic disorder. Breast-feeding infants delays the onset of symptoms of celiac disease and may minimize long-term gastrointestinal effects. The manifestations of celiac disease usually are not seen until 3–6 months following the introduction of grains into the infant's diet.

Clinical Manifestations

Diarrhea
Steatorrhea
Decreased urine output
Irritability
Apathy
Abdominal distention
Malnutrition (infant who is in 25th percentile for growth)
Anemia
Anorexia

Diagnostic Tests

Serum assay for the presence of antigliadin, antireticulin, and antiendomysial IgG and IgA antibodies
Intestinal biopsy
Breath hydrogen excretion tests
Enzyme tissue transglutaminase

Medical Management

The goal of medical management of celiac disease is to restore and maintain a homeostatic nutritional state, which is accomplished primarily by diet. Because dehydration is potentially life-threatening in children, immediate treatment is to provide intravenous fluid resuscitation, manage acidosis, and administer corticosteroids to decrease intestinal inflammation. Once homeostasis has been established, the lifelong management of celiac disease begins.

The diet prescribed is low in glutens even though it is usually referred to as gluten free. The primary sources of gluten are wheat, rye, barley, and oats and these are removed from the diet. Corn and rice are used as substitute grain sources. Processed foods must be consumed with caution because the gluten-containing grains frequently are used in these foods. Although celiac disease is considered to be a chronic condition, strict adherence to the prescribed diet usually minimizes exacerbations and prevents the most serious long-term effect—lymphoma.

Nursing Management

ASSESSMENT

1. Obtain history
2. Assess for manifestations of dehydration and acid-base imbalance requiring emergency care
3. Assess height and weight and plot on standardized growth chart
4. Perform physical assessment
5. Assess laboratory studies

Nursing Diagnoses (including but not limited to)

1. Imbalanced nutrition: less than body requirements R/T malabsorption
2. Deficient fluid volume (for child in celiac crisis) R/T diarrhea and malabsorption
3. Delayed growth and development R/T malabsorption
4. Deficient knowledge R/T child's condition, dietary management, and home care

Planning/Goals

1. Client will demonstrate weight gain and building of muscle mass as evidenced by achieving 50th percentile on standardized growth chart and anthropometric measurements.
2. Client will demonstrate fluid and electrolyte balance as evidenced by skin turgor, mucous membrane moistness, and urine output within defined limits (WDL).
3. Client will demonstrate characteristics of growth and development consistent with age.
4. Parents will demonstrate understanding of child's condition, dietary management, and home care.

NOC

1. Nutritional Status: Nutrient Intake
2. Electrolyte and Acid/Base Balance, Fluid Balance
3. Child Development
4. Knowledge: Disease Process, Diet, Health Promotion

Implementation

1. Nutrition
   a. Assess child's growth and compare to standardized growth chart
   b. Assess child's food preferences
   c. Provide age-appropriate eating environment
   d. Collaborate with dietician to provide foods low in gluten
   e. Institute gluten-free diet, providing appropriate instructions to parents
   f. Weigh daily
2. Fluid volume (for child in celiac crisis)
   a. Initiate and maintain patency of intravenous access device, monitoring hourly
   b. Administer intravenous fluids as prescribed
   c. Encourage oral fluids as tolerated
   d. Monitor acid-base balance
   e. Monitor serum electrolytes
   f. Monitor strict intake and output
   g. Monitor urine specific gravity
3. Growth and development
   a. Assess child's current level of growth and development
   b. Provide gluten-free diet
   c. Encourage participation in age-appropriate play activities
   d. Provide information to parents to foster child's growth and development

    4. Parent teaching

      a. Assess parents' current level of understanding of condition and treatment regimen

      b. Provide verbal and written information regarding:

        1) Celiac Disease Foundation

        2) Lifelong dietary avoidance of foods containing gluten

        3) Fostering of child's growth and development

        4) Other discharge instructions from health care provider

        5) Importance of follow-up with health care provider

        6) Contact information to maintain follow-up care and changes in child's condition

      c. Provide adequate time for teaching

      d. Document teaching and parental response

NIC

    1. Nutrition Management, Nutrition Monitoring

    2. Acid-Base Management, Fluid/Electrolyte Management, Fluid Monitoring

    3. Child Development Enhancement

    4. Teaching: Disease Process, Diet, Health Promotion

EVALUATION

    1. Client demonstrates weight gain and building of muscle mass as evidenced by achieving 50th percentile on standardized growth chart and anthropometric measurements.

    2. Client demonstrates fluid and electrolyte balance as evidenced by skin turgor, mucous membrane moistness, and urine output WDL.

    3. Client demonstrates characteristics of growth and development consistent with age.

    4. Parents demonstrate understanding of child's condition, dietary management, and home care.

References

Celiac Disease Foundation. (2007). *Celiac disease information.* Retrieved April 23, 2007, from http://www.celiac.org/cd-what.php

Hockenberry, M. J. (2005). *Wong's essentials of pediatric nursing* (7th ed.). St. Louis, MO: Mosby Elsevier.

National Institute of Diabetes and Digestive and Kidney Diseases. (2007). *Celiac disease.* Retrieved April 23, 2007, from http://digestive.niddk.nih.gov/ddiseases/pubs/celiac

Potts, N. L., & Mandleco, B. L. (2007). *Pediatric nursing: Caring for children and their families* (2nd ed.). Clifton Park, NY: Delmar Cengage Learning.

21

CEREBRAL PALSY (CP)

Definition

Cerebral palsy (CP) is a chronic, nonprogressive neurologic disorder resulting from insult (interruption in cerebral tissue perfusion) to the pyramidal motor system (motor cortex, basal ganglia, and cerebellum).

Pathophysiology

When the brain is deprived of oxygen, neurons die and their function is lost. Because of the damage to the motor cortex, the injury manifests itself as abnormal control of body movement and coordination of voluntary muscles (National Institute of Neurological Disorders and Stroke, 2007). As a result of neuron damage, approximately 50% of children with CP have concurrent cognitive impairment. Children with CP experience frequent respiratory infections due to lack of activity or aspiration secondary to gastroesophageal reflux disease, a common concurrent problem. Other dysfunctions that frequently accompany CP are visual and hearing impairments and seizures. United Cerebral Palsy (UPC) identifies different types or classifications of CP based on the manifestations of the disorder (United Cerebral Palsy, 2007).

Spastic CP is most common, affecting 70–80% of individuals. It is characterized by a period of hypotonia in the young infant and progresses to muscles that are stiff and eventually to permanently contracted muscles. This type is further classified according to the number of limbs affected (diplegia, triplegia, quadriplegia, or left or right hemiparesis).

Athetoid (dyskinetic) CP affects approximately 10–20% of individuals with CP and is characterized by "controlled, slow, writhing movements" (United Cerebral Palsy, 2007, p. 1). The parts of the body involved in these movements include the head, arms, legs, feet, and sometimes the face and tongue. When the face and tongue are affected, the client manifests drooling and grimacing. The movements increase when the infant/child is upset or stressed; movements decrease or disappear during sleep. Some clients experience lack of coordination of the muscles needed for speech (dysarthria).

Ataxic CP is a rare form (affecting 5–10% of individuals with CP) that affects the sense of balance and depth perception. To compensate for their poor coordination, these individuals walk with a wide-based gait, placing their feet unusually far apart. These individuals experience difficulty with precise movements such as writing and buttoning a shirt and frequently have what is termed intention tremors. These tremors begin when the individual attempts to reach for an object, causing a trembling of the limb being used. The trembling worsens as the individual gets closer to the object.

Finally, some individuals experience mixed forms of CP, exhibiting manifestations of more than one of the preceding three types. Although a combined spastic and athetoid type is most common, other combinations of the condition may occur (United Cerebral Palsy, 2007).

Complications

Contractures
Frequent respiratory infections
Cognitive impairment
Self-care deficits

Incidence

According to UCP, "It is estimated that some 764,000 children and adults in the United States manifest one or more of the symptoms of cerebral palsy. Currently, about 8,000 babies and infants are diagnosed with the condition each year. In addition, some 1,200–1,500 preschool age children are recognized each year to have cerebral palsy" (United Cerebral Palsy, 2007, p. 1).

This incidence translates into an "estimated 7 [cases] per 1,000 live births" (Potts & Mandleco, 2007, p. 1102). Low-birth-weight infants are at high risk for CP; and because more of these infants are surviving now, the rate of CP is increasing rather than decreasing (Potts & Mandleco, 2007).

Etiology

The causes of CP can be classified according to the time the insult to the brain occurs: prenatal, perinatal, or postnatal. Prenatal causes include maternal toxemia, maternal preeclampsia, exposure to toxic agents, genetics, blood Rh and type incompatibilities, intrauterine ischemia, toxoplasmosis, cytomegalovirus, rubella, and congenital brain malformations. Perinatal causes, or those occurring during the birthing process, include breech presentation, umbilical cord around the fetus's neck resulting in anoxia, low birth weight, asphyxia, precipitous delivery, birth trauma, intracranial bleeding, abruptio placenta, and placenta previa. CP can occur following the infant's birth resulting from shaken-baby syndrome, infections (bacterial meningitis or encephalitis), head injuries secondary to motor vehicle accidents or falls, and cerebrovascular accident (Potts & Mandleco, 2007).

Clinical Manifestations

Most frequent manifestation occurs before the child is 18 months old
and is not reaching expected gross motor developmental milestones
Lack of muscle coordination (ataxia)
Stiff or tight muscles
Exaggerated reflexes (spasticity)
Tendency to drag one foot or leg when walking
Tendency to walk on the toes
Crouched gait (National Institute of Neurological Disorders
and Stroke, 2007)
Hypotonia
Dyskinetic movements
Hemiplegia
Diplegia
Quadriplegia

Diagnostic Tests

Testing of infant's/toddler's gross motor skills
Reflexes
Computed tomography
Ultrasonography
Electroencephalogram
Magnetic resonance imaging

Medical Management

The goals of management are early detection and intervention to optimize the child's growth and development and to prevent complications secondary to inactivity. According to the National Institute of Neurological Disorders and Stroke, "Treatment may include physical and occupational therapy, speech therapy, and drugs to control seizures, relax muscle spasms, and alleviate pain; surgery to correct anatomical abnormalities or release tight muscles; braces and other orthotic devices; wheelchairs and rolling walkers; and communication aids such as computers with attached voice synthesizers" (National Institute of Neurological Disorders and Stroke, 2007, p. 1). Frequently, these children require alternative methods for obtaining nutrition, such as gastrostomy tubes. Seldom is parenteral nutrition required because the smooth muscle in the gastrointestinal tract is not affected directly by CP. Because of inactivity, pharmacological agents (kinetic agents and proton pump inhibitors or histamine 2 antagonists) may be required to assist with nutrition (Broyles, Reiss, & Evans, 2007).

A surgical intervention called a selective dorsal root rhizotomy, a procedure to sever nerves that are overactive and to provide reduction of muscles spasms or improvement of muscle tone, may be used. Cerebellar stimulation with the use of electrodes and stereotaxic thalamotomy are other symptomatic therapies.

As the child grows into adulthood, he/she may require support services such as "personal assistance services, continuing therapy, educational and vocational training, independent living services, counseling, transportation, recreation/leisure programs, and employment opportunities, all essential to the developing adult" (United Cerebral Palsy, 2007, p. 1).

Nursing Management

ASSESSMENT

1. Identify children at risk
2. Obtain history
3. Assess child's level of growth and development using standardized milestones
4. Assess for manifestations of CP
5. Assess alternative feeding methods used by parents
6. Obtain information about any assistive devices currently in use

NURSING DIAGNOSES (INCLUDING BUT NOT LIMITED TO)

1. Risk for injury R/T spastic movements, falls, and seizures
2. Impaired physical mobility R/T muscle spasms, hypotonicity
3. Imbalanced nutrition: less than body requirements R/T difficulty chewing and swallowing and decreased activity
4. Impaired verbal communication R/T neuromuscular impairment and difficulty with articulation
5. Delayed growth and development R/T neuromuscular dysfunction
6. Risk for infection R/T inactivity and risk for aspiration
7. Anxiety (parental) related to uncertainty of child's condition and future
8. Risk for caregiver role strain R/T having a child with complex needs
9. Deficient knowledge R/T child's complex needs, support services, medical management, and home care

PLANNING/GOALS

1. Client will remain free of injury.
2. Client will retain maximum ability of movement.
3. Client will achieve adequate nutrition for metabolic needs for growth and development as evidenced by nutritional intake, weight, and height within defined limits (WDL) within constraints of condition.

4. Client will express needs effectively through use of assistive devices.
5. Client will achieve highest level of growth and development as evidenced by achievement of milestones within constraints of condition.
6. Client will not experience infection or aspiration.
7. Parents will express feelings and concerns and demonstrate manifestations of decreased anxiety.
8. Parents (caregivers) will maintain emotional and physical health while providing care for child.
9. Parents will demonstrate understanding of child's complex needs, medical management, and home care and utilize available support services.

NOC

1. Risk Control, Safe Home Environment, Sensory Function Status
2. Coordinated Movement, Joint Movement
3. Nutritional Status: Food and Fluid Intake
4. Communication
5. Child Development
6. Risk Control
7. Anxiety
8. Caregiver Well-Being
9. Knowledge: Illness Care, Infection Control, Diet, Treatment Regimen, Health Resources

IMPLEMENTATION

1. Risk for injury
   a. Assess for potential injury risks
   b. Pad crib or bed rails
   c. Reposition every 2 hours
   d. Keep side rails of crib or bed in up position
   e. Assess caregiver's ability to provide safe care and prevent injury
   f. Position on right side after feedings to prevent aspiration injury
   g. Assist caregiver in problem solving regarding delegation of child's care to other family members
   h. Document caregiver interactions with child
2. Physical mobility
   a. Assess physical abilities
   b. Provide play activities within child's physical and growth and development abilities
   c. Turn every 2 hours if confined to bed
   d. Position for comfort and maintenance of alignment
   e. Provide passive range-of-motion exercises
   f. Collaborate with health care provider and physical therapist for exercise regimen
3. Nutrition
   a. Assess alternative feeding methods currently used
   b. Monitor intake and output
   c. Weigh daily
   d. Encourage caregiver to continue feeding schedule from home

    e. Evaluate caregiver's techniques of feeding or provide enteral nutrition

    f. Provide enteral tube care

    g. Administer medications as prescribed to maximize nutrition

    h. Elevate head of bed during enteral feedings

    i. Position on right side following feedings to facilitate stomach emptying

    j. Use pacifier to maintain infant's suck reflex if infant is not receiving oral feedings

4. Verbal communication

    a. Assess child's current level of communication

    b. Collaborate with caregiver to help communicate with child

    c. Collaborate with health care provider for referral for speech or occupational therapy

    d. Use nonverbal communication when possible to communicate caring affect

    e. Assess nonverbal cues to help meet child's needs

5. Growth and development

    a. Assess child's current level of growth and development

    b. Provide parents with information on age-appropriate play activities

    c. Plot weight and height on growth chart, comparing to standardized chart

    d. Encourage child's participation in age-appropriate activities as child's energy level allows

6. Risk for infection

    a. Assess breath sounds

    b. Monitor vital signs

    c. Assess gastric residual prior to initiating enteral feeding

    d. Administer enteral feedings slowly, preferably continuous versus bolus feedings

    e. Elevate head of bed during feedings

    f. Position on right side following feeding

7. Anxiety (parental)

    a. Assess for parental behaviors that indicate anxiety

    b. Facilitate parental expression of feelings and concerns

    c. Encourage parents to participate in child's care

    d. Facilitate parents in decision making concerning child's care

    e. Provide parents/caregivers with information about CP, support groups, and support services provided by community

8. Caregiver role strain

    a. Assess for indications of caregiver strain

    b. Encourage caregiver to express feelings and concerns

    c. Listen actively

    d. Provide information about community resources, respite care, and support groups

    e. Involve caregiver in child's care during hospitalization, considering needs of caregiver/child

    f. Involve caregiver in decision making concerning child's care

    g. Assist caregiver in problem solving regarding delegation of child's care to other family members

    h. Document caregiver's interactions with child

9. Parent/client teaching

    a. Assess parental level of understanding of complex care needs of child

    b. Provide verbal and written information regarding:

      1) Enteral feedings

      2) Prevention of aspiration

      3) Referral information

      4) Instruction review concerning assistive devices

      5) Community support services, national organizations, and respite care

      6) Physical therapy exercises

      7) Observations to report to health care provider immediately

      8) Contact numbers for reporting concerns and asking questions

      9) Importance of follow-up and long-term care

    c. Provide sufficient time for parental return demonstration of needed procedures and parental questions

    d. Document teaching and parental response

NIC

1. Risk Identification, Environmental Management: Safety
2. Exercise Therapy: Joint Mobility, Muscle Control
3. Nutritional Monitoring, Fluid Monitoring
4. Communication Enhancement
5. Developmental Enhancement
6. Risk Identification, Infection Control
7. Anxiety Reduction
8. Caregiver Support, Respite Care, Teaching: Individual
9. Teaching: Illness Care, Infection Control, Diet, Treatment Regimen, Health Resources

EVALUATION

1. Client remains free of injury.
2. Client retains maximum ability of movement.
3. Client achieves adequate nutrition for metabolic needs for growth and development as evidenced by nutritional intake, and weight and height WDL within constraints of condition.
4. Client expresses needs effectively through use of assistive devices.
5. Client achieves highest level of growth and development as evidenced by achievement of milestones within constraints of condition.
6. Client does not experience infection or aspiration.
7. Parents express feelings and concerns and demonstrate manifestations of decreased anxiety.
8. Parents (caregiver) maintain emotional and physical health while providing care for child.
9. Parents demonstrate understanding of child's complex needs, medical management, and home care and utilize available support services.

References

Broyles, B. E., Reiss, B. S., & Evans, M. E. (2007). *Pharmacological aspects of nursing care* (7th ed.). Clifton Park, NY: Delmar Cengage Learning.

National Institute of Neurological Disorders and Stroke (NINDS). (2007). *Cerebral palsy information page.* Retrieved December 27, 2007, from http://www.ninds.nih.gov/disorders/cerebral_palsy/cerebral_palsy.htm

Potts, N. L., & Mandleco, B. L. (2007). *Pediatric nursing: Caring for children and their families* (2nd ed.). Clifton Park, NY: Delmar Cengage Learning.

United Cerebral Palsy. (2007). *Cerebral palsy—facts & figures.* Retrieved December 27, 2007, from http://www.ucp.org/ucp_generaldoc.cfm/1/9/37/37-37/447

22

CHEMOTHERAPY

Definition

Chemotherapy is the use of chemical agents that exert a specific or toxic effect on the cause of a particular condition. The more common use of this term is to describe the pharmacotherapeutic agents used in the treatment of cancer (antineoplastics).

Types, Actions, and Adverse Effects

Chemotherapy acts by altering cellular growth of the neoplasm through interference with the cell cycle of growth. Each subclassification of antineoplastic agents has unique biochemical properties that exert a highly toxic effect on the growth of the cancer cells. The primary problem with these agents is that although they are lethally selective to some cancers more than others, they also interfere with the cell cycle of growth of normal functioning cells. Chemotherapy usually involves the use of combinations of agents from one or more of the subclassifications to provide more effective therapy.

The first subclassification of antineoplastics contains the alkylating agents. These act to inhibit DNA synthesis by changing the internal acid-base balance of the cell. They are effective in all phases of the cell cycle; and for this reason, one or more of these agents is used in almost all combination chemotherapy regimens. Examples of commonly used alkylating antineoplastic agents include carboplatin, carmustine, chlorambucil, cisplatin, cyclophosphamide, ifosfamide, and thiotepa. Cyclophosphamide is a common agent used in chemotherapy regimens for the treatment of leukemia. Carmustine and cisplatin are used in combination regimens in the treatment of brain tumors (Potts & Mandelco, 2007).

All of the alkylating agents cause myelosuppression, that is, suppression of the bone marrow and its production of blood cells. The greatest impact is on the production of white blood cells (leukocytes). Because neutrophils compose 57–67% of the leukocyte count, neutropenia (neutrophil count < 500 cells/mm^3) is one of the most frequent adverse effects of chemotherapy. The primary function of leukocytes is to protect the body from infection. Consequently, dramatic reductions in these cells place the person at high risk for infection, including potentially life-threatening infections. Platelets play a significant role in blood coagulation. The normal platelet count is 150,000–400,000 cells/mm^3. A reduction in circulating platelets places the individual at risk for thrombocytopenia and bleeding episodes. The primary function of erythrocytes is to carry oxygen and carbon dioxide in the blood necessary for adequate tissue perfusion. Therefore, myelosuppression results in anemia, resulting in a decreased tissue perfusion necessary for cellular function.

Because the action of these agents is most toxic to rapid-growing cells, hair follicles are quickly destroyed, resulting in alopecia, a temporary loss of hair that returns following cessation of chemotherapy. The gastrointestinal tract also is a site of rapid-growing cells, and the toxic effects on the gastrointestinal epithelium commonly result in nausea and vomiting. In addition, these agents destroy normal gastrointestinal flora, leading to extremely painful stomatitis (inflammation of the oral mucous membranes) and extending down the esophagus, causing esophagitis. Furthermore, because the liver is the primary detoxifying organ for the body, impaired hepatic function can result.

Central nervous system changes can occur due to the toxic nature of these agents and to the decrease in tissue perfusion secondary to myelosuppression because the central nervous system is most sensitive to a reduction in circulating oxygen supply. The kidneys are the primary organs for excretion of chemotherapy agents, so the drugs must be used with caution in children with impaired renal function. Hemorrhagic cystitis is a potentially life-threatening complication specific to use of the alkylating agents cyclophosphamide and ifosfamide.

Most antineoplastics are administered via intravenous infusion. Because of the small diameters of children's veins, the risk of extravasation is high. Extravasation is a very serious complication that occurs when the chemotherapeutic agents being infused escape from the vein into the surrounding tissues, resulting in rapid and severe tissue necrosis (Broyles, Reiss, & Evans, 2007). Because of this risk, pediatric antineoplastic infusions are administered via central venous access devices (CVAD).

Antimetabolite antineoplastics "are a diverse group of agents [with] the ability to interfere with various metabolic actions of the cell" (Broyles et al., 2007, p. 928). By blocking the synthesis of DNA and RNA, antimetabolites either directly cause cellular death or interfere with the cell's ability to replicate. These agents are particularly effective during the S phase of the cell cycle. Examples of these agents include cytarabine, fluorouracil, mercaptopurine, and methotrexate.

The use of antimetabolites also results in myelosuppression, nausea and vomiting, stomatitis, and esophagitis. Children receiving these drugs usually develop both thrombocytopenia and anemia. Methotrexate poses specific complications because of its action in increasing uric acid levels. Because this agent can result in renal damage, precautions are taken before, during, and after its administration to protect body tissues and the kidneys from damage. Methotrexate is a common agent used in chemotherapy regimens for the treatment of certain types of leukemias.

Antitumor antibiotics, another subclassification of antineoplastics, act by interfering with the synthesis of DNA and RNA in all phases of the cell cycle. Unlike antibiotics used to treat infections, these agents are not selectively toxic to bacteria, but rather disrupt the cellular function of human cells. Bleomycin, dactinomycin, daunorubicin, doxorubicin, and mitomycin are some of the most frequently used antibiotic antineoplastic agents. Virtually all of these antineoplastic agents cause myelosuppression, nausea and vomiting, and stomatitis. Cardiotoxicity is a specific complication associated with the use of doxorubicin, a drug commonly used in the treatment of acute leukemia. Antitumor antibiotics are frequently used in combination with other antineoplastics for the treatment of a variety of pediatric and adult cancers.

Mitotic inhibitor antineoplastics cause cellular death by preventing the cell division, or mitosis, during the M phase of the cell cycle. Agents in this group commonly are used as monotherapy and in combination chemotherapy in children with leukemias, Hodgkin's disease, and non-Hodgkin's lymphomas. Etoposide, teniposide, vinblastine, vincristine, and vinorebine are commonly used mitotic inhibitor antineoplastics. These agents also cause myelosuppression (neutropenia, thrombocytopenia, and anemia) and alopecia. The oldest of these agents, vincristine, is derived from the periwinkle plant (*Vinca rosea*). "Etoposide is derived from the Mayapple (*Podophyllum*) plant and appears to exert its primary effect at the G_2 part of the cell cycle" (Broyles et al., 2007, p. 928) as well as to interfere with mitosis. Etoposide is a common agent used in combination chemotherapy in the treatment of many pediatric cancers including acute lymphocytic and acute myelocytic leukemias, non-Hodgkin's lymphoma, Hodgkin's disease, Wilms' tumor, and neuroblastomas (Potts & Mandleco, 2007). Teniposide seems to act during the late S or early G_2 phase of the cell cycle.

Hormone antineoplastics are frequently used in the treatment of hormone-dependent cancers. These agents act by altering the hormone environment and are "capable of selectively suppressing the growth of certain tissues (cells) of the body without exerting a cytotoxic action" (Broyles et al., p. 930). Examples of these agents are further subdivided into classes that include androgens, antiandrogens, antiestrogens, estrogens, gonadotropin-releasing hormone analogs, and progestins.

Biological response modifiers are "products of recombinant DNA technology using strains of genetically engineered *Escherichia coli*" (Spratto & Woods, 2008, p. 807) that "enhance the immunological function of the host (client), destroy or interfere with the cellular activities of tumors, and promote the differentiation of stem cells" (Broyles et al., 2007, p. 930). These agents, such as interferon alfa-2a, interferon alfa-2b, interferon alfa-n3, and aldesleukin, enhance the client's immune system by suppressing cell proliferation, increase macrophagocytic activity, and intensify the destructive effects of leukocytes on target cells.

Miscellaneous antineoplastic agents include a large number of anticancer drugs that do not fit into the previously discussed classifications. Among these are asparaginase, altretamine, cladribine, denileukin, flutamide, imatinib, levamisole, pegaspargase, and porfimer sodium. Bone marrow suppression, nausea and vomiting, fatigue, and alopecia are common adverse effects of these agents; and peripheral neuropathy can occur with some of these drugs.

Corticosteroids such as prednisone and prednisolone are commonly used as adjuncts to antineoplastic therapy in the treatment of cancers that involve the lymphatics, such as lymphoblastic leukemia and malignant lymphomas, because of their action to depress lymphocyte production. In addition, corticosteroids provide symptomatic relief and a general sense of well-being.

New groups of antineoplastics including monoclonal antibodies and the protease inhibitor bortezomib continue to be developed for the treatment of cancers in adults. However, as research continues, these agents most likely will be found to have efficacy and safety in the treatment of children as well. Examples of monoclonal antibodies include alemtuzumab, bevacizumab, cetuximab, rituximab, tositumomab, and iodine-131 tositumomab.

Complications

Myelosuppression
Neutropenia
Thrombocytopenia
Anemia
Extravasation
Fluid and electrolyte imbalance
Mucositis
Alopecia
Hemorrhagic cystitis
Cardiotoxicity
Neuropathy
Hypersensitivity

Incidence

Chemotherapy is the first-line treatment for leukemias, lymphomas, Hodgkin's disease, and cancers transmitted through the lymphatics. It also is used in conjunction with surgery and radiation therapy in the combination treatment for most cancers.

Clinical Manifestations of Adverse Effects of Chemotherapy

Myelosuppression
Fever
Infections
Bruising

Petichiae
Bleeding tendencies
Fatigue
Pallor
Weakness
Dizziness
Nausea and vomiting
Alopecia
Hemorrhagic cystitis
Occult blood in urine
Gross blood in urine
Cardiotoxicity
Dysrhythmias
Heart failure
Hypersensitivity reactions
Urticaria
Edema
Dyspnea

Diagnostic Tests to Detect Adverse Effects

Complete blood count with differential
Serum electrolyte levels
Uric acid
Urine testing for blood, specific gravity, and pH
Methotrexate serum levels

Medical Management

The use of antineoplastic agents in the treatment of cancer is a medical management standard of care. The goals of management before, during, and after the use of chemotherapy are to effectively destroy the cancer's cellular structure and to prevent and control the adverse effects associated with the mode of therapy. Most chemotherapy regimens involve the use of multiple antineoplastic agents in a combination therapy because they have been shown to be most effective in achieving remission states. Chemotherapy is administered in phases: (1) induction, (2) consolidation or intensification, and (3) maintenance. Remission is the goal of the induction phase, and some cancers do not require the maintenance phase.

High-volume intravenous fluid administration is a standard of care before and after the parenteral administration of antineoplastics. These fluids help dilute the agents as they are excreted from the body as well as provide for rapid excretion of these agents. Almost all chemotherapeutic agents used in children are administered parenterally and involve the surgical placement of a CVAD. This type of access lessens the risk of extravasation from vesicant agents because the agents enter the subclavian veins and empty into the superior vena cava. These CVADs usually are tunneled catheters such as Hickman, Broviac, or Groshong catheters or are implanted accesses such as the Port-a-Cath. Refer to Figure 22-1 and Figure 22-2. Tunneled CVADs are used for long-term parenteral access for chemotherapy administration.

Adjuvant agents used in combination with intravenous chemotherapy include agents classified as rescue agents. Leucovorin helps rescue the body from potential toxic effects of methotrexate by binding with the same cells and causing the excretion of methotrexate. Leucovorin's first dose is administered intravenously immediately following the completion of the methotrexate dose and is continued in intravenous bolus dosages

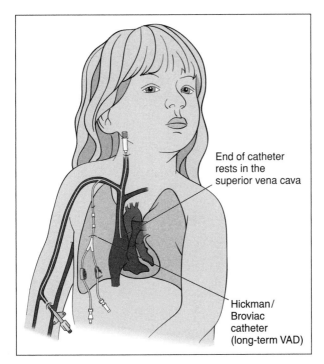

End of catheter
rests in the
superior vena cava

Hickman /
Broviac
catheter
(long-term VAD)

Figure 22-1: External Central Venous Catheters.

until the methotrexate level is below the toxic level. Intravenous hyperhydration prescribed before and after methotrexate also is focused on decreasing the uric acid levels by containing sodium bicarbonate in a dextrose solution. Mesna is a rescue agent used to prevent hemorrhagic cystitis associated with ifosfamide and cyclophosphamide. The total dose of mesna is 60% of the ifosfamide dose, administered intravenously in three equal doses with the first dose administered immediately following the completion of the ifosfamide or cyclophosphamide infusion.

Agents used to treat the myelosuppression associated with parenteral antineoplastics are recent adjuncts to chemotherapy. Among these agents are epoetin, a synthetic version of erythropoietin, used to stimulate red blood cell production in the bone marrow; filgrastim, a granulocyte colony-stimulating factor used to increase neutrophil production; and pegfilgrastim, a colony-stimulating factor that "is derived from filgrastim . . . that acts by binding to specific receptors on hematopoietic cell surfaces to proliferate, differentiate, commit, and activate cell function" (Broyles et al., 2007, p. 933).

One of the most important breakthroughs in caring for children and adults receiving chemotherapy has been the aggressive control of nausea and vomiting. The focus on managing this adverse effect (the one most dreaded by clients) of chemotherapy leads the way for the development of the newest classification of antiemetics—the serotonin-blocking agents, or serotonin antagonists. Ondansetron, granisetron, and dolasetron are the $5\text{-}HT_3$ antagonists that have proven to be the most effective antiemetics in children, with ondansetron remaining the gold standard. Lorazepam, a benzodiazepine, is the most commonly used drug for breakthrough chemotherapy-induced nausea in children.

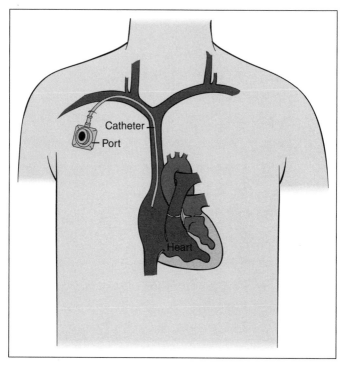

Figure 22-2: A Surgically Implanted Port-A-Cath.

Nursing Management
Adapted from Broyles et al., 2007, pp. 954–968.

ASSESSMENT
1. Obtain health history
2. Perform physical assessment
3. Assess laboratory data

NURSING DIAGNOSES (INCLUDING BUT NOT LIMITED TO)
1. Risk for infection R/T bone marrow suppression secondary to chemotherapy effects
2. Risk for injury, bleeding R/T bone marrow suppression secondary
   to chemotherapy effects
3. Risk for ineffective tissue perfusion R/T bone marrow suppression
   secondary to chemotherapy effects
4. Nausea R/T toxic effects on gastrointestinal epithelium from chemotherapy effects
5. Acute pain R/T mucositis secondary to chemotherapy effects
6. Imbalanced nutrition: less than body requirements R/T anorexia
   secondary to chemotherapy effects
7. Disturbed body image R/T alopecia secondary to chemotherapy effects
8. Risk for injury, uric acid neuropathy R/T use of methotrexate

9. Risk for injury, hemorrhagic cystitis R/T use of ifosfamide/cyclophosphamide

10. Risk for injury, cardiotoxicity R/T use of doxorubicin

11. Anticipatory grieving (parent/child) R/T diagnosis of cancer

12. Deficient knowledge R/T chemotherapy, adverse effects, and home care

PLANNING/GOALS

1. Client will not experience life-threatening infection; but if infection occurs, it will be promptly and effectively treated.

2. Client will not experience bleeding injury.

3. Client will not experience reduced tissue perfusion as evidenced by skin color, skin temperature, capillary refill, and peripheral oxygen saturation within defined limits (WDL).

4. Client will not experience nausea and vomiting; but if nausea occurs, it will be promptly and effectively treated.

5. Client will demonstrate pain control at a level acceptable to child, using an age-appropriate pain assessment tool.

6. Client will consume adequate age-appropriate nutrition as evidenced by weight within 50th percentile on standardized pediatric growth chart.

7. Parents/child (if age-appropriate) will demonstrate acceptance of alopecia.

8. Client will not experience uric acid neuropathy.

9. Client will not experience hemorrhagic cystitis.

10. Client will not experience cardiotoxicity.

11. Parents/child (if age-appropriate) will effectively work through anticipatory grieving as evidenced by verbalizations, active participation in child's care, and in age-appropriate activities for child.

12. Parents/child (if age-appropriate) will demonstrate understanding of chemotherapy, adverse effects, and home care.

NOC

1. Immune Status, Vital Signs Status

2. Risk Control, Vital Signs Status

3. Circulation Status, Vital Signs Status

4. Comfort Level, Nausea and Vomiting Control

5. Comfort Level, Pain Level

6. Nutrition Status

7. Body Image

8. Risk Control

9. Risk Control

10. Risk Control

11. Grief

12. Knowledge: Medications

IMPLEMENTATION

1. Infection
   a. Monitor temperature every 4 hours during hospitalization
   b. Monitor white blood cell count and differential
   c. Assess skin for reddened areas; if noted, notify health care provider immediately

    d. Maintain patency of intravenous access, monitoring hourly

    e. Administer antimicrobial agents as prescribed

    f. Maintain strict asepsis when caring for CVAD

    g. Obtain blood cultures as prescribed. *NOTE:* One of the most common sites of infection is the central venous catheter.

    h. Institute neutropenic precautions as indicated, following facility protocol

    i. Instruct parents and visitors about the importance of hand washing

    j. Instruct parents and visitors about neutropenic precautions

2. Bleeding

    a. Assess oral mucous membranes and nares for bleeding (epistaxis)

    b. Monitor platelet count

    c. Institute bleeding precautions if platelet count falls below 50,000 cells/mm^3 and administer platelets as prescribed

    d. Hemocult/guiac stools

    e. Monitor urine for blood each void

    f. Protect child from injury; provide for age-appropriate play activities

    g. Collaborate with health care provider for prophylactic prescription for stool softener, administering on scheduled basis

    h. Do not administer medications intramuscularly

3. Tissue perfusion

    a. Monitor complete blood count

    b. Institute falls precautions if hematocrit falls below 25%

    c. Administer blood products as prescribed, following facility protocols

    d. Monitor oxygen saturation via pulse oximetry

    e. Administer oxygen and titrate to prescribed oxygen saturation parameters

    f. *NOTE:* Monitor nares closely for bleeding if administering oxygen via nasal cannula or prongs

    g. Assess for manifestations of anemia

4. Nausea

    a. Premedicate child with antiemetics prior to administration of chemotherapy

    b. Administer serotonin antagonists as prescribed and on a scheduled basis for at least 24 hours following chemotherapy

    c. Administer lorazepam as prescribed for breakthrough nausea

    d. Eliminate offensive odors from environment

5. Pain

    a. Proactively manage child's pain

    b. Assess oral mucous membranes for signs of stomatitis

    c. Administer nystatin as prescribed (swish and spit)

    d. Administer nystatin (swish and swallow) as prescribed for esophagitis

    e. Assess pain level hourly using age-appropriate pain scale

    f. Administer morphine sulfate as prescribed via patient-controlled analgesia (PCA) using both continuous and PCA dosing

    g. Encourage oral intake of cool liquids

    h. Administer enteral feedings as indicated and prescribed if child has esophagitis

6. Nutrition
   a. Monitor strict intake and output
   b. Weigh daily
   c. Assess child's food preferences and collaborate with dietician to provide favorite foods
   d. Encourage high-calorie diet
   e. Provide age-appropriate environment for feedings
   f. Encourage parents to visit at mealtimes
   g. Administer enteral feedings if prescribed
   h. Monitor serum electrolyte levels

7. Body image
   a. Assess parents'/child's (if age-appropriate) knowledge of this adverse effect
   b. Stress that alopecia is temporary and that hair grows back after chemotherapy
   c. Inform parents/child that "[c]hildren with alopecia must protect their heads from cold weather and sunburn." (Potts & Mandleco, 2007, p. 929)
   d. Encourage parents and child (if needed) to express feelings
   e. Listen actively
   f. Encourage interaction of parents and child with other parents and children experiencing this issue
   g. For school-age or adolescent girls, encourage use of scarves or wigs

8. Uric acid neuropathy
   a. Administer prechemotherapy hydration (5% Dextrose and sodium bicarbonate) as prescribed
   b. Monitor urine pH with each void
   c. Notify health care provider if urine pH is < 5.5, and hold methotrexate
   d. Monitor serum uric acid levels
   e. Administer leucovorin as prescribed following methotrexate infusion
   f. Monitor methotrexate levels
   g. Administer allopurinol as prescribed
   h. Monitor renal function

9. Hemorrhagic cystitis
   a. Administer prechemotherapy hydration as prescribed
   b. Monitor urine for blood each void
   c. Monitor urine specific gravity each void
   d. Notify health care provider if urine specific gravity falls below 1.010
   e. Administer mesna as prescribed immediately following cyclophosphamide or ifosfamide infusions and at prescribed intervals for 24 hours

10. Cardiotoxicity
    a. Assess vital signs every 4 hours
    b. Initiate cardiorespiratory monitoring for child receiving doxorubicin

      c.   Auscultate heart sounds before and after doxorubicin infusion

      d.   Monitor continuous pulse oximetry

11. Anticipatory grieving

      a.   Encourage parents/child (if age-appropriate) to verbalize feelings

      b.   Listen actively to concerns

      c.   Provide for spiritual needs of family

      d.   Encourage parents to participate in child's care

      e.   Provide privacy for family unit as indicated or verbalized by parents

12. Parent/child teaching

      a.   Assess current level of knowledge about child's cancer and chemotherapy

      b.   Provide verbal and written information regarding:

          1) Monitoring of child's axillary temperature (rectal temperature should not be taken due to risk for injuring anal mucosa)

          2) Importance of avoiding crowds and teaching visitors about proper hand washing

          3) Importance of immunizing child on schedule

          4) Necessity of caring for central venous access device

          5) Adherence to neutropenic precautions (if indicated)

          6) Importance of follow-up monitoring of platelet count

          7) Importance of providing age-appropriate play activities with very low risk of injury

          8) Importance of monitoring for bruising and petechiae

          9) Necessity of seeking immediate medical care in event of uncontrolled bleeding

         10) Importance of using soft-bristled toothbrush

         11) Need to avoid nose-picking

         12) Need to avoid hot, spicy foods

         13) Importance of offering child frequent cool liquids and small feedings

         14) Necessity of administering medications as prescribed

         15) Signs and symptoms of adverse effects of medications

         16) Signs and symptoms to report immediately to health care provide

         17) Contact numbers to use for reporting to health care provider

         18) Contact numbers for community, state, and national support groups

         19) Importance of follow-up care

      c.   Provide adequate time for teaching and return demonstrations of skills required

      d.   Document teaching and parental response

NIC

1. Infection Control, Infection Protection, Vital Signs Monitoring
2. Bleeding Precautions, Surveillance Safety, Vital Signs Monitoring
3. Circulatory Care, Vital Signs Monitoring
4. Nausea Management, Medication Management

5. Pain Management, Analgesia Administration
6. Nutrition Management
7. Body Image Enhancement
8. Surveillance: Safety, Medication Administration
9. Surveillance: Safety, Medication Administration
10. Surveillance: Safety
11. Grief Work Facilitation
12. Teaching: Medication, Health Promotion

EVALUATION

1. Client does not experience life-threatening infection; but if infection occurs, it will be promptly and effectively treated.
2. Client does not experience bleeding injury.
3. Client does not experience reduced tissue perfusion as evidenced by skin color, skin temperature, capillary refill, and peripheral oxygen saturation WDL.
4. Client does not experience nausea and vomiting; but if nausea occurs, is will be promptly and effectively treated.
5. Client demonstrates pain control at a level acceptable to child, using an age-appropriate pain assessment tool.
6. Client consumes adequate age-appropriate nutrition as evidenced by weight within 50th percentile on standardized pediatric growth chart.
7. Parents/child (if age-appropriate) demonstrate acceptance of alopecia.
8. Client does not experience uric acid neuropathy.
9. Client does not experience hemorrhagic cystitis.
10. Client does not experience cardiotoxicity.
11. Parents/child (if age-appropriate) effectively work through anticipatory grieving as evidenced by verbalizations, active participation in child's care, and participation is age-appropriate play.
12. Parents/child (if age-appropriate) demonstrate understanding of chemotherapy, adverse effects, and home care.

References

Broyles, B. E., Reiss, B. S., & Evans, M. E. (2007). *Pharmacological aspects of nursing care* (7th ed.). Clifton Park, NY: Delmar Cengage Learning.

Potts, N. L., & Mandleco, B. L. (2007). *Pediatric nursing: Caring for children and their families* (2nd ed.). Clifton Park, NY: Delmar Cengage Learning.

Spratto, G. R., & Woods, A. L. (2008). *2008 edition PDR nurse's drug handbook*. Clifton Park, NY: Delmar Cengage Learning.

CLEFT LIP AND CLEFT PALATE

Definition

Clefts are fissures, or elongated openings, in body structures. "Clefts that occur in the oral-facial region often involve the lip, the roof of the mouth (hard palate) or the soft tissue in the back of the mouth (soft palate). Two major types of oral-facial clefts are cleft lip/palate and isolated cleft palate" (March of Dimes, 2007, p. 1). Refer to Figure 23-1.

Pathophysiology

During fetal development, the soft tissue of the lip and soft tissue and bone of the palate are supposed to close or fuse. The lip usually fuses by five to six weeks' gestation, and the palate closes by ten weeks. The fusion of the palate tissues separates the mouth from the nasal cavity. In cleft lip and cleft palate, fusion did not occur. Unilateral or bilateral cleft lip may occur with or without a cleft palate, and the severity of the fissure in the palate varies from a small notch to a complete cleft through the hard palate and the small palate extending into the nose. The extent of disfigurement and dysfunction of the mouth structures at the time of birth determines the surgical repair of this anomaly.

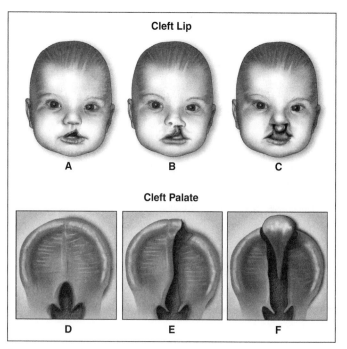

Figure 23-1: Cleft Lip: **(A)** Unilateral Incomplete, **(B)** Unilateral Complete, and **(C)** Bilateral Complete.
Cleft Palate: **(D)** Incomplete, **(E)** Unilateral Complete, **(F)** Bilateral Complete.

Cleft lip and cleft palate create numerous problems for the neonate, including risk for aspiration because of the connection between the nasal cavity (infants breathe through their noses) and the oral cavity. Difficulties with feedings occur with this anomaly because the neonate sucks by pressing its tongue against the palate. One of the greatest difficulties for the neonate's parents is the body image disturbance that cleft lip and palate present.

Complications

Risk for aspiration
Feeding difficulties
Risk for impaired parenting
Speech difficulties
Malocclusion problems
Hearing impairment

Incidence

Cleft lip or cleft palate occurs in 1.5 in 1,000 births (Potts & Mandleco, 2007). According to the March of Dimes, cleft lip/palate occurs more often among Asians, affecting approximately 1.7 per 1,000 births and among certain groups of American Indians, the incidence is more than 3.6 per 1,000 births. It occurs least frequently among African Americans, affecting approximately 1 per 2,500 births. Approximately 6,800 babies in the United States are born with oral-facial clefts annually, and about 4,200 babies are born each year with cleft lip/palate. Isolated cleft palate occurs less frequently, affecting approximately 2,600 babies each year with an incidence of 1 per 2,000 births. An isolated cleft palate is more common in females than males. Up to 13% of babies with cleft lip/palate have other birth defects (March of Dimes, 2007). Males are affected more often than girls (Family Doctor.org, 2006).

Etiology

The exact cause of cleft lip/cleft palate is not completely understood; however, both genetic and environmental factors have been associated with this anomaly. Environmental factors include maternal use of anticonvulsant medications, maternal alcohol use, infections, maternal illnesses, and possibly folic acid deficiency. Research studies supported by the National Institute of Dental and Craniofacial Research (NIDCR), part of the National Institutes of Health, "report that women who smoke during pregnancy and carry a fetus whose DNA lacks both copies of a gene involved in detoxifying cigarette smoke substantially increase their baby's chances of being born with a cleft lip and/or palate. According to the scientists, about a quarter of babies of European ancestry and possibly up to 60 percent of those of Asian ancestry lack both copies of the gene called GSTT1. Based on their data, published in the *American Journal of Human Genetics*, the scientists calculated that if a pregnant woman smokes 15 cigarettes or more per day, the chances of her GSTT1-lacking fetus developing a cleft increase nearly 20 fold" (National Institutes of Health, 2007, p.1).

Clinical Manifestations

Visual confirmation of cleft lip
    Notched upper lip border
    Nasal distortion
    Unilateral or bilateral cleft lip/palate
Visual confirmation of cleft palate
    Visible or palpable gap in uvula, soft palate, or hard palate
    Exposed nasal cavity
    Nasal distortion

Diagnostic Tests

Physical examination with visual inspection is sufficient for diagnosis.

Medical Management

The goals of management are to prevent aspiration, stabilize the neonate by providing alternative feeding techniques to allow for adequate intake and growth, and eventually to correct the anomaly surgically. The members of the treatment team include orthodontist, otolaryngologist, pediatrician, speech pathologist, pediatric surgeon, neurosurgeon, plastic surgeon, audiologist, and nurse. According to the circumstances and availability, the team also may include a psychologist, an ear-nose-throat specialist, and a genetic counselor.

Speech therapists assess the neonate with a cleft palate concerning its ability to consume oral feedings and then develop alternative feeding methods that include use of specialized elongated nipples (sometimes referred to as lamb's nipples) or breast shields that are very pliable and the ESSR (Enlarge nipple, stimulate Suck by rubbing nipple on lower lip, Swallow, Rest after each swallow to allow for complete swallowing) method. Feeding the infant in an upright position helps decrease gravity drainage of formula into the nasal cavity, lessening the risk of aspiration. Adjusting the amount of time it takes for the infant to eat is necessary. All of these techniques, including infant-child cardiopulmonary resuscitation procedures, are taught to the child's parents or caregivers. The more severe the anomaly, the more adjustments are required.

Cleft lips usually are surgically repaired when the infant is approximately 12 weeks of age or 12 pounds. The goal of repairing this early is to limit scarring and increase chances for normal facial development. Usually, an incision is made on either side of the cleft; then the surgeon turns down the outer portion of the cleft. The muscle and skin of the lip are sutured together to close the separation. According to the American Society of Plastic Surgeons, palate repair is usually done when the child is 9 to 18 months old because it is a more extensive surgery. "To repair a cleft palate, the surgeon will make an incision on both sides of the separation, moving tissue from each side of the cleft to the center or midline of the roof of the mouth. This rebuilds the palate, joining muscle together and providing enough length in the palate so the child can eat and learn to speak properly" (American Society of Plastic Surgeons, 2007, p. 1).

Nursing Management

ASSESSMENT

Assess airway and breathing

Assess cardiorespiratory status with cardiorespiratory monitor

Perform physical assessment

Assess for presence of other anomalies

Assess parental adjustment to neonate's condition

NURSING DIAGNOSES (INCLUDING BUT NOT LIMITED TO)

PREOPERATIVE

1. Risk for aspiration R/T abnormal connection between mouth and nasal passage
2. Risk for imbalanced nutrition: less than body requirements R/T feeding difficulties
3. Impaired parenting R/T interruption in bonding process
4. Deficient knowledge R/T neonate's condition, alternative feeding techniques, and home care

POSTOPERATIVE

5. Risk for injury and infection R/T surgical incision
6. Acute pain R/T surgical incision
7. Deficient knowledge R/T surgical treatment and long-term care

PLANNING/GOALS

1. Client will not experience aspiration.
2. Client will consume adequate nutritional intake for growth and development as evidenced by doubling birth weight by 6 months of age and tripling birth weight by 1 year of age.
3. Parents/caregivers will demonstrate bonding with infant and actively participate in care.
4. Parents/caregivers will demonstrate understanding of child's condition, alternative feeding techniques, and home care.
5. Client will not experience injury or infection postoperatively.
6. Client will demonstrate adequate pain management as evidenced by behavioral indicators.
7. Parents will demonstrate understanding of surgical treatment, postoperative course, and long-term care.

NOC

1. Aspiration Prevention
2. Nutritional Status
3. Child Development: Safe Home Environment
4. Knowledge: Child Safety
5. Risk Control
6. Pain Control
7. Knowledge: Illness Care, Health Promotion

IMPLEMENTATION

1. Risk for aspiration
   a. Assess respiratory status continuously using cardiorespiratory monitor
   b. Monitor continuous pulse oximetry if defect is severe
   c. Collaborate with speech therapist regarding infant feedings
   d. Feed neonate in upright position on lap using ESSR method
   e. Burp or bubble frequently
   f. Use alternative feeding devices including elongated nipple or breast shield
   g. Instruct parents about feeding techniques
2. Nutrition
   a. Assess degree of anomaly and infant's sucking ability
   b. Collaborate with speech therapist regarding infant feedings
   c. Feed neonate in upright position on lap using ESSR method
   d. Burp or bubble frequently
   e. Use alternative feeding devices including elongated nipple or breast shield
   f. Monitor intake and output. *NOTE:* Infant intake is usually 60–90 mL every 2–3 hours
   g. Weigh daily
   h. Monitor diapers. *NOTE:* Infant should have at least six to eight wet diapers every 24 hours

3. Parenting
   a. Assess parent-infant bonding process
   b. Encourage parents to express feelings and concerns
   c. Assess parental support systems and assist in their use
   d. Provide parents with pictures of other infants before and after corrective surgery
   e. Encourage parental touching, holding, cuddling, and bonding and involvement in care
   f. Discuss infant's positive features
   g. Express acceptance of infant to serve as role model for parents
   h. Discuss growth and development needs of infant
   i. Refer to community resources and parent support groups
4. Parent teaching preoperatively
   a. Assess parents' current level of knowledge about infant's condition and care needs
   b. Provide verbal, written, and demonstration instructions regarding:
      1) Alternative infant feeding techniques (ESSR)
      2) Infant cardiopulmonary resuscitation
      3) Infant positioning for sleeping
      4) Method of taking infant's axillary temperature
      5) Infant growth and development
      6) Infant monitoring
   c. Keep teaching as simple as possible
   d. Provide adequate time for teaching and parental return demonstration of skills
   e. Document teaching and parental response
5. Risk for injury and infection postoperatively
   a. Assess operative site hourly
   b. Place elbow restraints (No-Nose) to prevent infant from putting fingers in mouth
   c. Monitor axillary temperature every 4 hours
   d. Maintain patency of intravenous access device, monitoring hourly
   e. Encourage parental holding (restraints can be removed as long as infant is being held and is unable to put fingers in mouth)
   f. Resume preoperative feeding schedule and techniques as prescribed following lip repair
   g. Use short, soft nipples that do not rest on palatal sutures and offer infant foods mixed with water following palate repair
6. Acute pain
   a. Assess infant's pain level hourly using age-appropriate pain assessment tool
   b. Proactively provide for pain management
   c. Place infant on cardiorespiratory monitoring and pulse oximetry if using opioids for pain management
   d. Involve parents in decision making regarding pain management
7. Parent teaching postoperatively
   a. Assess parents' current level of knowledge regarding postoperative and home care

   b. Provide verbal and written instructions regarding:
       1) No straws, pacifiers, spoons, or fingers in or around mouth
          for 7–10 days postoperatively
       2) No oral temperatures; reinforce how to take axillary temperature
       3) Suture line care
       4) Advance feedings as tolerated from clear liquids to preopera-
          tive soft diet
       5) Post-palate repair: provide short nipples that do not rest on
          palatal sutures and increase fluid intake by adding water to
          soft food
       6) Signs and symptoms to report to health care provider
       7) Contact numbers of health care provider and referral contacts
   c. Provide adequate time for teaching and parents' questions
   d. Document teaching and parental response

NIC

1. Aspiration Precautions, Positioning
2. Nutritional Monitoring, Infant Feeding
3. Attachment Promotion, Newborn Care, Breastfeeding Assistance,
   Bottle Feeding
4. Teaching: Infant Safety
5. Surveillance: Safety, Infection Protection
6. Analgesic Administration
7. Teaching: Procedure/Treatment, Child Safety

EVALUATION

1. Client does not experience aspiration.
2. Client consumes adequate nutritional intake for growth and development as evidenced by doubling birth weight by 6 months of age
   and tripling birth weight by 1 year of age.
3. Parents/caregivers demonstrate bonding with infant and actively
   participate in care.
4. Parents/caregivers demonstrate understanding of child's condition,
   alternative feeding techniques, and home care.
5. Client does not experience injury or infection postoperatively.
6. Client demonstrates adequate pain management as evidenced by
   behavioral indicators of periods of restful sleep and absence of crying.
7. Parents demonstrate understanding of surgical treatment, postoperative course, and long-term care.

References

American Society of Plastic Surgeons. (2007). *Cleft lip or palate.* Retrieved December 27,
    2007, from http://www.plasticsurgery.org/patients_consumers/procedures/CleftLipPalate
    .cfm?CFID=69697605&CFTOKEN=63237509

Family Doctor.org. (2006). *Cleft lip and cleft palate.* Retrieved December 27, 2007, from
    http://familydoctor.org/034.xml

March of Dimes. (2007). *Cleft lip and cleft palate.* Retrieved December 27, 2007, from
    http://www.marchofdimes.com/professionals/14332_1210.asp

National Institutes of Health. (2007). *Scientists discover how maternal smoking can cause cleft lip and
    palate.* Retrieved December 27, 2007, from http://www.nih.gov/news/pr/jan2007/nidcr-03.htm

Potts, N. L., & Mandleco, B. L. (2007). *Pediatric nursing: Caring for children and their families*
    (2nd ed.). Clifton Park, NY: Delmar Cengage Learning.

24

COARCTATION OF THE AORTA

Definition

Coarctation of the aorta is stenosis, or narrowing, of the lumen of the arch (thoracic aorta) of the major artery exiting the left ventricle (LV) of the heart that carries blood into systemic circulation. "The most common position of the coarctation is opposite the insertion of the PDA [patent ductus arteriosus]" (Potts & Mandleco, 2007, p. 784). Refer to Figure 24-1.

Pathophysiology

Because the narrowing of the aorta in coarctation is at the left of the PDA, there is no obstruction to the blood flow out of the aorta in utero or after birth as long as the ductus remains open. As a result, these children frequently are asymptomatic other than a systolic murmur. Even though resistance within the ascending aorta is increased, resulting in higher coronary artery pressure, rarely does heart failure occur unless the stenosis is severe. In infants/children with severe coarctation, "an increase in left ventricular

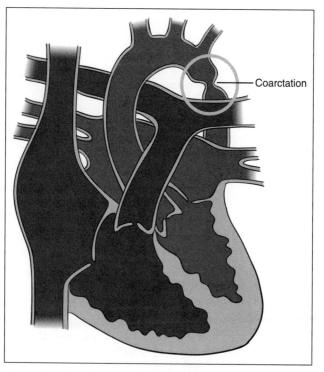

Figure 24-1: Coarctation of the Aorta.

pressure and work occurs with resulting LV [left ventricle] hypertrophy" (Potts & Mandleco, 2007, p. 785).

Complications

Increased coronary artery pressure

Patent ductus arteriosus

Left ventricular hypertrophy

Pulmonary edema

Altered gas exchange

Incidence

"Coarctation of the aorta occurs in about 6 to 8 percent of all children with congenital heart disease. Boys have the defect twice as often as girls do" (Congenital Heart Defects, 2006, p. 1). Coarctation of the aorta frequently is associated with other congenital heart defects.

Etiology

According to the American Heart Association, "Most of the time we do not know (what causes congenital heart defects). Although the reason defects occur is presumed to be genetic, only a few genes have been discovered that have been linked to the presence of heart defects. Rarely the ingestion of some drugs and the occurrence of some infections during pregnancy can cause defects" (American Heart Association, 2007, p. 1).

Clinical Manifestations

Systolic murmur

Dyspnea on exertion

Manifestations of left-sided heart failure

Diagnostic Tests

Chest radiography

Echocardiogram

Cardiac catheterization

Medical Management

Because most children with coarctation of the aorta are asymptomatic, no treatment is required; however, if the stenosis is severe, medical/surgical intervention should be initiated. Refer to Chapter 26: Congenital Heart Disease/Open Heart Surgery.

Nursing Management

Refer to Chapter 26: Congenital Heart Disease/Open Heart Surgery.

References

American Heart Association. (2007). *Coarctation of the aorta (CoA)*. Retrieved December 27, 2007, from http://www.americanheart.org/presenter.jhtml?identifier=1667

Congenital Heart Defects. (2006). *Types of CHD and their descriptions*. Retrieved December 27, 2007, from http://www.congenitalheartdefects.com/typesofCHD.html#Coarc

Potts, N. L., & Mandleco, B. L. (2007). *Pediatric nursing: Caring for children and their families* (2nd ed.). Clifton Park, NY: Delmar Cengage Learning.

25

COLIC

Definition

Colic is a condition in otherwise healthy infants less than 3 months old that is characterized by "recurrent episodes of unexplained crying and the inability to be consoled" (Potts & Mandleco, 2007, p. 222). The crying usually lasts more than 3 hours a day 3 times a week, continuing for more than 3 weeks (eMedicine Health, 2005).

Pathophysiology

Colic occurs in infants with a healthy suck reflex and appetite. Although the exact process is not completely understood, it is believed that colic symptoms occur from paroxysmal abdominal bowel spasms causing stimulation to the nerve receptors in the bowel and acute pain. These spasms can lead to gas production, regurgitation following feedings, and constipation. Colic is self-limiting, subsiding spontaneously by the time the infant is 4 months old.

Complications

Pain
Regurgitation following feedings
Constipation
Parental anxiety

Incidence

Colic may affect as many as 20% of neonates and infants under 3 months of age. Colic symptoms occur more frequently in infants receiving iron-fortified formulas (eMedicine Health, 2005).

Etiology

Although the exact etiology of colic has not been established and supported by research, a number of factors may contribute to colic. These include an infant's sensitive temperament, allergies, lactose intolerance, an immature digestive system, parental anxiety, differences in the way an infant is fed or comforted, and an immature nervous system. Research reveals that it is still unclear why some infants have colic and others do not (Mayo Clinic, 2007).

Other factors that produce colic symptoms include excessive swallowing of air, improper feeding techniques (overfeeding is a major contributor), food allergies, and maternal use of tobacco. With infants who consume breast milk, maternal intake of foods that have a high incidence of producing allergies or that are gas-producing may induce excess gas in the infant. Some of these foods include chocolate, beans, broccoli, cauliflower, cabbage, onion, garlic, collards, spices, dairy products, caffeine, and eggs. Iron-based infant formulas may be difficult for many infants to digest or are delayed in being excreted from the infant's intestines, which could lead to constipation and flatus, just as it does in adults. Psychological factors also may contribute to the development of colic—for instance, high stress in the parents or caregivers that is transferred to the infant through touch, muscle tightness, and elevation of the caregiver's heart rate (which the infant hears when being held).

Clinical Manifestations

Crying beginning suddenly and accompanied by some or all of the following:

    Arching the back

    Extending the legs

    Clenching fists

    Displaying a reddened face

    Belching

    Having excessive post-feeding regurgitation

    Expelling flatus

    Having difficulty passing stools

Diagnostic Tests

Focus is on ruling out underlying medical problems.

Medical Management

The goal of management is to support both the infant and the parents through this frustrating yet self-limiting condition. Many pediatricians prescribe simethicone drops for the relief of gas. Changing the infant's diet and feeding techniques are the standards of management. Evaluating the diet of the breast-feeding mother and eliminating foods that may produce allergic responses or gas in the infant are other options. Avoiding spicy foods, raw vegetables, dairy products, and caffeine is recommended. Less than 10% of all neonates are nutritionally deficient and require iron-based formulas. Changing from iron-based and milk-based formulas to whey- or soy-based or hypoallergenic formulas may decrease the duration of colic symptoms or completely resolve them. Carnation Good Start is a whey-based formula, Isomil and Enfamil ProSobee are soy-based formulas, and Enfamil Nutramigen and Alimentum are hypoallergenic formulas. These products contain more easily digestible proteins than milk-based formulas.

Nursing Management

ASSESSMENT

1. Obtain infant history
2. Auscultate bowel sounds
3. Obtain nutrition history including maternal diet if breast feeding
4. Obtain height and weight
5. Perform physical assessment

NURSING DIAGNOSES (INCLUDING BUT NOT LIMITED TO)

1. Acute pain R/T bowel spasms and gas production
2. Anxiety (parental) R/T inconsolable infant
3. Deficient knowledge R/T condition and home care

PLANNING/GOALS

1. Client will exhibit decreasing crying episodes.
2. Parents will demonstrate reduction in anxiety level as evidenced by verbal and nonverbal cues.
3. Parents will demonstrate understanding of condition and home care.

NOC

1. Comfort Level, Pain Level
2. Anxiety
3. Knowledge: Health Promotion

IMPLEMENTATION

1. Pain
   a. Assess infant behaviors for indications of pain
   b. Feed infant slowly, burping or bubbling frequently
   c. Position infant upright during feedings
   d. Swaddle infant
   e. Place infant in swing for 20 minutes following feeding
   f. Massage infant's back gently during rest times
   g. Reduce environmental stimulation during rest times
2. Parental anxiety
   a. Encourage parents to express feelings and concerns
   b. Assure parents that colic is self-limiting
   c. Encourage parental participation in infant care
   d. Assess parent support systems for respite care
   e. Provide parents with techniques to reduce colic symptoms
3. Parent teaching
   a. Assess parents' knowledge of techniques to cope with colic
   b. Provide verbal, written, and demonstration (when appropriate) information:
      1) Feed infant slowly, burping or bubbling frequently (at least every ¼ oz or 3 minutes during breastfeeding)
      2) If breastfeeding, avoid spicy and gas-producing foods
      3) Swaddle infant or place in front baby carrier
      4) Take infant for car ride (vibration and movement)
      5) Place infant in swing for 20 minutes following feeding
      6) Walk or rock baby, applying gentle pressure to infant's abdomen
      7) Gently massage infant's back when resting
      8) Provide white noise and dark environment for sleep
      9) Pick up infant after 20 minutes of crying if infant has not fallen asleep
   c. Provide support to parents and sufficient time for teaching
   d. Document teaching and parental response

NIC

1. Pain Management
2. Anxiety Reduction
3. Teaching: Health Promotion

EVALUATION

1. Client exhibits decreasing crying episodes and increasing periods of sleep undisturbed by crying.
2. Parents demonstrate reduction in anxiety level as evidenced by verbal and nonverbal cues.
3. Parents demonstrate understanding of condition and home care.

References

eMedicine Health. (2005). *Colic*. Retrieved April 23, 2007, from http://www.emedicinehealth.com/colic/article_em.htm

Mayo Clinic. (2007). *Colic*. Retrieved April 23, 2007, from http://www.mayoclinic.com/health/colic/DS00058/DSECTION=3

Potts, N. L., & Mandleco, B. L. (2007). *Pediatric nursing: Caring for children and their families* (2nd ed.). Clifton Park, NY: Delmar Cengage Learning.

CONGENITAL HEART DISEASE/ OPEN HEART SURGERY

Definition

Congenital heart defects are structural and functional abnormalities in the heart that are present at birth and occur during fetal development. Although these defects are discussed individually in this text, "[i]t is not uncommon for the infant to present with a combination of defects" (Potts & Mandleco, 2007, p. 771).

Pathophysiology

The pathophysiology of congenital heart defects varies according to the individual type and extent of structural or functional impact on the intake and output of blood from the heart. Congenital heart defects are classified or divided into types according to how each affects the blood flow to and from the chambers of the heart.

Left-to-right shunts result in increased pulmonary blood flow and include atrial septal defects (ASDs) (refer to Chapter 10: Atrial Septal Defect [ASD]), ventricular septal defects (VSDs) (refer to Chapter 108: Ventricular Septal Defect [VSD]), patent ductus arteriosus (PDA) (refer to Chapter 82: Patent Ductus Arteriosus [PDA]), combined atrioventricular septal defects, hypoplastic left heart syndrome (HLHS) (refer to Chapter 58: Hypoplastic Left Heart Syndrome [HLHS]/Heart Transplantation), and truncus arteriosus. These defects cause a shifting of blood from the left side to the right side of the heart due to an abnormal connection between the two sides. Because the pressure is greater in the left side of the heart than in the right and fluid moves from an area of greater pressure to lesser pressure, these abnormal connections result in the shunting of the blood from left to right. The shunting is heard as a murmur representing the abnormal leaking of blood through the shunt. With increased blood flow to the right ventricle, the right side of the heart experiences an increased workload and potential right ventricular hypertrophy. As the right ventricular muscle hypertrophies, the chamber becomes smaller and the muscle becomes a less efficient pump. This results in incomplete emptying of the right atrium into the right ventricle, the right atria's inability to accept the normal input from the systemic blood supply, and backup of blood in the systemic system.

ASD is an opening in the septum between the right and left atria, allowing blood to flow from the left atrium to the right atrium; VSD is an abnormal opening between the right and left ventricles, allowing blood in the left ventricle to pass into the right ventricle; and PDA occurs when the ductus arteriosus does not close at birth or within three months after birth, allowing blood to flow from the higher-pressure aorta to the pulmonary artery. These defects usually are referred to as acyanotic heart defects because although there is some mixing of oxygenated and deoxygenated blood, these defects generally do not cause systemic cyanosis.

Truncus arteriosus and HLHS are cyanotic heart defects. Truncus arteriosus results from the failure of the embryonic trunk of the great vessels to divide into the pulmonary artery, aorta, and coronary arteries. With this defect, the heart has only one arterial trunk, resulting in the mixing of oxygenated and deoxygenated blood and this mixture being ejected through the common trunk into systemic circulation. In HLHS, "secondary to atresia of the mitral valve [between the left atrium and ventricle] and resulting hypoplasia of the LV [left ventricle], blood cannot pass into the LV and must cross the patent foramen ovale into the RA [right atrium] via a left-to-right shunt. The only way blood can enter the aorta is through retrograde flow across the PDA" (Potts & Mandleco, 2007, p. 787).

Right-to-left shunts result in decreased pulmonary blood flow and include pulmonary stenosis [PS] (refer to Chapter 85: Pulmonary Stenosis [PS]), tetralogy of Fallot (TOF) (refer to Chapter 103: Tetralogy of Fallot [TOF]), transposition of the great arteries (TGA)—aorta and pulmonary artery, pulmonary atresia, and tricuspid atresia.

PS is the narrowing of the pulmonary artery that decreases blood flow between the right ventricle and the lungs. It will be addressed during the discussion of stenotic defects.

Both TOF and TGA result in systemic cyanosis because of the pumping of deoxygenated blood into the systemic system. Each of the cyanotic defects differs in the structural reason for pumping blood that has not been oxygenated by the lungs into the systemic supply. In TOF, the presence of an overriding aorta over a VSD and PS allows deoxygenated blood (that the pulmonary artery is attempting to carry into the lungs for oxygenation) to be shunted into the aorta. In TGA, the aorta exits the right ventricle of the heart instead of the left ventricle and the pulmonary artery exits the left ventricle instead of the right ventricle. As a result, deoxygenated blood entering the right ventricle from the right atria is pumped into systemic circulation and oxygenated blood in the left ventricle is recirculated through the lungs.

Pulmonary atresia is the lack of an opening into the pulmonary artery from the right ventricle. The presence of a VSD allows deoxygenated blood from the right ventricle to cross into the left ventricle and mix with oxygenated blood from the left atria. This mixture is ejected through the aorta.

In tricuspid atresia, there is an absence or complete closure of the tricuspid valve, resulting in a lack of connection between the right atria and ventricle. Returning systemic blood mixes with pulmonary venous return in the atria; and because it cannot enter the right ventricle, the pressure in the right atria maintains the foramen ovale, allowing the mixed blood to enter the left atria. Some blood can enter the lungs through the PDA; the rest is ejected into systemic circulation by the aorta.

Stenotic defects result in decreased blood flow from the heart. PS causes a reduced blood flow from the right side of the heart to the lungs for oxygenation. This occurs because stenosis causes narrowing of the lumen of the pulmonary artery and decreases the amount of blood that can pass through the lumen with each contraction of the right ventricle. This leads to right ventricular hypertrophy. HLHS, aortic stenosis (AS) (refer to Chapter 6: Aortic Stenosis), and coarctation of the aorta (refer to Chapter 24: Coarctation of the Aorta) result in obstruction of left ventricular outflow.

As previously noted, in HLHS, atresia of the mitral valve and resulting hypoplasia of the left ventricle do not allow blood to enter the left ventricle, forcing the blood to cross the patent foramen ovale into the right atria. The only blood that enters the aorta is through retrograde flow across the PDA.

Aortic stenosis is a narrowing of the aorta at the location of the aortic valve, and coarctation of the aorta is the narrowing of the aorta at the aortic arch. These defects decrease the amount of blood that can be pumped by the left ventricle into systemic circulation. Aortic stenosis and coarctation of the aorta result in left ventricular hypertrophy.

Complications

Congestive heart failure

Failure to thrive (refer to Chapter 44: Failure to Thrive [FTT])

Decreased cardiac output

Pulmonary edema

Hypoxemia

Complications associated with surgical repair of the defect(s)

Incidence

Approximately 1% of the world's population is born with heart disease (International Children's Heart Foundation, n.d.). According to the March of Dimes, approximately 40,000 infants (1 out of every 125) are born with heart defects annually in the United States (March of Dimes, 2007). The estimates by the American Heart Association suggest that about 1 million Americans have a congenital heart defect (American Heart Association, 2007). According to the National Heart Lung and Blood Institute, congenital heart defects are the most common congenital anomalies affecting 8 out of every 1000 neonates in the United States (National Heart Lung and Blood Institute, 2007). Each heart defect has its statistical incidence; and defects range from simple to highly complex, with few or no symptoms to life-threatening manifestations requiring surgical repair.

Etiology

According to the American Heart Association, most of the time the cause of congenital heart defects is unknown. Although the reason defects occur is presumed to be genetic, only a few genes discovered have been linked to the presence of heart defects. Heredity may play a role in congenital heart disease (CHD), as well as coexisting conditions such as Down syndrome or a mother contracting rubella during the first trimester of pregnancy. The use of alcohol and illicit drugs during pregnancy increases the fetus's risk for developing CHD (American Heart Association, 2007).

Clinical Manifestations

LEFT-TO-RIGHT SHUNTS

Murmur

Dyspnea on exertion

Growth retardation

Failure to thrive

Diaphoresis

Right ventricular hypertrophy

Right-sided heart failure

Loud click sound on auscultation and cyanosis (truncus arteriosus)

RIGHT-TO-LEFT SHUNTS

Murmur

Dyspnea on exertion

Cyanosis

Failure to thrive

Left ventricular hypertrophy

Pulmonary edema

Tachypnea

Left-sided heart failure

STENOTIC SHUNTS

Murmur

Dyspnea on exertion

Right- or left-sided heart failure and resulting systemic or pulmonary
manifestations

Diagnostic Tests

DIAGNOSTIC

Auscultation of a murmur

Pulse oximetry

Electrocardiogram
Holter monitor
Chest radiography
Echocardiogram
Cardiac catheterization

LABORATORY TESTS (PREOPERATIVE)

Complete blood count
Coagulation studies
Electrolyte levels
Arterial blood gases
Pulse oximetry
Cardiac enzymes
Urinalysis

Medical Management

The goals of medical management are to prevent irreversible heart damage and to restore and maintain sufficient cardiac output to meet metabolic and growth needs. For children who are asymptomatic except for the presence of a murmur, no medical or surgical intervention is required beyond monitoring. Infants and children who experience dyspnea on exertion or fatigue that interferes with meeting growth and development needs or who develop hypertension or other manifestations of potential cardiac damage require medical management and/or surgical intervention.

In the pediatric intensive care environment, certain medications are administered via continuous intravenous infusion in the presence of life-threatening heart defects. Among these agents are sympathomimetics including dopamine, dobutamine, and epinephrine that increase cardiac output and blood pressure; the result is improved tissue perfusion. Dopamine also increases the heart rate and renal blood flow, and epinephrine decreases renal blood flow and increases systemic vascular resistance in high doses. Milrinone and amrinone, phosphodiesterase inhibitors, increase cardiac output and decrease afterload, cardiac workload, and cardiac chamber filling pressures. Nitrates such as nitroglycerine and nitroprusside decrease systemic vascular resistance and afterload and increase cardiac output.

Digoxin is a potent cardiac glycoside used for its positive inotropic action in slowing and strengthening cardiac contractions. Furosemide is a loop diuretic that reduces preload by decreasing the reabsorption of sodium, chloride, and water. Propranolol, a beta-blocking agent, reduces cardiac oxygen demands by inhibiting catecholamine-induced tachycardia and hypertension. Angiotensin inhibitors such as captopril and enalapril dilate arteries and veins to decrease pulmonary vascular resistance and systemic vascular resistance, allowing the heart to pump blood into the blood vessels with less effort, thus reducing afterload. Losartan, an angiotensin II receptor blocker, is used to decrease systemic vascular resistance through vasodilation.

Some defects are being repaired by nonsurgical placement of a device during cardiac catheterization. This is the treatment of choice for smaller ASDs, and it is being used increasingly with small VSDs. The nonsurgical placement or use of coils may be all that is required to occlude a PDA. Balloon valvuloplasties are used for small- to moderate-sized PS and aortic stenosis. Balloon dilation may repair a small- to moderate-sized coarctation of the aorta, sparing these children the physiological stress of open-heart surgery.

OPEN-HEART SURGICAL MANAGEMENT

Surgical repair is required for some congenital heart defects and usually involves open-heart (open-chest) surgery and cardiopulmonary bypass during the surgery.

Many complex defects need staged repairs (or more than one surgery) to complete correction of the defect(s); however, even completion of multiple surgeries usually is accomplished by the time the child is 2 to 4 years of age. Repairs of defects that do not cause significant hemodynamic alteration may be delayed until the child is 2 to 3 years of age.

Regardless of the type of defect, the procedure used to enter the chest and placement on the cardiopulmonary bypass is basically the same just as reattachment of the major vessels of the heart from cardiopulmonary bypass, placement of chest tubes, and closure of the chest following the defect repair. The actual repair of the defect is what differentiates each surgery.

The basic procedure of open-heart surgery involves opening the skin over the sternum and, using a circular-type surgical saw, transecting the sternum and entering the chest. The superior vena cava and aorta are attached to cardiopulmonary bypass that serves to oxygenate the returning systemic blood and then pump the oxygenated blood into systemic circulation. This allows the heart to be stopped so the repair can be accomplished on a still organ and the lungs, which have collapsed during the entry into the chest cavity, can be bypassed. Usually, three chest tubes are placed: one to drain the left side of the pleural cavity of air and fluid, one to drain the right side of the pleural cavity, and one in the pericardial sac to drain blood and prevent cardiac tampanode. On infants, two chest tubes may be used: one for pleural drainage and one for pericardial drainage. The heart is stimulated to functional rhythm if needed; however, the heart may return to functional rhythm by itself after reattachment of the major vessels. The sternum is wired closed; the skin layers are sutured and stapled closed. Pacemaker wires are inserted for access in the event that postoperative dysrhythmias occur.

The repair for septal defects involves suture closure of the defect. If the opening is too large to be sutured closed, a graft may be required to provide a functional septum. For a large PDA that cannot be closed by coils, the defect is ligated, or tied off, during open-heart surgery.

With truncus arteriosus, the pulmonary arteries are separated from the common trunk and the hole in the trunk that remains is closed. The associated VSD is closed, and a valved homograft conduit is used to connect the pulmonary arteries to the right ventricle. This allows the return of a functional path for the blood entering the right atria and then the right ventricle to be pumped through the conduit into the pulmonary arteries. The oxygenated blood returns through the pulmonary venous system into the left atria to the left ventricle and is pumped through the truncal valve out the aorta into systemic circulation.

Surgically repairable tricuspid atresia (infants with no VSD and a hypoplastic right ventricle that cannot be completely corrected by surgery) involves staged open-heart surgery including the placement of a Blalock-Taussig (BT) shunt, followed several months later by a Glenn shunt (or bicaval anastomosis). The final procedure is the Fontan procedure, the creation of a connection from the inferior vena cava to the pulmonary artery, allowing all systemic venous return to be directed to the lungs for oxygenation.

For infants with transposition of the great vessels, surgery (arterial switch) resects the aorta from the aortic trunk, resects the pulmonary artery from the pulmonary trunk, and then switches the vessels. This provides complete anatomical correction.

Infants with TOF who experience frequent cyanotic spells may have a palliative procedure that involves placement of a BT shunt to reduce the symptoms and allows complete repair of the defect to be deferred until the infant is 3 to 12 months of age. At that time, the PS is repaired and the VSD is closed.

Postoperatively, children following open-heart surgery and use of cardiopulmonary bypass are placed on anticoagulant therapy to prevent thrombus formation secondary to red blood cell damage as the cells pass through the cardiopulmonary bypass device. This therapy also is used following valve replacement to prevent clot formation secondary to red blood cell damage as the cells are pumped through the artificial valve. Prophylactic antimicrobials are used prior to dental procedures. The child is placed on mechanical ventilation to improve body temperature, facilitate lung inflation, and maintain gas exchange. This usually is limited to 6 hours immediately following surgery. The chest tube drainage is monitored hourly. Following resolution of drainage from the pericardial sac, the pericardial chest tube is removed (usually within 24 hours following surgery); and after chest radiography determines resolution of lung inflation, the pleural chest tubes are removed. Pain management is required for 2 to 6 weeks postoperatively to control chest tube pain (until chest tubes are removed) and chest incision pain.

Nursing Management

ASSESSMENT

1. Assess vital signs
2. Auscultate heart and lung sounds
3. Obtain height and weight
4. Assess nutritional intake
5. Assess for history or current presence of dyspnea on exertion
6. Assess for manifestations of right- or left-sided heart failure

NURSING DIAGNOSES (INCLUDING BUT NOT LIMITED TO)

PREOPERATIVE

1. Imbalanced nutrition, less than body requirements R/T activity intolerance
2. Decreased cardiac output R/T ineffectiveness of cardiac pump
3. Ineffective tissue perfusion R/T decreased cardiac output
4. Excess fluid volume R/T ventricular overload and heart failure
5. Delayed growth and development R/T imbalanced nutrition, ineffective systemic tissue perfusion, and activity intolerance
6. Parental anxiety R/T child's condition and surgical treatment plan
7. Deficient knowledge R/T child's condition and treatment plan

POSTOPERATIVE

8. Ineffective thermoregulation R/T decreased environmental temperature of operating room during surgical procedure to decrease metabolic demands and allow for asystolic operative conditions
9. Risk for injury, dysrhythmias R/T surgical repair
10. Impaired gas exchange and ineffective airway clearance R/T intubation, open-heart surgical procedure, and atelectasis
11. Risk for infection R/T surgical procedure
12. Ineffective breathing pattern R/T acute pain following surgical procedure and presence of chest tubes
13. Acute pain R/T tissue trauma of surgery, incision, and presence of chest tubes
14. Risk for injury, thrombus formation R/T erythrocyte damage during cardiopulmonary bypass
15. Disturbed sleep pattern R/T pediatric intensive care environment
16. Deficient knowledge R/T postoperative care of child and home care

PLANNING/GOALS

PREOPERATIVE

1. Client will consume adequate nutrition to meet metabolic needs.
2. Client will regain and maintain adequate cardiac output as evidenced by warm, well-perfused extremities, strong peripheral pulses, vital signs within defined limits (WDL), cardiac rhythm WDL, and urine output of 1–2 mL/kg/hr.
3. Client will regain and maintain adequate tissue perfusion as evidenced by vital signs WDL, strong pulses in extremities, urine output WDL, and pulse oximetry readings within prescribed parameters.
4. Client will experience loss of excess fluid as evidenced by clear breath sounds and intake and output balance following increased urine output in response to diuretic therapy.
5. Client will participate in age-appropriate activities without dyspnea.
6. Parents will verbalize feelings and concerns about child's condition and changes in family processes due to child's condition.
7. Parents will verbalize understanding of child's condition, surgical procedure, and risks of surgery and what they will observe in child following surgery (equipment, monitors, etc.).

POSTOPERATIVE

8. Client's core body temperature will return to WDL within 6 hours following transfer to pediatric intensive care unit (PICU).
9. Client will remain free of cardiac dysrhythmias.
10. Client will maintain patent airway and adequate gas exchange as evidenced by oxygen saturation WDL.
11. Client will remain free of postoperative infection as evidenced by absence of temperature elevation indicative of infection; tachypnea; incision redness, swelling, and purulent drainage; and adventitious breath sounds.
12. Client will maintain effective breathing pattern as evidenced by respiratory rate and effort WDL and oxygen saturation WDL.
13. Client's pain level will be maintained at 1–2/10 on a 10-point scale with 10 being severe pain.
14. Client will not experience thrombus formation as evidenced by lack of thrombus manifestations.
15. Client will experience minimal sleep disturbances while in the PICU.
16. Parents will verbalize understanding of child's hospital postoperative care and home care.

NOC

PREOPERATIVE

1. Nutritional Status: Food and Fluid Intake
2. Cardiac Pump Effectiveness
3. Vital Signs
4. Fluid Balance, Fluid Overload Severity
5. Child Development
6. Anxiety Level
7. Knowledge: Medication, Treatment Procedure

POSTOPERATIVE

8. Thermoregulation
9. Cardiac Pump Effectiveness
10. Respiratory Status: Gas Exchange
11. Risk Control
12. Respiratory Status: Gas Exchange
13. Pain Control
14. Risk Control
15. Sleep
16. Knowledge: Illness Care, Health Promotion

IMPLEMENTATION

PREOPERATIVE

1. Nutrition
   a. Assess child's food preferences
   b. Monitor growth using standardized growth chart
   c. Create environment conducive to optimal nutritional intake
   d. Provide for frequent small feedings
   e. Breast-feed or formula-feed infants using smaller quantities every 2 hours
   f. Monitor intake and output
   g. Monitor caloric intake
   h. Weigh daily if hospitalized
   i. Encourage dietary sources high in protein, carbohydrates, fats, and calories
2. Cardiac output
   a. Monitor vital signs
   b. Auscultate heart sounds
   c. Assess for manifestations of congestive heart failure
   d. Administer diuretics as prescribed
   e. Monitor intake and output
   f. Weigh daily
   g. Monitor cardiac enzyme and electrolyte results
3. Tissue perfusion
   a. Keep child as free from stress as possible to conserve energy and oxygen demands
   b. Monitor capillary refill, heart sounds, and breath sounds
   c. Monitor vital signs
   d. Monitor peripheral pulses
   e. Collaborate with health care provider if alterations in tissue perfusion are assessed
   f. Administer propranolol as prescribed
   g. Monitor capillary blood glucose levels if child is nothing by mouth (npo) and receiving propranolol
   h. Monitor pulse oximetry
   i. Administer oxygen to maintain oxygen saturation within prescribed parameters
   j. Provide instructions for parents concerning manifestations of inadequate tissue perfusion

4. Fluid volume
   a. Monitor intake and output
   b. Weigh daily
   c. Administer diuretics as prescribed
   d. Administer antihypertensives as prescribed
   e. Monitor heart sounds and breath sounds
   f. Monitor for manifestations of congestive heart failure
   g. Assess skin turgor and color
5. Growth and development
   a. Assess child's current level of growth and development
   b. Compare findings to standardized assessment tool
   c. Assess parents' current level of knowledge regarding growth and development
   d. Provide parents with information on age-appropriate activities for their child that will promote growth and development while conserving energy (in the symptomatic child)
   e. Plot weight and height on growth chart
   f. Encourage child to participate in age-appropriate activities within child's energy level
6. Anxiety
   a. Assess parents for behaviors indicating anxiety
   b. Encourage parents to express feelings and concerns
   c. Listen actively to parents
   d. Encourage parents to participate in child's care
   e. Provide for multidisciplinary services (chaplain, social worker, etc.) as needed
7. Parent teaching
   a. Assess parents' current level of knowledge
   b. Assess parents' readiness to learn
   c. Provide brief, factual information sessions
   d. Encourage parents to ask questions and to express fears and concerns
   e. Provide information regarding child's particular heart defect(s), medication regimen, dietary alterations, and activity modifications
   f. Assess parents' level of understanding of new information
   g. Provide contact numbers for parents to call when questions and concerns arise
   h. Document teaching and parents' response

POSTOPERATIVE

8. Thermoregulation
   a. Place on mechanical ventilation upon arrival to PICU
   b. Monitor continuous skin temperature
   c. Provide warm blankets
   d. Monitor vital signs continuously
   e. Monitor respiratory status continuously for indications of hypothermia
   f. Monitor intravenous access site hourly
   g. Administer warmed intravenous fluids as prescribed, warming fluids by placing container in basin of warm water (do not microwave intravenous fluids)

9. Risk for dysrhythmias
    a. Place child on cardiopulmonary monitor with continuous pulse oximetry
    b. Administer oxygen to maintain oxygen saturation within prescribed parameters
    c. Administer volume resuscitation for hypovolemia
    d. Monitor strict intake and output and urine specific gravity
    e. Administer diuretics or afterload reducers as prescribed
    f. Monitor cardiac rate and rhythm continuously while in PICU
    g. Monitor ongoing losses through chest tubes, dressings, and urinary output
    h. Administer medications as prescribed
    i. Use temporary pacemaker as required
    j. Monitor calcium, magnesium, potassium, and sodium levels
    k. Administer electrolyte replacements as prescribed

10. Gas exchange
    a. Maintain on mechanical ventilation as prescribed until no longer experiencing postoperative hypothermia
    b. Ensure endotracheal tube security and verify placement every 2 hours
    c. Provide for adequate pharmacological interventions appropriate for mechanical ventilation
    d. Maintain continuous cardiopulmonary monitoring
    e. Monitor arterial blood gases via arterial line
    f. Monitor breath sounds
    g. Monitor intake and output
    h. Monitor chest and pericardial tube drainage at least hourly; if drainage exceeds prescribed volume parameters, report immediately to health care provider
    i. Maintain plastic or rubber-tipped hemostats at bedside while chest tubes are in place
    j. Monitor chest tube drainage device for indications of air leaks
    k. Encourage child to turn, cough, and deep-breathe every 2 hours once child no longer requires mechanical ventilation

11. Risk for infection
    a. Maintain and teach standard precautions and effective hand washing
    b. Monitor vital signs, especially temperature, every 2–4 hours
    c. Monitor heart and breath sounds
    d. Cleanse surgical incision per protocol
    e. Encourage high-protein, high-caloric diet

12. Breathing pattern
    a. Frequently assess breath sounds
    b. Assess pain level hourly using age-appropriate pain rating scales
    c. Administer analgesia proactively as prescribed
    d. Collaborate with health care provider for prescription changes if pain management is not adequate
    e. Monitor chest radiograph results
    f. Provide pulmonary toilet including chest physiotherapy
    g. Monitor arterial blood gases and pulse oximetry

    h. Administer oxygen to maintain oxygen saturation within pre-scribed parameters

13. Pain
    a. Assess pain level hourly using age-appropriate pain rating scale
    b. Position to avoid stress on chest tubes and incision
    c. Administer analgesia proactively as prescribed
    d. Administer analgesics (morphine sulfate) at scheduled intervals rather than p.r.n. basis
    e. Evaluate effectiveness of pain management interventions
    f. Address any concerns of parents regarding pain management

14. Risk for thrombus
    a. Assess for manifestations of thrombus formation
    b. Administer anticoagulants as prescribed
    c. Monitor laboratory values
    d. Monitor respiratory status for manifestations of embolus

15. Sleep
    a. Assess sleep pattern
    b. Cluster nursing activities to provide uninterrupted sleep
    c. Perform hourly assessments without waking child when possible
    d. Provide adequate pain management and control
    e. Maintain calm, quiet environment within constraints of the PICU setting

16. Parent teaching
    a. Assess parents' current level of understanding of child's hospital and home care
    b. Encourage parental participation in child's care during hospitalization
    c. Provide both verbal and written information regarding:
       1) Preventing infection (hand washing, which parents can return-demonstrate prior to the child's discharge)
       2) Administering medications, including information about medications (identification of each medication, drug action, route of administration, and adverse effects)
       3) Providing incision care
       4) Monitoring child's temperature and prescribed parameters for notifying the health care provider
       5) Stressing the importance of follow-up care and schedule for next appointment
       6) Discussing manifestations to report to health care provider
       7) Providing contact numbers
    d. Provide adequate time for teaching and parental questions
    e. Document teaching and parental response

NIC

PREOPERATIVE

1. Fluid Monitoring, Nutritional Monitoring
2. Medication Administration, Vital Signs Monitoring
3. Vital Signs Monitoring
4. Fluid Management, Hypervolemia Management
5. Developmental Enhancement: Child, Nutritional Monitoring

6. Anxiety Reduction
7. Teaching: Medication Administration, Treatment Procedure

POSTOPERATIVE

8. Temperature Regulation
9. Dysrhythmia Monitoring, Dysrhythmia Management
10. Oxygen Therapy, Ventilation Assistance
11. Risk Identification, Vital Signs Monitoring
12. Respiratory Monitoring, Pain Management
13. Pain Management
14. Risk Management
15. Sleep Enhancement
16. Health Education, Teaching

EVALUATION

PREOPERATIVE

1. Client consumes adequate nutrition to meet metabolic needs.
2. Client regains and maintains adequate cardiac output as evidenced by warm, well-perfused extremities, strong peripheral pulses, vital signs WDL, cardiac rhythm WDL, and urine output of 1–2 mL/kg/hr.
3. Client regains and maintains adequate tissue perfusion as evidenced by vital signs WDL, strong pulses in extremities, urine output WDL, and pulse oximetry readings within prescribed parameters.
4. Client experiences loss of excess fluid as evidenced by clear breath sounds and intake and output balance following increased urine output in response to diuretic therapy.
5. Client participates in age-appropriate activities without dyspnea.
6. Parents verbalize feelings and concerns about child's condition and changes in family processes due to child's condition.
7. Parents verbalize understanding of child's condition, surgical procedure, and risks of surgery what they will observe in child following surgery (equipment, monitors, etc.).

POSTOPERATIVE

8. Client's core body temperature returns to WDL within 6 hours following transfer to PICU.
9. Client remains free of cardiac dysrhythmias.
10. Client maintains patent airway and adequate gas exchange as evidenced by oxygen saturation WDL.
11. Client remains free of postoperative infection as evidenced by absence of temperature elevation indicative of infection; tachypnea; incision redness, swelling, and purulent drainage; and adventitious breath sounds.
12. Client maintains effective breathing pattern as evidenced by respiratory rate and effort WDL and oxygen saturation WDL.
13. Client's pain level is maintained at 1-2/10.
14. Client's does not experience thrombus formation as evidenced by lack of thrombus manifestations.
15. Client experiences minimal sleep disturbances while in the PICU.
16. Parents verbalize understanding of child's hospital postoperative care and home care.

References

American Heart Association. (2007). *Congenital cardiovascular defects*. Retrieved April 23, 2007, from http://www.americanheart.org/presenter.jhtml?identifier=4565

International Children's Heart Foundation. (n.d.). *Children and congenital heart defects*. Retrieved April 23, 2007, from http://www.ichf.org/doc/2354

March of Dimes. (2007). *Quick references and fact sheets: Congenital heart defects*. Retrieved January 24, 2008, from http://www.marchofdimes.com/professionals/14332_1212.asp

National Heart Lung and Blood Institute. (2007). *Congenital heart defects: What are congenital heart defects*. Retrieved January 24, 2007, from http://www.nhlbi.nih.gov/health/dci/Diseases/chd/chd_what.html

Potts, N. L., & Mandleco, B. L. (2007). *Pediatric nursing: Caring for children and their families* (2nd ed.). Clifton Park, NY: Delmar Cengage Learning.

27

CONGENITAL HIP DYSPLASIA/ DEVELOPMENTAL DYSPLASIA OF THE HIP

Definition

Congenital hip dysplasia, also called developmental dysplasia of the hip (DDH), is a congenital anomaly in which the head of the femur is not properly situated in the acetabulum, or hip socket, of the pelvis (Potts & Mandleco, 2007).

Pathophysiology

DDH can occur in one or both hips and includes three different conditions. An unstable hip is when the head of the femur is positioned in the acetabulum, but can be partially or completely luxated, or dislocated, with manual manipulation. When the head of the femur is partially positioned under the edge of the acetabulum, the DDH is called subluxation. Complete dislocation occurs when the femoral head is positioned completely outside the acetabulum. In addition to impairing physical mobility, DDH can place neuromuscular function at risk because of the malposition of the head of the femur, which can compress the tendons and ligaments attached to it. If untreated, DDH can result in osteoarthritis and pain by early adulthood (MedlinePlus, 2007).

Complications

Neuromuscular damage
Impaired physical mobility
Pain and osteoarthritis by early adulthood

Incidence

The incidence of DDH is variable and depends on many factors. Approximately 1 in 1,000 infants is born with a hip dislocation, and about 10 in 1,000 have hip subluxation (Storer & Scaggs, 2006). There is a higher incidence in girls than in boys, and it most often affects firstborn children. The risk is higher in Native Americans, "possibly due to swaddling of the infant that adducts the hips and brings them close together" (Potts & Mandleco, 2007, p. 1159). "The left hip is affected in 60 percent of children, the right hip in 20 percent, and both hips in 20 percent. The left hip is more commonly involved because it is adducted against the mother's lumbosacral spine in the most common intrauterine position" (Storer & Scaggs, 2006, p. 1).

Etiology

Various factors place an infant at risk for DDH, including breech presentation, female sex, positive family history for DDH, firstborn status, and oligohydramnios. Intrauterine position, gender, race, and positive family history are the most important risk factors. A family history of DDH is found in 12–33% of affected children. "The risk of DDH for a child has been documented at 6 percent when there is one affected sibling, 12 percent with one affected parent, and 36 percent if a parent and a sibling are affected. Eighty percent of children with DDH are females" (Storer & Scaggs, 2006, p. 1).

Clinical Manifestations

Asymmetry of gluteal folds

Limited range of motion in affected hip

Appearance of shortened femur on affected side

Asymmetric abduction of the affected hip

Diagnostic Tests

Barlow's test (maneuver)

Ortolani's test (maneuver)

Radiography of the hip

Ultrasound

Medical Management

The focus of management for DDH is early recognition and treatment to improve results and to decrease the risk of complications (Storer & Skaggs, 2006). For neonates, mild dysplasia can be treated through the use of double or triple diapering to maintain the hips in abduction and position the femoral head in the acetabulum. The standard of care for infants under the age of 6 months with mild to moderate dysplasia is wearing a Pavlik harness, an abduction device, for 1–2 months. Refer to Figure 27-1.

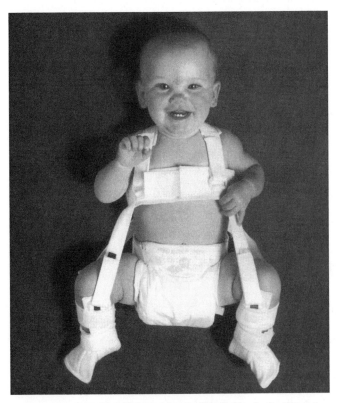

Figure 27-1: Infant with DDH in a Pavlik Harness. Courtesy of Wheaton Brace Co., Carol Stream, IL.

Skin traction or surgical repair is performed when the Pavlik harness is not successful in correcting the DDH or when the child is diagnosed after the age of 6 months. With the infant under anesthesia, manipulation and closed reduction of the dysplasia is the major method of treatment; however, open surgical reduction may be required. For both surgeries, the child must be placed in a spica cast postoperatively. Pain management and cast care are priorities following both reduction surgeries, and routine follow-up radiography determines when the cast can be removed.

Nursing Management

ASSESSMENT

1. Assess all neonates for possible DDH, especially females and all babies born in breech position
2. Assess neurovascular status of affected limb
3. Assess parental knowledge about condition, use of Pavlik harness, and postoperative home care
4. Assess skin of child in Pavlik harness or spica cast
5. Assess parental anxiety level and coping strategies

NURSING DIAGNOSES (INCLUDING BUT NOT LIMITED TO)

1. Impaired physical mobility R/T lack of continuity of femur and hip
2. Risk for ineffective peripheral tissue perfusion R/T compression of neuromuscular structures
3. Risk for injury R/T difficult positioning of child in infant-carrying devices (car seats and infant carriers)
4. Risk for impaired skin integrity R/T chafing of skin by Pavlik harness or edges of spica cast
5. Deficient knowledge R/T condition, treatment, and home care

PLANNING/GOALS

1. Client's hip will be maintained in abducted position until DDH is resolved as evidenced by radiography.
2. Circulation to client's feet and toes on affected side will remain adequate as evidenced by capillary refill, sensation, movement, and temperature within defined limits (WDL).
3. Client will not experience injury and will be safely restrained when traveling in motor vehicle.
4. Client's skin will remain intact.
5. Parents will demonstrate understanding of condition and treatment and care of child in Pavlik harness and spica cast.

NOC

1. Skeletal Function
2. Circulation Status
3. Risk Control
4. Tissue Integrity: Skin
5. Knowledge: Illness Care, Treatment, Health Promotion

IMPLEMENTATION

1. Physical mobility
   a. Assess every newborn for manifestations of DDH
   b. Notify health care provider if manifestations are noted

    c. Apply double or triple diapers as prescribed

    d. Be available for parents if diagnosis of DDH is made

2. Tissue perfusion

    a. Assess peripheral pulses, warmth and color of feet and toes, and pain after application of Pavlik harness, open reduction, and cast application

    b. Demonstrate application of Pavlik harness to ensure tissue perfusion

    c. Have parents return demonstration

    d. Assess tissue perfusion as stated previously every 30 minutes for 4 hours and then according to facility protocol if postoperative

    e. Handle cast with palms of hands (not fingers) until cast is dry

    f. Elevate casted lower extremities to decrease edema

    g. Encourage parents to participate in care

3. Risk for injury

    a. Assess parents' understanding of application of Pavlik harness or care of spica cast

    b. Stress importance of infant being in restraints when in motor vehicle

4. Skin integrity

    a. Assess skin under harness or spica cast

    b. Teach parents how to inspect skin and how to diaper infant without removing harness and the importance of frequent position changes

    c. Have parents return demonstration

    d. Encourage parents to participate in care

    e. Petal cast edges prior to discharging infant in spica cast from the hospital

5. Parent teaching

    a. Assess parents' current level of knowledge

    b. Provide verbal, written, and demonstration instructions regarding:

        1) Application of Pavlik harness

        2) Assessment of tissue perfusion

        3) Assessment of skin

        4) Diapering of infant in Pavlik harness or spica cast

        5) Importance of keeping skin dry

        6) Importance of reporting changes in tissue perfusion or skin integrity immediately to health care provider

        7) Importance of follow-up with health care provider

        8) Contact numbers for health care provider and any referrals

    c. Provide adequate time for teaching and parent return demonstration of skills

    d. Document teaching and parents' response

NIC

1. Positioning

2. Positioning

3. Surveillance Safety

4. Traction/Immobilization Care, Cast Care: Maintenance

5. Teaching: Illness Care, Treatment, Health Promotion

EVALUATION

1. Client's hip is maintained in abducted position until DDH is resolved as evidenced by radiography.
2. Circulation to client's feet and toes on affected side remains adequate as evidenced by capillary refill, sensation, movement, and temperature WDL.
3. Client does not experience injury and is safely restrained when traveling in motor vehicle.
4. Client's skin remains intact.
5. Parents demonstrate understanding of condition and treatment and care of child in Pavlik harness and spica cast.

References

MedlinePlus. (2007). *Developmental dysplasia of the hip.* Retrieved January, 24, 2007, from http://www.nlm.nih.gov/medlineplus/ency/article/000971.htm

Potts, N. L., & Mandleco, B. L. (2007). *Pediatric nursing: Caring for children and their families* (2nd ed.). Clifton Park, NY: Delmar Cengage Learning.

Storer, S. K., & Scaggs, D. L. (2006). Developmental dysplasia of the hip. *American Family Physician, 74*, 1310–1316. Retrieved April 23, 2007, from http://www.aafp.org/afp/20061015/1310.html

28

CONSTIPATION

Definition

"Constipation is defined as having a bowel movement fewer than three times per week" (National Institute of Diabetes and Digestive and Kidney Diseases, 2006, p. 1) and the difficult passage of dry, hard stools from the bowel.

Pathophysiology

Normally, when products of digestion move through the large intestines, fluid and electrolytes are extracted through the intestinal wall, changing the stool from a primarily liquid substance to a soft form shaped like the tubular colon. "Normal defecation occurs when stool moves into the rectum causing rectal distention and relaxation of the internal anal sphincter. The conscious awareness of the rectal distention results in the contraction of voluntary muscles of the external anal sphincter. Voluntary relaxation of the external sphincter and increased intra-abdominal pressure results [*sic*] in defecation" (Potts & Mandleco, 2007, p. 680).

Normal defecation is contingent on the presence of three factors: (1) adequate fluid intake, (2) physical activity, and (3) ingestion of dietary bulk. If any of these factors is inadequate or if an obstruction is present, intestinal peristalsis slows or stops, resulting in constipation. The presence of other factors can decrease peristalsis, including structural gastrointestinal disorders, metabolic and endocrine disorders, and neurogenic dysfunction. This can then lead to organic constipation.

The majority of children have functional constipation brought about by emotional stress, changes in a child's normal daily routine, a desire not to interrupt play, and excess milk or cheese intake. Some children choose not to defecate. If a child does not want to defecate, he/she tightens the external anal sphincter and the gluteal muscles, causing the feces to be pushed in the rectal vault, which reduces the urge to defecate. If this behavior is frequent, over time the rectum eventually stretches to accommodate the retained fecal mass and the propulsive power of the rectum is diminished (Biggs & Dery, 2006). When the child does defecate, it can be painful. Once overdistention of the rectum occurs and defecation becomes painful, the child can worsen the condition by voluntarily refusing to defecate because of the pain. Eventually, as the stool products remain in the rectum, forcing the rectum to become increasingly distended, anal fissures can develop from the strain the distention places on the sensitive mucous membranes lining the rectum. Furthermore, over time, the bulk of the stool can lead to rectal enlargement, loss of anal sphincter control, and encopresis (fecal incontinence). Encopresis occurs in 35% of girls and 55% of boys who have constipation (Biggs & Dery, 2006). According to the American Academy of Family Physicians, in spite of treatment, only 50–70% of children with functional constipation demonstrate long-term improvement (American Academy of Family Physicians, 2006).

If the child does not consume sufficient fluids, the products of digestion are less liquid and as they move through the large intestines and fluid and electrolytes are absorbed, the stool becomes dry and hard and less movable. As long as stool remains in the large intestines, more fluid is removed, causing the stool to become ever drier and harder. This causes the stool to become difficult and even painful to expel. Decreased activity leads to slowed peristalsis, and the same process occurs. Inadequate dietary bulk also decreases peristalsis.

Complications

Rectal distention

Painful defecation

Rectal fissures

Encopresis

Incidence

Constipation is a very common problem in children and accounts for 3–5% of all pediatric outpatient clinics visits and up to 35% of all pediatric gastroenterologist visits (Borowitz, 2006). "In general, over 4 million people in the United States have frequent constipation, accounting for 2.5 million health care provider visits annually" (National Institute of Diabetes and Digestive and Kidney Diseases, 2006, p. 1). Constipation is extremely common among infants and young children. Approximately 16% of toddlers experience constipation. Internationally, approximately 34% of children aged 4–7 years living in the United Kingdom had at least intermittent difficulties with constipation. Another study found that 28% of Brazilian children aged 8–10 years experienced constipation. Prior to puberty, the incidence is the same for boys and girls; but after puberty, females are more likely to develop constipation (Borowitz, 2006). Constipation is responsible for an estimated 3–5% of children's visits to pediatricians (Borowitz, 2006).

Etiology

For the majority of children, constipation is not related to structural physiological disorders. Rather, it is related to emotional stress (moving to a new home or parental discord); major changes in the child's daily routine (starting preschool or school); and inadequate fluid intake, excessive milk or cheese intake, and lack of dietary bulk. Constipation is a common adverse effect of surgical procedures as well as central nervous system pharmacological agents required for pain management following surgery. The most common adverse effect associated with the use of opioid analgesics is constipation (Broyles, Reiss, & Evans, 2007). Iron-fortified formula is a leading cause of constipation in infants. Examples of organic causes include gastrointestinal disorders (intussusception, Hirschsprung's disease, and appendicitis), metabolic and endocrine disorders (hypothyroidism), and neurogenic dysfunction (spina bifida). Constipation may be genetic in origin.

Clinical Manifestations

Abdominal cramping and pain

Infrequent passage of dry, hard stools

Large, palpable stool in the rectum

Nausea and vomiting

Malaise

"Liquid or solid, clay-like stool in the child's underwear—a sign that stool is backed up in the rectum" (National Institute of Diabetes and Digestive and Kidney Diseases, 2006, p. 1)

Anal fissure

Encopresis

Diagnostic Tests

Abdominal radiography

Computed tomography

Medical Management

The focus of management is to return the bowel to normal functioning. This involves combination therapy including determining the cause of the constipation, cleansing the bowel, changing dietary and fluid habits, and changing defecation habits. Mechanical or organic causes must be ruled out; then the team must determine what psychosocial issue is causing the constipation and develop an approach to overcome the problem. Communicating with the child using age-appropriate language is important when determining the etiology as well as planning the treatment regimen (Biggs & Dery, 2006).

Enemas, suppositories, and medications are used to empty the colon and cleanse the bowel. Dietary changes include increasing fluid intake, increasing intake of high-fiber foods, and limiting milk and cheese intake. Changing bowel patterns may be the greatest challenge; however, the use of stool softeners may help decrease the discomfort the child has experienced when defecating. Stool softeners and laxatives must be used with caution to prevent diarrhea and resulting dehydration and electrolyte imbalances. Having the child sit on the commode for 10–15 minutes after meals and providing a relaxed, nonhurried environment have been successful techniques.

Nursing Management

ASSESSMENT

1. Obtain nutritional history
2. Obtain bowel habit history
3. Assess for changes in child's routine or presence of emotional stressors
4. Obtain height and weight

NURSING DIAGNOSES (INCLUDING BUT NOT LIMITED TO)

1. Constipation R/T emotional stress, inadequate fluid and fiber intake, dramatic reduction in activity, and pain during elimination
2. Acute pain R/T defecation
3. Risk for impaired tissue integrity R/T incontinence, development of fissures
4. Deficient knowledge R/T condition, treatment regimen, and bowel health promotion

PLANNING/GOALS

1. Client will experience normal bowel function as evidenced by passage of soft, formed stools every 1–2 days.
2. Client will experience normal bowel function without pain.
3. Client's anal area will not exhibit skin/tissue breakdown.
4. Parents/child (if age-appropriate) will demonstrate understanding of condition, treatment regimen, and bowel health promotion.

NOC

1. Bowel Elimination
2. Comfort Level, Pain Level
3. Tissue Integrity
4. Knowledge: Illness Care, Treatment, Health Promotion

IMPLEMENTATION

1. Bowel elimination
   a. Assess fluid and fiber intake
   b. Assess child's food and fluid preferences

   c. Collaborate with parents and dietician to develop a diet high in fluids and fiber considering child's preferences as much as possible
   d. Increase fluid intake to 20 mL/kg until constipation is resolved
   e. Encourage child to sit (for 10–15 minutes) on commode 20–30 minutes after eating
   f. Create a calm, unhurried environment
   g. Encourage child to discuss any events that have been stressful
   h. Encourage parents to participate in discussion
   i. Administer enemas and suppositories as prescribed to cleanse bowel
   j. Administer stool softeners and gentle child laxative (MiraLAX) as prescribed
2. Painful defecation
   a. Discuss causes of painful defecation
   b. Administer stool softeners and gentle child laxative as prescribed, explaining to child that the hard stool caused the pain but that these medications will make the stool soft so there is no pain
   c. Encourage verbalization of concerns, fears, and anxieties
3. Tissue integrity
   a. Assess anal area for indications of skin/tissue breakdown
   b. Teach appropriate hygiene to keep area as clean as possible
   c. Apply topical medications as prescribed
4. Parent/client teaching
   a. Assess current level of understanding of constipation
   b. Provide verbal and written instructions regarding:
      1) Causes of constipation
      2) Prescribed fluid intake
      3) Prescribed dietary modifications—increased fiber including unrefined cereal grains, fresh fruits, whole wheat, vegetables, dried fruits (prunes, figs, and apricots), and unprocessed wheat bran.
      4) Modifications focused on overcoming withholding stool
      5) Medication administration if prescribed for home use
      6) Anal skin care
   c. Provide adequate time for teaching and questions
   d. Document teaching and parent/child response

NIC

1. Bowel Management
2. Pain Management
3. Skin Surveillance
4. Teaching: Illness Care, Treatment, Health Promotion

EVALUATION

1. Client experiences normal bowel function as evidenced by passage of soft, formed stools every 1–2 days.
2. Client experiences normal bowel function without pain.
3. Client's anal area does not exhibit skin/tissue breakdown.
4. Parents/child (if age-appropriate) demonstrate understanding of condition, treatment regimen, and bowel health promotion.

References

American Academy of Family Physicians. (2006). *Constipation: Keeping your bowels moving smoothly.* Retrieved April 23, 2007, from http://familydoctor.org/037.xml

Biggs, W. S., & Dery, W. H. (2006). *Evaluation and treatment of constipation in infants and children.* Retrieved January 24, 2007, from http://www.aafp.org/afp/20060201/469.html

Borowitz, S. (2006). *Constipation.* Retrieved January 24, 2007, from http://www.emedicine.com/ped/topic471.html

Broyles, B. E., Reiss, B. S., & Evans, M. E. (2007). *Pharmacological aspects of nursing care* (7th ed.). Clifton Park, NY: Delmar Cengage Learning.

National Institute of Diabetes and Digestive and Kidney Diseases. (2006). *Constipation.* Retrieved April 23, 2007, from http://digestive.niddk.nih.gov/ddiseases/pubs/constipation

Potts, N. L., & Mandleco, B. L. (2007). *Pediatric nursing: Caring for children and their families* (2nd ed.). Clifton Park, NY: Delmar Cengage Learning.

29

CROUP

Definition

Croup is an acute respiratory syndrome usually occurring after an acute viral infection of the respiratory system. Laryngotracheobronchitis (LTB) and spasmodic laryngitis (spasmodic croup) are the different types of croup.

Pathophysiology

The viral respiratory infection usually caused by parainfluenza results in inflammation that leads to edema of the mucosa, increased respiratory secretions, and spasms of the bronchial smooth muscle. The inflammation and the normal narrow pediatric airway result in varying amounts of obstruction as air flows through the larynx (Cincinnati Children's Hospital Medical Center, 2005). In addition, "the glottis tends to collapse during inspiration in response to edema and muscle spasms [and] further obstructs the airway" (Potts & Mandleco, 2007, p. 716). This obstruction leads to the characteristic stridor and barking cough. As the child struggles to inspire sufficient oxygen, varying degrees of respiratory distress can occur. As the respiratory rate increases, the child experiences an increase in insensible fluid loss. As the condition progresses, the child is at increased risk for a secondary bacterial infection, usually tracheitis. Croup in its most severe form, epiglottitis, is a medical emergency. (*NOTE:* Refer to Chapter 39: Epiglottitis.)

Complications

Respiratory distress
Bacterial tracheitis
Dehydration
Epiglottitis

Incidence

Viral croup is most common in young children ages 6 months to 5 years. Croup is rare in the first 6 months of life with the youngest reported child with croup being 3 months old (Desai & Greenberg, 2007). It accounts for approximately 15% of clinic and emergency department visits for pediatric respiratory infections. In the United States the incidence peaks in 2-year-olds at 5–6 cases per 100 children. Approximately 5% of children experience more than one episode, and it is most common in late fall and early winter (Molodow, 2007). Croup is more common in males than in females. Children who are born prematurely, have reactive airway disease (asthma), or have especially small airways are more prone to develop croup (Kids Health, 2005).

Etiology

Croup is a viral respiratory infection that is easily passed among children. The most common cause is parainfluenza, accounting for 75% of cases. Other etiologies include influenza, adenovirus, respiratory syncytial virus (RSV), rhinovirus, and measles (MedlinePlus, 2006).

Clinical Manifestations

Cough that sounds like a barking seal, particularly when a child is crying (MedlinePlus, 2006)

Low-grade fever

Nasal drainage

Coarse throat

Tachycardia

Tachypnea

Hoarseness

Difficulty swallowing

Stridor

Varying degrees of respiratory distress

Diagnostic Tests

Pulse oximetry

Bronchoscopy

Presence of steeple sign (visible upper airway narrowing)

Medical Management

The goals of treatment are to restore airway patency, support respiratory function, and treat any underlying bacterial infection. Most children with croup can be effectively treated at home with humidification, acetaminophen for fever, fluids, and rest. Over-the-counter cough preparations should be avoided.

If home care is not effective and the child has LTB, hospitalization usually is necessary. Humidified oxygen and cool mist environment are prescribed to moisten secretions and inflamed tissues to open the airway and soothe irritation. Children who do not respond to the mist tent are prescribed albuterol nebulizer treatments to decrease the swelling in the respiratory airway. Intravenous steroid therapy has been shown to be of benefit in children with moderate to severe croup. Intravenous antibiotics are prescribed to treat secondary bacterial infections.

Nursing Management

Assessment

1. Obtain history
2. Assess airway, breath, and circulation (ABC)
3. Assess for respiratory stridor, barking cough, and tachypnea
4. Obtain vital signs
5. Assess breath sounds
6. Assess hydration status

Nursing Diagnoses (including but not limited to)

1. Ineffective airway clearance R/T inflamed and edematous airway tissues
2. Deficient fluid volume R/T insensible fluid loss and inadequate intake
3. Anxiety (parent/child) R/T hospitalization, dyspnea
4. Deficient knowledge R/T condition, treatment plan, and home care

Planning/Goals

1. Client will experience return to baseline respiratory status as evidenced by a respiratory rate and breath sounds within defined limits (WDL) and absence of stridor and barking cough.

2. Client will regain and maintain fluid balance as evidence by fluid intake WDL for age and weight and urine output > 1 mL/kg/hr.

3. Parents/client will demonstrate reduced anxiety as evidenced by verbalizations, participation in child's care, and presence of nonverbal indicators of decreased anxiety.

4. Parents will demonstrate understanding of condition, treatment, and home care.

NOC

1. Respiratory Status: Airway Patency
2. Fluid Balance
3. Anxiety Level
4. Knowledge: Illness Care, Treatment, Health Promotion

IMPLEMENTATION

1. Airway
   a. Assess respiratory status and vital signs frequently
   b. Place on cardiorespiratory monitor and pulse oximetry monitoring
   c. Administer oxygen and titrate to prescribed level of oxygen saturation
   d. Administer nebulizers as prescribed
   e. Maintain cool mist environment
   f. Maintain patency of intravenous access, monitoring hourly
   g. Administer steroid therapy as prescribed
   h. Elevate head of child's bed
   i. Keep emergency equipment nearby
   j. Provide calm, supportive environment and frequent rest periods

2. Fluid balance
   a. Monitor strict intake and output
   b. Report urine output < 1 mL/kg/hr to health care provider
   c. Maintain patency of intravenous access, monitoring hourly
   d. Encourage oral fluid intake, monitoring closely for aspiration
   e. Involve parents in child's care

3. Anxiety
   a. Assess for indications of anxiety in parents/child
   b. Encourage verbalization of feelings, concerns, and questions
   c. Explain condition and all treatments and equipment
   d. Encourage child's involvement in age-appropriate play with toys that can be used in a high-humidity environment (bath toys)
   e. Encourage parental participation in taking care of child and personalizing child's room with comfort items from home

4. Parent/caregiver teaching
   a. Assess parent's current level of knowledge
   b. Provide verbal and written information regarding:
      1) Importance of adequate hydration
      2) Importance of hand washing and appropriate technique for prevention of respiratory infections
      3) Medication administration if child remains on nebulizer treatments and antibiotics
      4) Importance of treating fever with acetaminophen or PediaProfen
      5) Need for follow-up care

      6) Manifestations of worsening of child's condition

      7) Contact numbers to report observations and ask questions

  c. Provide adequate time for teaching and parental questions

  d. Document teaching and parental response

NIC

1. Airway Management, Vital Signs Monitoring, Medication Administration

2. Fluid Resuscitation, Fluid Monitoring

3. Anxiety Reduction

4. Teaching: Illness Care, Treatment, Health Promotion

EVALUATION

1. Client experiences return to baseline respiratory status as evidenced by a respiratory rate and breath sounds WDL and absence of stridor and barking cough.

2. Client regains and maintains fluid balance as evidenced by fluid intake WDL for age and weight and urine output > 1 mL/kg/hr.

3. Parents/client demonstrate reduced anxiety as evidenced by verbalizations, participation in child's care, and presence of nonverbal indicators of decreased anxiety.

4. Parents demonstrate understanding of condition, treatment, and home care.

References

Cincinnati Children's Hospital Medical Center. (2005). *Croup*. Retrieved April 23, 2007, from http://www.cincinnatichildrens.org/health/info/chest/diagnose/croup.htm

Desai, A., & Greenbery, S. B. (2007). *Croup*. Retrieved January 24, 2008, from http://www.emedicine.com/radio/topic199.htm

Kids Health. (2005). *Croup*. Retrieved April 23, 2007, from http://kidshealth.org/parent/infections/bacterial_viral/croup.html

MedlinePlus. (2006). *Croup*. Retrieved April 23, 2007, from http://www.nlm.nih.gov/medlineplus/ency/article/000959.htm

Molodow, R. E. (2007). *Croup*. Retrieved January 24, 2008, from http://www.emedicine.com/ped/topic510.htm

Potts, N. L., & Mandleco, B. L. (2007). *Pediatric nursing: Caring for children and their families* (2nd ed.). Clifton Park, NY: Delmar Cengage Learning.

30

Cystic Fibrosis (CF)/Lung Transplantation

Definition

Cystic fibrosis is an inherited (autosomal recessive) chronic, progressive multisystem disease of the body's exocrine glands. Lung transplantation is the surgical procedure for removing diseased lungs and replacing them with functional lungs from a human donor.

Pathophysiology

Cystic Fibrosis (CF)

The exocrine glands of the body are located primarily in the digestive, pulmonary, integumentary, and reproductive systems and are mucus-secreting glands. CF is characterized by the secretion of thick, tenacious mucus from these glands and by altered sweat electrolytes. The digestive and pulmonary systems are the most adversely affected by this thick mucus. The mucus obstructs the pancreatic ducts in the digestive system, prohibiting the pancreatic enzymes from passing into the small intestine. These enzymes—amylase, trypsin, and lipase—are necessary for the chemical digestion of carbohydrates, proteins, and fats. Without these enzymes, malabsorption of these macronutrients occurs. In the case of carbohydrates, they already have undergone chemical digestion in both the mouth and the stomach. For proteins, chemical digestion begins in the stomach. But for fats, chemical digestion begins in the duodenum; so they are most affected by lack of chemical digestion. As a result, fats are not available as a secondary source of energy. Decreased muscle mass occurs as protein is used for energy. The undigested fat is expelled through the bowel (steatorrhea), which creates a distinctive bulky, foul-smelling stool. The bulkiness of the stools leads to rectal prolapse, a common complication of CF. Obstruction of the pancreatic ducts also leads to pancreatitis and diabetes mellitus in children with CF (Broyles, 2005).

The tenacious mucus affects the integumentary system, resulting in "marked impermeability to chloride and an excessive reabsorption of sodium" (Potts & Mandleco, 2007, p. 740). This has a negative impact on fluid balance and increases the risk for dehydration. The increased secretion of these electrolytes through the skin results in the classic, and frequently initial, manifestation of the skin of infants and young children with CF "tasting salty" when kissed.

With CF, the alterations that occur in the reproductive system affect both males and females. Sterility occurs in 98% of males as a result of mucus obstruction of the ducts and seminal vesicles. Although sterility occurs, there is no evidence of impotence in these individuals. In females with CF, the beginning of menses is usually delayed and fertility is compromised because the thick cervical mucus impedes the travel of sperm (Broyles, 2005).

The most life-shortening and life-threatening changes occurring with CF are in the lungs. The alterations in electrolytes cause dehydration of the airway secretions. Although the cough reflex is active, the nature of the secretions inhibits expectoration, which leads to obstruction of the airway. The thick, tenacious secretions not only obstruct the airway but also serve as excellent media for bacterial growth. Over time, the majority of children with CF become colonized with multiple organisms such as *Haemophilus influenzae, Staphylococcus aureus, Pseudomonas aeruginosa, Pseudomonas cepacia, Serratia, Actinobacilli,* and *Klebsiella.* These bacterial infections cause the release of toxins and other products that lead to inflammation of the bronchi. Chronic infections (the most common cause of hospitalization in these children) and obstruction of the airway by the thick secretions cause the obstruction of bronchial epithelium and bronchiestasis, the irreversible dilation and deterioration of the bronchial walls (Potts & Mandleco, 2007).

In addition, these recurrent infections cause scarring (fibrosis) of the alveoli of the lungs, leading to impaired gas exchange. As the child works harder to compensate, the muscles of the thoracic cavity are stretched, resulting in another classic manifestation of CF, the barrel chest. Ultimately, these changes result in respiratory failure.

The obstruction in the lungs causes increased pulmonary resistance that leads to an increased workload on the heart, especially the right side. As the heart attempts to pump blood into the lungs against this resistance, right ventricular hypertrophy occurs, which eventually can result in cor pulmonale. Over time, congestive heart failure results.

LUNG TRANSPLANTATION

Although lung transplantation is considered a last resort for those experiencing respiratory failure due to CF, it is the only cure for the lung involvement of CF and is necessary to extend the lives of these children into adulthood. As with all transplants, the possibility of life-threatening infections secondary to immunosuppression (required to prevent organ rejection) is high and these infections are the leading cause of posttransplant death. Currently, survival rates are as high as 80% at one year following transplantation and 60% at four years (MedlinePlus, 2007).

To be considered a candidate for lung transplantation, the potential recipient must meet strict criteria, including severe end-stage pulmonary disease for which there is no alternative treatment, progressive disability, and life expectancy of two years or less. Donor requirements include a healthy organ for transplant, compatible blood type (same blood type as the recipient), donor who is free of infection and cancer, and donor who is less than 55 years of age. Lung transplant donors may be living or deceased. A complication unique to lung transplants is the development of obliterative bronchiolitis, an irreversible lung infiltration resolvable only with retransplantation and a complication that occurs in 10–50% of long-term survivors' experiences (MedlinePlus, 2007).

Complications

CYSTIC FIBROSIS

Malabsorption
Dehydration
Liver failure
Pancreatitis
Diabetes mellitus
Congestive heart failure
Cor pulmonale
Sterility
Life-threatening respiratory infections
Rib fractures (from severe coughing to expel secretions)
Respiratory acidosis
Respiratory failure
Death

LUNG TRANSPLANTATION

Life-threatening infections secondary to immunosuppression
Organ rejection
Obliterative bronchiolitis

Incidence

CYSTIC FIBROSIS

Until the advent of aggressive pulmonary therapy and lung transplantation, children with CF died in early childhood. Today people with CF often live into their thirties; some live even longer.

According to the Cystic Fibrosis Foundation and the March of Dimes, CF affects the lungs and digestive systems of about 30,000 children and adults in the United States (70,000 worldwide) (Cystic Fibrosis Foundation, 2007; March of Dimes, 2006). At least 40% of people with CF today are 18 years or older; and in 2005, the average age of survival was nearly 37 years (Cystic Fibrosis Foundation, 2007). CF affects Caucasian children more than any other race, with approximately 1 in 3,200 being affected. The incidence in Hispanic children is 1 in 9,500; in African-American children, the incidence is 1 in 15,000; and in Asian-American children, the incidence is 1 in 31,000. Approximately 1,000 new cases are diagnosed each year, usually before the child reaches three years of age (Potts & Mandleco, 2007).

LUNG TRANSPLANTATION

"According to the International Society of Heart and Lung Transplantation (ISHLT), 1245 lung or heart-lung transplants were performed in children as of 2003. In January 2005, 214 patients younger than 18 years were on the United Network for Organ Sharing (UNOS) waiting list for either lung or heart-lung transplants" (Faro & Visner, 2006, Section 2). According to UNOS, since 1988, approximately 500 lung transplants have been completed on children 17 years old and younger, with 49 transplants in the first half of 2006 (United Network for Organ Sharing, 2007).

Etiology

CYSTIC FIBROSIS

CF is an autosomal recessive genetic disorder; and according to the Cystic Fibrosis Foundation, "more than 10 million people in the United States, or 1 in 31, are symptomless carriers of the defective CF gene. An individual must inherit a defective copy of the CF gene—one from each parent—to have CF. Each time two carriers conceive a child, there is a 25% chance that the child will have CF, a 50% chance that the child will be a carrier, and a 25% chance that the child will be a noncarrier" (Cystic Fibrosis Foundation, n.d., p. 1).

LUNG TRANSPLANTATION

"In children aged 1–10 years, end-stage lung disease due to cystic fibrosis (CF) results in approximately 36% of all lung transplants. In adolescents, that number increases to approximately 60%. Chronic lung disease of infancy, bronchiolitis obliterans, congenital cardiac disease, and pulmonary fibrosis are other diagnoses that commonly lead to lung transplantation" (Faro & Visner, 2006, p. 1). As many as 90% of people with CF survive one year after transplantation, and 50% are alive after five years (Cystic Fibrosis Foundation, 2007).

Clinical Manifestations

CYSTIC FIBROSIS

Meconium ileus (occurs in about 20% of cases)
Rectal prolapse
Steatorrhea
Malabsorption
Thin, underweight, and lacking fat deposits

Protuberant abdomen

Biliary cirrhosis

Hyperglycemia

Hyponatremia

Hypochloremia

Infertility

Recurrent respiratory infections

Adventitious breath sounds including wheezing and crackles

Use of accessory muscles to breathe

Productive cough

Barrel chest

Heart failure

Pneumothorax, hemothorax, and atelectasis

Hemoptysis

Cor pulmonale

Diagnostic Tests

CYSTIC FIBROSIS

Sweat chlorides (definitive diagnostic test for CF)

Family history of CF

Prenatal chorionic villi sampling and DNA analysis

72-hour fecal fat

Liver enzymes

Fasting blood sugar

Chest X-ray

Sputum culture and sensitivity

Pulmonary function test

LUNG TRANSPLANTATION

Blood and tissue typing

Complete blood count

Serum chemistries

Blood coagulation studies

Urinalysis and culture and sensitivity

Pulmonary function tests

Ventilation-perfusion lung scan

Chest computed tomography (CT)

Liver function tests

Kidney function tests

Echocardiography

Electrocardiography

Medical Management

CYSTIC FIBROSIS

Management for CF is a lifelong process. The goals of treatment are to maintain respiratory function, prevent infection, and maintain nutrition consistent with metabolic needs. The primary focus of treatment is to maintain pulmonary function and prevent respiratory infections. The client with CF is placed on a strict regimen of chest physiotherapy (CPT), including percussion and postural drainage, two to four times a day depending on the severity of the disease, active cycle breathing exercises, positive expiratory pressure, and an individualized exercise program. Parents/family members are involved in the respiratory regimen, performing the percussion and postural drainage and ensuring that the exercises are routinely completed. Antibiotic therapy is essential in treating lung infections that are common with CF. This may require hospitalization for "pulmonary cleanout" using a 14-day regimen of intravenous medications including an aminoglycoside (gentamicin), vancomycin or tobramycin, and the cephalosporin ceftazidime. Ceftazidime has been shown to keep *Pseudomonas* pulmonary infections in check. Bronchodilators, anti-inflammatory agents, and mucolytics are all part of the maintenance regimen. Inhaled medications such as Pulmozyme (especially designed to thin mucus associated with CF), gentamicin, albuterol, and colistin are adjunctive medications also used to treat/prevent infections (Broyles, Reiss, & Evans, 2007).

Pancreatic enzymes (Pancrease) are taken with each high-calorie, high-carbohydrate, high-protein meal and snack to facilitate digestion and absorption. Supplemental fat-soluble vitamins (A, D, E, and K) are needed daily. If a child is not able to consume sufficient intake, the individual may require the surgical placement of a gastrostomy tube for overnight enteral feedings. This is most commonly needed during adolescence when growth is rapid (Broyles, 2005).

Gene therapy has been investigated since 1989, when the defective CF gene was discovered. Gene therapy has the potential for offering the best hope for providing a life-saving treatment that attacks the cause of CF, rather than just managing the symptoms. Clinical research continues to help refine gene delivery.

LUNG TRANSPLANTATION

If the child with CF has experienced a loss of over 50% pulmonary function, lung transplantation becomes a viable option. Although lung transplantation will not cure CF, it does cure the respiratory involvement because the transplanted lung(s) are free of the defective CF gene. Partial lung transplantation (transplanting individual lobes from live donors) has been used with success in pediatric clients.

The goal of lung transplantation is to provide healthy functional lungs that allow the recipient a longer life span and greater quality of life than the recipient would otherwise experience. A lung transplantation procedure lasts from 4 to 8 hours for single-lung transplants and from 6 to 12 hours to transplant both lungs. The surgery is performed only in medical centers that have the technology for such a procedure and for posttransplant care. In complicated cases, these time frames may be longer.

The procedure begins when the donor lung or lungs are delivered to the operating room. After the induction of general anesthesia, an indwelling urinary catheter, a nasogastric tube, a central venous access device (CVAD), and an arterial line are established. For a single-lung transplant, a lateral incision is made on the side where the transplant is to be performed. With double-lung transplants, an incision that crosses the entire chest is required. Cardiopulmonary bypass is generally not used except for heart-lung transplants. After the recipient's diseased lung is removed, the donor lung is placed in the pleural cavity, where the pulmonary artery and pulmonary vein and the bronchus of the donor lung are anastomosed to the recipient's airway. Chest tube(s) placement is completed to reinflate the donor lung, and the incision is closed. Multiple hemodynamic monitoring lines are established, and the recipient is transferred to the critical care unit or pediatric intensive care unit (PICU) and placed on mechanical ventilation. Mechanical ventilation not only maintains patency of the client's airway but also facilitates reexpansion of the lung(s) by increasing the pressure within the transplanted lung(s). The client usually remains on mechanical ventilation for one or two days depending on the child's condition, and the critical care stay varies depending on how extensive the surgery was and how well the donor lung functions after reinflation. Total hospital stay is usually 10–14 days.

Nursing Management of Cystic Fibrosis

Assessment

1. Obtain client history
2. Assess breath sounds and pulse oximetry
3. Measure weight, height, and body fat
4. Assess sweat chloride test results
5. Assess for the presence of indicators of CF including barrel chest and steatorrhea
6. Obtain baseline vital signs
7. Complete physical examination

Nursing Diagnoses (including but not limited to)

1. Ineffective airway clearance R/T tenacious and increased pulmonary secretions
2. Impaired gas exchange R/T air trapping in alveoli and alveolar fibrosis
3. Ineffective protection R/T tenacious secretions and impaired body defenses
4. Imbalanced nutrition: less than body requirements R/T impaired absorption
5. Ineffective family coping R/T chronic illness and potentially fatal disease
6. Deficient knowledge R/T condition, treatment, and lifelong home care

Planning/Goals

1. Client will be able to effectively remove pulmonary secretions and remain compliant with therapy.
2. Client will regain and maintain gas exchange as evidenced by oxygen saturation within prescribed limits.
3. Client will not experience signs of infection as evidenced by body temperature within defined limits (WDL), intravenous access site that is free of redness and swelling, nonpurulent sputum, decreased respiratory distress, and compliance with respiratory treatments. If infection occurs, it will be treated promptly and effectively.
4. Parents/client will be compliant with pancreatic enzyme therapy; high-calorie, high-carbohydrate, and high-protein diet; consumption of at least 80% of diet; and maintenance of normal body weight for height.
5. Client (if age-appropriate) and family will verbalize feelings and concerns and demonstrate positive coping strategies. Child will participate in age-appropriate activities.
6. Client (if age-appropriate) and family will demonstrate understanding of condition, treatment, and home care.

NOC

1. Respiratory Status: Airway Patency
2. Respiratory Status: Gas Exchange
3. Risk Control
4. Nutritional Status: Nutrient Intake, Food and Fluid Intake
5. Coping
6. Knowledge: Illness Care, Treatment, Health Promotion

IMPLEMENTATION

1. Airway
   a. Assess breath sounds before and after breathing treatments
   b. Assess respiratory status every 4 hours and as needed
   c. Explain importance of compliance with prescribed therapies
   d. Explain all equipment and procedures
   e. Administer nebulizers as prescribed prior to CPT
   f. Collaborate with physical therapy and respiratory therapy for respiratory treatments
   g. Organize CPT to be performed a minimum of 30 minutes before or after meals
   h. Collaborate with health care provider to prescribe peripherally inserted central catheter for 14-day administration of IV antibiotics
   i. Maintain patency of intravenous access device, monitoring hourly
   j. Administer mucolytics and antibiotics as prescribed
   k. Assess child's fluid likes and dislikes
   l. Encourage oral intake of favorite fluids and water
   m. Encourage family involvement in care

2. Gas exchange
   a. Refer to interventions for airway clearance
   b. Assess oxygen saturation by pulse oximetry and titrate routinely to maintain saturation within prescribed parameters
   c. Elevate head of bed to facilitate breathing
   d. Encourage use of cyclic breathing exercises according to home schedule
   e. Administer medications as prescribed
   f. Monitor arterial blood gases if in respiratory acidosis

3. Infection
   a. Assess vital signs every 4 hours
   b. Monitor breath sounds and respiratory status
   c. Obtain sputum for culture and sensitivity and monitor results
   d. Assess odor, color, and consistency of sputum and document
   e. Maintain good hand washing and universal (standard) precautions
   f. Monitor white blood cell count
   g. Administer antibiotics as prescribed. *NOTE:* Because of the potential irritation caused by infusing vancomycin through peripheral venous accesses (except peripherally inserted central venous catheters), it should be infused only through a CVAD.
   h. Obtain blood cultures as prescribed
   i. Place on respiratory precautions as indicated

4. Nutrition
   a. Monitor intake and output
   b. Assess client's food preferences and collaborate with dietician to incorporate these into diet
   c. Ensure that appropriate diet (high-calorie, high-carbohydrate, and high-protein) is prescribed, including double portions
   d. Administer pancreatic enzymes with each meal and snack
   e. Administer vitamin supplements as prescribed, providing discharge planning

      f.   Reinforce importance of dietary modifications

      g.   Weigh daily

      h.   Monitor glucose level daily

      i.   Administer enteral feedings throughout the night as prescribed

5. Coping

      a.   Assess client's/family's coping strategies

      b.   Assess for indicators of ineffective coping

      c.   Explain all procedures using age-appropriate explanations

      d.   Encourage client (if age-appropriate) and family to express feelings and concerns

      e.   Collaborate with client/family to develop positive coping strategies

      f.   Encourage client/family to participate in care

      g.   Instruct about home procedures

      h.   Provide nonthreatening environment to perform return demonstrations of home care procedures

      i.   Encourage questions, providing honest answers

      j.   Provide information about what support groups are available, including the Cystic Fibrosis Foundation, and how to retrieve information about other support groups via the Internet

6. Parent/client teaching

      a.   Assess client's (if age-appropriate) and family's current level of knowledge

      b.   Provide verbal and written information and demonstrations of equipment as needed regarding:

          1) CPT, postural drainage, and breathing treatments, stressing importance of compliance with this as lifelong therapy

          2) Medication administration including oral and inhalation medications, stressing importance of compliance with medication regimen and the fact that it is a lifelong therapy

          3) Signs and symptoms of adverse effects of medications

          4) Signs and symptoms of respiratory infections and need to report these to initiate antibiotic therapy promptly

          5) CVAD care if client receives frequent antibiotic therapy for recurrent infections

          6) Signs and symptoms of worsening of condition

          7) Contact phone numbers to report signs and symptoms

          8) Importance of regular hand washing and appropriate technique

          9) Importance of follow-up with health care provider

          10) Contact information for local and national CF support groups

      c.   Provide adequate time for client's/family's questions, answering honestly

      d.   Document teaching and client's/family's response

NIC

1. Airway Management, Medication Administration

2. Airway Management, Chest Physiotherapy, Respiratory Monitoring

3. Infection Control

4. Nutrition Management, Nutrition Monitoring

5. Coping Enhancement

6. Teaching: Illness Care, Treatment, Health Promotion

EVALUATION

1. Client is able to effectively remove pulmonary secretions and remains compliant with therapy.
2. Client regains and maintains gas exchange as evidenced by oxygen saturation within prescribed range.
3. Client experiences no signs of infection as evidenced by body temperature WDL, intravenous access site that is free of redness and swelling, nonpurulent sputum, decreased respiratory distress, and compliance with respiratory treatments. If infection occurs, it is treated promptly and effectively.
4. Parents/client is compliant with pancreatic enzymes therapy; high-calorie, high-carbohydrate, and high-protein diet; consumption of at least 80% of diet; and maintenance of normal body weight for height.
5. Client (if age-appropriate) and family verbalize feelings and concerns and demonstrate positive coping strategies. Child participates in age-appropriate activities.
6. Client (if age-appropriate) and family demonstrate understanding of condition, treatment, and home care.

Nursing Management for Lung Transplantation

ASSESSMENT

1. Obtain client history
2. Assess respiratory status
3. Assess results of diagnostic testing
4. Obtain baseline data including vital signs, height and weight, arterial blood gases, and serum blood values
5. Complete physical assessment

NURSING DIAGNOSES (INCLUDING BUT NOT LIMITED TO)

1. Impaired gas exchange R/T incisional pain, altered breathing pattern, impaired airway clearance, pulmonary edema, atelectasis, and potential lung rejection
2. Risk for injury; infection/rejection R/T surgical procedure, invasive lines and tubes, immunosuppression therapy, and donor organ
3. Acute pain R/T chest tube placement, tissue trauma, and surgical incision
4. Risk for ineffective tissue perfusion R/T hypoxia, hypovolemia, and tachydysrhythmias
5. Risk for imbalanced fluid volume R/T interstitial fluid shifts, hyper/hypovolemia
6. Risk for injury R/T complications of lung transplantation
7. Deficient knowledge R/T condition, treatment, rehabilitation, and home care

PLANNING/GOALS

1. Client will regain and maintain adequate gas exchange as evidenced by oxygen saturation/pulse oximetry, vital signs, and arterial pH WDL; absence of cyanosis and cardiac dysrhythmias; and ability to perform activities of daily living (ADL) without supplemental oxygen prior to discharge.
2. Client will not experience infection or organ rejection as evidenced by temperature WDL, no decrease forced expiratory ventilation or forced

vital capacity, vital signs WDL, white blood cell count WDL, urine output > 1–2 mL/kg/hr, and no increase in chest tube drainage.

3. Client will demonstrate pain control at a level of 1 on a scale of 5, with 5 being most severe or 2 on a scale of 1–10, as evidenced by lack of nonverbal indicators of pain, vital signs WDL, and verbalizations after mechanical ventilation is discontinued.

4. Client will demonstrate adequate tissue perfusion as evidenced by (a) MAP 80–120 mm Hg, urine output > 1–2 mL/kg/hr, heart rate and capillary refill WDL, and warm extremities during critical care stay and (b) vital signs WDL and heart rate with activity 20 beats higher than resting heart rate prior to discharge.

5. Client will experience fluid balance as evidenced by stable fluid and electrolyte balance, potassium level and magnesium levels WDL, chest tube drainage within prescribed parameters, mean arterial pressure and systolic blood pressure WDL, and urine output > 1–2 mL/kg/hr within 24 hours posttransplant.

6. Client will not experience complications associated with lung transplantation as evidenced by stable vital signs, absence of dyspnea, and oxygen saturation > 94%.

7. Client/family will demonstrate understanding of condition, treatment, rehabilitation, lifelong immunosuppressant therapy, and home care.

NOC

1. Respiratory Status: Gas Exchange
2. Infection Severity, Circulation Status
3. Comfort Level, Pain Level
4. Respiratory Status: Gas Exchange, Tissue Perfusion: Pulmonary, Circulation Status
5. Fluid, Electrolyte, and Acid-Base Balance
6. Risk Control
7. Knowledge: Illness Care, Health Promotion, Infection Control, Medication

IMPLEMENTATION

1. Gas exchange
   a. Assess chest tubes, ensuring that all connections and dressings are occlusive
   b. Maintain endotracheal intubation and place on mechanical ventilation according to prescribed settings
   c. Reposition every 2 hours when hemodynamically stable
   d. Perform endotracheal suction as indicated by client's condition
   e. Initiate and maintain continuous pulse oximetry
   f. Maintain oxygen saturation at prescribed level
   g. Monitor arterial blood gases through arterial line
   h. Maintain intravenous access patency, monitoring hourly
   i. Administer medications as prescribed to maintain pulmonary function and cardiac output
   j. Maintain hemodynamic monitoring
   k. Perform CPT every 2–4 hours as prescribed and indicated after weaning from mechanical ventilation

l. Assist with positioning for chest radiography (to determine lung reinflation)

m. Assess breath sounds at least every 2–4 hours prior to removal of chest tube

n. Maintain pain control at level of 1/5 or 1-2/10.

o. Ensure continuous cardiorespiratory monitoring while client is receiving opioid analgesia

p. Space nursing activities/interventions to minimize hemodynamic effects/distress

q. Assess and document client's response to activities/procedures

2. Infection/rejection

   a. Assess vital signs every 4 hours following critical care

   b. Report any temperature elevation to health care provider immediately

   c. Maintain compromised host or protective isolation using facility infection control guidelines

   d. Teach visitors appropriate hand washing technique and importance of washing hands before coming in contact with client

   e. Implement neutropenic precautions when neutrophils are less than 100 mm^3

   f. Maintain urinary indwelling catheter care protocol

   g. Administer immunosupressants as prescribed

   h. Monitor cyclosporine level

   i. Monitor white blood cell count and report to health care provider if it falls below prescribed parameter

3. Acute pain

   a. Assess pain hourly using age-appropriate pain assessment tool

   b. Administer opioid analgesics proactively

   c. Explain all equipment and procedures

   d. Collaborate with health care provider for patient-controlled analgesia (PCA) when client is able to use

   e. Assess need for and administer analgesics as prescribed prior to CPT and any other activities

   f. Position for comfort

   g. Maintain chest drainage integrity, avoiding strain on insertion site

   h. Assist with diversion, guided imagery, and relaxation techniques

4. Tissue perfusion

   a. Maintain hemodynamic monitoring

   b. Assess heart sounds every 2–4 hours

   c. Maintain patency of intravenous access, monitoring hourly

   d. Implement hemodynamic medication infusion protocol

   e. Wean drips to maintain hemodynamic parameters as prescribed

   f. Administer intravenous volume replacement and blood products as prescribed

   g. Monitor complete blood count

   h. Maintain continuous pulse oximetry

   i. Administer oxygen and titrate to maintain oxygen saturation within prescribed parameters

   j. Monitor hourly urine output

5. Fluid balance
    a. Maintain strict intake and output
    b. Monitor serum electrolyte levels
    c. Monitor for signs and symptoms of electrolyte imbalances
    d. Monitor chest tube drainage, reporting to health care provider if drainage is greater than prescribed parameters
    e. Weigh daily
    f. Advance diet as prescribed after bowel sounds return
    g. Replace electrolytes as indicated and prescribed
    h. Monitor vital signs every 4 hours following transfer from critical care
    i. Auscultate breath and heart sounds every 4 hours
    j. Assess client's food and fluid preferences
    k. Collaborate with dietician as needed
6. Risk for complications
    a. Assess swallow when fluids are taken
    b. Position with head of bed elevated when anything is taken by mouth
    c. Instruct client to take fluids and food slowly to prevent aspiration
    d. Monitor vital signs and breath sounds
    e. Assist with positioning for routine chest radiography
    f. Encourage gradual ambulation
    g. Schedule nursing care to allow for undisturbed sleep
    h. Encourage family to participate in all aspects of child's care in preparation for discharge
7. Family/client teaching
    a. Assess client's/family's current level of knowledge
    b. Provide verbal and written information regarding:
        1) Risk factors for infection related to immunosuppression and ways to avoid them
        2) Taking of oral or axillary temperature each day and whenever child appears feverish
        3) Importance of reporting elevations to health care provider immediately
        4) Medication administration, including importance of compliance with the prescribed medication regimen and lifelong immunosuppression
        5) Manifestations indicating adverse effects of medications
        6) Rehabilitation schedule and importance of compliance
        7) Manifestations of organ rejection
        8) Alterations in immunizations (use of dead viruses for immunizations)
        9) Contact phone numbers to report signs and symptoms
        10) Importance of regular hand washing and appropriate technique
        11) Importance of follow-up with health care provider
        12) Information about referrals made
    c. Provide sufficient time for client's/family's questions and return demonstrations (as needed)
    d. Document teaching and client/family response

NIC

1. Oxygen Therapy, Acid-Base Management, Ventilation Assistance, Respiratory Monitoring
2. Infection Protection, Infection Control, Circulatory Care
3. Analgesia Administration, Pain Management
4. Hemodynamic Regulation, Acid-Base Monitoring, Respiratory Monitoring
5. Fluid/Electrolyte Management, Acid-Base Management
6. Surveillance: Safety
7. Teaching: Illness Care, Health Promotion, Infection Control, Medication

EVALUATION

1. Client regains and maintains adequate gas exchange as evidenced by oxygen saturation/pulse oximetry, vital signs, and arterial pH WDL; absence of cyanosis and cardiac dysrhythmias; and ability to perform ADL without supplemental oxygen prior to discharge.
2. Client experiences no infection or organ rejection as evidenced by temperature WDL, no decrease forced expiratory ventilation or forced vital capacity, vital signs WDL, white blood cell count WDL, urine output > 1–2 mL/kg/hr, and no increase in chest tube drainage.
3. Client demonstrates pain control at a level of 1 on a scale of 5, with 5 being most severe or 2 on a scale of 1–10, as evidenced by lack of nonverbal indicators of pain, vital signs WDL, and verbalizations after mechanical ventilation is discontinued.
4. Client demonstrates adequate tissue perfusion as evidenced by (a) MAP 80–120 mm Hg, urine output > 1–2 mL/kg/hr, heart rate and capillary refill WDL, and warm extremities during critical care stay and (b) vital signs WDL and heart rate with activity 20 beats higher than resting heart rate prior to discharge.
5. Client experiences fluid balance as evidenced by stable fluid and electrolyte balance, potassium level and magnesium levels WDL, chest tube drainage within prescribed parameters, mean arterial pressure and systolic blood pressure WDL, and urine output > 1–2 mL/kg/hr within 24 hours posttransplant.
6. Client experiences no complications associated with lung transplantation as evidenced by stable vital signs, absence of dyspnea, and oxygen saturation > 94%.
7. Client/family demonstrates understanding of condition, treatment, rehabilitation, lifelong immunosuppressant therapy, and home care.

References

Broyles, B. E. (2005). *Medical-surgical nursing clinical companion.* Durham, NC: Carolina Academic Press.

Broyles, B. E., Reiss, B. S., & Evans, M. E. (2007). *Pharmacological aspects of nursing care* (7th ed.). Clifton Park, NY: Delmar Cengage Learning.

Cystic Fibrosis Foundation. (2007.). *About cystic fibrosis.* Retrieved January 24, 2008, from http://www.cff.org/AboutCF

Faro, A., & Visner, G. A. (2006). *Lung transplantation.* Retrieved April 23, 2007, from http://www.emedicine.com/ped/topic2844.htm

March of Dimes. (2006). *Cystic fibrosis.* Retrieved April 23, 2007, from http://www.marchofdimes.com/pnhec/4439_1213.asp

MedlinePlus. (2007). *Lung transplantation.* Retrieved April 23, 2007, from http://www.nlm.nih.gov/medlineplus/lungtransplantation.html

Potts, N. L., & Mandleco, B. L. (2007). *Pediatric nursing: Caring for children and their families* (2nd ed.). Clifton Park, NY: Delmar Cengage Learning.

United Network for Organ Sharing. (2007). *Lung transplants.* Retrieved April 23, 2007, from http://www.optn.org/data/

31

CYTOMEGALOVIRUS (CMV)

Definition

Cytomegalovirus (CMV) is a member of the herpes strain of viruses and is the leading cause of congenital viral infections in the United States.

Pathophysiology

The incubation period for congenital human CMV is unknown; but it is transmitted through blood and body fluids from mother to infant before, during, and after birth. No immunity is available at this time. It is most commonly transmitted to the pregnant mother who is exposed to urine and saliva of CMV-infected children, such as those in day care.

A trademark characteristic of CMV is the reappearance of symptoms throughout life, as the virus cycles through periods of dormancy and active infection (National Institute of Neurological Disorders and Stroke, 2007).

"Congenital CMV infection is one of the TORCH infections (toxoplasmosis, other infections including syphilis, rubella, CMV, and herpes simplex virus), which carry a risk of significant symptomatic disease and developmental defects in newborns. The clinical syndrome of congenital cytomegalic inclusion disease includes jaundice, splenomegaly, thrombocytopenia, intrauterine growth retardation, microcephaly, and retinitis" (Wills & Goodrich, Section 2, 2006).

Most infants with congenital CMV infection are asymptomatic at birth; however, as many as 5% have developed varying degrees of fetal damage including intrauterine growth retardation, jaundice, hepatitis, hepatosplenomegaly, brain damage, petechial rash, and retinitis (Potts & Mandleco, 2007). Neurologic devastation including microcephaly and mental retardation also can occur from congenital CMV. Infants can continue to shed the virus for up to five years and experience progressively worsening neurologic manifestations.

Complications

Intrauterine growth retardation
Cognitive impairment
Retinitis
Hearing impairments
Hepatosplenomegaly
Hepatitis

Incidence

Approximately 1% (range 0.5–2.5%) of all newborns is congenitally infected with CMV (Schleiss, 2005). According to the Centers for Disease Control and Prevention, "[e]very hour, congenital CMV causes one child to become disabled . . . [and] each year, about 40,000 children are born with congenital CMV infection" (Centers for Disease Control and Prevention, 2006, p. 1). "The cytomegalovirus (CMV) is a virus found universally throughout the world that infects between 50 to 80 percent of all adults in the United States by the age of 40. . . . Babies at the highest risk are those whose mothers have had their first CMV infection during pregnancy" (National Institute of Neurological Disorders and Stroke, 2007, p. 1). "About 10 to 15 percent of infected newborns show symptoms of CMV at birth. . . . Up to 20 percent of these babies die, and about 90 percent of survivors suffer from serious neurological defects, such as mental retardation" (March of Dimes, 2006, p. 1).

Etiology

The cause of congenital CMV infection usually is the transplacental transmission from an infected mother to the fetus. It also can occur during delivery or through breastfeeding, although infants who are infected during delivery or through breast milk rarely develop serious problems (March of Dimes, 2006).

Clinical Manifestations

Most infants are asymptomatic

Jaundice

Hepatosplenomegaly

Petechial rash

Lethargy

Seizures

Diagnostic Tests

IgG antibodies (Centers for Disease Control and Prevention, 2006)

Viral culture

Shell vial assay

Computed tomography of the brain

Medical Management

"There is no available vaccine for preventing congenital [present at birth] CMV disease" (Centers for Disease Control and Prevention, 2006, p. 1). The best course is prevention by using appropriate hand washing and avoiding blood and body fluids of infected individuals. Treatment usually is symptomatic and focuses on preserving the integrity of the central nervous system. Severe cases of CMV in immunocompromised individuals have been treated with ganciclovir; however, "safety and effectiveness of ganciclovir have not been established for . . . neonatal CMV disease" (Spratto & Woods, 2008, p. 694).

Nursing Management

ASSESSMENT

1. Obtain history
2. Assess for manifestations of CMV infection
3. Obtain baseline vital signs

NURSING DIAGNOSES (INCLUDING BUT NOT LIMITED TO)

1. Disturbed sensory perception R/T impact of congenital CMV infection
2. Risk for injury R/T neurologic deficits
3. Deficient knowledge R/T prevention of spread and treatment of manifestations

PLANNING/GOALS

1. Client will experience highest level of neurologic functioning.
2. Client will not incur injury due to sensorineural deficits.
3. Parents will demonstrate understanding of illness care, symptomatic treatment, prognosis, and transmission prevention.

NOC

1. Neurologic Status: Cranial/Sensory Motor Function
2. Risk Control
3. Knowledge: Illness Care, Treatment, Infection Control

IMPLEMENTATION

1. Neurologic development
   a. Assess presence of newborn reflexes
   b. Instruct parents of importance of follow-up monitoring for neurologic deficits
   c. Assess auditory nerve function
   d. Encourage parents to express feelings and concerns
   e. Encourage parents to participate in care
2. Risk for injury
   a. Monitor closely for neurologic deficits as child develops
   b. Instruct parents about environmental safety measures for child
3. Parent teaching
   a. Assess parents' level of understanding
   b. Provide verbal and written information regarding:
      1) CMV including its transmission, course (dormant/active states), symptomatic treatment, prognosis for child (follow-up to determine that this will take time to determine and measure against parameters and milestones of growth and development)
      2) Growth and developmental milestones
      3) Needs of newborn/infant (feeding, hygiene, holding, cuddling, and age-appropriate activities)
      4) Appropriate technique for hand washing and its importance in preventing transmission
      5) Clinical manifestations to report to health care provider
      6) Contact numbers for health care provider and community support services
   c. Provide adequate time for teaching and parental questions
   d. Document teaching and parental response

NIC

1. Neurologic Monitoring, Environmental Management: Safety, Surveillance: Safety
2. Environmental Management: Safety, Surveillance: Safety
3. Teaching: Illness Care, Treatment, Infection Protection

EVALUATION

1. Client experiences highest level of neurologic functioning.
2. Client does not incur injury due to sensorineural deficits.
3. Parents demonstrate understanding of illness care, symptomatic treatment, prognosis, and transmission prevention.

References

Centers for Disease Control and Prevention. (2006). *About CMV.* Retrieved April 23, 2007, from http://www.cdc.gov/cmv/facts.htm

March of Dimes. (2006). *Quick reference: Cytomegalovirus infection in pregnancy.* Retrieved April 23, 2007, from http://www.marchofdimes.com/professionals/14332_1195.asp

National Institute of Neurological Disorders and Stroke. (2007). *NINDS neurological consequences of cytomegalovirus infection information page.* Retrieved April 23, 2007, from http://www.ninds .nih.gov/disorders/cytomegalic/cytomegalic.htm

Potts, N. L., & Mandleco, B. L. (2007). *Pediatric nursing: Caring for children and their families* (2nd ed.). Clifton Park, NY: Delmar Cengage Learning.

Spratto, G. R., & Woods, A. L. (2008). *2008 edition PDR nurse's drug handbook.* Clifton Park, NY: Delmar Cengage Learning.

Wills, T.S., & Goodrich, J.M. (2006). *Cytomegalovirus.* Retrieved May 17, 2008, from http:// www.emedicine.com/med/topic504.htm

Diabetes Insipidus (DI)

Definition

Diabetes insipidus (DI) is a disorder in which there is an inadequate secretion of antidiuretic hormone (ADH) and dysfunctional water regulation (Broyles, 2005).

Pathophysiology

DI occurs when there is dysfunction of either the hypothalamus or the posterior pituitary. This creates a deficiency of the ADH vasopressin. Normally, the posterior pituitary stimulates the hypothalamus gland to secrete ADH in response to vascular fluid levels. ADH functions to concentrate urine by stimulating the reabsorption of water in the collecting tubules of the kidneys (National Institute of Diabetes and Digestive and Kidney Diseases, 2005). In DI, the deficiency of ADH results in an abnormal increase in urinary output and in sodium and potassium excretion. This creates problems with fluid and electrolyte balance, leading to dehydration, hypokalemia, and hyponatremia. The loss of the neurotransmitter potassium leads to risks for cardiac dysrhythmias. Hyponatremia results in risks for acid-base imbalance, fluid imbalance, and alterations in neurotransmission.

There are four different types of DI. According to Diabetes Insipidus Foundation, Inc., they are (1) neurogenic DI caused by a deficiency of the ADH vasopressin, (2) nephrogenic DI (NDI), also called vasopressin-resistant, caused by an insensitivity of the kidneys to vasopressin, (3) dipsogenic DI, the result of abnormal thirst and intake of water and other fluids, and (4) gestational DI, which occurs only during pregnancy (Robertson, 2006). If untreated in adults, DI does not cause death or reduce life expectancy unless the client does not have an adequate supply of drinkable water. However, if DI is not treated in children, it can lead to dehydration and shock, brain damage, impaired mental function, mental retardation, hyperactivity, short attention span, and/or restlessness (Lucile Packard Children's Hospital at Stanford, 2007).

Complications

Dehydration/hypovolemia
Hyponatremia
Hypokalemia
Acid-base imbalance
Cardiac dysrhythmias

Incidence

DI is a rare disorder affecting only 1 in 25,000 people; and for genetic DI, the incidence is 1 in 100,000 (Robertson, 2006).

Etiology

In children, DI most often occurs as a complication of head trauma or surgery to remove hypothalamic or pituitary tumors. Other causes include encephalitis, meningitis, vascular anomalies in the brain, and congenital DI resulting from a defect in the synthesis of ADH (Potts & Mandleco, 2007).

Three manifestations of DI are pituitary DI, central DI, and nephrogenic DI. "Nearly half the time, however, pituitary DI is 'idiopathic' and the underlying cause(s) is (are) still unknown. . . . The gene involved in familial DI depends on which type of DI it is. In CDI (central DI), the mutation is usually in the gene that directs the production of vasopressin and two associated proteins. This gene is on chromosome 20. However there is another type of familial CDI that is due to a recessive mutation in an as yet unidentified gene located on the x-chromosome. This type of CDI affects only males, but can be carried by females. In NDI (nephrogenic DI), the mutation is either a gene on the x-chromosome that encodes the vasopressin receptor or in a different gene on an autosome that encodes a protein known as aquaporin that forms water channels in the kidney" (Robertson, 2006, p. 1).

Clinical Manifestations

Excessive thirst

Polyuria

Dehydration

Poor feeding in infant

Irritability in infant

Inconsolable crying in infant

Failure to thrive in infant

Diagnostic Tests

Magnetic resonance imaging

Water deprivation test

Urine specific gravity

Serum electrolyte levels

Vasopressin stimulation test

Urinalysis

Medical Management

The goals of treatment are to control DI by replacing the action of ADH, prevent dehydration and electrolyte imbalances, and promote normal growth and development. As long as the child has a normal thirst and free access to water, treatment may not be required (Potts & Mandleco, 2007). For affected infants, a breast milk diet should be provided to decrease the solute load, with protein comprising 6% of the caloric intake. For children, 8% of their caloric intake should be protein. Infants and children with genetic DI should consume 0.7 mEq of sodium per kilogram of body weight per day (Chan & Roth, 2006).

Vasopressin, the pharmacological form of ADH, is administered parenterally and is used during acute episodes of DI. Desmopressin (DDAVP) is a synthetic vasopressin analog of ADH and is the first choice for long-term ADH replacement. DDAVP is administered intranasally (Broyles, Reiss, & Evans, 2007).

Nursing Management

ASSESSMENT

1. Obtain client history
2. Assess urine output and thirst level
3. Assess weight and height
4. Assess urine specific gravity
5. Perform physical examination to determine effects on body systems
6. Obtain serum electrolyte levels as prescribed

Nursing Diagnoses (including but not limited to)

1. Risk for deficient fluid volume R/T diuresis
2. Deficient knowledge (parents) R/T disease, treatment, and home care

Planning/Goals

1. Client will maintain fluid and electrolyte balance as evidenced by return of urine output to within defined limits (WDL) (2 mL/kg/hr in infants and young children) and sodium level of 139–146 mmol/L for infant and 138–145 mmol/L for child.
2. Parents will demonstrate understanding of DI, treatment, and home care.

NOC

1. Fluid Balance
2. Knowledge: Illness Care, Medications, Health Promotion

Implementation

1. Fluid balance
   a. Obtain baseline weight and height
   b. Maintain strict intake and output
   c. Measure urine specific gravity every void during acute episode
   d. Administer parenteral fluids as prescribed
   e. Administer antidiuretic pharmacological agents as prescribed
   f. Weigh daily
2. Parent teaching
   a. Assess parents' current level of knowledge
   b. Provide verbal and written information regarding:
      1) Medication effects and adverse effects
      2) Demonstration of DDAVP administration with parent return demonstration
      3) Importance of continued follow-up visits with child's health care provider
      4) Signs and symptoms to report to health care provider
      5) Information regarding national and community support organizations for DI
   c. Provide sufficient time for parents' questions, demonstrations, and return demonstrations
   d. Document teaching and parental response

NIC

1. Fluid Management
2. Teaching: Illness Care, Medications

Evaluation

1. Client maintains fluid and electrolyte balance as evidenced by return of urine output to WDL (2 mL/kg/hr in infants and young children) and sodium level of 139–146 mmol/L for infant and 138–145 mmol/L for child.
2. Parents demonstrate understanding of DI, treatment, and home care.

References

Broyles, B. E. (2005). *Medical-surgical nursing clinical companion.* Durham, NC: Carolina Academic Press.

Broyles, B. E., Reiss, B. S., & Evans, M. E. (2007). *Pharmacological aspects of nursing care* (7th ed.). Clifton Park, NY: Delmar Cengage Learning.

Chan, J. C. M., & Roth, K. S. (2006). *Diabetes insipidus.* Retrieved May 10, 2007, from http://www.emedicine.com/ped/topic580.htm

Lucile Packard Children's Hospital at Stanford. (2007). *Diabetes insipidus.* Retrieved May 10, 2007, from http://www.lpch.org/diseasehealthinfo/healthlibrary/diabetes/di.html

National Institute of Diabetes and Digestive and Kidney Diseases. (2005). *Diabetes insipidus.* Retrieved January 24, 2008, from http://kidney.niddk.nih.gov/kudiseases/pubs/insipidus/

Potts, N. L., & Mandleco, B. L. (2007). *Pediatric nursing: Caring for children and their families* (2nd ed.). Clifton Park, NY: Delmar Cengage Learning.

Robertson, G. L. (2006). *What is diabetes insipidus?* Retrieved May 10, 2007, from http://www.diabetesinsipidus.org/whatisdi.htm

33

DIABETES MELLITUS (DM)

Definition

Diabetes mellitus (DM) is a chronic disorder of carbohydrate, fat, and protein metabolism that results from a deficiency or complete lack of insulin.

Pathophysiology

Insulin is a hormone secreted by the beta cells in the islets of Langerhans of the pancreas. The primary function of insulin is to facilitate the transport of glucose into the cells for energy. Insulin is released in response to the serum blood glucose level; when the blood glucose, or "sugar," level rises, insulin is secreted; as the blood glucose level decreases, the pancreas decreases the amount of insulin it produces and secretes. This process is continuous and maintains blood glucose levels within defined limits (WDL) of 70–99 mg/dL. Insulin also promotes glycogen storage in the liver and storage of fat in adipose tissue. According to the American Diabetes Association (ADA), "with the FPG [fasting plasma glucose] test, a fasting blood glucose level between 100 and 125 mg/dL signals pre-diabetes. A person with a fasting blood glucose level of 126 mg/dL or higher has diabetes" (American Diabetes Association, n.d., p. 1).

There are four etiologic classifications of diabetes. Type 1 (previously known as insulin-dependent DM, or IDDM) results from the destruction or genetic lack of development of beta cells and most often results in complete insulin deficiency. The two subsets of type 1 are immune-mediated (most common) and idiopathic. Type 1 diabetes is the most common type affecting children. In those children with genetic predisposition, exposure to certain viruses or environmental chemicals initiates the immune-mediated process. T lymphocytes damage and destroy the beta cells of the pancreas by the development of isletcell antibodies, insulin autoantibodies, glutamic acid decarboxylase, and other beta cell-specific antibodies. The process of developing type 1 diabetes usually takes years; however, "the rate of beta-cell destruction . . . is quite variable" (National Diabetes Education Program, 2006, p. 4). Because of the body's compensatory mechanisms for supplying energy to the cells through fat and protein metabolism, by the time symptoms indicating hyperglycemia occur, approximately 90% of the beta cells have been destroyed.

Type 2 DM historically has accounted for only a small percentage (2–3%) of diabetes in children. However, in recent years, the incidence has shown a gradual increase, especially in ethnic minorities. The increase in type 2 diabetes (previously termed non-insulin-dependent DM, or NIDDM) has paralleled the rise in childhood obesity. The exact mechanism of action for type 2 diabetes in children is not understood, but theories relating it to obesity are currently being explored. In recent studies, as many as 16% of children with type 2 diabetes have met the criteria for obesity. According to 2005 statistics from the ADA, "[Type 2 diabetes is being seen] frequently in children and adolescents, particularly in American Indians, African Americans, and Hispanic/Latino Americans" (American Diabetes Association, n.d., p. 1). It is important to remember that when the body is stressed (trauma or infections), children with type 2 diabetes can become insulin-dependent, which may resolve after the stressors are removed, or the children may remain insulin-dependent indefinitely. Gestational diabetes occurs during pregnancy and increases the mother's risk of developing type 2 diabetes.

Iatrogenic-induced DM is caused by the administration of drugs, such as corticosteroids, diuretics, certain antimicrobials (levofloxacin), and some birth control pills. Children with other disorders that require the use of corticosteroids for treatment, including organ transplantation, chemotherapy, and autoimmune disorders, can develop this type of diabetes.

The National Diabetes Education Program of the National Institutes of Health further identifies "hybrid," or "mixed," diabetes. Although most children can be diagnosed with type 1 or type 2 diabetes, "some children have elements of both kinds of diabetes including insulin resistance associated with obesity and type II diabetes as well as antibodies against the pancreatic islet cells that are associated with autoimmunity and Type I diabetes" (National Diabetes Education Program, 2006, p. 3).

In the child with diabetes, the beta cells of the pancreas do not produce insulin or the insulin they do produce is ineffective in action (unable to enter the cells) or in amount to maintain blood glucose levels WDL. Inadequate insulin results in decreased uptake of glucose by the cells (glucogenesis). Instead, the glucose remains in vascular areas, resulting in an increase in the blood glucose level. As a result, the kidneys attempt to excrete excess glucose when the level reaches 150–180 mg/dL. This causes glycosuria as well as a loss of electrolytes (sodium, potassium, and chloride) and water. The loss of fluids stimulates the thirst center, causing polydipsia; and cellular lack of glucose causes polyphagia, or increased hunger.

Fats and proteins are mobilized for energy because the cells cannot utilize the glucose in the vascular compartment. The use of fats and proteins for energy results in less availability of these macronutrients for the development of subcutaneous fat and muscle mass. As the liver metabolizes fats for energy, ketone bodies (metabolic by-products of fat metabolism) bind with hydrogen ions to create metabolic acidosis. This is termed diabetic ketoacidosis (DKA). As the respiratory system attempts to compensate for the acidosis, the client begins to hyperventilate in an attempt to decrease carbon dioxide and resolve the acidosis. This breathing pattern in DKA is called Kussmaul's breathing and is characterized by rapid, deep respirations that contain an acetone smell due to the elevated ketone bodies in the bloodstream (Broyles, 2005).

DKA creates immediate problems due to the acidotic condition as well as the impact of elevated blood glucose and ketone bodies on neurons in the brain. This causes the characteristic "diabetic coma." In addition, as the kidneys continue to increase excretion of urine, dehydration and hypovolemia occur (Broyles, 2005).

Diabetes also is responsible for long-term changes in both the blood vessels and nerves of the body. Clients with type 1 diabetes are most likely to develop these long-term complications. Prolonged elevated blood glucose levels (> 140 mg/dL according to the American Diabetes Association) gradually result in micro- and macrovascular changes leading to the chronic luminal narrowing of the vessels. This eventually leads to necrosis and death to the tissues supplied by these vessels. Macrovascular complications include coronary artery disease (CAD), cardiomyopathy, and peripheral vascular disease (PVD). Changes in peripheral vessels lead to decreased blood supply to the feet and decreased healing power in the event of injury. Microvascular changes involve vessels in the retina (diabetic retinopathy), resulting in diabetes being the leading cause of blindness in individuals under 30 years of age. The renal vessels also experience microvascular changes, resulting in diabetes being the leading cause of chronic renal failure. Chronic elevated blood glucose levels cause peripheral neuropathy. This results as the myelin sheaths of the nerves that go to the extremities, abdomen, and back gradually deteriorate, leading to decreased nerve function. This can cause numerous symptoms from numbness to burning, tingling, and pain.

Complications

Hyperglycemia

Hypoglycemia

Hypokalemia

Hyponatremia

Cardiac dysrhythmias
DKA
Hypovolemia
Diabetic coma

Long-Term Complications

Diabetic foot ulcers
Blindness
Renal failure
Cardiovascular disease

Incidence

According to the ADA, "There are 20.8 million children and adults in the United States, or 7% of the population, who have diabetes. While an estimated 14.6 million have been diagnosed with diabetes, unfortunately, 6.2 million people (or nearly one-third) are unaware that they have the disease. . . . It is estimated that 5–10% of Americans who are diagnosed with diabetes have type 1 diabetes" (American Diabetes Association, n.d., p. 1). The annual incidence is 18 per 100,000 children under 20 years of age. The peak onset is 11 years of age in girls and 13 years of age in boys, with a significant drop in incidence after the age of 20 (Potts & Mandleco, 2007). In 2005 government statistics, 176,500 people, or 0.22% of all people under the age of 20, have diabetes. About 1 in every 400–600 children and adolescents has type 1 diabetes. Two million adolescents (or 1 in 6 overweight adolescents) aged 12–19 have prediabetes. Populations at greater risk for type 2 diabetes include African Americans, Hispanic Americans, Native Americans, obese individuals, and older adults (Fain, 2005).

Etiology

Although the exact cause of DM is unknown, a number of theories have been proposed. One of the most well known of these is the genetic-hereditary connection. A family history of diabetes increases the risk of future family members developing the disease. Another theory involves viral etiology. The diabetogenic virus destroys the beta cells and is most directly associated with type 1 diabetes. Environmental factors such as obesity and stress also are indicated in the development of type 2 DM. In addition, the newer theory that diabetes is an autoimmune disorder is encouraging further research in this area.

Clinical Manifestations

TYPE 1

Polyuria
Polydipsia
Polyphagia
Weight loss
Blurred vision
Fatigue
Persistent hyperglycemia
Possible progression to DKA

TYPE 2

Obesity
Fatigue
Blurred vision

Occurrence of frequent infections

Polyuria

Polydipsia

HYPOGLYCEMIA

Trembling

Tachycardia and palpitations

Diaphoresis

Anxiety

Polyphagia

Pallor

Headache

Changes in level of consciousness

Diagnostic Tests

FPG > 126 mg/dL

Random serum glucose > 200 mg/dL

C-peptide levels

Oral glucose tolerance test (OGTT)

Urine for glucose and ketones

Serum electrolytes

Insulin level

LDL, HDL, and triglyceride levels

Glycosylated hemoglobin (Hgb A_{1c})

Glycosylated serum proteins and albumin

Medical Management

Currently, there is no cure for diabetes. The goals of treatment for diabetes are to maintain a blood glucose level < 100 mg/dL and to prevent or minimize the long-term visual, vascular, renal, and neurologic complications of this disease. The basic elements of management are insulin administration (type 1 diabetes), nutrition management, physical exercise, blood glucose testing, and the avoidance of hypoglycemia. Management for type 2 diabetes in children consists of nutrition management, increased physical activity, blood glucose testing, and (if needed) the use of the oral hypoglycemic agent metformin. Intensive control is the standard of care and requires frequent monitoring of blood glucose levels and multiple injections of insulin daily to keep blood sugar between 85 and 100 mg/dL. Insulin therapy must be individualized to maintain blood glucose control and minimize the risk of hypoglycemia (Dow, 2005). At this time, long-term complications of type 1 diabetes cannot be prevented entirely, but the severity of these complications can be dramatically reduced through compliance with this interdependent treatment regimen.

INSULIN THERAPY

As noted, insulin therapy must be individualized to each child's needs. Some children are managed using fixed insulin doses of intermediate-acting insulin (NPH) injections subcutaneously twice a day and rapid-acting regular insulin injections titrated to serum glucose levels before meals and at bedtime. With this regimen, the child must have food given at the time of peak action of the insulin. A new agent, insulin glargine, has recently been approved by the FDA and is indicated for children (aged 6 and over) with type 1 diabetes and for children and adults with type 2 diabetes who require basal insulin (Spratto & Woods, 2008; Broyles, Reiss, & Evans, 2007).

External and implantable insulin pumps have been widely researched and are found to be very useful methods of achieving near normal blood glucose levels, as well. Insulin pumps have been available commercially since the 1980s and are designed to mimic the pancreas by injecting insulin in response to stimulation by serum glucose levels. Current available pumps are the size of a small cell phone, weighing 2.7–3.2 ounces. They contain a syringe that holds up to 300 units of insulin and deliver insulin through a small catheter that is placed in subcutaneous fat. The pump is programmed to release small amounts of insulin throughout the day and night as well as boluses of insulin when meals are consumed. The boluses are based on the child's plasma glucose level and the amount of carbohydrate consumed during the meal. These pumps have proven to be quite effective in reducing the number of hypoglycemic episodes in children (Potts & Mandleco, 2007). Research in this area continues.

The three sources of insulin are beef, pork, and humulin. The use of beef and pork insulins has declined over the past two decades because of the production of humulin and Novolin insulins, which do not carry the hypersensitivity risks of animal insulins. Humulin is the type prescribed for children. Insulin also is classified according to the onset, peak, and duration of action. Regular insulin is rapid-acting with an onset of 30 minutes to an hour, peak (most likely time to see a hypoglycemic reaction) of 2–3 hours, and duration of 4–6 hours. NPH insulin is an intermediate-acting insulin with an onset of 1–2 hours, a peak of 6–8 hours, and a duration of 12–24 hours. These are usually used as combination therapy. The safety and efficacy of Humalog insulin has not been determined in children under the age of 12 years.

The primary (and potentially life-threatening) complication associated with insulin therapy is hypoglycemia. This occurs when too much insulin is circulating in the body. Hypoglycemia can produce insulin shock and death if not recognized early and treated.

Other problems include lipodystrophy, allergic reactions, the Somogyi effect, and the dawn phenomenon. Lipodystrophy, the hypertrophy of subcutaneous tissues, occurs when subcutaneous injection sites for insulin are not rotated. This impacts insulin absorption. It is more closely associated with the use of pork and beef insulin. A much lower incidence occurs with humulin insulin.

The Somogyi effect is characterized by erratic levels of serum glucose. Blood sugar levels drop during the night and then rise quickly in the early morning hours. Then as counterregulatory hormones are released, lipolysis, gluconeogenesis, and glucolysis occur. This causes the blood glucose levels to rise sharply.

The dawn phenomenon also results in early morning hyperglycemia and is believed to be caused by the release of endogenous growth hormone or cortisol. Both of these act as counterregulatory hormone agents to insulin, thus decreasing insulin levels with resultant hyperglycemia.

DIET THERAPY

Nutritional care is the cornerstone of management for diabetes. This requires a coordinated effort based on age, growth and development, and activity level. The goals of diet therapy are to achieve and maintain (1) as near normal glucose levels as possible, (2) optimal lipid levels, (3) adequate calories for growth and development and activity level, (4) improvement of total health, and (5) aggressive treatment for acute and long-term complications. Limiting concentrated carbohydrates and simple sugars is the key to nutritional therapy. Nutritional guidelines include dividing caloric intake into 20–25% proteins and the remaining 75–80% divided between fats and carbohydrates. Alcohol consumption should be restricted due to the simple sugars prevalent in alcoholic beverages. This can present a challenge with the national health issue of alcohol use in adolescents.

EXERCISE

Because exercise aids in lowering blood glucose levels, it is an integral part of diabetes treatment. Exercise in children should be geared to the appropriate level of growth and development. Exercise also should be closely coordinated with dietary intake and monitoring of blood glucose levels to prevent hypoglycemia because of too much endogenous insulin. This can be especially challenging for children and adolescents involved in competitive sports such as football, basketball, soccer, baseball, and volleyball.

BLOOD GLUCOSE MONITORING

Self-monitoring combined with regular follow-up with health care providers has proven to be effective in controlling serum glucose levels. Using capillary blood glucose monitoring technology is the most reliable method for assessing serum glucose levels. The handheld machines use a drop of capillary blood, usually from the tip of the finger, and work by sensors or reflectance meters. These machines are widely available commercially, and many are now computerized. School-age children should be able to perform their own blood glucose monitoring.

MANAGEMENT OF DKA

Treatment for DKA includes insulin therapy, replacement of fluids using IV saline, electrolyte replacement, sodium bicarbonate ($NaHCO_3$) to treat the metabolic acidosis, and mechanical ventilation if the Kussmaul's respirations are compromising gas exchange. This treatment is usually administered in a critical care environment. As the client's blood glucose begins to lower, 5% dextrose solution is added to prevent a too rapid drop in blood glucose with resulting hypoglycemia.

Nursing Management

ASSESSMENT

1. Obtain client history focusing on development of symptoms
2. Assess weight and height
3. Obtain urine for glucose and ketone testing
4. Measure capillary blood glucose
5. Perform physical assessment to determine effects of diabetes on systems
6. Assess visual acuity
7. Assess psychosocial impact of diabetes on child/family
8. Assess current level of knowledge about diabetes

NURSING DIAGNOSES (INCLUDING BUT NOT LIMITED TO)

1. Imbalanced nutrition, less than body requirements R/T insulin deficit and hyperglycemia
2. Risk for injury R/T hypoglycemia and/or hyperglycemia
3. Risk for injury R/T chronic visual, cardiovascular, neurologic, and renal effects of diabetes
4. Deficient knowledge R/T disease, management, and long-term home care
5. Risk for ineffective health maintenance R/T nutrition, chronic nature of diabetes
6. Impaired adjustment R/T chronic health care needs of child with Type 1 diabetes

SPECIFIC FOR DKA

1. Deficient fluid volume R/T diuresis
2. Risk for injury R/T alteration in acid-base balance and electrolyte imbalance
3. Risk for ineffective cerebral tissue perfusion R/T cerebral edema secondary to resolving DKA

Planning/Goals

1. Client will regain and maintain optimal body weight for height, age, and activity level.
2. Client will not experience hypoglycemia and/or hyperglycemia.
3. Client will experience minimal long-term effects of diabetes as evidenced by maintaining follow-up medical management and receiving aggressive care of effects.
4. Client (if age-appropriate) and family will demonstrate understanding of DM, self-medication administration, glucose monitoring, signs and symptoms of hyper- and hypoglycemia, diet, exercise, foot care, and importance of follow-up medical management.
5. Client/family will demonstrate ability to manage diabetic condition through appropriate administration of insulin (type 1), compliance with diet and exercise, and monitoring of blood glucose levels as evidenced by serum glucose levels WDL.
6. Client/family will use adaptive coping skills and recognize areas of management that challenge them and use effective problem-solving skills to cope with these issues.

Specific for DKA

1. Client will regain and maintain fluid and electrolyte balance as evidenced by urine output and serum electrolyte values WDL.
2. Client will regain and maintain acid-base balance as evidenced by laboratory values WDL.
3. Client will not experience ineffective cerebral tissue perfusion as evidenced by neurologic status WDL.

NOC

1. Nutritional Status
2. Risk Control
3. Risk Control
4. Knowledge: Disease Process and Management
5. Knowledge: Health Promotion
6. Family Coping
7. Fluid Balance
8. Risk Control
9. Neurologic Status

Implementation

1. Nutrition
   a. Obtain baseline weight and height
   b. Perform nutritional assessment
   c. Consult with dietician if available
   d. Weigh daily
   e. Assess child's level of physical activity comparing to expected age-appropriate activity
   f. Monitor nutritional intake
   g. Refer to "Client teaching"
2. Hyperglycemia/hypoglycemia prevention/management
   a. Ensure that child and supervising adult:
      1) Have access to blood glucose monitoring equipment at all times
      2) Know that child must wear medical information

        3) Monitor capillary blood glucose levels as prescribed

        4) Administer morning and evening NPH insulin as prescribed

        5) Administer regular insulin per sliding scale (based on Accu-Check results as prescribed)

  b. Administer intravenous 0.9% normal saline and insulin as prescribed if client is admitted with DKA; add prescribed 5% dextrose and potassium to IV solution when glucose begins to drop

  c. Provide orange juice and perform Accu-Check immediately if client reports symptoms of hypoglycemia

  d. If client experiences symptoms of hyperglycemia, assess blood sugar level and administer insulin as prescribed

  e. Refer to "Client teaching"

3. Long-term effects of diabetes

  a. Assess peripheral pulses, skin color, skin integrity, and sensation

  b. Assess visual acuity and ask client about any visual changes experienced

  c. Assess cardiovascular status including carotid and apical pulses

  d. Ask client about any changes in bowel habits

  e. Monitor blood urea nitrogen (BUN) and creatinine levels

  f. Refer to "Client teaching"

4. Client teaching

  a. Assess client's/family's current level of knowledge

  b. Explain the basic pathophysiology of diabetes at client's/family's level of understanding

  c. Provide verbal, written, and demonstration instructions regarding:

        1) Self-monitoring of blood glucose, stressing importance of use according to manufacturer's instructions

        2) Diet instructions of the ADA exchange list and ways to adjust diet to activity level and illness

        3) Instructions on how to test urine for ketones if blood glucose level is higher than prescribed limits and written instructions on actions to take if ketones are present

        4) Signs and symptoms of hypoglycemia and hyperglycemia and actions to take if symptoms are present

        5) Importance of treating child with type 1 diabetes for hypoglycemia if child is found unconscious (most likely because of too much insulin; can be more easily reversed if problem is determined to be hyperglycemia)

        6) Storage, preparation, and administration of insulin and proper disposal of used syringes

        7) Subcutaneous sites and importance of rotating sites

        8) Preparation and administration of parenteral glucagon if client becomes unconscious due to hypoglycemia

        9) Procedure for performing daily inspections of feet and proper foot care:

           a) Wash feet daily

           b) Keep skin soft and smooth using skin lotion, skin cream, or petroleum jelly

      c) Smooth corns and calluses gently

      d) Trim toenails each week and as needed being careful not to injure skin

      e) Wear shoes and socks

      f) Protect feet from heat and cold

      g) Be active

  d. Stress importance of child visiting an ophthalmologist to undergo an annual eye examination

  e. Stress importance of routine medical follow-up with health care provider

  f. Provide information that must be shared with school nurse

  g. Provide adequate time for client/family return demonstrations and questions

  h. Document teaching and client/family response

5. Health maintenance

  a. Monitor capillary glucose levels before meals and at bedtime

  b. Monitor for signs and symptoms of hyperglycemia, DKA, and hypoglycemia

  c. Maintain strict intake and output

  d. Assess feet daily and provide foot care

  e. Assess respiratory status

  f. Administer insulin as prescribed, rotating sites and maintaining documentation

  g. Monitor dietary intake to prevent intake of concentrated or simple sugars

  h. Refer to "Client teaching"

6. Client/family adjustment

  a. Assess client/family for psychosocial and financial impact of disease

  b. Encourage client/family verbalization of feelings and concerns

  c. Discuss growth and development needs of child and importance of involving child in own care when developmentally ready

  d. Assist in identifying problem-solving strategies

  e. Provide information concerning diabetes support groups

Specific for DKA

1. Fluid volume

  a. Initiate and maintain peripheral vascular access as prescribed

  b. Administer 0.9% normal saline intravenously as prescribed

  c. Monitor serum glucose levels

  d. Follow critical care guidelines/protocols for titrating fluids and adding glucose and potassium to IV solution as serum glucose level decreases

  e. Maintain hemodynamic monitoring

  f. Monitor intake and output

  g. Assess urine pH and specific gravity

2. Acid-base and electrolyte balance

  a. Monitor respiratory status

  b. Place child on continuous cardiorespiratory monitoring

  c. Monitor arterial blood gases

  d. Monitor serum electrolyte levels

  e. Maintain intravenous access, monitoring at least hourly

    f. Administer sodium bicarbonate as prescribed

    g. Administer intravenous fluids as prescribed

    h. Assess for manifestations of acid-base imbalances

3. Cerebral tissue perfusion

    a. Monitor neurologic status

    b. Maintain intravenous access, monitoring at least hourly

    c. Administer osmotic diuretic (mannitol) as prescribed for manifestations of increased intracranial pressure

    d. Position with head of bed elevated 15–30 degrees as prescribed

    e. Monitor urinary output and urine specific gravity

    f. Monitor intracranial pressure readings as prescribed

    g. Avoid activities that could result in Valsalva's maneuver by client

    h. Sedate as prescribed

    i. Avoid use of restraints if possible

NIC

1. Nutrient Intake
2. Risk Identification, Surveillance, Safety
3. Risk Identification, Surveillance, Safety
4. Teaching: Disease Process and Management
5. Teaching: Treatment Regimen
6. Coping Enhancement
7. Fluid Management
8. Risk Identification, Surveillance, Safety
9. Cerebral Perfusion Promotion, Neurologic Monitoring

EVALUATION

1. Client regains and maintains optimal body weight for height, age, and activity level.
2. Client does not experience hypoglycemia and/or hyperglycemia.
3. Client experiences minimal long-term effects of diabetes as evidenced by maintaining follow-up medical management and receiving aggressive care of effects.
4. Client (if age-appropriate) and family demonstrate understanding of DM, self-medication administration, glucose monitoring, signs and symptoms of hyper- and hypoglycemia, diet, exercise, foot care, and importance of follow-up medical management.
5. Client/family demonstrate ability to manage diabetic condition through appropriate administration of insulin (type 1), compliance with diet and exercise, and monitoring of blood glucose levels as evidenced by serum glucose levels WDL.
6. Client/family use adaptive coping skills and recognize areas of management that challenge them and use effective problem-solving skills to cope with these issues.

SPECIFIC FOR DKA

1. Client regains and maintains fluid and electrolyte balance as evidenced by urine output and serum electrolyte values WDL.
2. Client regains and maintains acid-base balance as evidenced by laboratory values WDL.
3. Client does not experience ineffective cerebral tissue perfusion as evidenced by neurologic status WDL.

References

American Diabetes Association. (n.d.). *All about diabetes.* Retrieved February 8, 2007, from https://www.diabetes.org/about-diabetes.jsp

Broyles, B. E. (2005). *Medical-surgical nursing clinical companion.* Durham, NC: Carolina Academic Press.

Broyles, B. E., Reiss, B. S., & Evans, M. E. (2007). *Pharmacological aspects of nursing care* (7th ed.). Clifton Park, NY: Delmar Cengage Learning.

Dow, N. E. (2005). Tight insulin control: Making it work. *RN, 68*(7), 46–48.

Fain, J. A. (2005). Management of clients with diabetes mellitus. In J. M. Black & J. H. Hawks, *Medical-surgical nursing.* St. Louis, MO: Elsevier.

National Diabetes Education Program. (2006). *Overview of diabetes in children and adolescents.* Retrieved February 9, 2007, from http://www.ndep.nih.gov/diabetes/pubs/Youth_FactSheet.pdf

Potts, N. L., & Mandleco, B. L. (2007). *Pediatric nursing: Caring for children and their families* (2nd ed.). Clifton Park, NY: Delmar Cengage Learning.

Spratto, G. R., & Woods, A. L. (2008). *2008 edition PDR nurse's drug handbook.* Clifton Park, NY: Delmar Cengage Learning.

34

DIARRHEA

Definition

Diarrhea is defined as frequent watery stools. It can be acute or chronic, inflammatory or noninflammatory, or viral, bacterial, or paracytic in nature.

Pathophysiology

Diarrhea is not a disease, but a symptom or result of a large variety of diseases including respiratory infections (especially in children) and gastrointestinal disorders; it also can be an adverse effect of medications. Although initial pathophysiology may vary depending on the cause, diarrhea occurs when a causative factor increases intestinal motility. This results in rapid emptying of the bowel and impaired absorption of water and electrolytes by the colon. The most critical of these electrolytes are potassium and sodium. This malabsorption forces increased quantities of these electrolytes and fluids to be excreted, and fluid and electrolyte imbalances and metabolic acidosis result. Dehydration is particularly dangerous for infants and young children, who can die from it within a matter of days. Viruses directly damage the villi of the small intestines, resulting in a decrease intestinal surface area and increased motility (Guandalini & Frye, 2006).

Acute diarrhea is a sudden increase in the number and consistency of stools and is a leading cause of illness in children under the age of 5 years. It usually results from respiratory or urinary tract infections or medications. Chronic diarrhea is defined as diarrhea that lasts more than 2 weeks. Intractable diarrhea of infancy "occurs in the first few months of life, persists longer than 2 weeks with no recognized pathogens, and is refractory to treatment" (Hockenberry, 2005, p. 843). Chronic nonspecific diarrhea (CNSD), also termed irritable colon of childhood and toddlers' diarrhea, is a common cause of chronic diarrhea in children from 6 months to $4\frac{1}{2}$ years of age. This type of diarrhea does not appear to impact physical growth and development or nutritional status of these children (Hockenberry, 2005).

Complications

Hyponatremia
Dehydration
Hypokalemia
Hypocalcemia
Metabolic acidosis
Hypovolemia
Cardiac dysrhythmias due to hypokalemia and hypocalcemia

Incidence

Diarrhea is the leading cause of death and a major contributor to morbidity in children throughout the world. Approximately 10% of all acute care visits for children under 2 years old in the United States are due to diarrhea. In the United States, the estimate of incidence in children younger than 5 years of age is one episode per child annually, accounting for approximately 220,000 hospital admissions (about 10% of all admissions for children in this age range) and resulting in approximately 400 deaths per year. In addition, acute diarrhea is responsible for 20% of referrals to pediatric health care providers for children younger than 2 years and 10% for children younger than 3 years (Guandalini & Frye, 2006).

Etiology

Causes of diarrhea in children include bacteria (*Campylobacter jejuni, Salmonella,* certain strains of *Escherichia coli,* and *Shigella*), viruses, parasites (*Giardia lamblia* and *Cryptosporidium*), medications (especially antibiotics), food allergies, enzyme deficiencies (as in lactose intolerance), and functional disorders (Crohn's disease and ulcerative colitis). Because these pathogens are expelled in the stool, diarrhea is easily transmitted from person to person. Infection with the rotavirus is the most common cause of acute childhood diarrhea (National Institute of Diabetes and Digestive and Kidney Diseases, 2007). It is responsible for an estimated 500,000 visits to health care providers' offices and 160,000 visits to emergency rooms by children each year in the United States (Stöppler & Lee, 2007).

Clinical Manifestations

Frequent watery stools
Manifestations of dehydration
Signs and symptoms of hypokalemia and hyponatremia
Abdominal cramping
Fever
Dry skin and mucous membranes

Diagnostic Tests

Stool cultures
Stool pH, leukocytes, glucose, and presence of blood
Urine specific gravity
Serum electrolyte levels
Computed tomography (CT) of the abdomen
Tests specific to pathophysiologic causes for diarrhea

Medical Management

The goals of management are to treat the cause, restore fluid and electrolyte balance, restore normal bowel function, and prevent spread if diarrhea is infectious. The cause of the diarrhea and the fluid and electrolyte imbalances that result from the diarrhea are treated concurrently. In the presence of mild to moderate dehydration, oral rehydration therapy (ORT) currently is the most common treatment modality in use and is recommended by the American Academy of Pediatrics, World Health Organization, and Centers for Disease Control and Prevention. ORT contains fluids and nutrients and includes products such as Pedialyte, Ceralyte, and Infalyte. In mild to moderate dehydration, the recommended ORT is 50 mL/kg every 4 hours. In children with severe dehydration, parenteral fluids are administered. The isotonic solution 0.9% normal saline is the initial fluid of choice. After the child voids, the solution is changed to 5% dextrose and 0.45% normal saline. Parenteral electrolyte replacements (especially potassium) are used in the event of symptomatic electrolyte imbalances. Antidiarrheal medications are not recommended for infants because of the adverse effects associated with them, including the risk of bowel obstruction. In older children, antidiarrheal agents should be used with caution and only under the direction of the child's health care provider (Broyles, Reiss, & Evans, 2007).

The BRAT (bananas, rice, applesauce, and toast) diet has been recommended for years when dietary intake is resumed; however, "no evidence shows that this diet is useful" (Guandalini & Frye, 2006, Section 6). The poor protein content of this diet may contraindicate its use. Research indicates that resumption of the prediarrhea diet "is perfectly safe and must be encouraged, obviously respecting any (usually temporary) lack of appetite" (Guandalini & Frye, 2006, Section 6).

Nursing Management

ASSESSMENT

1. Obtain client history including allergies to food and medications
2. Assess weight and height
3. Assess bowel sounds and stools
4. Obtain stool for culture and ova and parasite testing
5. Perform physical assessment to determine effects on body systems

NURSING DIAGNOSES (INCLUDING BUT NOT LIMITED TO)

1. Diarrhea R/T passage of frequent liquid stools
2. Deficient fluid volume R/T loss of body fluids and electrolytes
3. Imbalanced nutrition: less than body requirements R/T diarrheal losses, inadequate nutrient intake
4. Risk for infection R/T transmission of infectious microorganisms invading gastrointestinal tract
5. Risk for impaired skin integrity R/T frequent liquid stools
6. Deficient knowledge R/T diarrhea, treatment, prevention, and home care

PLANNING/GOALS

1. Client's diarrhea will resolve without complications.
2. Client will regain and maintain fluid and electrolyte balance as evidenced by urine output and electrolyte levels within defined limits (WDL).
3. Client will regain and maintain nutrition adequate to maintain appropriate weight for age.
4. Client and others will not exhibit manifestations of gastrointestinal infection.
5. Client's skin will remain intact.
6. Client (if age-appropriate) and family will demonstrate understanding of diarrhea, management, prevention, and home care.

NOC

1. Bowel Elimination, Electrolyte and Acid/Base Balance
2. Electrolyte and Acid/Base Balance
3. Nutritional Status: Food & Fluid Intake
4. Infection Severity
5. Tissue Integrity: Skin
6. Knowledge: Disease Process, Management

IMPLEMENTATION

1. Diarrhea
   a. Assess bowel sounds at least every shift
   b. Record number and description of stools when they occur
   c. Provide skin care to prevent rectal breakdown
   d. Collect stool specimens as prescribed for diagnostic tests
   e. Maintain intravenous access, monitoring hourly
   f. Administer intravenous fluids as prescribed
2. Fluid and electrolyte balance
   a. Obtain baseline weight and height
   b. Maintain strict intake and output (weigh infant diapers)

    c. Weigh daily

    d. Assess skin and mucous membranes

    e. Measure urine specific gravity every void

    f. Initiate and maintain patency of intravenous access, monitoring hourly

    g. Administer parenteral fluids as prescribed

    h. Provide for ORT as prescribed

    i. Encourage family involvement in infant's/child's care

3. Nutrition

    a. Encourage mother to continue breast-feeding infant

    b. Encourage age-appropriate prediarrhea diet as prescribed

    c. Assess and document feeding tolerance

    d. Weigh daily

    e. Maintain intake and output

4. Infection transmission

    a. Implement standard precautions

    b. Maintain careful hand washing

    c. Teach parents proper technique for hand washing and the importance of washing hands after changing infant's diaper

    d. Apply infant's diaper snugly

    e. Apply extra-absorbent diapers

    f. Attempt to keep infant's/children's hands from contaminated area

    g. Teach proper hand washing and monitor if child is age-appropriate

5. Skin integrity

    a. Assess skin with each diaper change

    b. Avoid wipes that contain alcohol

    c. Wash perineal area with mild soap and rinse with water after each stool

    d. Apply zinc-based ointment

    e. Expose slightly reddened intact skin to air as often as possible

    f. Assess perineal area for manifestations of fungal infections

    g. Apply antifungal topical agents as prescribed for fungal infections

6. Client/family teaching

    a. Assess client (if age-appropriate) and family's current level of knowledge

    b. Explain all procedures

    c. Provide written and verbal instructions regarding:

        1) ORT

        2) Effects of medication and any adverse effects

        3) Importance of follow-up with infant's/child's health care provider

        4) Signs and symptoms to report to health care provider

        5) Importance of adequate fluid intake

    d. Provide adequate time for teaching

    e. Document teaching and client/family response

NIC

1. Bowel Management, Diarrhea Management, Fluid/Electrolyte Management

2. Fluid/Electrolyte Management

3. Nutritional Monitoring, Nutrition Management
4. Infection Control, Infection Protection
5. Skin Surveillance
6. Teaching: Disease Process, Management

EVALUATION

1. Client's diarrhea resolves without complications.
2. Client regains and maintains fluid and electrolyte balance as evidenced by urine output and electrolyte levels WDL.
3. Client regains and maintains nutrition adequate to maintain appropriate weight for age.
4. Client and others do not exhibit manifestations of gastrointestinal infection.
5. Client's skin remains intact.
6. Client (if age-appropriate) and family demonstrate understanding of diarrhea, management, prevention, and home care.

References

Broyles, B. E., Reiss, B. S., & Evans, M. E. (2007). *Pharmacological aspects of nursing care* (7th ed.). Clifton Park, NY: Delmar Cengage Learning.

Guandalini, S., & Frye, R. E. (2006). *Diarrhea.* Retrieved May 11, 2007, from http://www.emedicine.com/ped/topic583.htm

Hockenberry, M. J. (2005). *Wong's essentials of pediatric nursing* (7th ed.). St. Louis, MO: Elsevier Mosby.

National Institute of Diabetes and Digestive and Kidney Diseases. (2007). NIH Publication No 04-2749. Retrieved May 11, 2007, from http://digestive.niddk.nih.gov/ddiseases/pubs/diarrhea/#children

Stöppler, M. C., & Lee, D. (2007). *Moms uninformed about rotovirus infection.* Retrieved May 11, 2007, from http://www.medicinenet.com/script/main/art.asp?articlekey=55474

35

DISSEMINATED INTRAVASCULAR COAGULATION (DIC)

Definition

Disseminated intravascular coagulation (DIC) is a complex and life-threatening bleeding disorder characterized by simultaneous proliferation of clotting factors and massive bleeding. It is not a disease, but the manifestation of an underlying condition.

Pathophysiology

DIC is a complication that can result from a number of physical disorders considered life-threatening, including sepsis (especially gram-negative bacterial), severe tissue injury (burns and head trauma), necrotizing enterocolitis, severe viral infections, severe fungal infections in immunosuppressed children, anaphylaxis, shock, cardiopulmonary arrest, venomous snake bites, pancreatitis, liver disease, cancer (acute promyelocytic leukemia and mucinous adenocarcinomas), and transplant rejection. Obstetrical complications such as abruptio placenta, amniotic fluid embolus, septic abortion caused by gram-negative bacteria, and retained fetus also can lead to the cascading effects of DIC (Daniels, Nosek, & Nicoll, 2007; Potts & Mandleco, 2007). In sepsis, the systemic inflammation leads to "the generation of proinflammatory cytokines that, among other things, orchestrate coagulation and fibrinolytic activation" (Zeerleder, Hack, & Wuillemin, 2005, p. 2865).

Once DIC is triggered by predisposing conditions, the pathophysiologic process is basically the same regardless of the cause. The process begins with endothelial cell damage causing extreme stimulation of clotting mechanisms. This initially enhances the normal coagulation; but as DIC progresses, the mechanisms proliferate out of control. Intrinsic or extrinsic clotting pathways or both are activated; and within a short time, these regulatory factors (including antithrombin III, protein C, and protein S) are depleted, causing a massive release of thrombin (Daniels et al., 2007). This activation results in widespread intravascular coagulation resulting in a depletion of clotting factors. The uncontrolled intravascular coagulation causes microvascular occlusions that lead to tissue ischemia. Also activated are the body's fibrolytic pathways, inhibiting coagulation that results in widespread bleeding. If DIC is not corrected, the individual dies from hypovolemic or hemorrhagic shock (Daniels et al., 2007). Refer to Figure 35-1.

Complications

Hemorrhage
Tissue ischemia
Hypovolemic shock
Death

Incidence

The true incidence of DIC in children in the United States is unknown. "The overall mortality rate for children with sepsis-related DIC is 13–40%" (Kanwar, Galardy, & Grabowski, 2006, p. 1). According to one study, DIC may be found in 25–50% of clients with sepsis (Zeerleder et al., 2005, p. 2865).

Etiology

Refer to "Pathophysiology."

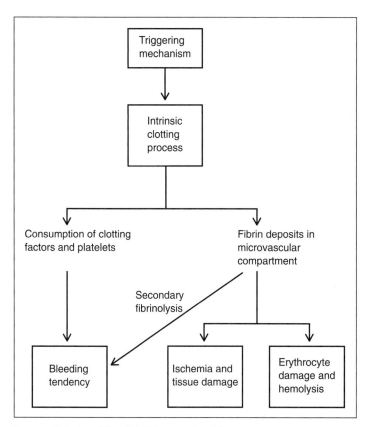

Figure 35-1: Mechanisms of Disseminated Intravascular Coagulation.

Clinical Manifestations

Presence of predisposing condition

Bleeding manifestations

Ecchymosis

Epistaxis

Spontaneous bleeding

Hematoma formation

Petechiae

Purpura

Dyspnea

Tachypnea

Hemoptysis

Manifestations of shock

Nausea

Vomiting

Abdominal pain

Hematemesis

    Rectal bleeding
    Decreased level of consciousness (LOC)
    Seizures
    Pain
  Thrombolytic manifestations
    Acute respiratory distress syndrome
    Oliguria
    Cardiac dysrhythmias
    Venous distention
    Paralytic ileus
    Manifestations of multiple organ dysfunction

Diagnostic Tests

Complete blood count
Prothrombin time
Partial thromboplastin time
Serum fibrinogen level
Fibrin degradation products (FDP) or fibrin split products (FSP)

Medical Management

The goals of treatment are to effectively treat the initiating disorder and to control bleeding and reestablish coagulation pathways. "The most important therapeutic maneuver is treating the initiating disorder. Without this, supportive measures ultimately fail" (Kanwar et al., 2006, p. 1). Children with DIC should be treated in the pediatric intensive care unit with supportive measures including ventilatory support, vascular volume support, and pressor therapy if the child is hypotensive, as well as close monitoring of neurologic and renal function. Units of fresh frozen plasma and units of platelets are administered intravenously to control bleeding. Cryoprecipitate is used to replace factor VIII and fibrinogen (Broyles et al., 2007). In clients with serious bleeding, packed red blood cells are transfused to improve blood oxygen carrying capacity. Children who develop shock and respiratory failure require mechanical ventilation support. If DIC results from trauma requiring surgery, a pediatric surgeon should be involved.

A pediatric hematologist, oncologist, neurologist, and nephrologist may be required to assist in the child's care. Renal thrombosis and decreased renal perfusion (secondary to shock) as well as central nervous system (CNS) thrombosis, infarction, or hemorrhage may occur. The use of heparin in the treatment of children with DIC is controversial and is indicated primarily in children who have not responded to treatment of the underlying cause of the DIC or to replacement therapy. If heparin is used, it should be in conjunction with further clotting factor replacement therapy. The child should remain in the critical care environment until the underlying condition is successfully treated and the DIC is under control.

Nursing Management

ASSESSMENT

    1. Obtain client history with focus on possible predisposing factors for DIC
    2. Assess airway, breath, and circulation (ABC)
    3. Obtain baseline vital signs
    4. Perform rapid initial physical assessment
    5. Assess for presence of clinical manifestations
    6. Obtain needed blood samples for laboratory testing as prescribed

NURSING DIAGNOSES (INCLUDING BUT NOT LIMITED TO)

1. Ineffective protection R/T widespread bleeding/hemorrhage
2. Ineffective tissue perfusion R/T blood loss and decreased circulation secondary to thrombus formation
3. Decreased cardiac output R/T fluid volume deficit and decreased mean arterial pressure secondary to blood loss
4. Impaired gas exchange R/T altered breathing pattern and loss of oxygen carrying capacity secondary to hemorrhage
5. Risk for injury R/T transfusion of blood products
6. Acute pain R/T tissue ischemia secondary to thrombus formation and tissue hypoxia
7. Anxiety R/T fear of the unknown, disease process, critical care environment, and treatment
8. Deficient knowledge R/T condition, treatment, and home care

PLANNING/GOALS

1. Client will be free of bleeding 48–72 hours after initiation of treatment.
2. Client will regain and maintain tissue perfusion as evidenced by pulses +2 on a scale of 0–4, brisk capillary refill, color within defined limits (WDL), urine output > 1–2 mL/kg/hr for infants and small children and > 30 mL for older children, and stable vital signs.
3. Client will regain and maintain adequate cardiac output as evidenced by laboratory values WDL, oxygen saturation/pulse oximetry > 94%, and hemodynamic values WDL.
4. Client will regain and maintain adequate gas exchange as evidenced by oxygen saturation/pulse oximetry > 94%, pH 7.35–7.45, PaCO$_2$ 35–45 mm Hg, and respirations WDL for client.
5. Client will not experience transfusion reaction or fluid overload.
6. Client will demonstrate pain control as determined by client within 2 hours of initiation of treatment.
7. Client (if age-appropriate) and family will verbalize fears, concerns, and feelings and demonstrate decreased tenseness in body posture, more relaxed facial features, and other nonverbal indicators.
8. Client (if age-appropriate) and family will demonstrate understanding of condition, treatment, and home care.

NOC

1. Blood Coagulation, Immune Status
2. Vital Signs
3. Blood Loss Severity
4. Respiratory Status: Gas Exchange
5. Risk Control
6. Pain Control
7. Anxiety
8. Knowledge: Illness Care, Disease Process, Treatment

IMPLEMENTATION

1. Protection
   a. Monitor coagulation studies
   b. Protect from injury
   c. Monitor vital signs and hemodynamics

  d. Initiate and maintain patency of intravenous access, monitoring at least hourly

  e. Administer medications as prescribed, monitoring for effectiveness and adverse effects

  f. Use soft-bristle toothbrush for oral care

  g. Assess mucous membranes for bleeding

  h. Monitor closely for increase in petechiae, bruising, and purpura

  i. Maintain bedrest during active bleeding

  j. Monitor neurologic status

  k. Draw labs from central venous access device (CVAD) when possible

  l. Monitor for signs of emboli

  m. Avoid rectal temperatures

  n. Protect from infection by meticulous hand washing

2. Tissue perfusion

  a. Assess vital signs as condition warrants and continue hemodynamic monitoring

  b. Maintain patency of intravenous access, monitoring at least hourly

  c. Monitor urine output every hour and as condition warrants

  d. Maintain strict intake and output

  e. Administer intravenous fluids as prescribed to increase intravascular volume

  f. Administer medications as prescribed, monitoring for effectiveness and adverse effects

  g. Weigh daily

  h. Monitor complete blood count

  i. Administer blood products as prescribed

  j. Assess apical and peripheral pulses

  k. Assess for signs of impending shock

  l. Monitor for decreased cardiac output and pulmonary perfusion

  m. Carefully reposition every 2 hours

3. Cardiac output

  a. Monitor vital signs as condition warrants and hemodynamics continuously

  b. Maintain hemodynamic monitoring

  c. Monitor cardiac output

  d. Maintain patency of intravenous access, monitoring at least hourly

  e. Administer medications as prescribed, monitoring for effectiveness and adverse effects

  f. Administer intravenous fluids as prescribed

  g. Monitor urine output hourly

4. Gas exchange

  a. Monitor respiratory status and breath sounds every 2 hours and as condition warrants

  b. Monitor for dyspnea

  c. Monitor chest X-ray results

  d. Monitor continuous oxygen saturation per pulse oximetry

  e. Monitor arterial blood gas results

  f. Administer oxygen as prescribed, titrating to pulse oximetry and client response

      g. Encourage coughing and deep-breathing if not on mechanical ventilation and if age-appropriate

      h. Institute inhalation respiratory therapy as prescribed

      i. Monitor for manifestations of pulmonary embolus

      j. Assess for changes in LOC

      k. Monitor for paradoxical respiratory activity

5. Risk for injury

      a. Adhere to facility protocol for blood products administration

      b. Check with another licensed person regarding blood to be administered

      c. Obtain pretransfusion vital signs

      d. Verify blood products, client identification, blood expiration date, blood type, and blood unit number

      e. Monitor continuously during initial 15–30 minutes of transfusion

      f. Stop transfusion immediately if transfusion reaction occurs, while maintaining patency of intravenous access with 0.9% normal saline, and notify health care provider

      g. Administer medications as prescribed; use intravenous access other than the one infusing blood if medications are administered intravenously

      h. Monitor for fluid overload

      i. Obtain posttransfusion vital signs

      j. Monitor posttransfusion blood studies

6. Acute pain

      a. Assess pain level hourly

      b. Maintain patency of intravenous access, monitoring at least hourly

      c. Administer analgesics as prescribed on an "around-the-clock" schedule

      d. Place infant/young child on cardiorespiratory monitor while receiving opioid analgesics

      e. Monitor vital signs for indications of inadequate pain control

      f. Monitor for effectiveness of pain control measures

      g. Position for comfort

      h. Maintain body alignment

      i. Administer medications slowly, flushing before and after with normal saline to protect peripheral intravenous access from irritation

7. Anxiety

      a. Assess for manifestations of anxiety

      b. Explain all equipment and procedures to client (if age-appropriate) and family

      c. Encourage family involvement in child's care within constraints of critical care environment

      d. Maintain client's call bed in reach (if age-appropriate for child)

      e. Encourage client (if age-appropriate) and family to express feelings and concerns

      f. Encourage questions and answer them honestly

      g. Initiate referrals for pastoral care or facilitate family contacting its own spiritual leader

8. Client/family teaching
   a. Assess client's/family's current level of knowledge
   b. Provide verbal and written information regarding:
      1) Risk factors for developing DIC
      2) Signs and symptoms of bleeding and ineffective tissue perfusion
      3) Medication administration including importance of complying with prescribed medication regimen
      4) Signs and symptoms of adverse effects of medications
      5) Importance of adequate age-appropriate fluid intake
      6) Signs and symptoms of worsening of condition
      7) Contact phone numbers to report signs and symptoms
      8) Importance of follow-up with health care provider
   c. Provide sufficient time for client/family questions
   d. Document teaching and client/family response

NIC

1. Bleeding Precautions, Infection Protection
2. Hemodynamic Regulation, Vital Signs Monitoring
3. Bleeding Reduction, Hemorrhage Control, Shock Management: Volume
4. Acid-Base Monitoring, Oxygen Therapy, Respiratory Monitoring
5. Risk Identification, Safety Surveillance
6. Medication Management, Pain Management
7. Anxiety Reduction
8. Teaching: Illness Care, Disease Process, Treatment

EVALUATION

1. Client is free of bleeding 48–72 hours after initiation of treatment.
2. Client regains and maintains tissue perfusion as evidenced by pulses +2 on a scale of 0–4, brisk capillary refill, color WDL, urine output 1–2 mL/kg/hr for infants and young children and > 30 mL/hr for older children, and stable vital signs.
3. Client regains and maintains adequate cardiac output as evidenced by laboratory values WDL, oxygen saturation/pulse oximetry > 94%, and hemodynamic values WDL.
4. Client regains and maintains adequate gas exchange as evidenced by oxygen saturation/pulse oximetry > 94%, pH 7.35–7.45, $PaCO_2$ 35–45 mm Hg, and respirations WDL for client.
5. Client does not experience transfusion reaction or fluid overload.
6. Client demonstrates pain control as determined by client within 2 hours of initiation of treatment.
7. Client (if age-appropriate) and family verbalize fears, concerns, and feelings and demonstrate decreased tenseness in body posture, more relaxed facial features, and other nonverbal indicators.
8. Client (if age-appropriate) and family demonstrate understanding of condition, treatment, and home care.

References

Broyles, B. E., Reiss, B. S., & Evans, M. E. (2007). *Pharmacological aspects of nursing care* (7th ed.). Clifton Park, NY: Delmar Cengage Learning.

Daniels, R., Nosek, L. J., & Nicoll, L. H. (2007). *Contemporary medical-surgical nursing.* Clifton Park, NY: Delmar Cengage Learning.

Kanwar, V. S., Galardy, P. J., & Grabowski, E. (2006). *Consumption coagulopathy.* Retrieved May 11, 2007, from http://www.emedicine.com/ped/topic473.htm

Potts, N. L., & Mandleco, B. L. (2007). *Pediatric nursing: Caring for children and their families* (2nd ed.). Clifton Park, NY: Delmar Cengage Learning.

Zeerleder, S., Hack, C. E., & Wuillemin, W. A. (2005). *Disseminated intravascular coagulation in sepsis.* Retrieved May 11, 2007, from http://www.chestjournal.org/cgi/content/abstract/128/4/2864

36

DOWN SYNDROME/MENTAL RETARDATION

Definition

Down syndrome, also referred to as trisomy 21, is a congenital condition resulting from the genetic presence of an extra #21 X chromosome. Down syndrome is named after John Langdon Down, an English physician in the late 1800s who was the first to publish an accurate description of an individual with Down syndrome (National Down Syndrome Society, 2007).

Pathophysiology

Normally, chromosomes are present in 23 pairs. The condition results from an error in cell division called nondisjunction. Prior to or at the time of conception, a pair of 21st chromosomes in either the sperm or the egg fails to separate. As embryogenesis occurs and the embryo develops, the extra chromosome is replicated in every cell of the body. This error in cell division is responsible for 95% of all cases of Down syndrome. According to the National Down Syndrome Society, "Down syndrome also encompasses two other genetic conditions: 1) mosaicism and 2) translocation. Mosaicism occurs when nondisjunction of chromosome 21 occurs in one of the initial cell divisions after fertilization, causing an individual to have 46 chromosomes in some of his/her cells and 47 in others. Mosaicism is the least common form of Down syndrome, accounting for only 1 to 2 percent of all cases. Translocation occurs when part of chromosome 21 breaks off during cell division and attaches to another chromosome, usually chromosome 14. While the total number of chromosomes in the cells remains 46, the presence of an extra part of chromosome 21 causes the characteristics of Down syndrome. Translocation accounts for 3 to 4 percent of cases of Down syndrome" (National Down Syndrome Society, 2007, p. 1).

This presence of 47 chromosomes appears to alter the normal processes that regulate embryogenesis. It is responsible for numerous changes associated with the syndrome, including hypotonicity of the chest and abdominal muscles, alterations in connective tissue and facial features, and varying degrees of cognitive impairment (Potts & Mandleco, 2007). Further, it is related to other multisystem anomalies including congenital heart defects (present in 30–40% of children with Down syndrome); hearing and visual impairments; a narrow and short eustachian tube; and gastrointestinal abnormalities including a tracheoesophageal fistula, an atrioventricular canal, Hirschsprung's disease, and imperforate anus. Instability of the cervical spine resulting from atlantoaxial deformity, leukemia, and hypothyroidism are consequences of the disorder. It also is believed that the extra chromosome alters neurotransmitter function in the cholinergic system, resulting in premature aging and Alzheimer's disease.

The cognitive impairment associated with Down syndrome bears other names, including mental retardation (MR) and developmental delay. Regardless of the terminology used, some degree of impairment is present in these children.

According to the American Association on Intellectual and Developmental Disabilities, the definition of MR is "a disability characterized by significant limitations both in intellectual functioning and in adaptive behavior as expressed in conceptual, social, and practical adaptive skills. This disability originates before age 18" (American Association on Intellectual and Developmental Disabilities, 2005, p. 1). In addition to Down syndrome, a number of other conditions can result in cognitive impairment. These include other genetic conditions such as fragile X syndrome, Prader-Willi syndrome, and phenylketonuria (PKU); anoxia, maternal drug and alcohol use, toxemia of pregnancy, placental insufficiency, and maternal infections (rubella, toxoplasmosis, or cytomegalovirus) during fetal development; asphyxia during birth, prematurity, and low birth weight; certain diseases such as pertussis, measles, and meningitis; and exposure to poisons including lead and mercury. Accidents resulting in head trauma or any condition that sufficiently decreases oxygen available to the brain can cause MR (National Dissemination Center for Children with Disabilities, 2006; Sebastian, 2006).

According to the American Psychiatric Association (APA), there are four classifications of MR based on intelligence quotients (IQs). The normal IQ is defined as 100 or above. Mild MR is the most common type and is defined as an IQ of 50–55 to 70; moderate MR is an IQ level of 35–40 to 50–55; severe MR is an IQ of 20–25 to 35–40; profound MR is an IQ less than 20–25 (American Psychiatric Association, 2000). Children with Down syndrome usually achieve a level of cognitive functioning consistent with mild MR. Developmental characteristics of these types are located in Table 36-1.

Table 36-1 | Characteristics of Mental Retardation According to Types

Type	IQ	Developmental Characteristics
Mild	50–55 to 70	Is slower to walk, feed self, and talk Can acquire reading and math skills at a third- to sixth-grade level Has a psychosocial development of an 8- to 12-year-old Has social and vocational abilities Can adjust to marriage but not child rearing
Moderate	35–40 to 50–55	Has noticeable delays in motor and speech development Can learn simple communication, basic self-care skills (dressing and brushing hair and teeth), and safety habits Can learn basic counting and letter recognition consistent with a first grader Achieves a psychosocial developmental level of a 3- to 7-year-old Participates in simple tasks and activities Is unable to function independently

(continues)

Table 36-1 | Characteristics of Mental Retardation According to Types (*continued*)

Type	IQ	Developmental Characteristics
Severe	20–25 to 35–40	Has little or no communication skills Is usually able to walk but may continue to have an unsteady gait Functions best with systematic repetitive training Achieves the cognitive developmental level of a toddler Requires supervision in a protective environment
Profound	Less than 20–25	Has minimum functional capacity Has basic emotional responses Achieves a developmental level of an infant May walk, but basically requires custodial care

Complications

Cognitive impairment
Hearing impairment
Visual impairment
Nasopharyngeal alterations
Flaccid musculature
Tracheoesophageal fistula
Atrioventricular canal
Imperforate anus
Obesity in childhood
Hypothyroidism
Premature aging
Alzheimer's disease

Incidence

"According to a report released January 6, 2006 by the Centers for Disease Control (CDC), the occurrence of Down syndrome in the United States may be more common than previously thought, estimated at one case for every 733 live births" (National Down Syndrome Society, 2007, p. 1). More than 350,000 people in the United States have Down syndrome. As one of the most frequently occurring chromosomal abnormalities, Down syndrome affects individuals of all ages, races, and economic levels. Because of the increasing incidence of Down syndrome, "All pregnant women should be offered screening for Down syndrome, regardless of their age, according to new guidelines from the American College of Obstetricians and Gynecologists (ACOG)" (McCoy, 2007, p. 1).

In a statement released in 2006 by the CDC, "Children with Down syndrome are living longer, according to a new study, 'Survival in Infants with Down Syndrome, Metropolitan Atlanta, 1979–1998,' published in the June 2006 issue of *The Journal of Pediatrics*. The study examined the survival of 645 infants with Down syndrome in the Atlanta metropolitan area. It showed that nearly 93 percent of infants with Down syndrome now survive the first year and nearly 90 percent of affected infants survive the first 10 years" (Centers for Disease Control and Prevention, 2006, p. 1).

Etiology

As noted previously in "Pathophysiology," Down syndrome is the result of an error in cell division called nondisjunction. According to the National Down Syndrome, "A 35-year-old woman has a one in 350 chance of conceiving a child with Down syndrome. By age 45, the incidence has increased to one in 30. However, because younger women have higher fertility rates, 80 percent of babies with Down syndrome are born to women under the age of 35. Once a woman has given birth to a baby with Down syndrome, the chance of having a second child with Down syndrome is about 1 in 100" (National Down Syndrome Society, 2007, p. 1). According to the CDC, citing a study by the National Center for Birth Defects and Developmental Disabilities, both maternal cigarette smoking and use of contraceptives increase the risk of giving birth to a child with Down syndrome (Centers for Disease Control and Prevention, 2005).

Clinical Manifestations

Growth failure
Cognitive impairment
Flat back of the head
Low-set ears
"Loops" on the finger tips
Single deep crease across the center of the palm of the hand
(simian crease)
Short broad hands
Unilateral or bilateral absence of one rib
Muscle flaccidity
Flat facial profile
Small, short nose
Depressed bridge of the nose
Upward slant to the eyes
Hyperextension of the joints
Small skin folds on the inner corner of the eyes
(epicanthic eyelid)
Excessive space between large and second toe
Small and arched palate
Large wrinkled tongue
In older children
    Overweight
    Visual impairment
    Hearing impairment
    Cognitive impairment

Diagnostic Tests

Maternal serum testing for levels of alpha-fetoprotein and the hormones estriol and human chorionic gonadotropin (HCG)

Prenatal ultrasonography

Chorionic villus sampling (CVS)

Amniocentesis

Percutaneous umbilical blood sampling (PUBS)

Karyotyping

Following birth, the presence of the Down syndrome features initiate diagnostic testing for commonly associated anomalies

Medical Management

There is no cure for Down syndrome, so the goals of management are to manage associated anomalies and to facilitate the child's reaching his or her highest level of growth and development and wellness. During the neonatal period, the focus of care is on thermoregulation; feeding; and detection and monitoring of cardiac, gastrointestinal, and craniofacial abnormalities. Cardiac and gastrointestinal defects can be corrected by surgery.

As these children grow, they should take part in enrichment programs for infants, toddlers, and preschoolers. These programs can be pursued in stimulation programs outside the home or in one-on-one interactions at home. The transneuronal attachments in all infants, including those with Down syndrome, are abundant; therefore, early intervention is critical because these attachments decrease and disappear if not used. After preschool, many of these children are mainstreamed into the public school system. Special needs programs are available in many schools, and parents may need guidance in choosing the right school for their child (Potts & Mandleco, 2007). Health care guidelines are available from the National Down Syndrome Society—addressing neonatal, infant, childhood, adolescence, and adulthood needs.

Management for these children includes monitoring their growth and development using specialized growth charts. A child with Down syndrome should be screened for thyroid dysfunction; visual impairment (ocular cataract); and hearing impairment (including recurrent otitis media) annually throughout the childhood years. Another common problem is constipation, which can be addressed with the use of stool softeners. In children susceptible to subacute bacterial endocarditis, prophylaxis with antimicrobial therapy should be initiated and maintained.

Adolescents with Down syndrome should be screened for obstructive sleep apnea resulting from the short, thick structure of their necks. As their bodies mature sexually, adolescents with Down syndrome require consultation for sexuality issues. In addition, smoking, drug, and alcohol education is necessary. By the age of 16 years, functional transition planning including monitoring of the level of independent functioning should be addressed (National Down Syndrome Society, 2007).

Nursing Management

ASSESSMENT

1. Monitor temperature stabilization
2. Assess for feeding difficulties
3. Assess for presence of cardiac abnormalities
4. Assess for gastrointestinal abnormalities
5. Assess parents' current level of knowledge regarding neonatal care and parental skills

6. Assess as child grows for cognitive and developmental skills, hearing and vision status, child's ability to communicate, motor skills, and parental/family adjustment to diagnosis and child's needs

7. Assess sexuality, drug and alcohol use, and smoking issues in adolescents

Nursing Diagnoses (including but not limited to)

1. Ineffective thermoregulation R/T muscle flaccidity and extended posture of neonate

2. Imbalanced nutrition: less than body requirements R/T feeding difficulties secondary to protruding tongue and high arched palate

3. Ineffective family coping R/T increased financial and emotional stress of caring for a cognitively impaired child and chronic illness

4. Impaired social interaction R/T developmental delay

5. Delayed growth and development R/T cognitive impairment

6. Deficient knowledge R/T child's condition, treatment modalities for accompanying congenital anomalies, education needs, and home care

Planning/Goals

1. Client will maintain body temperature within defined limits (WDL) and will not experience respiratory compromise associated with hypothermia.

2. Client will consume adequate nutrition as evidenced by weight gain WDL and manifestations of adequate hydration including six to eight wet diapers per day, elastic skin turgor, moist mucous membranes, capillary refill < 2 seconds, and urinary output 1–2 mL/kg/hr.

3. Family will identify effective coping strategies and utilize community support services.

4. Client will demonstrate adequate social interaction skills, interacting appropriately with peers, engaging in developmentally appropriate play activities, and participating in group activities.

5. Client will master basic academic tasks for kindergarten, including letter and number recognition, simple word recognition, counting, simple writing, and simple math.

6. Family will demonstrate understanding of child's condition, treatment modalities for accompanying congenital anomalies, education needs, and home care.

NOC

1. Thermoregulation
2. Nutritional Status: Food & Fluid Intake, Nutrient Intake
3. Acceptance: Health Status
4. Social Involvement
5. Child Development, Knowledge: Parenting
6. Knowledge

Implementation

1. Thermoregulation
   a. Place neonate on warmer after birth until temperature rises to WDL
   b. Monitor temperature hourly for first 8 hours after birth, then every 4 hours until discharge

    c. Wrap neonate in warm blankets

    d. Monitor for increased respiratory rate, mottling, and other indicators of cold stress

    e. Teach parents to bundle-wrap infant at home and to avoid drafts

2. Nutrition

    a. Assess infant's sucking ability

    b. Assess nipple softness (use preemie nipple) as needed

    c. Sit infant upright for feedings if formula-fed

    d. Teach breastfeeding mother to keep infant wrapped during feedings

    e. Monitor for choking and aspiration continuously during feedings

    f. Instruct parents about appropriate feeding techniques

    g. Support parents during feedings and assist as needed

    h. Weigh daily while in hospital

3. Coping

    a. Encourage parents to verbalize feelings and concerns

    b. Provide supportive environment

    c. Assess parental bonding with infant

    d. Be an active listener

    e. Provide role modeling when interacting with infant and family

    f. Encourage active participation of parents in infant care

    g. Facilitate referrals to appropriate community services

    h. Teach parents about normal growth and development during infancy, emphasizing the need to follow up with nurse in health care provider's office

4. Social interactions

    a. Encourage parents to provide peer interactions during preschool stage and later growth and development stages

    b. Encourage parents to teach child important social language (*please* and *thank-you*)

    c. Encourage parents to be active in child's education, such as becoming class tutors, room parents, and field trip chaperones

    d. Encourage child advocacy

    e. Provide parents with information concerning community services

    f. Encourage involvement in after-school recreational programs (Boy/Girl Scouts, YMCA, swimming, soccer, etc.)

    g. Encourage parents to set aside time each evening to assist with homework assignments

    h. Encourage parents to make use of hospital school teachers and to provide for someone to pick up homework assignments if child is hospitalized for surgery to repair coexisting congenital anomalies

    i. Encourage any older siblings to assist child with school work

    j. Suggest conferences with teacher at bimonthly intervals during school year

    k. Provide parents with information about tutors and summer school programs

5. Growth and development

    a. Provide parents with information about how to facilitate child's growth and development

    b. Assess child's current level of growth and development at each health care provider's office visit

    c. Encourage parents to discuss child's mastering of developmental skills

    d. Suggest conferences with teachers at bimonthly intervals during school year

    e. Encourage parents and siblings to be active in child's growth and development

    f. Provide parents with information about tutors and summer school programs

    g. Provide positive reinforcement to parents/child for skill mastery

    h. Assist parents/child to expect success in school, socialization, and self-care skills

6. Family/client teaching

    a. Assess parents' level of understanding about child's condition

    b. Provide verbal and written information regarding:

        1) Prevention of hypothermia

        2) Appropriate feeding techniques

        3) Weight and activity management as child grows older to prevent obesity

        4) Importance of follow-up care

        5) Educational involvement previously addressed in this care plan

        6) Medication administration if needed

        7) Manifestations that need to be reported to health care provider

        8) Referral information and information concerning community resources

        9) Information concerning National Down Syndrome Society

        10) Contact phone numbers needed

    c. Provide adequate time for teaching and reinforcement of material

    d. Document teaching and parental responses

NIC

1. Temperature Regulation
2. Nutritional Monitoring
3. Coping Enhancement, Emotional Support
4. Socialization Enhancement, Teaching: Individual
5. Developmental Enhancement: Child
6. Teaching

EVALUATION

1. Client maintains body temperature WDL and does not experience respiratory compromise associated with hypothermia.

2. Client consumes adequate nutrition by doubling birth weight by 6 months and tripling birth weight by 1 year of age and shows manifestations of adequate hydration including six to eight wet diapers per day, elastic skin turgor, moist mucous membranes, capillary refill < 2 seconds, and urinary output 1–2 mL/kg/hr.

3. Family identifies effective coping strategies and utilizes community support services.

4. Client demonstrates adequate social interaction skills, interacting appropriately with peers, engaging in developmentally appropriate play activities, and participating in group activities.

5. Client masters basic academic tasks for kindergarten, including letter and number recognition, simple word recognition, counting, simple writing, and simple math.

6. Family demonstrates understanding of child's condition, treatment modalities for accompanying congenital anomalies, education needs, and home care.

References

American Association on Intellectual and Developmental Disabilities. (2005). *Definition of mental retardation.* Retrieved May 12, 2007, from http://www.aamr.org/Policies/faq_mental_retardation.shtml

American Psychiatric Association. (2000). *Diagnosis and statistical manual of mental disorders* (4th ed.). Washington, DC: Author.

Centers for Disease Control and Prevention. (2005). *Risk factors for Down syndrome (trisomy 21): Maternal cigarette smoking and oral contraceptive use in a population-based case-control study.* Retrieved May 11, 2007, from http://www.cdc.gov/ncbddd/bd/ds.htm

Centers for Disease Control and Prevention. (2006). *Down syndrome survival rate increasing: Racial disparities exist in a large metropolitan area.* Retrieved May 11, 2007, from http://www.cdc.gov/od/oc/media/pressrel/r060630.htm

McCoy, K. (2007). *Down syndrome screening recommended for all expectant moms.* Retrieved May 11, 2007, from http://www.spine-health.com/news/pregnancy/art600519.html

National Dissemination Center for Children with Disabilities. (2006). *Mental retardation.* Retrieved May 12, 2007, from http://www.nichcy.org/pubs/factshe/fs8txt.htm#whatis

National Down Syndrome Society. (2007). *CDC's new study on the prevalence of Down syndrome.* Retrieved May 11, 2007, from http://www.ndss.org/index.php?option=com_content&task=view&id=1622&Itemid=194

Potts, N. L., & Mandleco, B. L. (2007). *Pediatric nursing: Caring for children and their families* (2nd ed.). Clifton Park, NY: Delmar Cengage Learning.

Sebastian, C. S. (2006). *Mental retardation.* Retrieved May 12, 2007, from http://www.emedicine.com/med/topic3095.htm

37

DUODENAL ATRESIA

Definition

Duodenal atresia is the complete lack of the lumen of the first segment of the small intestine. Duodenal stenosis is a stricture in the duodenal lumen.

Pathophysiology

The duodenum is the first intestinal segment to receive stomach contents and is responsible for the majority of nutritional absorption. The current theory about duodenal atresia is that it occurs due to inadequate endodermal proliferation or failure of the duodenal lumen to recanalize. Regardless of why it occurs, the proximal and distal intestinal segments always end in a blind pouch. During the third through the seventh week of embryonic development, the gastrointestinal system is evolving, including active proliferation of the duodenal lumen. During this time, the active proliferation completely obliterates the lumen of the duodenum. This is followed by recanalization of the first portion of the duodenum, and the hollow lumen is reestablished. "The second part of the duodenum is the last to recanalize. The early-forming biliary system consists of 2 channels arising from the embryonic duodenum. This structure creates a narrow segment of bowel, approximately 0.125 mm in length that is interposed between the 2 biliary channels. This narrow region is the area most prone to problems, with recanalization and atresia formation. The ampulla of Vater usually is immediately adjacent to or traverses the medial wall of the diaphragm. The presence of a bifid biliary system, or the insertion of one duct above and one duct below the atresia, is rare and occurs when both biliary duct anlagen remain patent. The presence of bile above and below the atresia indicates a bifid biliary system" (Mandell, 2007, Section 2). The inability of the duodenum to function leads to electrolyte and acid-base imbalances, especially hypokalemia, hypochloremia, and metabolic acidosis. Duodenal atresia frequently accompanies Down syndrome and is usually associated with other structural defects including other gastrointestinal anomalies and cardiac defects.

There are three types of duodenal atresia, with each type having specific characteristics. The most common type is type 1, which is formed by a membrane composed of mucosa and submucosa that traverses the internal diameter of the duodenum. "The duodenum and stomach proximal to the obstruction are dilated and hypertrophied. The duodenum distal to the obstruction is narrowed. A variation of this occurs when the membrane is elongated in the shape of a windsock, and the site of origin of the membrane is proximal to the level of obstruction" (Lewis & Glick, 2006, Section 4). The second type (type 2) is characterized by a fibrous cord that connects the ends of the duodenum where the atresia is located. Finally, type 3 is when "complete separation of the atretic segments occurs. Most of the biliary duct anomalies associated with duodenal atresia are observed in type 3 defects" (Lewis & Glick, 2006, Section 4).

Complications

Electrolyte imbalances including hypokalemic/hypochloremic metabolic
   alkalosis
Bowel obstruction

Prematurity

Presence of other structural anomalies including cardiac defects

Postoperative intestinal motility problems and gastroesophageal reflux
(MedlinePlus, 2005)

Incidence

Congenital duodenal atresia occurs in 1 in 5,000–10,000 live births (Lewis & Glick, 2006). "In approximately 40% of cases, the anomaly is encountered in an infant with trisomy 21 [Down syndrome]" (Calkins & Karrer, 2006, p. 1). Similar international statistics are congruent with those of the United States. There are no differences in incidence due to race or gender.

Etiology

Duodenal atresia is considered to be the result of a developmental error that takes place during early gestation because it usually occurs in conjunction with other anomalies of structures developing during the same gestational period. "A few cases of duodenal atresia have been inherited as an autosomal recessive genetic trait" (National Organization for Rare Disorders, 2003, p. 1).

Clinical Manifestations

Vomiting soon after birth

Scaphoid abdomen

Dehydration

Weight loss

Hypokalemia

Hypochloremia

Metabolic alkalosis

Diagnostic Tests

Prenatal ultrasonography

Erect and recumbent plain radiography of the abdomen

Serum electrolytes

Urinalysis

Chromosome analysis (to detect trisomy 21)

Medical Management

The goals of treatment are to reestablish electrolyte and acid-base balance and surgically repair the atresia. No medical therapies are available for duodenal atresia or stenosis. The most common surgical procedure is a duodenostomy. As long as the diagnosis is verified within the first 24 hours and no other anomalies require more urgent repair, the procedure can be performed as soon as possible after birth. Intravenous fluid replacement and correction of electrolyte imbalances should be completed. An orogastric tube is placed, and intravenous replacement of gastric secretions is performed usually with 0.5 mL of 0.9% normal saline with potassium chloride for each milliliter of gastric contents. Cardiac and respiratory stability need to be established prior to surgery.

During surgery, special attention is paid to preventing hypothermia in the neonate. Infants with coexisting gastric-associated malrotation should undergo a Ladd procedure at the time of duodenal repair. Following the repair, a small transanastomotic feeding tube (5F silastic nasojejunal feeding tube) is placed across the anastomosis to facilitate postoperative enteral feeding. The orogastric tube remains in place for gastric decompression (Calkins & Karrer, 2006). Further recommended is "placing a peripheral intravenous central catheter (PICC) or central intravenous catheter at the time of operation because of the expected prolonged ileus and the need for parenteral nutrition" (Calkins & Karrer, Section 6). The orogastric tube remains until the infant passes stool.

Nursing Management

ASSESSMENT

1. Perform neonatal assessment
2. Assist with diagnostic examinations
3. Assess body temperature continuously until stable
4. Assess parental response to diagnosis

NURSING DIAGNOSES (INCLUDING BUT NOT LIMITED TO)

1. Risk for aspiration R/T vomiting
2. Deficient fluid volume R/T vomiting and structural anomaly
3. Risk for ineffective thermoregulation R/T prematurity and surgical procedure
4. Imbalanced nutrition: less than body requirements R/T inadequate intake and malabsorption
5. Anticipatory grieving (parental) R/T presence of congenital anomalies
6. Deficient knowledge R/T infant's condition, treatment modalities, and home care

PLANNING/GOALS

1. Client will not experience aspiration as evidenced by respiratory status within defined limits (WDL).
2. Client will regain and maintain fluid, electrolyte, and acid-base balance as evidenced by hydration indicators, serum electrolyte values, and acid-base values WDL.
3. Client will maintain thermoregulation as evidenced by body temperature WDL for neonate.
4. Client will regain and maintain adequate nutrition for weight gain and growth and developmental needs.
5. Parents will verbalize positive coping strategies and utilize support systems.
6. Parents will demonstrate understanding of infant care, infant's condition, treatment modalities, and home care.

NOC

1. Aspiration Prevention
2. Electrolyte and Acid/Base Balance, Fluid Balance
3. Risk Control, Thermoregulation: Newborn
4. Nutritional Status
5. Coping
6. Knowledge: Infant Care, Illness Care, Health Promotion

IMPLEMENTATION

1. Aspiration
   a. Assess respiratory status every hour and more often as indicated by neonate's condition
   b. Place neonate on continuous cardiorespiratory monitor
   c. Position with head of bed elevated
   d. Maintain nothing by mouth (npo) status

   e.   Place orogastric tube and maintain prescribed suction for decompression
   f.   Suction airway as needed
   g.   Monitor for emesis
   h.   Monitor vital signs
2. Fluid balance
   a.   Weigh daily
   b.   Maintain strict intake and output
   c.   Replace gastric contents with intravenous fluids as prescribed
   d.   Monitor vital signs
   e.   Monitor serum electrolyte values
   f.   Monitor acid-base status
   g.   Maintain intravenous access, monitoring a minimum of hourly
   h.   Administer intravenous fluids as prescribed
   i.   Administer electrolytes as prescribed and according to electrolyte values
   j.   Monitor neurologic status
3. Thermoregulation
   a.   Control environment temperature
   b.   Monitor continuous skin temperature
   c.   Place in infant warmer as needed to maintain body temperature WDL
   d.   Wrap neonate in warm blankets after removal from infant warmer
   e.   Monitor intake and output
   f.   Monitor vital signs
4. Nutrition
   a.   Monitor intake and output
   b.   Weigh daily
   c.   Administer enteral or parenteral feedings as prescribed
   d.   Supply infant with pacifier to preserve suck reflex
   e.   Teach parents how to perform enteral or parenteral feeding if it is to be continued at home
   f.   Encourage parents' participation in infant's feedings
5. Anticipatory grieving
   a.   Encourage parents to express feelings and concerns
   b.   Be an active listener
   c.   Assist parents in identifying positive coping strategies and support systems
   d.   Provide information concerning infant's condition
   e.   Encourage participation in infant's care preoperatively and postoperatively
6. Parent education
   a.   Assess parents' current level of understanding about infant's condition and care
   b.   Provide verbal and written information regarding:
        1) Infant's condition
        2) Alternative feeding techniques
        3) Medication administration as prescribed

4) Neonate care

5) Referrals and community resources

6) Manifestations to report to health care provider

7) Contact numbers for health care provider and community resources

c. Provide adequate time for teaching, demonstrations, and return demonstrations

d. Document teaching and parental response

NIC

1. Aspiration Precautions

2. Acid-Base Management, Fluid/Electrolyte Management

3. Risk Identification, Temperature Regulation, Newborn Care

4. Nutrition Management

5. Coping Enhancement

6. Teaching: Parent Education: Infant, Illness Care, Health Promotion

EVALUATION

1. Client does not experience aspiration as evidenced by respiratory status WDL.

2. Client regains and maintains fluid, electrolyte, and acid-base balance as evidenced by hydration indicators, serum electrolyte values, and acid-base values WDL.

3. Client maintains thermoregulation as evidenced by body temperature WDL for neonate.

4. Client regains and maintains adequate nutrition for weight gain and growth and developmental needs.

5. Parents verbalize positive coping strategies and utilize support systems.

6. Parents demonstrate understanding of infant care, infant's condition, treatment modalities, and home care.

References

Calkins, C. M., & Karrer, F. (2006). *Duodenal atresia.* Retrieved May 12, 2007, from http://www.emedicine.com/ped/topic2776.htm

Lewis, N., & Glick, P. L. (2006). *Duodenal atresia and stenosis: Surgical prospective.* Retrieved February 13, 2008, from http://www.emedicine.com/ped/topic2949.htm

Mandell, G. (2007). *Duodenal atresia.* Retrieved February 13, 2008, from http://www.emedicine.com/radio/topic223.htm

MedlinePlus. (2005). *Duodenal atresia.* Retrieved May 12, 2007, from http://www.nlm.nih.gov/medlineplus/ency/article/001131.htm

National Organization for Rare Disorders. (2003). *Duodenal atresia or stenosis.* Retrieved February 13, 2008, from http://www.rarediseases.org/search/rdbdetail_abstract.html?disname=Duodenal+Atresia+or+Stenosis

38

ELECTROLYTE IMBALANCES

Definition

Electrolyte imbalances reflect abnormal concentrations of the electrically charged particles in the body cells.

Pathophysiology

Body fluids are present in two fluid compartments: (1) intracellular (inside the cells) and (2) extracellular (outside the cells). The most abundant body fluid is water, and electrolytes are the electrically charged particles in the fluids. Electrolytes influence the presence and absence of fluids, and each electrolyte serves vital functions. The major electrolytes that influence fluid balance are sodium, potassium, and chloride. Other vital electrolytes include calcium, phosphorous, and magnesium. Fluid and electrolyte balance is different in neonates and children than in adults. The body fluid composition in neonates is 75% compared to 60% in adults, placing children at higher risk for fluid and electrolyte imbalances. In the preterm infant, the fluid composition is even higher. Preterm neonates born at 25–30 weeks' gestation have a fluid composition of approximately 84% water, and they may lose 5–15% of their birth weight in fluid compared to term neonates who usually lose 5–10% of their birth weight (Ambalavanan, 2006). Refer to Figure 38-1.

Sodium, a positively charged ion (cation), is the major extracellular electrolyte that is necessary for the maintenance of fluid osmolarity, cellular permeability, and acid-base balance. Osmolarity is "the concentration of solute within a solution measured by the

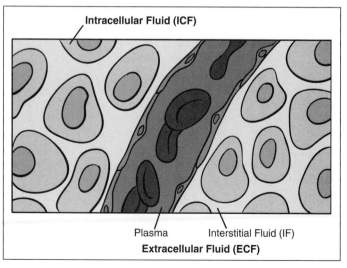

Figure 38-1: Body Fluid Compartments.

number of moles per liter of water" (Potts & Mandleco, 2007, p. 589). Normal serum sodium levels range from 136–146 mmol/L. Hyponatremia occurs when the blood serum level of sodium falls below 136 mmol/L. This can occur as a result of a deficient intake of sodium or an excess intake of water. This results in negative sodium balance, which leads to fluid imbalance and insufficient neurotransmission and inadequate muscle contraction and relaxation. In severe cases, hyponatremia can result in hypovolemia and hypovolemic shock. As a neurotransmitter, decreased sodium levels cause nerve and muscle tissues to be less responsive to normal stimuli. This is most critical in the heart because excitable tissues of the heart are most sensitive to sodium fluctuations.

"Hyponatremia leads to decreased exchange of hydrogen ions in the renal tubules allowing hydrogen levels to increase resulting in metabolic acidosis. The respiratory, neuromuscular, CNS, gastrointestinal, and renal systems also are impacted. The cardiac muscles lack adequate stimulation, but the pulse rate increases to compensate for the hypovolemia. Hypovolemia causes the blood pressure to decrease leading to decreased tissue perfusion. Pulmonary edema interferes with gas exchange that also leads to acidosis. Lack of electrical muscle stimulation causes generalized muscle weakness and diminished deep tendon reflexes. The gastrointestinal tract experiences increased motility and diarrhea, which further complicates the reduced sodium level. Sodium loss is mainly through the kidneys with some losses through the skin and respirations" (Broyles, 2005, p. 784). Hyponatremia causes neuronal cell edema, resulting in irritability and changes in level of consciousness.

Hypernatremia occurs when the blood serum level of sodium exceeds 146 mmol/L. There is a decreased concentration difference of sodium between the extracellular fluid and the intracellular fluid, resulting in increased cell excitability, requiring less intense stimuli for the excitable tissues to depolarize (contraction in muscle cells). This leads to unpredictable and inappropriate contraction of the muscle cells. Further, the osmolarity of the extracellular fluid increases, causing movement of fluid from the cells into the extracellular fluid, resulting in cell dehydration. Hypernatremia causes increased neural activity in the central nervous system (CNS) reflected in agitation, confusion, and seizures. The changes that occur with hypernatremia depend a great deal on how rapidly the sodium levels increase. For instance, if sodium levels rise suddenly, severe consequences occur, especially in the sensitive cardiac cells. This leads to decreased myocardial contractility and subsequent decreased cardiac output (Broyles, 2005).

Potassium, a positively charged ion and the major intracellular fluid electrolyte, works with sodium to maintain fluid and electrolyte balance. Its major function is as a neurotransmitter determining the excitability of neurons and muscles. Hypokalemia occurs when the blood serum level of potassium falls below 3 mmol/L in children less than 2 years of age or is less than 3.5 mmol/L in children older than 2 years. When the potassium level drops below normal limits, the functions of potassium decrease, the most critical being neurotransmission and muscle contraction and relaxation. In hypokalemia, the excitability of the cells decreases, causing nerve and muscle tissues to be less responsive to normal stimuli. The cardiac muscle is of most concern because insufficient potassium results in cardiac muscles lacking adequate stimulation, cardiac dysrhythmias, and decreased cardiac output. Peripheral pulses weaken, respirations are inadequate to maintain gas exchange due to weakened skeletal muscles of the chest, skeletal muscles throughout the body are weakened, and smooth muscle of the gastrointestinal tract is affected. The kidneys are less able to concentrate urine. This results in the inability to eliminate by-products of metabolism that are normally excreted through urine. Fluid loss, however, is increased.

Hyperkalemia occurs when the blood serum level of potassium exceeds 6 mmol/L in children less than 2 years of age or exceeds 5 mmol/L in children over the age of 12 years. "This decreases the concentration difference of potassium between the intracellular fluid and the extracellular fluid causing increased cell excitability. The result is that excitable tissues require less intense stimuli for them to depolarize (contract) leading to sporadic, unpredictable, and inappropriate depolarization of the muscle cells. If the extracellular potassium levels increase rapidly, the potential for life-threatening cardiac dysrhythmias is great as well as the decrease in cardiac output" (Broyles, 2005, p. 666).

Chloride is a negatively charged ion (anion) and is primarily responsible for maintaining "electroneutrality" (Potts & Mandleco, 2007, p. 590) in the extracellular fluid with sodium. The relationship of chloride and sodium is directly proportional. Chloride ions in combination with hydrogen ions maintain acid-base balance and are the major components of gastric juices (hydrochloric acid). The primary impact of changes in chloride levels is reflected in the concurrent loss of sodium ions (hyponatremia) or rise in sodium levels (hypernatremia) and in the state of acid-base balance. Hypochloremia is associated with metabolic alkalosis and dehydration; hyperchloremia can lead to metabolic acidosis and fluid overload. Hypochloremia occurs when the serum chloride levels falls below 98 mmol/L; hyperchloremia occurs when the serum chloride level is greater than 106 mmol/L.

Calcium is a cation with primary responsibilities for bone and teeth formation and maintenance, blood coagulation, muscle contraction, and nerve excitation. Because calcium is most concentrated in the skeletal system, which contains 99% of the body's calcium, adequate intake of calcium is especially significant during periods of bone growth in childhood (Broyles, 2005). Hypocalcemia occurs when the blood serum level of calcium falls below 9 mg/dL in the newborn or 8.8 mg/dL in all other children (Pagana & Pagana, 2007). The most critical functions affected by hypocalcemia are neurotransmission and muscle contraction and relaxation. Decreased calcium levels increase the permeability of excitable membranes to sodium, leading to sporadic, unpredictable, and inappropriate depolarization of the muscle cells. Although effects of hypocalcemia occur throughout the body, the most significant area of concern is the heart. Inadequate calcium can result in muscle spasticity and cardiac atony and life-threatening dysrhythmias. Cardiac output decreases, which can lead to cardiogenic shock. Hypocalcemia causes prolonged clotting, which can lead to bleeding complications. Hypercalcemia occurs when the blood serum level of calcium exceeds 10.8 mg/dL. Elevated calcium levels decrease the permeability of excitable membranes to sodium, requiring increasing stimuli to function. Hypercalcemia causes neuromuscular deficiencies, changes in mental status, renal calculi, cardiac dysrhythmias, hypertension, and more rapid coagulation.

Phosphorous, existing in the body in the form of phosphate, is a major component of bone, with 80–90% of the body's phosphorous used in the development of bones and teeth and linked closely to calcium. It further serves as a general body metabolizer, playing a crucial role in cellular metabolism and as a major renal buffer for hydrogen. Hypophosphatemia occurs when the blood serum level of phosphate falls below 4.3 mg/dL in newborns and below 4.5 mg/dL in children older than the neonate (Pagana & Pagana, 2007). There is an inversely proportional relationship between phosphorous and calcium; so when phosphate levels decrease, the serum levels of calcium rise. The resulting hypercalcemia creates risk of cardiac dysrhythmias from decreased excitability and responsiveness of muscle cells to normal stimuli. Stroke volume and cardiac output decrease. Peripheral pulses slow and weaken, resulting in decreased tissue perfusion. Decreased energy metabolism is especially evident in the myocardial cells; contractions are weak and can eventually lead to progressive but reversible cardiac muscle damage. Metabolic acidosis occurs as a result of increased hydrogen levels. Finally, reduced phosphate levels cause decreased platelet aggregation and increased bleeding risks.

Hyperphosphatemia occurs when the blood serum level of phosphate exceeds 9.3 mg/dL in neonates and 6.5 mg/dL in children (Pagana & Pagana, 2007). As with hypophosphatemia, most pathological effects of excessive phosphate result from the decreasing calcium levels associated hyperphosphatemia. Increased phosphate levels, in and of themselves, do not cause major problems. However, because of the decreased calcium levels, tetany and cardiac dysrhythmias are potential complications (Broyles, 2005).

"Magnesium is a mineral in the body, 70% of which is combined with calcium and phosphorous in the bone. Although less than an ounce is present in the body, it acts as a coenzyme in all cells, activating energy metabolism and building tissue protein. It aids in smooth muscle activity and neuromuscular excitability as a cofactor in the sodium/potassium activity" (Broyles, 2005, p. 524). Hypomagnesemia occurs when the blood serum level of magnesium falls below 1.4 mEq/L (Pagana & Pagana, 2007). As magnesium levels decrease, acetylcholine secretion increases, causing increased transmission between the nerves and skeletal muscle. This is reflected in hyperactivity in skeletal muscles, including deep tendon reflexes, painful parenthesia, and tetany in muscle contractions. Hypomagnesemia can lead to seizure activity because of the increase in activity from neuron to neuron in the CNS. Increased contractility in the heart is manifested in tachydysrhythmias, and vasoconstriction leads to hypertension.

Hypermagnesemia occurs when the blood serum level of magnesium rises above 2 mEq in the neonate and above 1.7 mEq in children (Pagana & Pagana, 2007). Related to magnesium's role as a membrane stabilizer, excesses in magnesium cause excitable membranes to be less sensitive to normal stimuli, requiring more stimuli to elicit a response. If the level of magnesium is too excessive, the membranes may not respond at all. When this occurs, reduced amounts of acetylcholine are released at neuromuscular junctions, resulting in muscle weakness. Muscle weakness can impair respiratory function, resulting in respiratory failure. Inability of cardiac muscle to respond to stimuli causes ineffective ventricular contractions, with the possibility of cardiac arrest. Decreased transmission of impulses in the CNS leads to decreased level of consciousness (Broyles, 2005).

Complications

Sodium
    Fluid imbalance
    Acid-base imbalance
    Cardiac dysrhythmias
    Altered mental status
Potassium
    Cardiac dysrhythmias
    Fluid imbalance
Chloride
    Acid-base imbalance
    Fluid imbalance
Calcium
    Cardiac dysrhythmias
    Altered blood clotting
    Disturbances in bone and teeth formation
Phosphorous
    Disturbances in utilization of calcium
Magnesium
    Cardiac failure
    Respiratory failure
    Altered mental status

Incidence

The exact incidence of electrolyte imbalances is not known because of the variety of causes of the imbalances.

Etiology

Causes of hyponatremia are factors that result in excessive sodium loss or dilution of serum sodium. Most common causes in children include vomiting; diarrhea; major burns or trauma; and medications including diuretics (loop or thiazide), the cardiac glycoside digoxin, or the anticonvulsant carbamazepine (Tegretol). Factors that cause dilution of serum sodium in children include near drowning, nephrotic syndrome, and hyperglycemia. Children involved in activities that increase their loss of fluid and sodium, including sports such as football, track, baseball, soccer, and basketball, are at risk for hyponatremia.

Hypernatremia is usually the result of decreased sodium excretion as in renal failure or increased water loss that occurs with fever, hyperventilation, and dehydration. Fluid administration in infants with respiratory distress syndrome can lead to sodium imbalances. "If the infants receive excessive fluids, hyponatremia and fluid volume excess occur" and can worsen their pulmonary condition. Inadequate fluid administration leads to hypernatremia and dehydration (Ambalavanan, 2006, Section 2).

Causes of hypokalemia that result in excessive potassium loss include the use of diuretics, the cardiac glycoside digoxin, and corticosteroids; alkalosis; hyperinsulinemia; diarrhea; vomiting; prolonged gastrointestinal decompression; excessive diaphoresis; diabetes insipidus; or excessive loss of body fluids secondary to burns or major trauma. The most common cause of hyperkalemia in children is renal failure; however, hyperkalemia also can result from the use of potassium-sparing diuretics (spironolactone).

Hypochloremia in children is usually the result of vomiting. Hyperchloremia occurs during periods of increased fluid loss such as fever, excessive diaphoresis, dehydration, and diarrhea.

Hypocalcemia in children occurs as a result of a deficiency in calcitonin due to inadequate thyroid function, diarrhea, malabsorption, burns, hypomagnesemia (secondary to cisplatin therapy for certain cancers), hyperphosphatemia (commonly present in renal failure), vitamin D deficiency, AIDS, medications such as loop diuretics, and anticonvulsants such as phenytoin and phenobarbital. Hypercalcemia results from hyperthyroidism, renal transplantation, and drugs such as thiazide diuretics.

Hypophosphatemia results from factors that cause excessive phosphate loss, including malnutrition, increased excretion of phosphates as with hypercalcemia, intracellular fluid shifts resulting from hyperglycemia or uncontrolled diabetes mellitus, and respiratory alkalosis. Causes of hyperphosphatemia include conditions that result in increased phosphate absorption, inadequate phosphate excretion, or shifts in intracellular to extracellular fluid. Inadequate phosphate excretion in children is usually associated with renal insufficiency or renal failure. Fluid shifts occur in acute acidosis and insulin deficiency.

Hypomagnesemia occurs as a result of insufficient magnesium intake, increased magnesium excretion, or intracellular movement of magnesium. Conditions that cause inadequate magnesium intake include malnutrition, diarrhea, steatorrhea (fatty stools as seen in children with cystic fibrosis), Crohn's disease, and celiac disease. Drugs such as amphotericin B, cisplatin, cyclosporine, diuretics, and aminoglycoside antibiotics can cause hypomagnesemia. In addition, hyperglycemia, sepsis, and alkalosis can result in increased intracellular movement of magnesium. Hypermagnesemia is very rare in children.

Clinical Manifestations

Adapted from Broyles, 2005.

Hyponatremia
  Tachycardia
  Weak peripheral pulses
  Orthostatic hypotension
  Rapid, shallow respirations
  Decreased breath sounds
  Generalized muscle weakness and hyporeflexia
  Diarrhea
  Nausea
  Irritability
  Altered mental status with decreasing level of consciousness
  Polyuria
  Decreased urine specific gravity
  Headache
Hypernatremia
  Tachydysrhythmias
  Dyspnea and moist respirations
  Generalized muscle twitches
  Decreased level of consciousness
  Polydipsia
  Increased deep tendon reflexes
  Dry mucous membranes
  Decreased urinary output
Hypokalemia
  Irregular heart rate
  Weak peripheral pulses
  Orthostatic hypotension
  Shallow, ineffective respirations
  Decreased breath sounds
  Hypoactive bowel sounds
  Constipation
  Paralytic ileus
  Nausea
  Vomiting
  Altered mental status
  Generalized muscle weakness and hyporeflexia
  Polyuria with decreased urine specific gravity
Hyperkalemia
  Cardiac dysrhythmias
  Elevated T waves, widened QRS complexes, and eventually prolonged
    PR interval on ECG tracing
  Generalized muscle cramps and spasms accompanied by some
    paresthesia
  Hyperactive bowel sounds
  Diarrhea
Hypochloremia
  Metabolic alkalosis

Moist breath sounds
Edema
Weight gain

Hyperchloremia
Dry skin and mucous membranes
Metabolic acidosis
Pallor
Weight loss

Hypocalcemia
Circumoral and peripheral parenthesia
Laryngeal spasms
Facial and extremity muscle spasms
Positive Trousseau's sign
Positive Chvostek's sign
Hypotension
Bradycardia
Ventricular tachycardia
Peticheae
Ecchymosis
Altered mental status
Seizures

Hypercalcemia
Fatigue
Muscle weakness
Depressed deep tendon reflex
Constipation
Nausea
Vomiting
Bradydysrhythmias
Hypertension
Increased risk of clot formation
Altered mental status
Polyuria
Polydipsia

Hypophosphatemia
Weak apical and peripheral pulses
Shallow, slow respirations
Muscle weakness and hyporeflexia
Irritability
Seizures
Increased bleeding
Immunosuppression

Hyperphosphatemia
Tachycardia
Muscle weakness
Muscle spasms, tetany, and hyperreflexia
Anorexia
Nausea
Vomiting

Hypomagnesemia
  Tachydysrhythmias
  Hypertension
  Shallow, ineffective respirations
  Decreased breath sounds
  Hypoactive bowel sounds
  Constipation
  Paralytic ileus
  Nausea
  Vomiting
  Altered mental status
  Muscle twitching, parenthesia, and tetany
  Positive Trousseau's sign
  Positive Chvostek's sign (if hypocalcemia is present)
  Seizures
  Irritability
Hypermagnesemia
  Bradydysrhythmias
  Hypotension
  Widened pulse pressure
  Lethargy
  Hypoactive or absent deep tendon reflexes
  Generalized muscle weakness including respiratory muscles

Diagnostic Tests

Serum electrolyte levels
Urine pH and specific gravity
Cardiac enzymes
Cardiac echocardiography

Medical Management

The goals of treatment are to correct the underlying cause of the electrolyte imbalance, achieve fluid and electrolyte balance, and prevent potential life-threatening complications of electrolyte imbalances. In electrolyte deficiencies, intravenous replacement of electrolytes is the standard of care. With electrolyte excesses, medications or intravenous fluids can decrease the electrolyte levels. Hypotonic intravenous solutions such as 0.45% and 0.225% normal saline are used to treat hypernatremia. Diuretics (loop or thiazide) may be used to decrease sodium and potassium levels. Hypertonic intravenous fluids and/or sodium polystyrene sulfonate may be used to lower potassium levels. Hyperchloremia is usually treated with the same intravenous solutions as hypernatremia. Intravenous 0.9% normal saline and loop diuretics are administered to treat hypercalcemia because sodium increases the excretion of calcium and loop diuretics increase urine output. In severe cases, dialysis may be required in the presence of life-threatening cardiac dysrhythmias. Agents that increase calcium levels are the standard of care for hyperphosphatemia because of the inverse relationship between calcium and phosphorous. In renal failure, dialysis and dietary modifications assist in decreasing phosphate levels.

Finally, to treat hypermagnesemia, agents that increase magnesium excretion, including loop diuretics (furosemide), are administered (Spratto & Woods, 2008). If cardiac effects of elevated magnesium need to be reversed, calcium supplements may be used. Because of cardiac involvement with most electrolyte imbalances, continuous cardiac monitoring is necessary during replacement therapy or treatment to decrease electrolyte levels.

Nursing Management

ASSESSMENT

1. Obtain client history
2. Perform physical assessment
3. Evaluate serum electrolyte levels
4. Obtain baseline vital signs and height and weight

NURSING DIAGNOSES (INCLUDING BUT NOT LIMITED TO)

1. Imbalanced fluid volume R/T alterations in electrolyte levels
2. Risk for decreased cardiac output R/T alterations in electrolyte levels
3. Risk for ineffective tissue perfusion R/T alterations in electrolyte levels
4. Risk for injury R/T alterations in mental status secondary to altered electrolyte levels
5. Deficient knowledge R/T condition, causes, treatment, and home care

PLANNING/GOALS

1. Client will regain and maintain fluid and electrolyte balance as evidenced by serum electrolyte levels within defined limits (WDL) and resolution of symptoms of electrolyte imbalance.
2. Client will maintain adequate cardiac output as evidenced by cardiac status, urinary output, vital signs, and level of consciousness WDL.
3. Client will maintain effective tissue perfusion as evidenced by heart sounds, breath sounds, bowel sounds, and level of consciousness WDL.
4. Client will maintain neurologic integrity and sustain no injury.
5. Parents will demonstrate understanding of condition, causes, treatment, and home care.

NOC

1. Electrolyte and Acid/Base Balance, Fluid Balance
2. Risk Control, Cardiac Output Effectiveness
3. Circulation Status
4. Risk Control
5. Knowledge: Illness Care, Treatment, Health Promotion

IMPLEMENTATION

1. Fluid and electrolyte balance
   a. Monitor serum electrolyte levels
   b. Monitor lab values related to specific electrolyte imbalance
   c. Monitor intake and output
   d. Weigh daily
   e. Initiate and maintain intravenous access, monitoring at least hourly
   f. Administer intravenous fluids as prescribed
   g. Administer medications as prescribed
   h. Monitor for effectiveness of therapy
   i. Monitor urine specific gravity
   j. Monitor cardiac status
   k. Monitor closely for overcorrection of electrolyte imbalance
   l. Maintain dietary alterations as prescribed

2. Cardiac output
    a. Monitor vital signs
    b. Monitor oxygen saturation using pulse oximetry
    c. Monitor peripheral pulses
    d. Monitor capillary refill
    e. Monitor heart sounds
    f. Monitor breath sounds
    g. Maintain hemodynamic monitoring if condition warrants
    h. Prepare client for cardioversion if severe alterations in cardiac rhythm occur
    i. Explain all equipment and procedures to parents and child (if age-appropriate)
3. Tissue perfusion
    a. Monitor vital signs
    b. Monitor oxygen saturation with pulse oximetry
    c. Monitor peripheral pulses
    d. Monitor capillary refill
    e. Monitor for manifestations of ineffective tissue perfusion
4. Risk for injury
    a. Monitor neuromuscular status
    b. Monitor level of consciousness
    c. Assist with activities as needed
    d. Encourage parents to actively participate in child's care
    e. Control potential environmental hazards
    f. Anticipate needs
5. Parent/client teaching
    a. Assess parents' and child's (if age-appropriate) level of understanding
    b. Provide verbal and written information regarding:
        1) Medication administration if needed
        2) Dietary modifications if needed
        3) Manifestations of electrolyte imbalance to report to health care provider
        4) Referral information if needed
        5) Importance of follow-up care
        6) Contact phone numbers
    c. Provide adequate time for teaching and encourage questions
    d. Document teaching and parent/client responses

NIC

1. Acid-Base Management, Electrolyte Management, Fluid Management
2. Surveillance: Safety, Electrolyte Management
3. Intravenous Therapy, Acid-Base Management
4. Risk Identification, Environmental Management: Safety
5. Teaching: Illness Care, Treatment, Health Promotion

Evaluation

1. Client regains and maintains fluid and electrolyte balance as evidenced by serum electrolyte levels WDL and resolution of symptoms of electrolyte imbalance.

2. Client maintains adequate cardiac output as evidenced by cardiac status, urinary output, vital signs, and level of consciousness WDL.
3. Client maintains effective tissue perfusion as evidenced by heart sounds, breath sounds, bowel sounds, and level of consciousness WDL.
4. Client maintains neurologic integrity and sustains no injury.
5. Parents demonstrate understanding of condition, causes, treatment, and home care.

References

Ambalavanan, N. (2006). *Fluid, electrolyte, and nutrition management of the newborn.* Retrieved May 12, 2007, from http://www.emedicine.com/ped/topic2554.htm

Broyles, B. E. (2005). *Medical-surgical nursing clinical companion.* Durham, NC: Carolina Academic Press.

Pagana, K. D., & Pagana, T. J. (2007). *Mosby's diagnostic and laboratory test reference* (8th ed.). St. Louis, MO: Mosby Elsevier.

Potts, N. L., & Mandleco, B. L. (2007). *Pediatric nursing: Caring for children and their families* (2nd ed.). Clifton Park, NY: Delmar Cengage Learning.

Spratto, G. R., & Woods, A. L. (2008). *2008 edition PDR nurse's drug handbook.* Clifton Park, NY: Delmar Cengage Learning.

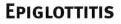

EPIGLOTTITIS

Definition

"Acute epiglottitis, sometimes classified as a croup syndrome, is a life-threatening bacterial infection that can lead to complete airway obstruction" (Potts & Mandleco, 2007, p. 716).

Pathophysiology

The epiglottis, aryepiglottic folds, and surrounding structures become inflamed and edematous due to overwhelming infection. Bacteria directly invade the mucous membranes of the epiglottis in the area where the submucosa is loosely attached. Secretions pool in the larynx and hyopharynx, resulting in progressive swelling that makes the child unable to swallow. The epiglottis becomes so swollen that it completely covers the glottis and obstructs the airway. The onset of this process is sudden; and the progressive airway obstruction can result in hypoxia, respiratory acidosis due to inability to expel carbon dioxide on expiration, and death within 2–6 hours after onset. The airway obstruction and hypoxia cause increased anxiety in the child. This can lead to reflex laryngospasm, further worsening the condition even more rapidly.

Complications

Airway obstruction
Hypoxia
Respiratory acidosis
Death due to respiratory failure

Incidence

Since the introduction of the Hib vaccine in the United States in 1985, the incidence of epiglottitis has decreased significantly. The peak incidence in children is between the ages of 2 and 6 years (MedlinePlus, 2006) with the mean age of 36 months (Kahn & Mahl, 2006).

Etiology

"Epiglottitis is usually caused by infectious agents including *H [aemophilus] influenzae* type b and group A *S. pneumoniae, H. parainfluenzae, S. aureus,* and beta-hemolytic streptococci (group A, B, or C)" (Kahn & Mahl, 2006, Section 1). The most common microorganism is *H. influenzae.*

Clinical Manifestations

Abrupt onset of fever, sore throat, and dysphagia
Four *D*s: drooling, dysphasia, dysphonia, and distressed inspiratory
    efforts
Stridor
Lethargy
Anxiety
Tachypnea
Nasal flaring, retractions, and use of accessory muscles

Pallor

Edematous, cherry red epiglottis. *NOTE:* Tongue blade should not be used because it can stimulate spasms.

Diagnostic Tests

Laryngoscopy

Lateral neck radiography

Complete blood count

Medical Management

The goals of treatment are to maintain a patent airway, support ventilation, and effectively treat the infection. Immediate hospitalization is required whenever a child is suspected of having epiglottitis because of the danger of sudden and unpredictable airway obstruction. The priority is maintaining a patent airway. Visual examination of the throat with a tongue blade is contraindicated because of the risk of laryngospasms and complete airway obstruction (Potts & Mandleco, 2007). Placing the child in a dimly lit room with a parent holding the child, humidified oxygen, and continuous monitoring may initially decrease the child's anxiety if the airway is not obstructed on admission. An intravenous access is established, and intravenous fluids and antibacterial agents (cephalosporins and aminoglycosides) are initiated. Treatment with systemic corticosteroids may be beneficial as an early course of management (Potts & Mandleco, 2007; Hockenberry, 2005).

If the child is experiencing airway obstruction, a laryngoscope and artificial airway are inserted. In severe cases, a tracheostomy and mechanical ventilation may be required. Rapid improvement is usually as dramatic as the onset of epiglottitis itself. Extubation routinely occurs within 48 hours following initiation of systemic antimicrobial therapy. The child may be discharged within three to seven days following admission. Discharge antibiotics are prescribed.

Nursing Management

ASSESSMENT

1. Assess airway patency
2. Assess for presence of four *D*s
3. Assess for inspiratory stridor and increased work of breathing
4. Perform a rapid physical assessment
5. Obtain vital signs

NURSING DIAGNOSES (INCLUDING BUT NOT LIMITED TO)

1. Ineffective airway clearance R/T edema of epiglottis
2. Impaired gas exchange R/T airway obstruction
3. Anxiety R/T hypoxia and increased work of breathing
4. Deficient knowledge R/T child's condition, treatment, and home care

PLANNING/GOALS

1. Client will regain and maintain patent airway as evidenced by respiratory status within defined limits (WDL).
2. Client will maintain adequate gas exchange as evidenced by acid-base balance and respiratory status WDL.
3. Parents and client (if age-appropriate) will use positive coping strategies to reduce anxiety.
4. Parents will demonstrate understanding of child's condition, treatment plan, and home care.

NOC

1. Respiratory Status: Airway Patency
2. Respiratory Status: Gas Exchange
3. Anxiety
4. Knowledge: Disease Process, Treatment, Health Promotion

IMPLEMENTATION

1. Airway
   a. Never leave child unattended
   b. Maintain a tracheostomy insertion set at the bedside
   c. Keep child as calm as possible
   d. Encourage parental involvement
   e. Administer oxygen titrated to oxygen saturation/pulse oximetry
   f. Have emergency intubation equipment ready in operating room
   g. Report any decline in respiratory status to health care provider immediately
   h. Suction as needed if child has been intubated,
   i. Tape tube in place securely to prevent dislodgement if child has endotracheal tube
   j. Perform tracheostomy care and suctioning if child has tracheostomy
   k. Maintain intravenous access, monitoring at least hourly
   l. Administer antibiotics as prescribed
   m. Administer systemic corticosteroids as prescribed

2. Gas exchange
   a. Follow interventions for airway patency
   b. Place on continuous pulse oximetry
   c. Titrate oxygen therapy to maintain prescribed oxygen saturation
   d. Place on continuous cardiorespiratory monitor
   e. Monitor arterial blood gases if arterial line has been established
   f. Administer antipyretics to reduce fever
   g. Maintain nothing by mouth (npo) status

3. Anxiety
   a. Encourage parents to express feelings and concerns
   b. Avoid unnecessary procedures
   c. Explain all equipment and procedures
   d. Maintain calm, reassuring environment
   e. Encourage continuous presence of parents
   f. Encourage parental participation in child's care as soon as condition allows

4. Parent teaching
   a. Assess current level of understanding
   b. Provide verbal and written information regarding:
      1) Importance of Hib immunizations
      2) Antibiotic administration, stressing the importance of completing entire prescription
      3) Signs and symptoms to report to health care provider
      4) Use and administration of (acetaminophen) for fever
      5) Contact numbers for health care provider
      6) Importance of follow-up care

   c. Provide sufficient time for teaching and parents' questions

   d. Document teaching and parents' responses

NIC

1. Airway Management, Respiratory Monitoring, Ventilation Assistance
2. Oxygen Therapy, Ventilation Assistance
3. Anxiety Reduction
4. Teaching: Disease Process, Treatment, Health Promotion

EVALUATION

1. Client regains and maintains patent airway as evidenced by respiratory status WDL.
2. Client maintains adequate gas exchange as evidenced by acid-base balance and respiratory status WDL.
3. Parents and child (if age-appropriate) use positive coping strategies to reduce anxiety.
4. Parents demonstrate understanding of child's condition, treatment plan, and home care.

References

Hockenberry, M. J. (2005). *Wong's essentials of pediatric nursing* (7th ed.). St. Louis, MO: Elsevier Mosby.

Kahn, F. H., & Mahl, E. (2006). *Pediatrics, epiglottitis.* Retrieved May 12, 2007, from http://www.emedicine.com/emerg/topic375.htm

MedlinePlus. (2006). *Epiglottitis.* Retrieved May 12, 2007, from http://www.nlm.nih.gov/medlineplus/ency/article/000605.htm

Potts, N. L., & Mandleco, B. L. (2007). *Pediatric nursing: Caring for children and their families* (2nd ed.). Clifton Park, NY: Delmar Cengage Learning.

EPISPADIAS/HYPOSPADIAS

Definition

Epispadias is the congenital placement of the urethral meatus on the dorsal aspect of the penile shaft. Hypospadias is the congenital placement of the urethral meatus on the ventral aspect (the underside) of the penile shaft. The position of the urethral opening may occur at any point along the penile shaft or the scrotum. Refer to Figure 40-1.

Pathophysiology

Beginning during the fifth week of embryonic development, the genital tubercle, genital folds, and genital swelling begin to develop into specific female or male genitalia. Although the default developmental pathway is female, the presence of the male hormones testosterone and dihydrotestosterone (DHT) secreted by the male embryo alters the pathway to the development of male genitalia. These hormones cause the genital swelling that creates the scrotum, the genital folds fuse together to become the shaft of the penis, and the genital tubercle forms the glans, or tip, of the penis. Normally in male development, the fusion of the genital folds is complete by the 14th week of gestation so that the penis fully surrounds the urethra all the way to the tip. However, when the folds fail to completely fuse appropriately, hypospadias/epispadias results as the urethra does not reach all the way to the tip of the penis (Hypospadias and Epispadias Association, 2006). Epispadias causes impotentia coeundi, which results from the dorsal curvature of the penile shaft, and impotentia generandi, which results from the incomplete urethra. Hypospadias may be associated with chordee (downward curvature of the penis and incomplete foreskin).

Although this does not impact urinary function, it interferes with positioning during urination and creates the risk of body image issues. In severe cases, fertility risks due to the inability to ejaculate forward into the female reproductive anatomy are present if the hypospadias or epispadias is not surgically repaired. Hypospadias and epispadias that have not been repaired also are associated with frequent infections of the prostate, bladder, and kidneys.

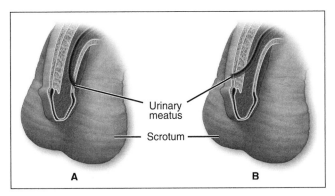

Figure 40-1: **(A)** Hypospadias; **(B)** Epispadias.

Complications

Difficulty urinating while standing
Disturbance of body image
Fertility risks in severe cases
Increased risk of renal, bladder, and prostate infections

Incidence

Epispadias occurs with a prevalence of one case in 10,000–50,000 persons (Santanelli & Grippaudo, 2005a). Epispadias may be seen in the presence of bladder exstrophy, the failure of the abdominal wall to fuse during fetal development, leaving the urinary bladder exposed at birth (Potts & Mandleco, 2007).

Hypospadias occurs in 1 in 350 live male births in the United States and is the most frequent malformation of the genitourinary tract. Infants with hypospadias have an increased incidence of concurrent cryptorchidism (undescended testes) and inguinal hernia (Santanelli & Grippaudo, 2005b).

Etiology

According to the Centers for Disease Control and Prevention, the cause of most hypospadias cases is unknown. Genetic factors contribute to approximately 25% of cases. Rates are highest among Caucasians, with an intermediate rate of occurrence in African Americans; the lowest rate is among Hispanics (Center for Disease Control and Prevention, 2007). Another risk factor is the maternal consumption of certain drugs during pregnancy. Finasteride is a drug used to treat benign prostatic hypertrophy (BPH) and male pattern baldness. Dutasteride is an androgen hormone inhibitor also used to treat BPH. Pregnant women who come in contact with either of these agents experience an increased risk of hypospadias or epispadias in their developing fetuses (Broyles, Reiss, & Evans, 2007).

Unlike hypospadias, the cause of epispadias is apparent and is associated with a defective migration of the paired primordia of the genital tubercle that fuse on the midline to form the genital tubercle at the fifth week of embryologic development. Epispadias and exstrophy of the bladder are considered varying degrees of the same condition (Santanelli & Grippaudo, 2005a).

Clinical Manifestations

Ventral or dorsal placement of the urethral opening at birth

Diagnostic Tests

Visual inspection
Complete blood count
Abdominal ultrasonography

Medical Management

The goals of treatment are to surgically repair the chordee and placement of the urethral meatus and to facilitate normal positioning for urination and the development of positive body image. Corrective surgery usually is completed prior to the age of 18 months, before toilet training begins. The surgery involves reconstruction to elongate the urethra extending it to the tip of the penis and straightening the chordee. The foreskin frequently is "used as a graft whereby it is rolled into a tube and fashioned into a urethra" (Potts & Mandleco, 2007, p. 636). Circumcision should not be performed on the neonate so that the foreskin is available for grafting. Postoperatively, a urethral stent or indwelling catheter may be used to facilitate graft healing and to prevent urinary obstruction secondary to operative site edema. Use of either of these usually is determined by the severity of the defect and the extent of correction required.

Nursing Management

Assessment

1. Perform neonatal assessment
2. Monitor for initiation of urinary output
3. Collaborate with health care provider to provide parental education
4. Assess parents' understanding of condition

Nursing Diagnoses (including but not limited to)

1. Acute pain R/T surgical tissue trauma
2. Deficient knowledge R/T condition, treatment, postoperative care, and home care
3. Risk for infection R/T surgical incision and presence of indwelling catheter or stent

Planning/Goals

1. Client will achieve adequate pain management as determined by client using age-appropriate pain assessment tool, achieving a pain level of 1 on a scale of 1–5 with 5 being the most severe pain as further evidenced by engaging in age-appropriate activities.
2. Parents will demonstrate understanding of condition, treatment, postoperative care, and home care.
3. Client will not experience postoperative infection.

NOC

1. Pain Level
2. Knowledge: Health Promotion, Illness Care, Infection Control
3. Infection Severity

Implementation

1. Acute pain
   a. Assess pain level hourly
   b. Administer analgesics proactively as prescribed
   c. Position for comfort
   d. Encourage parental involvement in care
   e. Discontinue indwelling catheter as prescribed as soon as possible postoperatively
   f. Encourage oral intake of fluid
   g. Encourage involvement in age-appropriate activities
2. Parent teaching
   a. Assess parents' current level of knowledge
   b. Provide verbal and written information regarding:
      1) Preoperative care including perineal hygiene and normal growth and development for neonate and infant
      2) Importance of follow-up with pediatrician and urology surgeon
      3) Postoperative care including perineal hygiene, stent care (if needed), proactive pain management, and age-appropriate activities to foster growth and development
      4) Signs of postoperative infection
      5) Importance of reporting signs of infection to health care provider
      6) Contact numbers for health care provider

   c. Provide sufficient time for teaching and parental questions
   d. Document teaching and parental response
3. Infection
   a. Maintain intravenous access, monitoring at least hourly
   b. Administer intravenous fluids as prescribed
   c. Encourage oral intake
   d. Monitor intake and output
   e. Assess urine specific gravity after each void
   f. Monitor urine for presence of infection
   g. Administer prophylactic antimicrobial agents if prescribed for child with stent or indwelling catheter
   h. Monitor vital signs
   i. Discontinue indwelling catheter as prescribed as soon as possible postoperatively
   j. Provide pain management to prevent child from withholding urine because of fear of pain upon urination

NIC

1. Pain Management, Medication Administration
2. Teaching: Health Promotion, Illness Care, Infection Protection
3. Infection Control

EVALUATION

1. Client achieves adequate pain management as determined by client using age-appropriate pain assessment tool, achieving a pain level of 1 on a scale of 1–5 with 5 being the most severe pain as further evidenced by engaging in age-appropriate activities.
2. Parents demonstrate understanding of condition, treatment, postoperative care, and home care.
3. Client does not experience postoperative infection.

References

Broyles, B. E., Reiss, B. S., & Evans, M. E. (2007). *Pharmacological aspects of nursing care* (7th ed.). Clifton Park, NY: Delmar Cengage Learning.

Centers for Disease Control and Prevention. (2007). *Hypospadias trends in two US surveillance systems.* Retrieved February 19, 2007, from http://www.cdc.gov/od/oc/media/pressrel/hypospad.htm

Hypospadias and Epispadias Association. Glossary of hypospadias and epispadias related terms. (2006). Retrieved February 13, 2008, from http://www.hypospadias.net/10.html

MedlinePlus. (2006). *Epispadias.* Retrieved May 12, 2007, from http://www.nlm.nih.gov/medlineplus/ency/article/001285.htm

Potts, N. L., & Mandleco, B. L. (2007). *Pediatric nursing: Caring for children and their families* (2nd ed.). Clifton Park, NY: Delmar Cengage Learning.

Santanelli, F., & Grippaudo, F. R. (2005a). *Urogenital reconstruction: Penile epispadias.* Retrieved February 19, 2007, from http://www.emedicine.com/plastic/topic528.htm

Santanelli, F., & Grippaudo, F. R. (2005b). *Urogenital reconstruction: Penile hypospadias.* Retrieved May 12, 2007, from http://www.emedicine.com/plastic/topic495.htm

ESOPHAGEAL ATRESIA/
TRACHEOESOPHAGEAL FISTULA

Definition

Esophageal atresia is a congenital anomaly of the esophagus ending in a blind pouch before it reaches the stomach. Tracheoesophageal fistula (TEF) is a form of esophageal atresia where the esophagus terminates in a fistula that forms an abnormal connection with the trachea. These can occur concurrently or can be isolated. Refer to Figure 41-1.

Pathophysiology

During embryonic development, the trachea and esophagus are foregut derivatives and originate as one single tube (Lucile Packard Children's Hospital at Stanford, 2007). During the fourth week of gestation, lateral mesodermal ridges form in the proximal esophagus and then fuse in the midline to separate the esophagus from the trachea. Alterations in the rate of cellular growth and proliferation in the embryonic foregut result in defective separation of the trachea and the esophagus. Also of concern is that during this time of development, a number of other structures and systems are forming, including the remainder of the intestinal tract, heart, kidneys, ureters, and skeletal system, leading to a higher risk of additional developmental anomalies (Kronemer & Snyder, 2006). Over 30% of neonates with esophageal atresia will experience additional anomalies (MedlinePlus, 2006). As a result, the acronym VACTERL has been established to describe other anomalies seen in infants with TEF. These include (1) **v**ertebral defect, (2) **a**norectal malformation, (3) **c**ardiac defects, (4) **t**racheoesophageal fistula, (5) **e**sophageal atresia, (6) **r**ectal anomalies, and (7) **l**imb defects (Potts & Mandleco, 2007).

Because of the lack of connection between the esophagus and the stomach, neonates with esophageal atresia are unable to clear oral and esophageal secretions, causing continuous drooling and risk of aspiration. If not diagnosed prior to the neonate being fed, regurgitation of feedings occur. In addition, with TEF, the reflux of secretions and food may enter the tracheobronchial tree through the fistula, leading to atelectasis and pneumonia. Further, when the infant with TEF strains, cries, or coughs, air enters the stomach through the fistula, causing the stomach and small intestines to dilate. This, in turn, results in an elevation of the diaphragm and causes difficulty breathing due to decreased lung capacity, resulting in respiratory distress.

Complications

Pneumonia
Atelectasis
Aspiration

Incidence

In the United States, the frequency of esophageal atresia is 1 case in 3,000 live births; and internationally the incidence is approximately 0.4–3.6 cases per 10,000 live births in different regions of the world. There appear to be no racial differences; however, males have a slightly higher incidence than females (Kronemer & Snyder, 2006). TEF is the most common congenital anomaly occurring in 1 of every 2,000–4,000 births (Sharma & Duerksen, 2006).

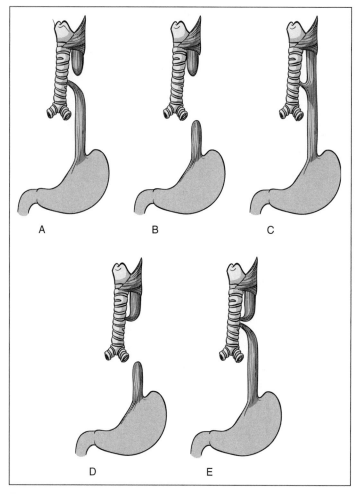

Figure 41-1: Types of Esophageal Atresia: **(A)** Esophageal Atresia with Distal TEF; **(B)** Isolated Esophageal Atresia; **(C)** TEF without Esophageal Atresia; **(D)** Esophageal Atresia with Proximal TEF; **(E)** Esophageal Atresia with Proximal and Distal TEF.

Etiology

The causes of esophageal atresia remain unknown; however, a number of theories about their origins have been proposed. Among them are notochord abnormalities, desynchronous esophageal mesenchymal and epithelial growth rates, neural crest cell involvement, and incomplete tracheoesophageal separation due to a lack of apoptosis. Other complications specifically associated with TEF are incomplete tracheoesophageal septation, lateral ridge fusion failure, and the proximity of the trachea and esophagus. Other contributing factors that have been theorized to explain why esophageal atresia and TEF occur are embryonic vascular insufficiencies; genetic factors; vitamin deficiencies; drug and alcohol exposure; and viral, chemical, and physical external events. Although the exact etiology has not been definitively determined, the basic premise is an alteration in the rate and timing of cell growth and proliferation in the embryonic foregut prior to 34 days' gestation (Kronemer & Snyder, 2006). TEF has been associated with genetic anomalies such as trisomy 18, 21, and 13 (Sharma & Duerksen, 2006).

Clinical Manifestations

Maternal polyhydramnios occurs in 95% of neonates with esophageal atresia without TEF and 35% in neonates with esophageal atresia and distal TEF.

Three Cs: coughing, choking, and cyanosis

Excessive drooling

Excessive oral secretions

Regurgitation

Abdominal distension

Diagnostic Tests

Maternal ultrasonography

Radiography

Computed tomography

Magnetic resonance imaging

Medical Management

The goals of treatment are prevention of respiratory complications and surgical correction of the anomaly. Prior to the first surgical repair of esophageal atresia/TEF in 1939, this condition was fatal. The procedure for surgical repair depends on the type of esophageal atresia and the neonate's condition at birth. If no other anomalies are present and the neonate is healthy, the surgical repair can be performed during the first days of life. However, if other anomalies exist or the neonate is premature, has a low birth weight, or has aspiration pneumonia, the procedure is usually performed in stages (Potts & Mandleco, 2007). The procedure involves closing the fistula, anastomosing the esophagus and the stomach, and creating the esophageal sphincter.

"The repair is performed via right thoracotomy in the left lateral decubitus position, and the head of table is elevated to avoid gastric reflux. A posterolateral thoracotomy incision is made through the fourth intercostal space, and a retropleural exposure is obtained. During the dissection, the azygos vein is divided and the vagus nerve is identified. The distal esophagus is identified and dissected distal to the TEF. The fistula is divided and closure is performed with stay sutures. Dissection is carefully performed to avoid interruption of blood supply or the branches coming off the vagus nerve. Tracheal suture line may be covered with a flap of mediastinal pleura. Prior to esophageal anastomosis, the proximal pouch of the trachea is mobilized. If a fistula lies between the esophageal pouch and trachea, it is divided and closed. The esophageal anastomosis is performed in 1–2 layers and is covered with mediastinal pleura. A nasogastric feeding tube is placed through the esophagus into the stomach prior to the chest closure, and a chest tube is placed in the retropleural space" (Sharma & Duerksen, 2006, Section 6). Because the sphincter is surgically created, the infant is at risk for developing gastro-esophageal reflux.

Nursing Management

ASSESSMENT

1. Perform neonatal assessment
2. Monitor for excessive oral secretions and drooling

3. Assess for indications of respiratory distress
4. Assess breath sounds

Nursing Diagnoses (including but not limited to)

1. Risk for aspiration R/T congenital malposition of trachea and esophagus and presence of fistula
2. Impaired gas exchange R/T surgical repair and need for chest tube placement
3. Imbalanced nutrition: less than body requirements R/T restricted intake preoperatively and altered feeding methods postoperatively
4. Risk for infection R/T surgical incision and neonatal immune status
5. Acute pain R/T surgical incision and chest tube placement
6. Parental anxiety R/T neonatal emergency condition requiring surgery
7. Deficient knowledge R/T neonate's condition, treatment, and home care

Planning/Goals

1. Client will not experience aspiration as evidenced by respiratory status within defined limits (WDL) for neonate.
2. Client will experience adequate gas exchange as evidenced by oxygen saturation WDL for neonate, clear breath sounds, and lack of respiratory distress.
3. Client will regain and maintain adequate nutrition as evidenced by weight gain consistent with doubling of birth weight by 6 months of age and tripling of birth weight by 12 months of age.
4. Client will not experience infection.
5. Client will experience adequate pain control as evidenced by behavioral indicators.
6. Parents will demonstrate use of effective coping strategies.
7. Parents will demonstrate understanding of neonate's condition, treatment, and home care.

NOC

1. Aspiration Prevention, Respiratory Status: Ventilation
2. Respiratory Status: Gas Exchange
3. Nutritional Status
4. Infection Severity: Newborn
5. Pain Control
6. Anxiety
7. Knowledge: Illness Care, Treatment, Health Promotion

Implementation

1. Risk for aspiration
   a. Preoperatively
      1) Provide warmth and humidified oxygen
      2) Place on and maintain nothing by mouth (npo) status
      3) Place on continuous cardiorespiratory monitor
      4) Place on continuous pulse oximetry
      5) Administer oxygen as prescribed to maintain oxygen saturation within prescribed parameters
      6) Monitor thermoregulation

       7) Place neonate on chalasia board to maintain head of bed elevated at 30 degrees

       8) Place suction catheter into proximal pouch and suction as needed

   b. Postoperatively

      1) Monitor respiratory status continuously

      2) Maintain thermoregulation

      3) Monitor chest tube placement and drainage

      4) Monitor for nasal flaring, sternal retractions, and changes in skin color

2. Gas exchange

   a. Place on cardiorespiratory monitor and monitor continuously

   b. Assess breath sounds

   c. Monitor chest tube placement and drainage

   d. Monitor continuous pulse oximetry

   e. Maintain thermoregulation

   f. Monitor chest tube placement and drainage

   g. Administer oxygen as prescribed, titrating to oxygen saturation parameters

   h. Maintain mechanical ventilation as prescribed

   i. Instruct parents about infant cardiopulmonary resuscitation (CPR) for discharge

3. Nutrition

   a. Monitor intake and output

   b. Weigh daily

   c. Maintain intravenous access, monitoring at least hourly

   d. Assess hydration status: fontanels and urine specific gravity

   e. Administer enteral feedings or parenteral nutrition as prescribed

   f. Elevate head of bed

   g. Provide pacifier to satisfy sucking needs of neonate and to maintain sucking reflex

   h. Provide oral feedings when there is evidence of swallow reflex and when prescribed

4. Risk for infection

   a. Monitor vital signs frequently

   b. Maintain continuous cardiorespiratory monitoring

   c. Provide enteral tube care

   d. Maintain strict asepsis when caring for central venous access for parenteral nutrition

5. Pain

   a. Assess for behavioral pain indicators (crying and inability to sleep)

   b. Provide intravenous analgesics proactively as prescribed

   c. Maintain continuous cardiorespiratory monitoring

   d. Administer analgesics at prescribed intervals around the clock for first 24–48 hours postoperatively

   e. Encourage parents to hold and cuddle infant

   f. Explain all equipment and procedures to parents to decrease anxiety and to prevent transmitting anxious feelings to infant

6. Anxiety
   a. Encourage parents to express feelings and concerns
   b. Listen actively to parents
   c. Facilitate parent/infant bonding
   d. Explain all equipment and procedures
   e. Assist identification of positive coping strategies and support providers

7. Parent teaching
   a. Assess parents' current level of understanding
   b. Provide verbal and written information regarding:
      1) Postoperative home care
      2) Pain management and medication administration
      3) Schedule for infant immunizations
      4) Infant CPR
      5) Infection protection
      6) Neonate care and feeding
      7) Referral information such as home health and monitor company as needed
      8) Enteral feedings if necessary
      9) Use of pacifier to maintain suck response if infant is receiving enteral feedings
      10) Enteral tube assessment and care
      11) Manifestations to report to health care provider
      12) Contact numbers for health care provider and referral contact people
   c. Provide sufficient time for teaching, including demonstrations and parental return demonstrations (infant CPR), monitoring, and enteral feedings
   d. Document teaching and parental responses

NIC

1. Aspiration Precautions
2. Oxygen Therapy, Ventilation Assistance
3. Nutrition Management, Weight Gain Assistance
4. Infection Control, Infection Protection
5. Pain Management, Analgesic Administration
6. Coping Enhancement
7. Teaching: Illness Care, Treatment, Health Promotion

EVALUATION

1. Client does not experience aspiration as evidenced by respiratory status WDL for neonate.
2. Client experiences adequate gas exchange as evidenced by oxygen saturation WDL for neonate, clear breath sounds, and lack of respiratory distress.
3. Client regains and maintains adequate nutrition as evidenced by weight gain consistent with doubling of birth weight by 6 months of age and tripling of birth weight by 12 months of age.
4. Client does not experience infection.

5. Client experiences adequate pain control as evidenced by behavioral indicators.
6. Parents demonstrate use of effective coping strategies.
7. Parents demonstrate understanding of neonate's condition, treatment, and home care.

References

Kronemer, K. A., & Snyder, A. (2006). *Esophageal atresia/tracheoesophageal fistula.* Retrieved February 19, 2007, from http://www.emedicine.com/radio/topic704.htm

Lucile Packard Children's Hospital at Stanford. (2007). *Digestive and liver disorders: Tracheoesophageal fistula and esophageal atresia.* Retrieved May 12, 2007, from http://www.lpch.org/DiseaseHealthInfo/HealthLibrary/digest/tracheo.html

MedlinePlus. (2006). *Esophageal atresia.* Retrieved February 19, 2007, from http://www.nlm.nih.gov/medlineplus/ency/article/000961.htm

Potts, N. L., & Mandleco, B. L. (2007). *Pediatric nursing: Caring for children and their families* (2nd ed.). Clifton Park, NY: Delmar Cengage Learning.

Sharma, S., & Duerksen, D. (2006). *Tracheoesophageal fistula.* Retrieved February 19, 2007, from http://www.emedicine.com/med/topic3416.htm

42

EWING'S SARCOMA

Definition

Ewing's sarcoma is a malignant bone tumor that represents one third of all malignant childhood bone cancers (Potts & Mandleco, 2007). It was first described by James Ewing in 1921 (Strauss, 2007).

Pathophysiology

Ewing's sarcoma arises from small round blue primitive undifferentiated cells resulting from embryonic chromosomal rearrangement that alters the position and function of genes and results in an abnormal genetic fusion transcript. In Ewing's sarcoma, when chromosomes are viewed under a microscope, a piece of chromosome 11 has moved to chromosome 22 and a piece of chromosome 22 has moved to chromosome 11, resulting in 11:22 translocation. As a result, there is new genetic information from the recombination of two unrelated genes (Cancer Index, 2003). According to the American Cancer Society, Ewing's sarcoma is part of the Ewing family of tumors that shares this genetic abnormality and includes peripheral primitive neuroectodermal tumor, or PNET (American Cancer Society, 2006).

Most often Ewing's sarcoma invades the soft tissue surrounding the femur, pelvis, ribs, spine, and humerus. As it imbeds into the midshaft of the bone, it competes with normal cells for nutrients, oxygen, and metabolic products, resulting in the crowding out and ultimate death of the normal cells. Although malignant, gross metastasis seldom is present at the time of diagnosis. However, as the disease progresses, metastasis occurs and usually involves the lungs, bones, and bone marrow. Once metastasis occurs, the prognosis is poor. Although tissue and organ failure result if Ewing's sarcoma is not treated, most complications are associated with the chemotherapy and radiation used to treat the disease. Therefore, the complications are iotragenic in nature.

Complications

Immunosuppression
Pain
Nausea and vomiting

Incidence

Ewing's sarcoma is the second most common malignant bone tumor of children and young adults, accounting for approximately 1% of all childhood tumors. About 90% of clients with Ewing's sarcoma are under the age of 30, and about 70% are under 20 with an incidence of 4.6 per 1 million children in those 15–19 years of age (Strauss, 2007). In the United States, approximately 200 children and adolescents are diagnosed with Ewing's sarcoma annually (Potts & Mandleco, 2007). Fewer than 30 children each year in the United Kingdom develop this cancer (Cancerbackup, 2007). The peak incidence is between 10 and 20 years of age. The highest rates occur during adolescence, and over 50% of these children are under 15 years of age at diagnosis. The tumor is rare before the age of 3 years with an incidence of 0.3 per 1 million children. During adolescence, the rate of incidence in boys is slightly higher than in girls. It is seldom seen in African-American, African, and Chinese children (MedlinePlus, 2006).

Etiology

The etiology of the majority of Ewing's sarcomas is a chromosome rearrangement between chromosomes 11 and 22. This alters both the position and function of genes, resulting in a fusion of genes referred to as a fusion transcript. Over 90% of individuals with Ewing's sarcoma have an abnormal fusion transcript involving two genes known as EWS and FLI1. As in the cases of osteogenic sarcoma, Ewing's sarcoma can arise at sites that previously experienced trauma or injury. However, it is believed that the injury is not causal but rather results in an awareness of the Ewing's sarcoma (Loyola University Health Systems, 2005).

In addition, some research has led health care providers to believe that Ewing's sarcoma belongs to a family of PNETs that arise from embryonic tissue that develops into nerve tissue. There appears to be a relationship between bone growth and the onset of Ewing's, which is believed to be associated with an increased vulnerability of the rapidly growing bone cells during adolescence.

Clinical Manifestations

Pain around the site of the tumor
Soft tissue swelling and/or redness around the site of the tumor
Fever
Weight loss and decreased appetite
Fatigue
Paralysis and/or incontinence (if the tumor is in the spinal region)
Symptoms related to nerve compression from tumor (numbness, tingling, and paralysis)

Diagnostic Tests

Radiography
Radionuclide bone scan
Magnetic resonance imaging
Computerized tomography
Serum chemistry
Bone biopsy
Bone marrow aspiration/biopsy

Medical Management

The goals of treatment are to cure the cancer and to limit both disease and treatment-based complications. With improvements in combination therapy, most children with Ewing's sarcoma can be cured; and even if the tumor returns, additional treatment with surgery, chemotherapy, and/or radiation therapy can be successful.

The treatment is individualized and involves a multidisciplinary approach. Most of the protocols for the treatment of Ewing's sarcoma originated with the Pediatric Intergroup Ewing's Sarcoma Study Group and the Children's Oncology Group (National Cancer Institute, 2006). Combination therapy that includes antineoplastics, surgery, and/or radiation is the current standard of care. The current chemotherapy regimen includes vincristine, doxorubicin, and cyclophosphamide, alternating with ifosfamide and etoposide (Broyles, Reiss, & Evans, 2007). Although study results favor the use of doxorubicin instead of dactinomycin, dactinomycin still is included in some European protocols. Chemotherapy usually is run in 14–17 cycles with the two chemotherapy regimens (National Cancer Institute, 2006).

Surgery and/or radiation are used for local tumor control. Surgery is preferred when the lesion is small, peripheral, and respectable, whereas more central tumors usually are treated with radiation. A group of 39 children who were treated at St. Jude Children's

Research Hospital with both surgery and radiation was followed; the study showed the eight-year local failure rate was 5% for children with negative surgical margins and 17% for children with positive margins (Krasin et al., 2004). In very young children, however, surgery may produce less morbidity than the standard six weeks of daily radiation therapy because of the growth retardation that occurs with radiation. European researchers continue to study whether treatment intensification (high-dose chemotherapy with stem cell rescue [SCR]) will improve outcome for clients with a poor histologic response to radiation (National Cancer Institute, 2006).

Radiation therapy should be used for children who do not have a surgical option that preserves function and should be used for children who have been treated surgically but did not achieve adequate margins. Radiation therapy should be administered in a setting in which stringent planning techniques are used by those experienced in the treatment of the Ewing family of tumors, as this approach will result in local control of the tumor with the fewest adverse effects. Although individualized, radiation generally is administered in fractionated doses totaling approximately 5,580 cGy to the prechemotherapy tumor volume. However, even with this dosing, some children need surgical resection following radiation therapy. Children older than 14 years of age with tumors greater than 8 cm in length have a higher rate of failure with local radiation (National Cancer Institute, 2006).

Nursing Management

Refer to Chapter 22: Chemotherapy, Chapter 87: Radiation Therapy, and Chapter 100: Surgical Client.

References

American Cancer Society. (2006). *What is the Ewing family of tumors?* Retrieved May 12, 2007, from http://www.cancer.org/docroot/CRI/content/CRI_2_4_1X_What_is_Ewings_Family_of_tumors_48.asp

Broyles, B. E., Reiss, B. S., & Evans, M. E. (2007). *Pharmacological aspects of nursing care* (7th ed.). Clifton Park, NY: Delmar Cengage Learning.

Cancerbackup. (2007). *Ewing's sarcoma in children.* Retrieved May 12, 2007, from http://www.cancerbackup.org.uk/Cancertype/Childrenscancers/Typesofchildrenscancers/Ewings sarcoma

Cancer Index. (2003). *Ewing's sarcoma.* Retrieved May 12, 2007, from http://www.cancerindex.org/ccw/faq/ewings.htm#q5

Krasin, M. J., Rodriguez-Galindo, C., Davidoff, A. M., Billups, C. A., Fuller, C. E., Neel, M. D., Kun, L. E., & Merchant, T. E. (2004, September). Efficacy of combined surgery and irradiation for localized Ewings sarcoma family of tumors. *Pediatric Blood Cancer, 43*(3). Retrieved May 12, 2007, from http://www.ncbi.nlm.nih.gov/entrez/query.fcgi?cmd=Retrieve&db=PubMed&list_uids=15266406&dopt=Abstract

Loyola University Health Systems. (2005). *Ewing's sarcoma.* Retrieved February 13, 2008, from http://loyolauniversity.adam.com/content.aspx?productId=105&pid=1&gid=001302

MedlinePlus. (2006). *Ewing's sarcoma.* Retrieved May 12, 2007, from http://www.nlm.nih.gov/medlineplus/ency/article/001302.htm

National Cancer Institute. (2006). *Ewing family of tumors treatment.* Retrieved May 12, 2007, from http://www.cancer.gov/cancertopics/pdq/treatment/ewings/healthprofessional/allpages

Potts, N. L., & Mandleco, B. L. (2007). *Pediatric nursing: Caring for children and their families* (2nd ed.). Clifton Park, NY: Delmar Cengage Learning.

Strauss, L. G. (2007). *Ewing sarcoma.* Retrieved February 13, 2008, from http://www.emedicine.com/radio/topic275.htm

43

Exstrophy of the Bladder

Definition

Exstrophy of the bladder is a congenital anomaly of the urinary system characterized by improper fusion of the abdominal cavity resulting in the urinary bladder protruding through the abdominal wall. Frequently, this presents with epispadias and is called bladder exstrophy-epispadias complex.

Pathophysiology

Exstrophy of the urinary bladder is an uncommon birth defect in which the bladder is exposed inside out and protrudes through the abdominal wall (MedlinePlus, 2006). During the 4–11th week of embryonic development, there is a maldevelopment of the cloacal membrane, mesoderm, and lower abdominal wall. The nature of this maldevelopment is not completely understood; however, there are two theories as to why it occurs. One theory suggests that during this early folding, fusing, and separating, something causes the cloacal membrane not to close, causing the bladder to develop outside the abdominal wall. A second theory proposes that the skin that forms over the bladder during this early stage of development is thin, leading to a rupture that causes the bladder to evert and communicate with the amniotic fluid (Association for Bladder Exstrophy Community, 2007). The bladder is flattened; and the mucosa at birth is thin, reddened, and very susceptible to injury (Potts & Mandleco, 2007).

This anomaly involves many systems in the body, including the urinary tract, bones and skeletal muscles, and reproductive system. Other anomalies include epispadias, vesicoureteral reflux, decreased bladder capacity, absent bladder neck and sphincter, and widening of the symphysis pubis resulting in separation of the pelvic bones. Infertility related to malformation of the vagina can occur.

If left untreated, bladder exstrophy results in complete bladder incontinence, sexual dysfunction, and increased risk of developing bladder cancer. Even though the kidneys of a child with bladder exstrophy develop normally, vesicoureteral reflux and pyelonephritis can occur following reconstructive surgery.

Complications

Infection within urinary system
Complete urinary incontinence
Vesicoureteral reflux
Pyelonephritis
Long-term:
    Sexual dysfunction
    Increased risk of bladder cancer

Incidence

Bladder exstrophy occurs in 3.3 out of 100,000 live births with a 2.3:1 male:female ratio and is more common in Caucasians (Yerkes & Rink, 2006). The risk of a family having more than one child with this condition is approximately 1 in 100, and children born to a parent with exstrophy have a risk of approximately 1 in 70 of having the condition. Recent published evidence suggests that the risk of bladder exstrophy in children born as a result of assisted fertility techniques is 7 times greater than in children conceived naturally (John Hopkins University, 2007).

Etiology

The cause of bladder exstrophy is uncertain. There are no identifiable inherited factors although the incidence is higher in children of a parent with exstrophy. As previously noted, infertility treatments increase the fetal risk of developing exstrophy (Yerkes & Rink, 2006).

Clinical Manifestations

Exposed bladder mucosa
Displaced anal opening
Widened symphysis pubis
External rotation of lower extremities
Triangular-shaped abdominal muscles
Epispadias
Narrow vaginal opening
Wide labia
Shortened urethra

Diagnostic Tests

Fetal ultrasonography
Renal ultrasonography
Voiding dystourethrogram
Radiography of the symphysis pubis

Medical Management

The goals of treatment are surgically to close the bladder and pelvis, reconstruct the male penis and female external genitalia, and achieve urinary continence and renal function. The surgery involves stages with the separation of the exposed bladder from the abdominal wall and closure of the bladder during the neonatal period. This includes placement of a suprapubic urinary catheter and an indwelling urethral catheter. Because the pelvic bones are separated, the child also will have the pelvic bones surgically attached to each other. After surgery, the child is placed in a lower body cast or sling to promote healing of the bones. This surgery involving the pelvic bones may be done with the first surgery or delayed for weeks or months (MedlinePlus, 2006).

Epispadias repair may be performed between the ages of 6 months and 1 year or done at the time of bladder neck surgery during the preschool years (ages 3–5 years). Waiting allows the bladder to reach sufficient capacity and the muscles to develop control continence. Further surgeries for bladder reconstruction and augmentation often are needed as well as procedures to improve the external genitalia. Prophylactic antimicrobials are used routinely; and when a child develops a fever, urinary tract infection should be ruled out first.

The results of staged reconstruction have been well documented; and as long as the bladder develops sufficient capacity, continence can be achieved in up to 90% of cases. Even in the presence of poor quality bladders at birth that are not suitable for closing, it is exceptionally rare for a child to reach adolescence without achieving continence.

Nursing Management

Also refer to Chapter 100: Surgical Client.

ASSESSMENT

1. Assess condition of the exposed bladder mucosa
2. Assess urinary output
3. Assess parental understanding and adaptation to the infant's condition

NURSING DIAGNOSES (INCLUDING BUT NOT LIMITED TO)

1. Impaired tissue integrity R/T exposed bladder mucosa
2. Risk for infection R/T exposed bladder mucosa and surgical repair
3. Parental anxiety R/T infant's condition and need for surgery
4. Deficient knowledge R/T infant's condition, surgical treatment, and home care

PLANNING/GOALS

1. Client will maintain integrity of exposed bladder mucosa evidenced by tissue that is smooth, moist, red, and intact.
2. Client will not experience infection.
3. Parents will demonstrate use of positive coping strategies and support systems.
4. Parents will demonstrate understanding of infant's condition, treatment, and home care.

NOC

1. Tissue Integrity: Skin and Mucous Membranes
2. Infection Control
3. Anxiety
4. Knowledge: Illness Care, Treatment, Health Promotion

IMPLEMENTATION

1. Tissue integrity
   a. Assess condition of exposed bladder mucosa
   b. Immediately cover exposed bladder mucosa with sterile saline-soaked gauze
   c. Assess wound hourly
   d. Rehydrate or change sterile saline-soaked gauze as prescribed
   e. Keep area clean of urine
   f. Do not apply diaper
   g. Prepare neonate for surgery as prescribed
2. Risk for infection
   a. Monitor lab values
   b. Assess bladder mucosa for signs of infection
   c. Assess vital signs hourly after birth and then every 4 hours and as needed
   d. Use meticulous hand washing
   e. Teach hand washing technique to parents
   f. Provide suprapubic and urethral catheter care per facility protocol
   g. Demonstrate catheter care, emptying of drainage bags, recording of urinary output, and axillary temperature
   h. Provide time for return demonstration of skills
3. Anxiety
   a. Encourage parents to express feelings and concerns
   b. Listen actively

   c. Foster parent/child bonding

   d. Assist parents in identifying positive coping strategies and support systems

   e. Collaborate with health care provider for referrals as needed

   f. Address parents' spiritual needs

   g. Have parents accompany neonate to surgical hold area

   h. Keep parents informed during and after surgery

   i. Encourage parents to visit neonate in postanesthesia care unit

   j. Encourage parental participation in neonate's care

4. Parental teaching

   a. Assess parents' current level of understanding

   b. Provide verbal and written information regarding:

     1) Skin care

     2) Catheter care

     3) Emptying of catheter drainage bags and measuring of output

     4) Neonatal and infant care

     5) Infant feeding and bathing techniques

     6) Procedure for taking axillary temperature

     7) Medication administration as prescribed, stressing the importance of compliance with care

     8) Signs and symptoms to report to health care provider

     9) Referral information as needed

     10) Contact numbers for health care provider and referral contacts

   c. Provide adequate time for teaching, demonstrating catheter care and emptying, and allowing parents' return demonstrations

   d. Document teaching and parents' response

NIC

1. Wound Care
2. Infection Precautions
3. Anxiety Reduction
4. Teaching: Illness Care, Treatment, Health Promotion

EVALUATION

1. Client maintains integrity of exposed bladder mucosa as evidenced by tissue that is smooth, moist, red, and intact.
2. Client does not experience infection.
3. Parents demonstrate use of positive coping strategies and support systems.
4. Parents demonstrate understanding of infant's condition, treatment, and home care.

References

Association for Bladder Exstrophy Community. (2007). *Frequently asked questions.* Retrieved February 13, 2008, from http://www.bladderexstrophy.com/faq.htm#C_AtWhatStage

John Hopkins University. (2007). *Classic bladder exstrophy.* Retrieved May 12, 2007, from http://urology.jhu.edu/pediatric/diseases/DEx1.php

MedlinePlus. (2006). *Bladder exstrophy repair.* Retrieved February 27, 2007, from http://www.nlm.nih.gov/medlineplus/ency/article/002997.htm

Potts, N. L., & Mandleco, B. L. (2007). *Pediatric nursing: Caring for children and their families* (2nd ed.). Clifton Park, NY: Delmar Cengage Learning.

Yerkes, E. B., & Rink, R. C. (2006). *Exstrophy and epispadias.* Retrieved May 12, 2007, from http://www.emedicine.com/ped/topic704.htm

FAILURE TO THRIVE (FTT)

Definition

Failure to thrive (FTT) is a term used for a child who experiences inadequate growth, falling below the third to fifth percentile on a standardized growth chart (Potts & Mandleco, 2007). Growth charts are available from the Centers for Disease Control and Prevention (Centers for Disease Control and Prevention, 2007).

FTT is defined as "the failure to maintain an established pattern of growth and development that responds to the provision of adequate nutritional and emotional needs of the patient" (Sirotnak, 2006, p. 1).

Pathophysiology

FTT is classified as organic or inorganic depending on the etiology. Organic FTT results from physiological factors that interfere with ingestion, absorption, or metabolism of nutritional intake leading to inadequate weight gain appropriate for height and level of development. Organic causes include malabsorption syndromes such as cystic fibrosis (the most common physiological cause), celiac disease (second most common), and short bowel syndrome (small gut syndrome). Other causes are congenital heart defects and endocrine disorders (hyperthyroidism, growth hormone deficiency, and diabetes mellitus). The exact pathophysiology depends on the organic etiology. For instance, cystic fibrosis interferes with absorption of nutrients in the duodenum because of blockage of pancreatic digestive enzymes; celiac disease disrupts absorption due to decreased functional intestinal villa for absorption; and in the child with small bowel syndrome, there is a dramatic decrease in the absorption surface of the intestines. Congenital heart defects cause fatigue and respiratory insufficiency during exertion that for the infant with a congenital heart defect, interferes with the quantity of nutritional intake because of fatigue during feedings. Hyperthyroidism increases the metabolic rate of the child, resulting in excess burning of calories.

Nonorganic FTT is caused by psychosocial factors and is suspected after organic disease has been ruled out. The most common nonorganic cause is lack of bonding or attachment between the neonate/infant and the primary caregiver. Other reasons for nonorganic FTT include poverty; inadequate social support; family stress; insufficient breast milk; errors in formula preparation; lack of caregiver knowledge related to nutritional needs of child; and maternal psychopathology including mood disorders, anxiety, and substance abuse (Potts & Mandleco, 2007). Nonorganic FTT also is a manifestation of child abuse (Schnitzer & Ewigman, 2005; Sirotnak, 2006).

FTT leads to malnutrition. In addition to delayed growth and development and vitamin and mineral deficiencies, the immune system is compromised, leading to recurrent infections. Developmental delays are both physical and psychosocial in nature. In the presence of malnutrition, the brain can experience lack of development in brain size, a decreased number of neurons, and synaptic complexity.

Complications

Delayed growth and development
Recurrent respiratory infections
Recurrent gastrointestinal infections
Iron-deficiency anemia

Vitamin deficiencies

Cognitive impairment

Emotional behavior

Incidence

In the United States, approximately 10% of children experience manifestations of FTT. International rates are higher, especially in underdeveloped countries (Bassali & Benjamin, 2006). Other estimates imply a higher incidence considering approximately "20% of children live in poverty, and the inability to obtain adequate food is directly related to such conditions" (Sirotnak, 2006, Section 2).

Etiology

As noted in the discussion of pathophysiology, causes for FTT are organic or nonorganic.

Clinical Manifestations

Growth less than third to fifth percentile on standardized growth chart

Sudden and rapid deceleration in growth curve

Failure to accomplish milestones for growth and development

Loss of subcutaneous fat

Decreased muscle mass and tone

Apathy and lethargy

Infrequent urination and stools

Manifestations of neglect

Flattening of occiput from remaining in supine position

Avoidance of eye contact

Lack of interaction with caregiver

Diagnostic Tests

First, organic causes are ruled out

Developmental screening

Urinalysis

Complete blood count

Sweat chloride level

Thyroid panel

Serum electrolyte levels

Analysis of stool

Tuberculin test

Chest X-ray

Electrocardiography

Gastrointestinal studies

Bone scan

Bowel and muscle biopsies

Medical Management

The goals of treatment are to provide adequate nutritional intake and enhance development. In the presence of suspected child abuse, securing the child's safety is a priority. A multidisciplinary approach is necessary for treatment because FTT is a complex condition. Nurses, health care providers, dieticians, occupational therapists, recreation therapists, physical therapists, and mental health professionals (for nonorganic FTT) are necessary members of this team. Nutritional supplementation is a standard of care for these children regardless of the type of FTT the child is experiencing, and it is used in conjunction with treatment of the cause. Nutritional therapy is designed to facilitate growth that is 2–3 times the average rate for age (catch-up growth). It involves the child receiving 150% of the recommended daily caloric intake and supplementation with vitamins and minerals. Recreational therapists are helpful in identifying developmental lapses and providing measures to facilitate the child's growth and development (Potts & Mandleco, 2007).

Nursing Management

ASSESSMENT

1. Obtain complete history
2. Obtain a thorough diet history
3. Obtain height and weight and plot on growth chart
4. Assess oral mucous membranes and tooth condition
5. Assess caregiver/infant interactions

NURSING DIAGNOSES (INCLUDING BUT NOT LIMITED TO)

1. Imbalanced nutrition: less than body requirements R/T inadequate intake, digestion, or absorption and metabolism of nutrients
2. Delayed growth and development R/T factors influencing FTT
3. Deficient knowledge (parental/caregiver) R/T nutritional needs of child, treatment, and home care

PLANNING/GOALS

1. Client will consume adequate nutritional intake to experience growth and developmental within defined limits (WDL) for age and gender.
2. Client will demonstrate achievement of developmental milestones.
3. Parents will demonstrate understanding of child's nutritional needs, treatment, and home care.

NOC

1. Nutritional Status
2. Child Development
3. Knowledge: Diet, Parenting

IMPLEMENTATION

1. Nutrition
   a. Provide for consistency in nursing care provided
   b. Assess and document child's eating habits
   c. Assess and document parent–child interaction
   d. Encourage parents to discuss positive and negative feelings about caring for child
   e. Monitor intake and output
   f. Obtain daily weights
   g. Act as role model for parents during interactions with child
   h. Provide food on demand
   i. Increase intake as tolerated
   j. Offer high-protein, high-calorie foods and snacks
   k. Offer frequent small portions
   l. Encourage parental involvement in feedings
   m. Provide nutrition information to parents, stressing importance nutrition plays in child's growth and development
   n. Collaborate with health care provider to initiate referrals as needed

2. Growth and development
   a. Assess level of growth and development
   b. Collaborate with recreation therapist for age-appropriate activities
   c. Act as role model for parents during interactions with child
   d. Provide specific times during the day to play with child
   e. Assess changes in level of growth and development after interventions
3. Parent/caregiver teaching
   a. Assess parents' current level of knowledge
   b. Provide verbal and written information regarding:
      1) Child's dietary needs
      2) Prescribed supplements
      3) Child's need for schedules and routines
      4) Need to plan three meals and three snacks a day
      5) Importance of eating with child
      6) Importance of allowing child to feed self
      7) Importance of avoiding force feeding
      8) Importance of mealtimes being family time
      9) Need to provide relaxing interactions during meals and to avoid rushing
      10) Referral information including contact numbers
      11) Importance of compliance with care and follow-up with health care provider and other health professionals involved in care
      12) Contact numbers to use for asking questions or reporting difficulties
   c. Provide adequate time for teaching and parents' questions
   d. Document teaching and parental response

NIC

1. Nutrition Management, Weight Gain Assistance
2. Developmental Enhancement: Child, Parenting Promotion
3. Teaching: Prescribed Diet, Parent Education, Health Education

EVALUATION

1. Client consumes adequate nutritional intake to experience growth and developmental WDL for age and gender.
2. Client demonstrates achievement of developmental milestones.
3. Parents demonstrate understanding of child's nutritional needs, treatment, and home care.

References

Bassali, R. W., & Benjamin, J. (2006). *Failure to thrive.* Retrieved May 12, 2007, from http://www.emedicine.com/ped/topic738.htm

Centers for Disease Control and Prevention. (2007). *Clinical growth charts.* Retrieved May 12, 2007, from http://www.cdc.gov/nchs/about/major/nhanes/growthcharts/clinical_charts.htm

Potts, N. L., & Mandleco, B. L. (2007). *Pediatric nursing: Caring for children and their families* (2nd ed.). Clifton Park, NY: Delmar Cengage Learning.

Schnitzer, P. G., & Ewigman, B. G. (2005). Child deaths resulting from inflicted injuries: Household risk factors and perpetrator characteristics. *Pediatrics, 116*(5). Retrieved May 12, 2007, from http://pediatrics.aappublications.org/content/vol116/issue5/index.shtml

Sirotnak, A. P. (2006). *Child abuse & neglect: Failure to thrive.* Retrieved May 12, 2007, from http://www.emedicine.com/ped/topic2647.htm

FOREIGN BODY ASPIRATION (FBA)

Definition

Foreign body aspiration (FBA) is the lodging of an object or substances in the airway.

Pathophysiology

For several reasons, children are more prone than adults to aspirate foreign material. Children have a decreased ability to chew food adequately because they the lack molar teeth and thus leave larger pieces of food to be swallowed. Children also are likely to talk, laugh, run, or play when eating. This increases their risk of inhaling food. Although possible at any age, FBA usually is experienced by infants, toddlers, and preschoolers (Bye, 2007).

The objects may be small toys, balloons, and food. Food items easily aspirated include raisins, nuts, hot dogs, little sausages, and small foods such as grapes. Usually, the cough reflex expels an object and protects the airway. However, aspirated foreign bodies can become lodged in the larynx or trachea; or if small enough, they can pass through the larynx or trachea and become lodged in the bronchial tree. The right bronchus is the most common point of obstruction because of the smaller angle of the bifurcation from the trachea into the bronchi. Aspiration can result in damage to the tissue lining of the airway, leading to swelling and decreasing of the airway lumen. A foreign body aspirated into the lung can cause aspiration pneumonia. Atelectasis occurs in 63% of childhood FBA (Munter, 2007).

Obstruction may cause partial or complete obstruction. Partial obstruction can result in atelectasis and hyperexpansion of the alveoli, leading to respiratory distress. Complete obstruction causes hypoxia, brain injury that occurs within 3–6 minutes following obstruction and hypoxia, and death (Potts & Mandleco, 2007).

Complications

Aspiration pneumonia
Airway trauma
Atelectasis
Alveolar hyperexpansion
Hypoxia
Brain injury
Death

Incidence

FBA is most common in children 6 months to 4 years of age (Potts & Mandleco, 2007). By age 5, children are able to sit and eat; so the incidence declines after this point. In a 2000 study, FBA accounted for more than 17,000 emergency department visits and over 160 deaths in children younger than 14 years (Bye, 2007). There is a higher incidence in the United States of FBA in boys; however, in studies performed outside the United States, females usually have a higher incidence (Munter, 2007).

Etiology

Children's normal active state and lack of molar teeth as well as their normal curiosity and the oral phase of development (1–3-year-olds) place them at risk for aspirating any object small enough to put into their mouths (Munter, 2007). Over half of the cases of FBA occurred in unsupervised children. Peanuts are the most commonly aspirated foreign body. Other commonly inhaled foods in children are seeds and popcorn (MedlinePlus, 2007). "The most common etiology of aspiration deaths in children is a toy, with balloons accounting for 29% of deaths" (Munter, 2007, Section 2). Latex balloons are especially dangerous because of the flexibility of the fiber in balloons allowing them to expand over the airway during inspiration attempts and then deflate again to completely block the airway. The aspiration of baby powder can be particularly dangerous because the infant can experience a symptom-free period before suffocation (Munter, 2007).

Clinical Manifestations

IMMEDIATE RESPONSES

Sudden, violent coughing
Gagging
Wheezing
Brief periods of apnea
Vomiting
Circumoral cyanosis
Anxiety

LARYNGEAL OR TRACHEAL OBSTRUCTION

Croupy cough
Hoarseness
Stridor
Dyspnea with wheezing
Cyanosis
Anxiety
Respiratory arrest with complete tracheal obstruction

BRONCHIAL OBSTRUCTION

Deep, dry cough
Wheezing
Decreased breath sounds unilaterally
Stridor
Anxiety
Respiratory arrest

Diagnostic Tests

Completed blood count
Erythrocyte sedimentation rate (ESR)
Radiography
Fluoroscopy
Computed tomography
Bronchoscopy

Medical Management

The goal of treatment is to remove the foreign body and preserve respiratory function. If the child experiences a complete obstruction, the Heimlich maneuver should be performed for infants and children too large to straddle the rescuer's arm or thigh for back blows and chest thrusts. Flexible bronchoscopy can locate and identify the aspirated foreign body, but a rigid bronchoscopy performed under anesthesia is needed to remove the object. Surgical removal of the object may be required for larger objects.

Prophylactic antimicrobial agents usually are prescribed to prevent infection from the encounter of a foreign object in the respiratory tract.

Nursing Management

ASSESSMENT

1. Assess airway, breathing, and circulation (ABC)
2. Obtain history while performing rapid assessment
3. Obtain height, weight, and vital signs
4. Assess psychosocial impact on parents
5. Prepare child for bronchoscopy

NURSING DIAGNOSES (INCLUDING BUT NOT LIMITED TO)

1. Ineffective airway clearance R/T aspiration of foreign body
2. Anxiety R/T child's difficulty breathing and urgency of care
3. Risk for infection R/T aspiration of foreign body
4. Deficient knowledge R/T prevention, treatment, and home care

PLANNING/GOALS

1. Client will regain and maintain airway patency, and foreign body will be successfully extracted.
2. Parents/caregivers will demonstrate use of positive coping strategies.
3. Client will not experience infection related to FBA.
4. Parents, caregivers, and child (if age-appropriate) will demonstrate understanding of aspiration prevention, treatment, and home care.

NOC

1. Respiratory Status: Airway Patency
2. Anxiety
3. Infection Control
4. Knowledge: Child Physical Safety, Treatment, Health Promotion

IMPLEMENTATION

1. Airway clearance
   a. Assess respiratory status continuously during acute period
   b. Initiate rescue measures for obstructed airway with complete obstruction
   c. Monitor and place in position to facilitate breathing with partial obstruction
   d. Place on continuous cardiorespiratory monitor and pulse oximetry
   e. Administer oxygen as prescribed, titrating to oxygen saturation
   f. Monitor breath sounds
   g. Monitor child's vital signs
   h. Monitor status according to facility postprocedure protocol following removal of object during bronchoscopy or surgery
   i. Hold fluids until object is removed and gag reflex returns
2. Anxiety
   a. Assess parents/child for manifestations of anxiety
   b. Explain all procedures and equipment
   c. Encourage verbalization of feelings and concerns
   d. Assist in identifying positive coping strategies
   e. Stay with child until transfer to bronchoscopy personnel

3. Risk of infection
   a. Monitor vital signs per child's condition and facility protocol
   b. Initiate and maintain intravenous access device, monitoring at least hourly
   c. Administer prophylactic antimicrobials as prescribed
   d. Explain medications to parents and child (if age-appropriate)
4. Parent/caregiver/client teaching
   a. Assess current level of knowledge
   b. Provide verbal and written information regarding:
      1) Aspiration prevention including avoiding foods inappropriate for toddlers and preschoolers; properly positioning and feeding infant; keeping small objects away from children under the age of 3 years; and not allowing children to run, talk, or laugh with food in their mouth
      2) Medication administration and importance of completing entire prescription of antimicrobials
      3) Growth and development activities of infant, toddler, and preschooler
      4) Signs and symptoms to report to health care provider immediately
      5) Contact number for health care provider
      6) Importance of follow-up with health care provider
   c. Provide adequate time for teaching and parental questions
   d. Document teaching and parental response

NIC

1. Airway Management, Respiratory Monitoring
2. Coping Enhancement
3. Infection Precautions
4. Teaching: Infant/Toddler/Preschooler Safety, Treatment, Health Promotion

EVALUATION

1. Client regains and maintains airway patency, and foreign body is successfully extracted.
2. Parents/caregivers demonstrate use of positive coping strategies.
3. Client does not experience infection related to FBA.
4. Parents, caregivers, and child (if age-appropriate) demonstrate understanding of aspiration prevention, treatment, and home care.

References

Bye, M. R. (2007). *Airway foreign body.* Retrieved February 13, 2008, from http://www.emedicine.com/ped/topic286.htm

MedlinePlus. (2007). *Foreign object—inhaled or swallowed.* Retrieved February 13, 2008, from http://www.nlm.nih.gov/medlineplus/ency/article/000036.htm

Munter, D. W. (2007). *Foreign bodies, trachea.* Retrieved February 13, 2008, from http://www.emedicine.com/emerg/topic751.htm

Potts, N. L., & Mandleco, B. L. (2007). *Pediatric nursing: Caring for children and their families* (2nd ed.). Clifton Park, NY: Delmar Cengage Learning.

46

FRACTURES, CASTS, AND TRACTION

Definition

A fracture is an interruption in the continuity of a bone in the body. Casts are fiberglass or plaster material used to immobilize extremity fractures; and traction is a device to immobilize fractures of the spine, pelvis, or hip.

Pathophysiology

Fractures result when more stress is placed on the bone than it can absorb, and they occur frequently during early childhood due to the porous nature of immature bones (Potts & Mandleco, 2007). Fractures can occur in any bone of the body and result in damage not only to the bone but also to soft tissue surrounding the bone at the site of the break. In addition, fractures may affect the blood vessels and nerves at the site of the break. Pain is the universal manifestation of a fracture. Immediately after the break occurs, the inflammatory response is initiated and fibrin clots are formed. Calluses or tissue masses form at the fracture site to connect the two bones. Also, osteoblasts converge in large numbers to create a new bone matrix between the two bone fragments, while calcium salts are deposited to provide stability to the forming matrix (Broyles, 2005). Osteoblasts continually form new bones, while osteoclasts remodel the bone at the fracture site, creating a compact bone mass that resembles uninjured bone (Potts & Mandleco, 2007). Children have a greater remodeling potential than adults because bone healing occurs more rapidly as a result of increased bone production (Wilkins, 2006).

Fractures are classified according to characteristics and severity. A simple or closed fracture is characterized by the skin surface over the break remaining intact. A compound or open fracture involves the broken bone protruding through the skin surface. Complete fractures are total breaks through the entire bone. Incomplete fractures involve breaks that do not extend completely through the bone, leaving it marginally intact. "Spontaneous or pathological fractures occur in the presence of diseased or weakened bone when pressure or force is present that would not have fractured a healthy bone" (Broyles, 2005, p. 339).

Other classifications describe the type of break. For instance, a transverse fracture is characterized by the fracture lines being at right angles to the long axis of the bone. It occurs on the bone shaft and results from a sharp, direct blow or prolonged stress. When the fracture line is slanting or diagonal across the bone, it is described as an oblique fracture. A spiral fracture is circular and twists the bone; it is commonly seen in victims of child abuse. Greenstick fractures are breaks in the periosteum and bone on one side while the other side of the bone only bends. This is a type of incomplete fracture (Potts & Mandleco, 2007). Refer to Figure 46-1.

Epiphyseal growth plate fractures are described using the Salter-Harris classification (Potts & Mandleco, 2007; Moore & Smith, 2007). Refer to Figure 46-2.

Stress fractures are common in older school-age children and adolescents who play sports. A stress fracture "is an overuse injury resulting from repetitive submaximal forces that are directed to weight bearing bones. These types of injuries occur when the stress to that area increases too quickly before the bone has a chance to adapt to changes. The bone weakens and pain develops. Lower leg and foot stress fractures are common among runners; [they] often occur in the tibia or fibula" (Columbus Children's Hospital, 2007, p. 1).

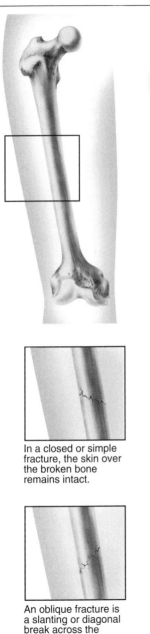

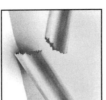

In an open or compound fracture, the broken bone protrudes through the skin.

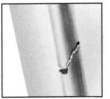

A spiral fracture is circular and twists around the bone shaft.

In a closed or simple fracture, the skin over the broken bone remains intact.

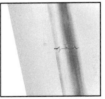

A transverse fracture occurs at a right angle to the long axis of the bone.

An oblique fracture is a slanting or diagonal break across the bone.

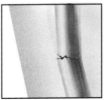

A greenstick fracture is a break through the periosteum and bone on one side while the other side only bends.

Figure 46-1: Common Childhood Fractures.

Comminuted fractures are seen in children who have experienced trauma, as in motor vehicle accidents. A comminuted fracture is characterized by splintering or excessive fragmentation of the bone.

Infection can occur from microorganisms entering the wound, especially in the presence of an open fracture. Compartment syndrome is a condition of bleeding into the

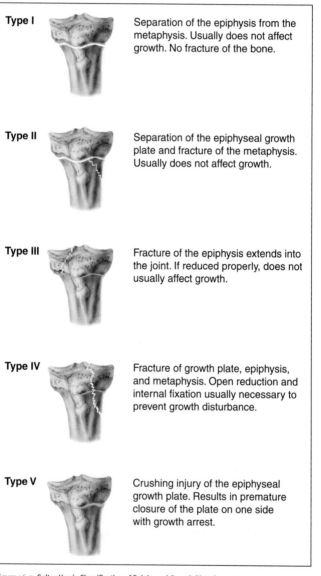

Type I — Separation of the epiphysis from the metaphysis. Usually does not affect growth. No fracture of the bone.

Type II — Separation of the epiphyseal growth plate and fracture of the metaphysis. Usually does not affect growth.

Type III — Fracture of the epiphysis extends into the joint. If reduced properly, does not usually affect growth.

Type IV — Fracture of growth plate, epiphysis, and metaphysis. Open reduction and internal fixation usually necessary to prevent growth disturbance.

Type V — Crushing injury of the epiphyseal growth plate. Results in premature closure of the plate on one side with growth arrest.

Figure 46-2: **Salter-Harris Classification of Epiphyseal Growth Plate Fractures.**

muscle at the site of the break. This is very painful and can result in damage to blood vessels and nerves at the site. Damage to the structures surrounding the break can occur, such as a hemothorax or pneumothorax secondary to rib fractures or paralysis secondary to spinal fractures.

Complications

Impaired physical mobility
Growth plate injuries
Infection
Compartment syndrome
Neurovascular damage
Hemothorax
Pneumothorax
Spinal cord injuries

Incidence

Approximately 25% of the population experiences some type of musculoskeletal injury annually. Areas that are frequently involved in children are the upper and lower extremities. "Children have a 42% higher incidence of arm fractures as compared to 30 years ago" (Potts & Mandleco, 2007, p. 1144).

Etiology

Motor vehicle accidents, all-terrain vehicles (ATVs), falls from playground equipment or other structures, in-line skating, horseback riding, and sports injuries are the leading causes of fractures in children. The porous nature of their immature bones places children at higher risks. Epiphyseal growth plate fractures are common in children because this plate is the weakest part of the long bone (Potts & Mandleco, 2007).

Clinical Manifestations

Pain at the fracture site
Obvious deformity of the affected area
Immobility or decreased range of motion
Crepitus
Ecchymosis
Hematoma
Erythema
Edema
Inability to bear weight
Inability or unwillingness to move area
Presence of bone protruding through skin and open wound

Diagnostic Tests

Radiographic studies are most definitive
Computed tomography (CT)
Magnetic resonance imaging (MRI)

Medical Management

The goals of treatment include immobilization of the fracture to prevent complications, pain management, and prevention teaching. Pain management is accomplished by the use of analgesics and anti-inflammatory agents, which should begin as soon as possible following the injury.

Immobilization is the standard of care for fractures. At the scene of the accident, the injury should be immobilized in the position found. Untrained attempts to reduce the fracture can result in permanent neurovascular injuries. Once the child has received professional medical help, a decision is made concerning how to reduce the fracture. Closed reduction with the use of fluoroscopy may be accomplished with some uncomplicated fractures. For more complex fractures, open reduction and internal fixation (ORIF) may be required. This surgical procedure involves realigning or reducing the bone fragments into their normal position and placing metal screws, rods, or plates to the surface of the bone to secure the anatomical alignment. Although ORIF can realign the fracture fragments precisely, risks associated with surgery result in this procedure being used only when the pediatric orthopedic surgeon considers open reduction the best therapy for restoring the fractured bone(s) to normal function. Open compound fractures of a long bone may require open reduction with the placement of external fixators. External fixation is a procedure where pins or screws are placed in the broken bone above and below the fracture site and then repositioned to realign the bones. The pins or screws are connected to a metal bar or bars outside the skin (Broyles, 2005). The primary problem associated with external fixators is the risk of infection at the pin site. Percutaneous pin fixation in forearm fractures is currently used with the same results as the placement of plates for these fractures. In this procedure, flexible intramedullary nails are used to manage open forearm fractures with Grade I puncture wounds. Because these pins are placed under the skin, they can remain in place throughout the healing process. This procedure also is appropriate for children with large soft tissue swelling at the site of the fracture in which cast pressures could be detrimental (Wilkins, 2006).

Following closed reduction or ORIF of the fracture, immobilization provides support to the broken bone and keeps the broken ends in proper position for healing. The type of immobilization device depends on the location and severity of the fracture. Immobilization using a plaster or fiberglass material is the most common type of fracture treatment, especially for extremity fractures. A functional cast or brace may be indicated for spinal fractures; and rib belts may be used to control the movement of the ribs, but not immobilize them. The use of rib belts involves close monitoring of the child's respiratory status.

Traction may be indicated as a preliminary treatment (spinal fractures) or for areas where casting is impractical (pelvis and hip). "Traction is used to align a bone or bones by a gentle, steady pulling action. Traction may be skeletal (metal pin through a bone) or skin (skin tapes or Velcro)" (Broyles, 2005, p. 340). Halo traction involves cranial pins attached to a metal structure that rests on the client's shoulders to allow for mobility in the presence of cervical fractures. Refer to Figure 46-3 and Figure 46-4.

Education focusing on accident prevention and bone strengthening should be part of any fracture treatment. It should include information about the importance of adequate nutrition and exercise in increasing and maintaining bone strength.

Nursing Management

ASSESSMENT

1. Assess child's airway, breathing, and circulation
2. Obtain history of injury
3. Assess injury site
4. Assess neurovascular status below the site of the injury
5. Perform physical assessment
6. Assess pain level

NURSING DIAGNOSES (INCLUDING BUT NOT LIMITED TO)

1. Risk for injury, neurovascular compromise, bleeding, and compartment syndrome R/T vessel and nerve damage at site of fracture
2. Acute pain related to tissue trauma secondary to fracture

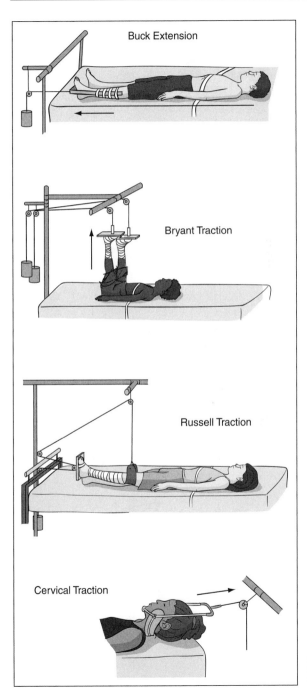

Figure 46-3:
Types of Skin
Traction.

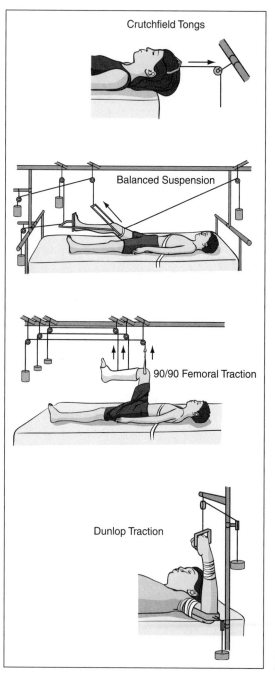

Figure 46-4: Types of
Skeletal Traction.

3. Risk for injury, complications related to traction, or cast placement

4. Deficient knowledge related to condition, treatment, and home care

PLANNING/GOALS

1. Client will not experience neurovascular complications secondary to fracture.

2. Client will demonstrate pain management as determined by client using age-appropriate pain assessment tool within 20 minutes following administration of analgesics.

3. Client will not experience injury secondary to surgery or application of traction or cast.

4. Parents and client (if age-appropriate) will demonstrate understanding of condition, treatment, prevention, and home care.

NOC

1. Risk Control

2. Comfort Level, Pain Level

3. Risk Control

4. Knowledge: Illness Care, Accident Prevention, Treatment, Health Promotion

IMPLEMENTATION

1. Risk for complications of fracture
   a. Assess for manifestations of arterial damage and bleeding
      1) Pain
      2) Swelling
      3) Pallor or cyanosis
      4) Variable or absent pulse distal to fracture
      5) Abnormal capillary return distal to fracture
      6) Coolness of extremity
      7) Paralysis or sensory loss
   b. Assess for manifestations of compartment syndrome
      1) Severe pain (ischemic pain)—pain not relieved by opioid analgesics
      2) Pain with passive stretch
      3) Pins-and-needles sensation progressing to sensory loss at site
      4) Weakened or absent pulses distally
      5) Coolness and pallor of extremity
   c. Monitor vital signs continuously during acute phase and every 4 hours after stabilization
   d. Monitor complete blood count
   e. Document and report any abnormal findings to health care provider

2. Pain
   a. Assess pain hourly
   b. Use age-appropriate pain assessment tool
   c. Position for comfort
   d. Assess cast borders for skin irritation
   e. Assess skin around pins (if external fixator is present)
   f. Administer analgesics and anti-inflammatory agents proactively as prescribed

    g. Administer analgesics at equal intervals during first 24 hours after fracture/surgery

    h. Apply ice to fracture site first 24 hours postoperatively

    i. Encourage parents/client to be proactive with pain management

    j. Collaborate with health care provider for patient-controlled analgesia if pain control is not adequate

3. Risk for injury from traction/cast

    a. If client is in traction:

        1) Assess traction to ensure prescribed weight is present and hanging free

        2) Assess traction to ensure pulleys and rope hang free

        3) Position client to facilitate traction and comfort

        4) Assess for skin irritation because of contact with traction

        5) Monitor neurovascular status of extremity distal to traction every shift

        6) Provide pin care every shift and as needed for clients in skeletal traction

        7) Change weights as prescribed by health care provider

        8) Monitor pain level at least hourly

        9) Change linen from top to bottom of bed

        10) Use fracture bedpan for elimination

        11) Provide age-appropriate diversionary play activities

        12) Provide bed trapeze to facilitate movement

        13) Perform range of motion, assist with range of motion, or encourage active range of motion to all joints except those immediately proximal and distal to the fracture

        14) Assess breath sounds every shift

        15) Encourage coughing and deep breathing

        16) Monitor intake and output

        17) Collaborate with health care provider for prophylactic stool softeners to prevent constipation

    b. If client is placed in cast:

        1) Assess cast for indentations

        2) Assess color, warmth, movement, and sensation distal to cast every 2 hours after cast is applied

        3) Use only palms of hands to move or position cast until it dries

        4) Promote drying of cast

        5) Cover areas not casted to promote warmth

        6) Elevate casted extremity on pillows to above level of heart

        7) Monitor neurovascular status of casted limb

        8) Monitor for manifestations of nerve damage increasing or for persistent pain, parenthesia, or numbness or tingling distal to cast

        9) Monitor for infection ("hot spot" on cast, drainage, odor, or fever)

        10) Monitor cast for drainage

        11) Ensure for leg that is casted that foot is supported at a 90 degree angle to prevent foot drop

        12) Perform range of motion, assist with range of motion, or encourage active range of motion to all joints except those immediately proximal and distal to the fracture

    c. Encourage fluids

    d. Collaborate with recreation therapy for diversionary activities

4. Parent/client teaching

    a. Assess parents'/child's current level of understanding

    b. Provide verbal and written information regarding:

        1) Accident prevention

        2) Cast care, assessment of skin, and pin care

        3) Importance of never placing anything under cast to "scratch" the skin

        4) Medication administration including proactive use of analgesics and importance of completing prescribed medication regimen of anti-inflammatory agents or antibiotics

        5) Signs and symptoms of adverse effects of medications

        6) Signs and symptoms of worsening of condition (fever or neurovascular changes)

        7) Contact phone numbers to use for reporting signs and symptoms

        8) Referral information and contact numbers if applicable

        9) Importance of follow-up with health care provider and prescribed physical therapy

    c. Provide adequate time for teaching and parents'/child's questions

    d. Document teaching and parent/child response

NIC

1. Risk Identification, Surveillance: Safety
2. Pain Management, Analgesic Administration
3. Risk Identification, Surveillance: Safety
4. Teaching: Illness Care, Accident Prevention, Treatment, Health Promotion

EVALUATION

1. Client does not experience neurovascular complications secondary to fracture.
2. Client demonstrates pain management as determined by client using age-appropriate pain assessment tool within 20 minutes following administration of analgesics.
3. Client does not experience injury secondary to surgery or application of traction or cast.
4. Parents and client (if age-appropriate) demonstrate understanding of condition, treatment, prevention, and home care.

References

Broyles, B. E. (2005). *Medical-surgical nursing clinical companion.* Durham, NC: Carolina Academic Press.

Columbus Children's Hospital. (2007). *Stress fractures.* Retrieved May 12, 2007, from http://www .columbuschildrens.org/GD/Templates/Pages/Childrens/SportsMed/SportsMedLongContent .aspx?page=4243

Moore, W., & Smith, T. H. (2007). *Salter-Harris fractures.* Retrieved May 12, 2007, from http://www.emedicine.com/radio/TOPIC613.HTM

Potts, N. L., & Mandleco, B. L. (2007). *Pediatric nursing: Caring for children and their families* (2nd ed.). Clifton Park, NY: Delmar Cengage Learning.

Wilkins, K. (2006). *Overview of children's fractures.* Retrieved May 12, 2007, from http://www.fracturesinchildren.org/overview_of_children_fracture.htm

47

GASTROESOPHAGEAL REFLUX (GER)

Definition

Physiologic gastroesophageal reflux (GER) is the backflow of stomach contents through the lower esophageal sphincter (LES) into the esophagus. Pathologic GER, also referred to as gastroesophageal reflux disease, or GERD, occurs in the presence of an incompetent LES. Refer to Figure 47-1.

Pathophysiology

The LES is a structure of smooth muscle that surrounds the distal end of the esophagus and normally prevents the backflow of stomach contents into the esophagus. It is innervated by vagal nerves and stimulated by multiple organs. As food enters the esophagus, the lining secretes mucus that facilitates food's travel down the esophagus. As the food approaches, the LES opens to allow the food to enter the stomach. At this time, the LES closes to prevent the food bolus from being forced back up into the esophagus when the stomach contracts during digestion and when the stomach is ready to expel the chyme into the small intestines for final digestion.

The LES may be weak in infants and not form a tight seal, allowing food to backflow through the LES into the esophagus. Physiologic GER is common in healthy infants, resulting in "spitting up, wet burps, or wet hiccups." It usually resolves when the infant is 6–12 months of age due to elongation of the esophagus resulting in the movement of the LES below the level of the diaphragm and maturation of the musculature (Potts & Mandleco, 2007).

Pathologic GER or GERD and an incompetent esophageal sphincter is most common in preterm infants and in infants/children with neurologic impairments such as cerebral palsy, Down syndrome, seizure disorders, hydrocephalus, and head injury

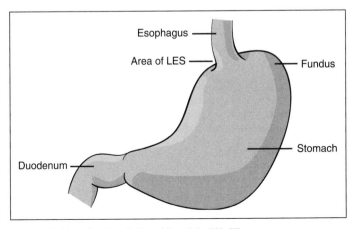

Figure 47-1: Food Regurgitates from the Stomach through the LES in GER.

because of a defect in neural control that allows the LES to relax spontaneously. In the presence of pathologic GER (but also with physiologic GER), the leaking of food combined with gastric secretions that backflow into the esophagus can cause esophageal inflammation (esophagitis), a burning sensation in the epigastric area. If the gastric contents leak into the throat, the infant/child will spit up. Esophagitis can be very painful and decreases the desire to eat. Severe esophagitis can lead to bleeding from the inflamed portion of the esophagus that is comprised of very vascular smooth muscle. If the inflammation is present long enough as in children with neurologic impairments, scar tissue can form inside the lower esophagus, forming a stricture. This can reduce the lumen of the esophageal opening and make swallowing difficult (Pediatric/Adolescent Gastroesophageal Reflex Association, 2007).

The primary differentiations between physiologic and pathologic GER are that (1) physiologic GER resolves without medication but pathologic GER requires medical and/or surgical intervention and (2) physiologic GER is not associated with weight loss but children with pathologic GER do experience weight loss. Failure to thrive and even aspiration leading to respiratory infections also can occur, especially in premature infants and neurologically compromised children. Pathologic GER can lead to recurrent otitis media related to the pooling of secretions in the nasopharynx while the infant sleeps. Reflux is considered a cause of sinus infections, and gastric acid can cause dental problems resulting in tooth decay and tooth enamel erosion. Anemia can occur in the presence of esophageal bleeding. Regardless of which type of GER the infant has, aspiration is the complication of greatest concern.

Complications

Aspiration (both physiologic and pathologic GER)
Recurrent pneumonia
Recurrent otitis media
Esophagitis
Esophageal stricture
Failure to thrive
Anemia
Dental problems

Incidence

"GER is known to occur in 5 in 1,000 live births. Boys are affected three times more frequently than girls" (Potts & Mandleco, 2007, p. 677). "Epidemiology estimates in 2005 indicate that as many as seven million children in the US may suffer from GERD" (Pediatric/Adolescent Gastroesophageal Reflux Association, 2007, p. 1). As many as "85% of infants vomit during the first week of life, and another 10% have symptoms by 6 weeks of age" (Schwarz & Hebra, 2008, Section 2). "Nearly all infants have some degree of GER. This reflux is transient and does not cause any morbidity" (Garza & Jaksic, 2006, Section 2). Pathologic GER occurs in approximately 2–10% of infants (Schwarz & Hebra, 2008).

Etiology

The exact cause of physiologic GER is not known, but it is common in healthy infants and resolves by 6–12 months of age due to elongation of the esophagus resulting in the movement of the LES below the level of the diaphragm and maturation of the musculature (Potts & Mandleco, 2007). GERD is most common in premature infants and children with neurologic deficits and is associated with a defect in neural control that allows the LES to relax (Schwarz & Hebra, 2008).

Clinical Manifestations

BOTH PHYSIOLOGIC AND PATHOLOGIC GER

Frequent spitting up with and after feedings

"Wet burp" or "wet hiccup" sounds

PATHOLOGIC GER

Pain

Inconsolable crying

Irritability

Constant or sudden crying

Frequent spitting up or vomiting

Emesis, or spitting up, more than one hour after eating

Not outgrowing the spitting-up stage

Refusing to eat or accepting only a few bites even when hungry

Poor sleep habits with frequent waking

Sunken fontanels (dehydration)

Chronic cough (Children's Digestive Health and Nutrition
Foundation 2007)

Neck tilting

Diagnostic Tests

Fluoroscopy

24-hour pH probe

Abdominal computed tomography

Abdominal ultrasonography

Intralumen impedance monitor

Electrogastrogram

Medical Management

The goals of treatment are to prevent aspiration, maintain hydration, and maintain nutritional intake to meet the child's growth and development needs. Medical management for physiologic GER includes upright positioning and thickened feedings with small, more frequent feedings for up to several months. Most healthy infants respond to this treatment or outgrow GER and do not require surgical intervention.

With pathologic GER, the upright positioning and thickened feedings are combined with the addition of meclopramide, proton pump inhibitors, or histamine-2 antagonists. Premature infants usually are prescribed elemental formulas that are more easily digested, such as Progestamil or Nutramigen. In older children, especially those with neurologic deficits, the risk of complications from this type of GER is increased; so medical treatment is not used for more than 6–8 weeks before surgical intervention is considered.

Indications for surgical treatment without initially attempting medical therapy include the presence of esophageal narrowing (or strictures), a near-fatal (SIDS) event, and severe aspiration. The other indication for surgical treatment is when medical therapy is employed and fails. The surgical placement of a gastrostomy tube frequently is used in the treatment of neurologically impaired children to provide for their nutritional needs before and after the surgical repair until the site heals.

A number of surgical procedures have been employed in the surgical management of infants and children with GER, including the Nissen fundoplication, the anterior (Thal) fundoplication, the Boix-Ochoa procedure, and the posterior (Toupet) fundoplication (Garza & Jaksic, 2006). The Nissen fundoplication is the most frequently used procedure in the United States (Potts & Mandleco, 2007).

"The Nissen fundoplication is a full 360-degree wrap, whereas the Thal fundoplication is an anterior 270-degree partial wrap. Cited disadvantages of the Nissen procedure are the inability to vomit, trouble with swallowing, and the development of stomach gas bloating. Potential gas bloat seems to occur less frequently in children than in adults. Although the Thal fundoplication has a higher incidence of recurrent reflux compared with the Nissen fundoplication, it does not have the associated postoperative problems of swallowing difficulties and bloating. The Nissen fundoplication lends itself best to the laparoscopic approach and is the most commonly performed laparoscopic fundoplication in the world" (American Pediatric Surgical Association, 2008, p. 1).

The Nissen and Thal procedures may be performed laparoscopically; and the laparoscopic fundoplication has been well studied in adults, with results equivalent to the open surgery methods. Findings from early follow-up studies suggest that laparoscopic fundoplication in children has shown comparable results with the open surgery and that laparoscopic fundoplication is associated with a shorter hospital stay (Garza & Jaksic, 2006).

Recurrence of GER and the development of postoperative intestinal obstruction following fundoplication have been concerns because of recurrence rates of 10% for the Nissen procedure and 15–20% for the Thal operation. The most common reason for recurrence with the Nissen fundoplication is migration of the wrap into the chest from the abdomen followed by breakdown of the wrap. Postoperative intestinal obstruction, occurring in 15–25% of cases after an open surgical fundoplication, is rare following the laparoscopic procedure (American Pediatric Surgical Association, 2008).

Nursing Management

ASSESSMENT

1. Obtain history including amount and frequency of feedings, positioning during and after feedings, and any recent changes in infant formula or breastfeeding
2. Assess frequency, pattern, and characteristics of regurgitation
3. Perform infant physical assessment
4. Obtain height, weight, and head circumference measurements compared to standardized chart
5. Assess fontanels for manifestations of dehydration
6. Assess family for psychosocial impact of infant's/child's condition

NURSING DIAGNOSES (INCLUDING BUT NOT LIMITED TO)

1. Risk for aspiration R/T backflow of food from stomach
2. Fluid volume deficit R/T regurgitation and emesis
3. Imbalanced nutrition: less than body requirements R/T decreased intake and emesis
4. Deficient knowledge R/T condition, treatment, home management, and home care

PLANNING/GOALS

1. Client will maintain a patent airway and will not experience aspiration or other respiratory complications as evidenced by clear breath sounds and respiratory status within defined limits (WDL).
2. Client will regain and maintain fluid balance as evidenced by urine output > 1–2 mL/kg/hr or 6–8 wet diapers/day.
3. Client will maintain normal growth pattern as evidenced by weight gain compared to standardized chart and adequate intake of calories.
4. Parents will demonstrate understanding of condition, treatment, and home management and care.

NOC

1. Aspiration Prevention
2. Fluid Balance
3. Nutrition Status
4. Knowledge: Illness Care, Treatment, Health Promotion

IMPLEMENTATION

1. Risk for aspiration
   a. Assess infant during and after feedings
   b. Position upright on lap for feedings
   c. Elevate head of crib 30–60 degrees after feedings
   d. Assess breath sounds and respiratory status
   e. Maintain on cardiorespiratory monitor at night
   f. Administer medications for GER as prescribed
   g. Encourage parental involvement in feeding and medication administration
   h. Offer frequent, small feedings
   i. Thicken feedings as prescribed
   j. Encourage frequent burping or bubbling during feedings
   k. Discourage breastfeeding mother from consuming chocolate or caffeine
2. Fluid balance
   a. Maintain intake and output
   b. Weigh diapers to obtain accurate urine output
   c. Assess mucous membranes, fontanels, and skin turgor
   d. Provide frequent, small feedings
   e. Offer fluid between feedings
   f. Weigh daily
   g. Monitor urine specific gravity
3. Nutrition
   a. Weigh daily if hospitalized
   b. Encourage parents to take infant for follow-up weights at health care provider's office or clinic
   c. Monitor intake and output
   d. Provide feedings with adequate caloric content
   e. Offer age-appropriate foods
   f. Provide elemental formulas as prescribed
4. Parent teaching
   a. Assess parents' current level of understanding
   b. Provide verbal and written information regarding:
      1) Infant feedings including positioning during and after feedings, types of feedings, and thickening of formula as prescribed
      2) Medication administration and compliance with medications prescribed
      3) Signs and symptoms of adverse effects of medications
      4) Signs and symptoms of worsening of condition
      5) Importance of notifying health care provider of adverse effects of medications or worsening of condition
      6) Contact number for health care provider

       7) Importance of follow-up with health care provider

       8) Reinforcement of infant care

  c. Provide adequate time for teaching and parental questions

  d. Document teaching and parental response

NIC

1. Aspiration Precautions; Positioning
2. Fluid Management
3. Nutrition Management
4. Teaching: Illness Care, Treatment, Health Promotion

EVALUATION

1. Client maintains a patent airway and does not experience aspiration or other respiratory complications as evidenced by clear breath sounds and respiratory status WDL.
2. Client regains and maintains fluid balance as evidenced by urine output > 1–2 mL/kg/hr or 6–8 wet diapers/day.
3. Client maintains normal growth pattern as evidenced by weight gain compared to standardized chart and adequate intake of calories.
4. Parents demonstrate understanding of condition, treatment, and home management and care.

References

American Pediatric Surgical Association. *Gastroesophageal reflux and other disorders of esophageal function.* (2008). Retrieved February 13, 2008, from http://www.eapsa.org/parents/resources/GER.cfm

Children's Digestive Health and Nutrition Foundation. *GER: Signs and symptoms and diagnosis.* (2007). Retrieved February 13, 2008, from http://gerd.cdhnf.org/cms/en/PatientsAndFamilies/Infants/Patients/Patients_Infants_SignsSymptomsDiagnosis.aspx?menu=patientsinfant

Garza, J., & Jaksic, T. (2006). *Gastroesophageal reflux: Surgical perspective.* Retrieved February 13, 2008, from http://www.emedicine.com/ped/topic2957.htm

Pediatric/Adolescent Gastroesophageal Reflux Association. (2007). Retrieved May 14, 2007, from http://www.reflux.org/Reflux/webdoc01.nsf/(vwWebPage)/WhoWeAre.htm?OpenDocument

Potts, N. L., & Mandleco, B. L. (2007). *Pediatric nursing: Caring for children and their families* (2nd ed.). Clifton Park, NY: Delmar Cengage Learning.

Schwarz, S. M., & Hebra, A. (2008). *Gastroesophageal reflux.* Retrieved February 13, 2008, from http://www.emedicine.com/ped/topic1177.htm

48

GASTROSCHISIS

Definition

Gastroschisis is a congenital anomaly of the gastrointestinal tract where a defect in the abdominal wall to the right of the umbilicus permits abdominal contents to herniate through the abdominal wall (National Organization for Rare Disorders, 2007). In contrast to an omphalocele (herniation contents are covered by a peritoneal sac), with gastroschisis, the contents lie openly on the abdomen. Refer to Figure 48-1.

Pathophysiology

Gastroschisis is a full-thickness abdominal fusion defect resulting in the small and/or large intestines floating freely in amniotic fluid. The bowel is not rotated or fixed to the posterior peritoneal wall and is not contained within the abdomen cavity and covered by abdominal viscera and musculature. It results from a failure of the mesoderm to replace the body stalk during fetal development; and in "50% of cases, the liver, spleen, and ovaries or testes accompany the extruded midgut" (Glasser, 2006, Section 2). Gastroschisis usually occurs on the right side (National Organization for Rare Disorders, 2007). "Prune-belly syndrome (abdominal wall dysplasia) . . . occurs as a result of increased apoptotic cell death in the body-wall placode, which leads to insufficient deposition of mesodermal cells" (Glasser, 2007, Section 2).

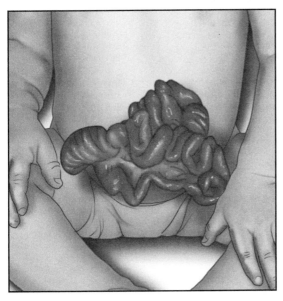

Figure 48-1: Gastroschisis.

Gastroschisis usually is diagnosed by the second trimester through prenatal ultrasound although exactly when the defect occurs is not completely understood because the intestines appear initially to be normal in size and structure. However, later in fetal development, irritation to the exposed bowel by contact with amniotic fluid results in alterations to the bowel structure and function.

One theory of why gastroschisis occurs is that there is an abnormal involution of the right umbilical vein causing the anterior abdominal wall to rupture at an area of weakness in the wall. Other researchers believe that it results from rupture of an exomphalos or premature interruption of the right omphalomesenteric artery leading to ischemic injury to the anterior abdominal wall through which herniation of abdominal contents occurs (Khan & Thomas, 2005; Glasser, 2006). It may result from an "incomplete folding of the embryonic disc" (Potts & Mandleco, 2007, p. 698). This would allow the bowel to herniate.

Later during fetal development, bowel dilatation, bowel obstruction, peritonitis, bowel perforation, and restrictions to fetal growth can occur. Intrauterine growth restrictions (IUGRs) occur in up to 77% of these fetuses as a result of nutrient loss through the exposed bowel (Khan & Thomas, 2005).

Gastroschisis is considered an open fetal defect because it is not covered by skin. As a result, alpha-fetoprotein (AFP) diffuses from fetal circulation into the amniotic fluid. This causes the AFP levels to elevate as much as 200–300 times the normal level. Maternal serum AFP levels are higher in gastroschisis than omphalocele (a closed fetal defect), causing researchers to believe that the amnion is a significant barrier that prevents the AFP in the amniotic fluid from diffusing into maternal circulation (Khan & Thomas, 2005). After birth, if the gastroschisis is not repaired, the neonate faces a high risk of bowel necrosis and life-threatening peritonitis.

Complications

Bowel dysfunction including short bowel (gut) syndrome

Bowel necrosis

Peritonitis

Ventral hernia

Incidence

The incidence of gastroschisis is 1.75–2.5 cases per 10,000 live births in the United States and around the world (Khan & Thomas, 2005). Females are 5 times more likely to experience abdominal wall defects as males, and the survival rate in these infants now is over 90% compared to 60% in the 1960s (Glasser, 2007).

Etiology

Although a number of theories have evolved over the years, the exact cause of gastroschisis is unknown. Some researchers believe that gastroschisis is "an omphalocele that ruptures before the somatic components of the anterior abdominal wall become folded" (Khan & Thomas, 2005, Section 2). Risk factors include young maternal age and low gravidity.

Clinical Manifestations

Protrusion of the intestines outside the abdominal wall

Small for age

Diagnostic Tests

Prenatal AFP levels

Prenatal ultrasonography (usually diagnosed during second trimester)

Medical Management

The goals of treatment are prevention of hypothermia, immediate (within 24 hours) surgical closure of the abdominal wall, and prevention of complications of the anomaly and low birth weight. If gastroschisis is diagnosed prenatally, a cesarean section is recommended to avoid damage to the abdominal contents that can occur during vaginal delivery. Delivery, however, is not performed prior to term unless fetal distress occurs. Immediately following delivery, any exposed organs are covered with warm, sterile saline-soaked gauze. Usually, a nasogastric (NG) tube is inserted to provide gastric decompression to prevent aspiration of gastric contents. As soon as the neonate is stable, surgery is performed.

During surgery, the intestines are examined closely for signs of damage and any defective areas are excised and the intestinal sections anastomosed together. The exposed intestines are placed into the abdomen, and the abdominal wall defect is repaired. If there is not sufficient space in the abdominal cavity to return the organs without causing excess pressure against the diaphragm, leading to respiratory compromise, a synthetic material is used to create a pouch or sac to protect the intestines that are gradually pushed into the abdomen over seven to ten days (MedlinePlus, 2006; Potts & Mandleco, 2007).

Following surgery, the neonate is transferred to the neonatal intensive care unit (NICU) where thermoregulation, intravenous fluids, antimicrobial agents, pain management, and oxygen are standards of care. Mechanical ventilation frequently is required for these neonates to maintain gas exchange following general anesthesia during the surgical repair. Gastric decompression continues until bowel function resumes, and then feedings are started very slowly. If the infant does not tolerate oral feedings, enteral feedings are used. For all infants receiving enteral feedings, a pacifier should be used to stimulate and maintain the suck reflex.

Nursing Management

ASSESSMENT

1. Assess neonate's airway, breathing, and circulation (ABC)
2. Perform rapid neonatal assessment
3. Assess exposed abdominal contents
4. Assess parental response to neonate's condition

NURSING DIAGNOSES (INCLUDING BUT NOT LIMITED TO)

1. Ineffective thermoregulation R/T environmental adjustment of the neonate
2. Risk for infection R/T exposed abdominal contents
3. Ineffective breathing pattern R/T high intra-abdominal pressure secondary to return of intestinal contents to a closed abdominal cavity
4. Risk for deficient fluid volume R/T gastric decompression and inadequate intake
5. Risk for imbalanced nutrition: less than body requirements R/T gastric decompression and inadequate intake
6. Anxiety (parental/caregiver) R/T critical nature of neonate's condition and surgery
7. Deficient knowledge R/T neonate's condition, treatment, and home care

PLANNING/GOALS

1. Client will maintain thermoregulation as evidenced by body temperature within defined limits (WDL).
2. Client will not experience infection.

3. Client will regain/maintain respiratory status WDL.

4. Client will maintain adequate hydration as evidenced by urine output > 1–2 mL/kg/hr.

5. Client will regain and maintain adequate nutrition for growth according to standardized growth chart.

6. Parents/caregivers will verbalize concerns and feelings and use positive coping strategies.

7. Parents/caregivers will demonstrate understanding of neonate's condition, treatment, and home care.

NOC

1. Thermoregulation: Newborn
2. Risk Control
3. Respiratory Status: Ventilation, Vital Signs
4. Fluid Status
5. Nutritional Status
6. Anxiety
7. Knowledge: Illness Care, Treatment, Health Promotion

IMPLEMENTATION

1. Thermoregulation
   a. Place neonate in infant warmer
   b. Monitor continuous skin temperature
   c. Avoid drafts in delivery room and nursery
   d. Assess skin for mottling
   e. Assess continuous respiratory status

2. Risk for infection
   a. Use sterile technique for care of exposed intestines
   b. Cover exposed intestines immediately with sterile saline-soaked gauze in delivery room
   c. Monitor continuous skin temperature. *NOTE:* Temperature elevation may be masked by neonate's lowered body temperature immediately after birth.
   d. Minimize manipulation of exposed intestines
   e. Use sterile technique for maintenance of central venous access device
   f. Following surgery, use sterile technique for surgical dressing changes
   g. Monitor complete blood count

3. Breathing pattern
   a. Assess respiratory status
   b. Place on continuous cardiorespiratory monitoring
   c. Place on continuous pulse oximetry
   d. Administer oxygen, titrating to neonate's oxygen saturation as prescribed
   e. Monitor vital signs at least hourly
   f. Position to maximize ventilatory efforts
   g. Monitor temperature, peripheral pulses, capillary refill, and skin color
   h. Monitor for increased respiratory rate, nasal flaring, and sternal retractions
   i. Support ventilatory efforts with mechanical ventilation as prescribed

4. Fluid balance
   a. Assess oral mucous membranes
   b. Monitor strict intake and output
   c. Weigh diapers for accurate urine output
   d. Weigh daily
   e. Assess fontanels, skin turgor, and mucous membranes for dehydration
   f. Monitor serum electrolyte levels
   g. Maintain central venous access, monitoring at least hourly
   h. Administer intravenous fluids as prescribed
   i. Maintain NG tube for gastric decompression
   j. Replace gastric output with intravenous boluses as prescribed
   k. Offer pacifier (holding pacifier in neonate's mouth for sucking as normal tongue movement will push pacifier out of mouth)

5. Nutrition
   a. Monitor daily weight
   b. Monitor for return of bowel sounds
   c. Monitor strict intake and output
   d. Maintain intravenous access, monitoring at least hourly
   e. Offer oral fluids slowly after return of bowel function
   f. Offer nipple feeding and then whatever prescribed amount of feeding is not consumed orally, administer via enteral feeding

6. Parental/caregiver anxiety
   a. Assess parents for manifestations of anxiety
   b. Encourage parents/caregivers to verbalize feelings and concerns
   c. Listen actively
   d. Assist parents/caregivers in identifying positive coping strategies and support systems
   e. Collaborate with members of health care team to provide answers to parental questions
   f. Assist with parent-infant bonding
   g. Encourage parents/caregivers to visit infant in NICU
   h. Explain all equipment and procedures
   i. Provide for spiritual needs

7. Parent/caregiver teaching
   a. Assess parents' current level of knowledge
   b. Provide verbal and written information regarding:
      1) Wound care
      2) Infant feedings
      3) Infant care
      4) Infant's developmental needs
      5) Importance of holding, cuddling, and bonding with neonate
      6) Infection precautions
      7) Medication administration if needed
      8) Manifestations of complications (bowel obstruction, infection, or feeding intolerance)
      9) Contact information for reporting manifestations to health care provider

10) Contact information for nutrition support if applicable

11) Importance of follow-up care

12) Referral information and contact numbers as needed

c. Provide adequate time for teaching, demonstrations, and return demonstrations

d. Document teaching and parental response

NIC

1. Temperature Regulation, Newborn Care

2. Infection Control, Infection Precautions

3. Ventilation Assistance, Respiratory Monitoring, Vital Signs Monitoring

4. Fluid Management, Fluid Monitoring

5. Nutrition Management, Nutrition Monitoring

6. Anxiety Reduction, Coping Enhancement

7. Teaching: Illness Care, Treatment, Health Promotion

EVALUATION

1. Client maintains thermoregulation as evidenced by body temperature WDL.

2. Client does not experience infection.

3. Client regains/maintains respiratory status WDL.

4. Client maintains adequate hydration as evidenced by urine output > 1–2 mL/kg/hr.

5. Client regains and maintains adequate nutrition for growth according to standardized growth chart.

6. Parents/caregivers verbalize concerns and feelings and use positive coping strategies.

7. Parents/caregivers demonstrate understanding of neonate's condition, treatment, and home care.

References

Glasser, J. G. (2007). *Omphalocele and gastroschisis*. Retrieved February 13, 2008, from http://www.emedicine.com/ped/topic1642.htm

Khan, A. N., & Thomas, N. (2005). *Gastroschisis*. Retrieved May 14, 2007, from http://www.emedicine.com/radio/topic303.htm

MedlinePlus. (2006). *Gastroschisis repair*. Retrieved March 1, 2007, from http://www.nlm.nih.gov/medlineplus/ency/article/002924.htm

National Organization for Rare Disorders (NORD). (2007). *Gastroschisis*. Retrieved May 14, 2007, from http://www.rarediseases.org/search/rdbdetail_abstract.html?disname=Gastroschisis

Potts, N. L., & Mandleco, B. L. (2007). *Pediatric nursing: Caring for children and their families* (2nd ed.). Clifton Park, NY: Delmar Cengage Learning.

49

GLOMERULONEPHRITIS

Definition
Glomerulonephritis is inflammation in the small functional filtering structures in the body of the kidneys. Refer to Figure 49-1.

Pathophysiology
The glomeruli are responsible for supplying blood to the nephrons for filtering body fluids and wastes (Potts & Mandleco, 2007). Inflammation of the glomeruli in children usually occurs following a streptococcal upper respiratory infection and is considered an immune complex disorder (Hahn, Knox, & Forman, 2005; Lucile Packard Children's Hospital at Stanford, 2007). As the antigen-specific antibodies to the streptococcal antigens pass through the kidneys to be excreted, they localize on the renal capillary walls and activate immunologic complex resulting in glomerular edema. In addition, the glomeruli become infiltrated with polymorphonuclear leukocytes that occlude the glomerular capillary vessels. These changes cause decreased plasma filtration resulting in water and sodium retention that is reflected in increased interstitial fluid volume and edema. Circulatory congestion occurs leading to hypertension.

There are eight basic types of glomerulonephritis including poststreptoccocal glomerulonephritis, diabetic nephritis, IgA nephropathy, focal segmental glomerulonephritis,

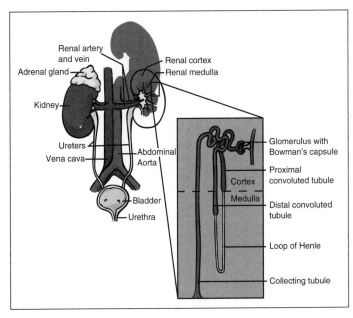

Figure 49-1: Genitourinary Anatomy with Inset of a Nephron.

Goodpasture's syndrome, IgM mesangial proliferative glomerulonephritis, crescentic glomerulonephritis, and lupus nephritis. Glomerulonephritis in children usually is acute poststreptococcal glomerulonephritis (APSGN) that occurs following a group A streptococcal infection. The clinical course is predictable with the edema usually resolving within 5–10 days, hypertension resolving within 2–3 weeks, and gross hematuria usually disappearing in 1–3 weeks. The chemotactic plasma-activated complement 3 (C3) concentration returns to normal level by 6–8 weeks after onset in more than 95% of clients (Schacht, Kim, & Travis, 2006).

Glomerulonephritis also can be chronic, involving renal deterioration over 10–30 years and leading to acute and chronic renal failure. This usually happens when the glomerulonephritis is caused by a systemic immune disease or chromosomal gene defect.

Complications

Edema

Hematuria

Hypertension

Chronic glomerulonephritis can lead to acute and chronic renal failure

Incidence

Glomerulonephritis "occurs with the greatest frequency in children aged 4–12 years, with a peak prevalence in individuals aged approximately 5–6 years" (Schacht et al., 2006, Section 2). It is more common in males (Penn State Hershey Medical Center, 2007; Schacht et al., 2006).

Etiology

The most common cause of acute glomerulonephritis in children is a previous streptococcal upper respiratory infection. Systemic immune diseases such as systemic lupus erythematosus (SLE), polyarteritis nodosa, Wegener's vasculitis, and Henoch-Schönlein purpura can lead to glomerulonephritis. It also can result from an X chromosome gene passed from mothers (carriers) to their male children, who are affected with the disorder approximately 50% of the time (National Institute of Diabetes and Digestive and Kidney Diseases, 2006).

Clinical Manifestations

Pharyngitis

Skin rash

Sore throat

Decreased urinary output

Fatigue

Dark brown-colored urine

Gross hematuria

Abdominal pain

Flank pain

Lethargy

Dyspnea

Headache

Hypertension

Purpural rash, especially over the buttocks and legs

Anorexia

Weight loss

Joint pain

Pallor

Facial and peripheral edema

Diagnostic Tests

Urinalysis for presence of blood and protein

Complete blood count with differential

Blood culture

Computed tomography of the abdomen

Renal ultrasonography

24-hour urine for glomerular filtration rate (GFR)

Blood urea nitrogen (BUN) levels

Serum electrolyte levels

Serum antistreptolysin O (ASO) titer

Erythrocyte sedimentation rate (ESR)

Renal biopsy

Medical Management

The goals of management for acute glomerulonephritis are to treat the streptococcal infection successfully with appropriate antimicrobial agents and to provide supportive care for the clinical manifestations. If residual infection is suspected, antimicrobial therapy may be needed; agents of choice include penicillin, azithromycin, and erythromycin In the presence of circulatory complications (edema and hypertension), medications (diuretics and antihypertensives) and dietary modifications (restricted sodium and fluid) usually are prescribed. Daily fluid restrictions are generally based on 24-hour urine output but must be prescribed with great care when dealing with children because of the fragile fluid balance in pediatric clients. In the event that uremia occurs and cannot be controlled, dialysis may be required. In the presence of systemic immune conditions, plasmapheresis may be used to remove antibodies (Broyles, 2005).

Nursing Management

ASSESSMENT

1. Obtain client history with focus on recent streptococcal infection
2. Obtain vital signs including blood pressure
3. Assess for presence of clinical manifestations during physical assessment

NURSING DIAGNOSES (INCLUDING BUT NOT LIMITED TO)

1. Ineffective protection R/T upper respiratory streptococcal infection
2. Fluid volume excess R/T retention of fluid and sodium
3. Deficient knowledge R/T child's condition, treatment, and home care

PLANNING/GOALS

1. Client will experience complete recovery from glomerulonephritis within six weeks following the initiation of treatment with antibiotics.
2. Client will regain and maintain fluid balance as evidenced by absence of edema and hypertension.
3. Client (if age-appropriate) and parents will demonstrate understanding of condition, treatment, and home care.

NOC

1. Immune Status
2. Fluid Balance
3. Knowledge: Illness Care, Treatment, Health Promotion

IMPLEMENTATION

1. Ineffective protection
   a. Monitor temperature every 4 hours if hospitalized
   b. Administer antibiotics as prescribed
   c. Monitor for adverse effects of antimicrobial therapy
   d. Teach child/parents to complete entire antibiotic prescription even if symptoms appear to resolve before then
2. Fluid volume excess
   a. Monitor intake and output
   b. Weigh daily
   c. Auscultate lung sounds for evidence of pulmonary edema
   d. Monitor respiratory status
   e. Protect edematous skin through position changes
   f. Elevate edematous extremities
   g. Maintain dietary alterations
   h. Administer diuretics and antihypertensives as prescribed
   i. Monitor blood pressure every 4 hours if hospitalized
3. Client/parent teaching
   a. Assess client's/family's current level of knowledge
   b. Provide verbal and written information regarding:
      1) Risk factors for developing glomerulonephritis and necessary instructions to avoid risk factors
      2) Dietary and fluid intake modifications and importance of compliance
      3) Medication administration including importance of completing the prescribed medication regimen
      4) Signs and symptoms of adverse effects of medications (primarily hypersensitivity reactions)
      5) Signs and symptoms of worsening of condition
      6) Contact phone numbers for reporting signs and symptoms
      7) Importance of regular hand washing and appropriate technique
      8) Importance of keeping scheduled appointments with health care provider for blood pressure monitoring and follow-up care

NIC

1. Infection Protection, Nutrition Therapy
2. Fluid Monitoring, Fluid Management
3. Teaching: Illness Care, Treatment, Health Promotion

EVALUATION

1. Client experiences complete recovery from glomerulonephritis within six weeks following the initiation of treatment with antibiotics.
2. Client regains and maintains fluid balance as evidenced by absence of edema and hypertension.
3. Client (if age-appropriate) and parents demonstrate understanding of condition, treatment, and home care.

References

Broyles, B. E. (2005). *Medical-surgical nursing clinical companion.* Durham, NC: Carolina Academic Press.

Hahn, R. G., Knox, L. M., & Forman, T. A. (2005). *Evaluation of poststreptococcal illness.* Retrieved May 15, 2007, from http://www.aafp.org/afp/20050515/1949.html

Lucile Packard Children's Hospital at Stanford. (2007). *Genitourinary and kidney disorders: Glomerulonephritis.* Retrieved March 3, 2007, from http://www.lpch.org/DiseaseHealthInfo/ HealthLibrary/urology/glomerul.html

National Institute of Diabetes and Digestive and Kidney Diseases. (2006). *Glomerular diseases.* Retrieved May 15, 2007, from http://kidney.niddk.nih.gov/kudiseases/pubs/glomerular/ index.htm

Penn State Hershey Medical Center. (2007). *Glomerulonephritis.* Retrieved March 3, 2007, from http://www.hmc.psu.edu/healthinfo/g/glomerulonephritis.htm

Potts, N. L., & Mandleco, B. L. (2007). *Pediatric nursing: Caring for children and their families* (2nd ed.). Clifton Park, NY: Delmar Cengage Learning.

Schacht, R. G., Kim, Y. S., & Travis, L. (2006). *Acute poststreptococcal glomerulonephritis.* Retrieved May 15, 2007, from http://www.emedicine.com/ped/topic27.htm

50

HEAD TRAUMA

Definition

Head trauma is "any pathologic process occurring to the scalp, skull, or brain parenchyma resulting from a mechanical force" (Potts & Mandleco, 2007, p. 1086). Traumatic brain injury (TBI) is a severe physical wound to the large soft mass of nerve tissue in the cranium that is caused by external force and disrupting neurologic functioning (Olsen, 2006; Broyles, 2005). Injuries are classified as open or closed.

Pathophysiology

Head trauma with TBI is the leading cause of death in children under the age of 15 years (Potts & Mandleco, 2007). TBI occurs when the head forcefully hits an object such as a dashboard or tree when the child is thrown from a motor vehicle or all-terrain vehicle (ATV), for example, or hits a motor vehicle when the child is a pedestrian or in the event a bullet pierces the brain. This results in bleeding and inflammation that causes edema and increased intracranial pressure (ICP). Damage occurs at the site of the blunt force or puncture injury, but also results from brain tissue shifting, the movement back and forth of the brain against the cranium.

The Head Injury Interdisciplinary Special Interest Group of the American Congress of Rehabilitation Medicine classifies TBI as mild, moderate, and severe with identifiable criteria for each. Each group of criteria includes Glasgow Coma Scale scores. Criteria for mild TBI are "any period of loss of consciousness, any loss of memory for events immediately before or after the accident, any alteration in mental state at the time of the accident, and focal neurologic deficits, which may or may not be transient" (Dawodu, 2007, Section 2). Other criteria for classifying a TBI as mild TBI include a Glasgow Coma Scale score of 13–15, no abnormalities on computed tomography (CT) scan, no operative lesions, and length of hospitalization less than 48 hours. The criteria for moderate TBI include Glasgow Coma Scale score between 9 and 12 or higher, abnormal CT scan findings, and presence of operative intracranial lesion. The National Institutes of Health (NIH) sponsored the Traumatic Coma Data Bank (TCDB) that determined that severe TBI is indicated when the Glasgow Coma Scale score is below 9 within 48 hours of the injury (Dawodu, 2007).

The frontal lobe receives the most damage because it frequently is the site of the original injury. The frontal lobes of the brain contain nerve tissue associated with impulse control, judgment, language, memory, motor function, problem solving, sexual behavior, socialization, and spontaneity. These lobes also assist in planning, coordinating, controlling, and executing behavior. Because the occipital lobe, which controls all aspects of vision, is opposite the frontal lobes, it frequently sustains collateral damage related to brain shifting. The temporal lobes are situated in pockets of the skull that allow more brain shifting (Olsen, 2006).

Brain tissue dies because of lack of oxygen and nutrients resulting from interruption in blood supply and impaired tissue perfusion. This occurs from compression of the vessels by increased ICP resulting from cerebral edema or from direct damage to the vessels that supply oxygen to the involved tissues. "Because nerve cells do not regenerate, death of brain cells is permanent. Consequently, whatever particular function the damaged or destroyed brain cells performed is lost. . . . Damage to or loss of control of any of the functions of the brain can occur including loss of speech and use of language, balance, coordination, muscle use, consciousness, concentration, memory, cognition, hearing, smell, taste, and vital functions (respiratory and cardiovascular)" (Broyles, 2005, p. 383).

Most injuries actually cause focal brain damage. However, increased ICP and the extent of brain cell death determine the clinical manifestations and disabilities seen in children with TBI. In addition to cerebral edema, malignant brain edema may occur. Unique to children, this is the hyperemic or vascular reaction to impaired blood supply.

Brain injuries can vary in severity from mild and/or temporary neurologic dysfunction to severe brain tissue death leading to permanent disabilities and even death. A concussion, usually considered temporary, is a stretching, compression, or tearing of nerve fibers without gross structural damage to the brain (Potts & Mandleco, 2007). A brain contusion or bruising usually does not cause permanent damage once the edema and bruising resolve.

Skull fractures occur in approximately 7% of all head injuries and are treated as neurologic conditions; TBI usually accompanies the fracture. More severe TBI includes subdural hematoma (SDH), epidural hematoma, subarachnoid hemorrhage (SAH), and intracerebral bleeding.

The SDH results from bleeding between the dura and the arachnoid in the subdural space and usually occurs in infants 6 months old and younger as a result of shaken-baby syndrome (SBS) or in the neonate from birth trauma. The SDH is due to damage to the bridging veins so that it develops more slowly than arterial bleeds. The hematoma causes increased ICP from the pressure of the hematoma against the brain tissue (Broyles, 2005). Refer to Figure 50-1.

An epidural hematoma (EDH) is bleeding into the space between the dura and the skull that frequently accompanies a skull fracture and results from arterial damage. Increased ICP occurs rapidly, as does neurologic deterioration. This type of injury is considered a medical emergency because of the risk of the rapidly rising ICP causing herniation of the brain through the foramen magnum (Broyles, 2005; Potts & Mandleco, 2007). These children may experience a short period of consciousness that is followed by deterioration as blood accumulates and ICP rises. Refer to Figure 50-2.

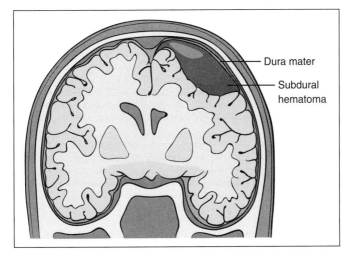

Dura mater

Subdural hematoma

Figure 50-1: Subdural Hematoma.

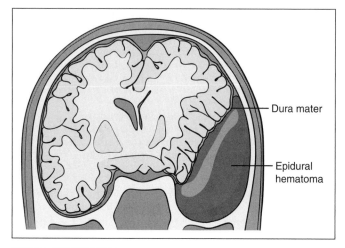

Figure 50-2: Epidural Hematoma.

SAH is associated with severe head trauma and involves bleeding from the cerebral artery into the area between the pia mater and the arachnoid, the protective membrane of the brain. The onset and course of the bleeding is rapid, frequently with neurologically devastating results.

As previously noted, herniations can occur as a result of TBI. These involve a portion of the brain protruding through openings within the intracranial cavity due to increased ICP. "When a herniation occurs, it causes compression, destruction, and lacerations of the vascular system of the brain that further results in ischemia, cellular necrosis, and death. Among the more common herniation syndromes are cingulate herniation, uncal herniation, transtentorial (central) herniation, and transcranial (extracranial) herniation. Cingulate herniation compresses the cerebral artery and internal cerebral vein causing further increase in intracranial pressure. An uncal herniation is a life-threatening situation occurring when the wound or lesion of the temporal fossa expands forcing the temporal lobe to the midline. Through its protrusion over the tentorium cerebelli, the oculomotor nerve and the posterior cerebral artery are compressed" (Broyles, 2005, p. 383). This causes physical damage to the nerve and vessel and a further increase in ICP. A transtentorial herniation may be an extension of a cingulated or uncal herniation that occurs when the tissue of the frontal, occipital, or parietal lobes expands causing the basal ganglia, diencephalons, thalamus, and hypothalamus to herniate through the tentorium cerebelli, resulting in compression of the midbrain and posterior cerebral arteries. Finally, a transcranial herniation occurs when intracranial contents are forced through an opening in the cranial vault, such as a wound, skull fracture, or surgical incision (Broyles, 2005).

Posturing is an indicator of severe brain injury. Decorticate ("to the core") posturing is represented by rigid flexion of the arms, wrists, and fingers accompanied by internal rotation of the legs and plantar flexion. Decorticate posturing indicates bilateral hemisphere damage, which interrupts corticospinal pathways. Rigid extension of the arms and legs, pronation of the arms, and opisthotonos are characteristics of decerebrate posturing and are associated with trauma to the brain stem and a poor prognosis (Potts & Mandleco, 2007). Refer to Figure 50-3.

The extent of neurologic dysfunction depends on factors such as the child's personality, abilities prior to the injury, and the location or severity of damage

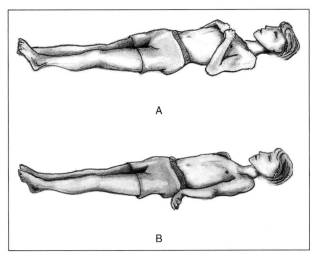

Figure 50-3: Motor System Dysfunction **(A)** Decorticate Posturing; **(B)** Decerebrate Posturing.

to the brain. Complications from moderate to severe TBI and the accompanying increase in ICP include impairment of (1) physical mobility, (2) cognitive abilities, (3) communication, (4) sensory abilities, (5) autonomic nervous system function, and (6) respiratory function. Other complications are pulmonary edema, respiratory distress syndrome (RDS), meningitis, diabetes insipidus, neurogenic shock, and even death.

Complications

SHORT-TERM

Increased ICP
Seizures
RDS
Pulmonary edema
Neurogenic shock
Meningitis and diabetes insipidus
Syndrome of inappropriate antidiuretic hormone (SIADH)
Muscle spasms

LONG-TERM

Immobility
Alterations in communication
Cognitive dysfunction
Sensory impairments
Speech and language impairments
Muscle spasms
Gastrointestinal bleeding secondary to immobility
Autonomic nervous system complications
Death

Incidence

Among children under the age of 14 years, TBI results in an estimated 2,685 deaths, 37,000 hospitalizations, and 435,000 emergency department visits each year in the United States (Centers for Disease Control and Prevention, 2008). Over 1 million children experience brain injuries each year and over 30,000 of these children have permanent disabilities as a result of the brain injury (National Dissemination Center for Children with Disabilities, 2006). The incidence of TBI is higher among children aged 0–4 years, and the death and hospitalization rates are highest among black children aged 0–9 years when compared with whites in motor vehicle-related accidents (including motor vehicle versus pedestrian) resulting in TBI (Centers for Disease Control and Prevention, 2007). Boys are 1.5 times as likely to experience head trauma as girls (Centers for Disease Control and Prevention, 2008).

SBS affects 1,200–1,400 infants annually, resulting in death to 1 out of every 4 infants. Male infants comprise approximately two thirds of victims of SBS. The majority (up to 90%) of the perpetrators in 65–90% of cases of SBS are males, most often either the infant's father or the mother's boyfriend and frequently in his late teens or early 20s (National Center on Shaken Baby Syndrome, n.d.: Nakagawa, 2004).

Etiology

Increased ICP usually occurs as a result of TBI and most commonly involves motor vehicle accidents (MVAs) including motor vehicles hitting children who are walking, bicycling, skate boarding, or in-line skating. Children as passengers in motor vehicles or adolescent drivers are frequent victims of TBI as a result of alcohol-related MVAs. Other causes include falls, firearms, ATV accidents, and SBS. Unfortunately there are not good statistics on SBS. "Until a method for collecting such statistics is established, the true incidence will not be known. It is recognized, however, that it is the most common cause of mortality and accounts for the most long-term disability in infants and young children due to physical child abuse. Based on a North Carolina research project published in the Journal of the American Medical Association in August of 2003, approximately 1,300 U.S. children experience severe or fatal head trauma from child abuse every year. The same study revealed that approximately 30 per 100,000 children under age 1 suffered inflicted brain injuries" (The National Center on Shaken Baby Syndrome, n.d., p. 1).

Clinical Manifestations

INCREASED ICP

> In infants: bulging fontanels, separated cranial sutures, distended scalp veins, setting-sun sign, increased occipitofrontal head circumference, and shrill cry (later sign)
>
> Irritation
>
> Decreasing level of consciousness (confusion, irritability, stupor, or coma)
>
> Changes in vital signs (increased blood pressure, decreased pulse, or erratic respirations)
>
> Vomiting
>
> Headache
>
> Impaired speech and language
>
> Decreased coordination and muscle strength
>
> Paresthesia
>
> Altered sensory function
>
> Changes in equilibrium
>
> Changes to pupil (dependent on type and extent of injury)

High-pitched cry

Retinal hemorrhages

Extraocular palsies

Posturing

MANIFESTATIONS DEPENDING ON THE AREAS OF THE
BRAIN INJURED

Pain (skull fracture)

Decreasing level of consciousness

Visual changes (occipital lobe)

Decreased coordination (cerebellum)

Impaired hearing and balance (temporal lobe or Wernicke's area)

Leakage of cerebrospinal fluid (CSF) from ears (otorrhea), eyes, or nose
(rhinorrhea)

Decreased muscle strength

Diagnostic Tests

Skull radiography

CT

Brain scan

Electroencephalogram

Cervical spine radiography

Magnetic resonance imaging (MRI)

Magnetic resonance arteriography (MRA)

Cerebral angiography

Evoked responses

Analysis of CSF

Complete blood count

Serum electrolytes and osmolality

Medical Management

The goals of treatment for TBI in children are to maintain a patent airway and effective breathing pattern, reduce ICP, and minimize complications secondary to brain tissue injury. To achieve these goals requires a multidisciplinary approach including health care professionals, nursing, physical therapy, occupational therapy, nutritional support, pharmacotherapeutics, psychosocial support for client and family members, social services, rehabilitation, home health, and community services. The initiation and coordination of these services is the combined responsibility of health care professionals.

Placement of an artificial airway and endotracheal intubation or immediate surgical intervention may be required to establish a patent airway (tracheostomy). Mechanical ventilation may be necessary depending on the client's ability to maintain adequate spontaneous ventilation and perfusion. Additional surgical procedures may be required, such as evacuation of lesions (epidural, subdural, and intracranial hematomas), placement of ICP monitoring system, debridement of wounds and brain tissue, repair of dural tears and lacerated cranial vessels, and removal of portions of the cranium to control increasing ICP. Nondepressed skull fractures usually do not require treatment. However, depressed skull fractures require removal of wound debris and bone fragments and closure of the dura. Children with depressed skull fractures also need to be monitored for encephalitis and meningitis resulting from the introduction of microorganisms into the wound at the time of the accident.

Management of ICP is a priority of care, and interventions to control its rise usually are initiated in concert with maintaining respiratory function. Initially, monitoring of the dynamics of ICP must be performed continuously in clients suspected of having head injuries that result in increased ICP. If ICP increases above 20 mm Hg, measures are taken to decrease the pressure before brain cell damage occurs. ICP can be reduced through the placement of an intraventricular or ventriculostomy system and drainage of CSF. To prevent herniation when these systems are used, the CSF drainage collection bag must be maintained at the level of the tragus of the ear or higher. Positioning with head of bed elevated 15–30 degrees is standard practice.

A first-line therapy to decrease ICP is administration of the osmotic diuretic mannitol (Broyles, Reiss, & Evans, 2007; Olsen, 2006) at an intravenous pediatric dose of 250 mg/kg that can be repeated every 5 minutes as the child's condition indicates. The loop diuretic furosemide should be administered at a dose of 1 mg/kg before and along with mannitol doses (Gahart & Nazareno, 2008). These drugs are used to reduce cerebral edema by extracting fluid from the intracellular compartment of the brain. The child must be monitored closely for dehydration. In addition, dexamethasone is a steroidal anti-inflammatory agent used to decrease cerebral inflammation. Its use is a standard of care for decreasing ICP.

Adequate gas exchange must be secured to maintain cerebral oxygenation. Oxygen therapy administered through a delivery system appropriate for the child's condition is accomplished by a variety of means–from nasal cannula (for children requiring < 40% oxygen) to mechanical ventilation (for children requiring 100% oxygen and experiencing ineffective spontaneous ventilation) (Potts & Mandleco, 2007).

Pain management is critical in the management of ICP. Pain increases ICP as well as metabolic demands. Unfortunately, treatment for pain in clients with head trauma lacks adequacy in many cases because of an outdated philosophy that pain control will "mask symptoms" of neurologic damage. Currently, pain management is better in children than in adults with TBI. Medications commonly used include the benzodiazepine midazolam, opioid analgesics such as fentanyl citrate and morphine sulfate, and pancuronium to provide pain management and produce sedation to decrease demands so that cerebral blood supply can maintain cerebral function. A pediatric benefit of midazolam over other benzodiazepines is its short half-life (Broyles et al., 2007).

Also, during the acute phase of TBI, interventions to prevent complications associated with TBI (seizures, neurologic deficits, impaired physical mobility, disuse syndrome, nutritional deficits, gastrointestinal bleeding, and immobility) are initiated. The anticonvulsant phenytoin is considered the first-line agent both in the prevention and treatment of seizures (Olsen, 2006). Because of its toxicity to the veins when administered peripherally, intravenous phenytoin should always be administered through a central venous access device. The serum levels of phenytoin should be monitored closely because of "the narrow margin of error between therapeutic and toxic dose" (Gahart & Nazareno, 2008, p. 1056).

Muscle relaxants such as dantrolene may be used to prevent muscle spasms that can result in pain and contractures. Histamine-2 antagonists, proton pump inhibitors such as lansoprazole, and the GI stimulant metoclopramide (Reglan) are used to prevent the hyperacidity and gastric ulcer formation (Curling's ulcers) associated with enteral feedings and immobility. Increased nutritional requirements from the TBI and pediatric growth needs and inability to take nutrition orally warrant the use of either enteral feedings or total parenteral nutrition (Broyles, 2005).

Once acute medical and surgical conditions have been stabilized, "the child who has a TBI is usually transferred to a specialized unit or facility for intensive rehabilitation aimed at maximizing independent functioning by reducing impairment and disability" (Blackman, 2005, p. 2). The goals of acute inpatient rehabilitation are to help restore the child's independence in mobility, communication, and self-care (feeding, grooming, and toileting). When the child has reached these goals or has reached a plateau in the rate of improvement, discharge to a pediatric rehabilitation facility or home for outpatient rehabilitation may be considered. Inpatient rehabilitation usually requires

1–2 months of intensive therapy of "at least three hours of physical, occupational, and speech therapy a day; cognitive retraining; and a variety of other treatment modalities, including recreation therapy, augmentative technology, and education . . . to have the greatest impact on reestablishing or facilitating alternate neural pathways as soon as possible after injury" (Blackman, 2005, p. 2).

Nursing Management

Refer to Chapter 61: Increased Intracranial Pressure.

References

Blackman, J. A. (2005). *Severe brain injury: Helping patient and family on the long road back.* Retrieved May 15, 2007, from http://www.modernmedicine.com/modernmedicine/article/articleDetail.jsp?id=143316

Broyles, B. E. (2005). *Medical-surgical nursing clinical companion.* Durham, NC: Carolina Academic Press.

Broyles, B. E., Reiss, B. S., & Evans, M. E. (2007). *Pharmacological aspects of nursing care* (7th ed.). Clifton Park, NY: Delmar Cengage Learning.

Centers for Disease Control and Prevention. (2007). *Facts about traumatic brain injury.* Retrieved February 21, 2008, from http://www.cdc.gov/ncipc/tbi/FactSheets/Facts_About_TBI.pdf.

Centers for Disease Control and Prevention. (2008). *What is traumatic brain injury?* Retrieved February 21, 2008, from http://www.cdc.gov/ncipc/twbi/TBI.htm

Dawodu, S. T. (2007). *Traumatic brain injury: Definition, epidemiology, pathophysiology.* Retrieved May 15, 2007, from http://www.emedicine.com/pmr/topic212.htm

Gahart, B. L., & Nazareno, A. R. (2008). *2008 intravenous medications* (22nd ed.). St. Louis, MO: Elsevier Mosby.

National Center on Shaken Baby Syndrome. (n.d.). *Shaken baby syndrome fact sheet.* Retrieved February 21, 2008, from http://www.dontshake.com/Subject.aspx?categoryID=24&PageName=FactSheet.htm

National Dissemination Center for Children with Disabilities. (2006). *Traumatic brain injury.* Retrieved March 1, 2007, from http://www.nichcy.org/pubs/factshe/fs18txt.htm

Olsen, D. A. (2006). *Head injury.* Retrieved March 2, 2007, from http://www.emedicine.com/neuro/topic153.htm

Potts, N. L., & Mandleco, B. L. (2007). *Pediatric nursing: Caring for children and their families* (2nd ed.). Clifton Park, NY: Delmar Cengage Learning.

51

HEARING IMPAIRMENT

Definition

Hearing impairment is the decreased acuity of perceiving sound.

Pathophysiology

The normal ear, developed at birth, is divided into three parts: external ear, middle ear, and inner ear. Each part contains special structures. Refer to Figure 51-1. The external ear is comprised of the auricle and ear canal. Because of its unique construction, the auricle is designed to seize incoming sound waves and funnel them down the external auditory canal to the middle ear structures. The middle ear is comprised of the tympanic membrane, malleus, incus, stapes, and middle ear space. The sound waves vibrate the tympanic membrane, causing motion in the malleus and incus. This causes a pistonlike motion of the stapes. The inner ear is comprised of the cochlea, semicircular canals, and internal auditory canals. The motion of the stapes results in inner ear fluid being pushed around the two and one-half turns of the cochlea. At this point, fluid movements are frequency-specific within the cochlea, leading to movement of the organ of Corti and resulting in bending of the sterocilia in the inner ear. Then the auditory message is

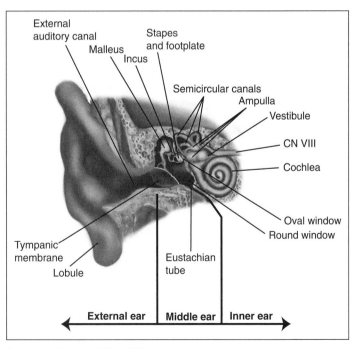

Figure 51-1: Ear Structures of a Young Child.

depolarized, and it travels to the brain via the auditory nerve. The brain processes the information and interprets the data into an organized auditory message.

There are four basic classifications of hearing impairment: (1) conductive, (2) sensorineural, (3) mixed conductive-sensorineural, and (4) central. Conductive hearing loss results from damage to the middle ear structures. This prevents sound from being "conducted" through these structures and may be caused by cerumen (wax), foreign bodies, excess fluid, or perforation or rupture of the tympanic membrane. Conductive hearing loss usually is reparable. The most common cause of this type of hearing loss is chronic inflammation, which usually is the result of recurrent otitis media.

Sensorineural hearing loss is due to damage or malformation of the auditory nerve resulting in interference with transmission of sound from the middle ear to the brain. This leads to distortions in sound discrimination and comprehension and usually is permanent. The most common causes of this type of hearing impairment are preterm birth, ototoxicity, congenital defect, and exposure to loud noises.

Mixed conductive-sensorineural hearing loss "results from interference with transmission of sound in the middle ear and along neural pathways" (Potts & Mandleco, 2007, p. 1023). This produces interferences with conduction and discrimination/comprehension of sound along neural pathways. Although the conductive hearing impairment is reparable, the sensorineural loss is permanent.

Finally, central hearing impairment is the result of "damage that interrupts sound transmission between the brain stem and the cerebral cortex, resulting in difficulty in sound discrimination" (Potts & Mandleco, 2007, p. 1023). Hearing impairment during the first years of life can cause delays in speech, language, and cognitive development. Speech and language delays secondary to hearing loss are preventable. Developmental safety concerns exist because if the child has a hearing impairment, he/she may not perceive dangerous situations. In addition, children experiencing decreased hearing may be labeled a behavior problem because the behavior is interpreted as inattentiveness.

Complications

Developmental safety issues
Psychosocial or behavioral problems
Speech, language, and cognitive delays

Incidence

Annually in the United States, as many as 12,000 neonates are born with hearing impairment (Centers for Disease Control and Prevention, 2007). In the 2002–2003 school year, nearly 72,000 children aged 6–21 years received special education services under the "hearing impairment" category in the United States (Centers for Disease Control and Prevention, 2004). In their article, Shaw and Lotke (2007) cite the incidence of hearing loss as 10 per 1,000 children in the United States, with approximately 1 in 1,000 of these children experiencing profound hearing loss and 3–5 per 1,000 having mild to moderate hearing loss that may affect language development unless assistance with hearing and/or language is available. "The prevalence of hearing loss requiring intervention in neonatal intensive care unit (NICU) graduates is 1%–4% or 10–40 per 1000" (Lotke, 2004, Section 2). Internationally, the prevalence of sensorineural hearing loss is 9–27 per 1,000 children. Significant hearing loss occurs in 1 or 2 per 1,000 newborns, with 4,000 children born each year having profound deafness. Hearing loss in early childhood deafness occurs in 2 per 1,000 children (Potts & Mandleco, 2007). Nearly all children will develop some hearing loss related to ear infections during the period from birth to 11 years of age.

Etiology

Causes for hearing impairment in children are classified as congenital or acquired. Congenital causes include genetic disorders with as many as 50% of all cases of congenital hearing loss in children resulting from genetic factors. Since the adoption of Early Detection & Hearing Intervention (EHDI) programs, "more than 70 hearing impairment genes have been identified. Mutations in two of these genes, which code for proteins known as connexin 26 (GJB2 and GJB6) account for over half of the cases of genetic hearing loss in some populations" (National Institute on Deafness and Other Communication Disorders, 2007, p. 1). Family history of childhood hearing impairment increases the neonate's risks of being born with hearing impairment, although as many as 90% of children with congenital hearing loss are born to hearing parents who may have passed on the condition by being carriers of recessive genes.

Nongenetic congenital causes include perinatal infections such as maternal rubella, rubeola, cytomegalovirus (CMV), toxoplasmosis, herpes, syphilis, and bacterial meningitis; metabolic disease; prenatal asphyxia; Rh incompatibility; ototoxic agents; radiation; anoxia; birth trauma; and preterm birth or low birth weight (Potts & Mandleco, 2007). Congenital CMV "is a leading cause of progressive hearing loss in children in the United States. Approximately 10%–15% of children with congenital CMV infection have some degree of hearing loss that has delayed onset and worsens during childhood" (National Institute on Deafness and Other Communication Disorders, 2007, p. 1).

Causes for acquired hearing loss include head trauma or childhood infections such as meningitis, measles, mumps, otitis media, or chicken pox. Otitis media may result in temporary hearing loss except if the child experiences recurrent otitis media, which can cause permanent hearing impairment if not treated. Certain medications such as antimicrobials (streptomycin and aminoglycosides) also result in pediatric hearing impairment. In addition, neoplastic disorders, metabolic disorders, NICU noise, and environmental noise can damage the auditory structures.

Clinical Manifestations

Infant

Absence of startle or blink response to sound

Failure to awaken to loud environmental noises

Absence of babbling by 7 months of age

Generalized indifference to sound

Lack of eye contact or response when spoken to

Children

Poor school performance

Intense staring at the mouth of the person speaking

Tilting head to listen

Facial expressions indicating lack of understanding conversation

Failure to respond or inappropriately responding when spoken to

Failing to develop easily understood speech by 18–24 months

Consistently screeching or yelling to express happiness

Talking loudly

Sitting close to the television, radio, or audio-computer programs

Avoiding social contacts

Asking to have words or phrases repeated

Not responding when spoken to if speaking person is not facing the child

Diagnostic Tests

Brainstem auditory evoked response (BAER)

Otoacoustic emission (OAE) test

Crib-o-Gram

Rinne test

Weber test

Audiometry

Otoscopy

Magnetic resonance imaging

Medical Management

Prevention of hearing impairment is the primary focus of health professionals. This is followed by early detection and treatment before language and behavior problems develop. Early childhood screening for hearing impairment is the most important step in detection. "All infants should be screened for hearing loss before 1 month of age. It is best if they are screened before leaving the hospital (as a neonate)" (Centers for Disease Control and Prevention, 2007, p. 1). Furthermore, "every state has an Early Hearing Detection and Intervention (EHDI) program that works to identify infants and children with hearing loss and promotes timely follow-up testing and services for any family whose child has a hearing loss" (Centers for Disease Control and Prevention, 2007, p. 1).

Many ear infections can be prevented by simple actions and health education. Infants who are formula-fed should never be put down to sleep with a bottle of formula or juice. This encourages drainage from the throat up the short eustachian tube, resulting in otitis media. Infants and children should not be exposed to secondhand smoke as this dries the cilia, decreasing the drainage of fluid from the ear. Children should not be exposed to loud noises including industrial noise, loud music, or entertainment noise. Children's ears should not be cleaned with cotton swabs or applicators. Small children should not have access to small toys that the children could insert in their ears. Parents and children should be taught not to put anything smaller than their elbow in the ear.

Treatment options for children with hearing impairment depend on the etiology. The underlying cause is addressed whenever possible and as soon as possible. In 2004, the American Academy of Pediatrics and the American Academy of Family Physicians convened a committee that developed guidelines for the treatment of acute otitis media (AOM). According to the committee, AOM "is the most common infection for which antibacterial agents are prescribed for children in the United States" (American Academy of Family Physicians, 2004, p. 2). The antibacterial treatment guideline is the use of amoxicillin 80–90 mg/kg/day in children aged 2 months through 12 years with uncomplicated AOM. For children with severe AOM (moderate to severe otalgia or a temperature of 39°C [102.2°F] or higher), amoxicillin/potassium clavulanate (90 mg/kg/day of amoxicillin and 6.4 mg/kg/day of clavulanate in two divided doses) is recommended (Spratto and Woods, 2008). In addition, for children who have developed organisms resistant to amoxicillin, amoxicillin/potassium clavulanate is the agent of choice. Impacted cerumen is removed using wax emulsifiers such as carbamide peroxide 0.5% (Broyles, Reiss, & Evans, 2007).

Ototoxic drugs that can result in reversible hearing loss should be discontinued if alternative therapy is available. The most commonly used ototoxic antimicrobials are aminoglycosides. The chronic, high-dose therapy using gentamycin is routinely employed in the treatment of severe respiratory infections associated with cystic fibrosis. Unfortunately, this is part of an effective three-antibiotic regimen to treat these children, with no alternative therapy as effective.

Surgical procedures for children with complications of otitis media include tympanoplasty (reconstruction of the tympanic membrane) and myringotomy (placement of a pressure equalization tube to drain the middle ear in a child with recurrent otitis media) (Broyles, 2005).

Amplification devices (hearing aids) are recommended for children with mild bilateral sensorineural hearing loss or chronic conductive hearing loss. Cochlear implants are an option for children with profound bilateral hearing loss who do not benefit from traditional amplification. Cochlear implants deliver electrical stimulation to the auditory nerve (acoustic nerve or cranial nerve VIII). This allows nerve impulses to be transmitted to the brain as normal sounds. The brain then can organize and interpret the sound (Broyles, 2005). Speech and language development usually is required for children with profound hearing impairment.

Nursing Management

ASSESSMENT

1. Obtain client and family history (for risk factors)
2. Perform physical assessment
3. Assess hearing acuity
4. Assess child's developmental behavior
5. Assess parents'/child's understanding of how to prevent hearing impairment

NURSING DIAGNOSES (INCLUDING BUT NOT LIMITED TO)

1. Disturbed auditory sensory perception R/T hearing impairment
2. Risk for impaired verbal communication R/T hearing impairment
3. Delayed growth and development R/T inability to hear verbal communication
4. Deficient knowledge (child if age-appropriate and parent) R/T hearing impairment prevention techniques, child's condition, treatment, and home care

PLANNING/GOALS

1. Client will use and interpret speech cues.
2. Client will use communication aids as recommended.
3. Client will engage in appropriate activities for level of development.
4. Client (if age-appropriate) and parents will demonstrate understanding of prevention of hearing impairment, child's condition, treatment, and home care.

NOC

1. Communication: Receptive, Sensory Function: Hearing
2. Communication: Expressive
3. Child Development
4. Knowledge: Illness Care, Treatment, Health Promotion

IMPLEMENTATION

1. Auditory impairment
   a. Assess hearing acuity
   b. Teach parents the importance of timely treatment for child's otitis media
   c. Encourage parents to participate actively in planning and implementing care
   d. Minimize background noise
   e. Stand so child can see face when speaking
   f. Speak facing child
   g. Speak clearly and in a normal tone
   h. Avoid chewing gum or covering mouth when speaking
   i. Use appropriate hand gestures
   j. Provide adequate light to facilitate lip reading if child has profound hearing impairment

    k. Do not avoid child with hearing loss

    l. Encourage use of amplification devices as recommended

    m. Teach proper care of amplification devices

    n. Provide postoperative tympanoplasty care

        1) Keep child flat with operative ear up for prescribed postoperative period

        2) Follow postoperative protocol

        3) Assess pain level hourly using age-appropriate pain scale

        4) Medicate to maintain optimal pain control

        5) Monitor ear canal for bleeding

        6) Reinforce dressing (if present) as prescribed

        7) Administer prophylactic antibiotics as prescribed

        8) Teach postoperative instructions from health care provider

    o. Provide postoperative stapendectomy care

        1) Instruct child/parents that improvement in hearing may take up to six weeks

        2) Follow postoperative care protocol

        3) Assess pain level hourly using age-appropriate pain scale

        4) Medicate to maintain optimal pain control

        5) Assess for complications of surgery (facial nerve damage, muscle weakness, changes in sensation or taste, vertigo, nausea, and vomiting)

        6) Administer antibiotics as prescribed

        7) Encourage child to rise slowly from lying or sitting position

        8) Review postoperative instructions from health care provider

    p. Provide postoperative cochlear implant care

        1) Follow postoperative care protocol

        2) Maintain integrity of ear shield

        3) Assess pain level hourly using age-appropriate pain scale

        4) Medicate proactively to maintain pain control

        5) Avoid loud noises in child's presence

2. Verbal communication

    a. Assess history of verbal skills development

    b. Assess verbal communication skills

    c. Use developmentally appropriate skills measurement

    d. Involve parents in planning and implementation of care

    e. Collaborate with health care provider for referral to appropriate speech and language therapists

3. Growth and development

    a. Assess parents' current level of understanding about growth and development

    b. Assess child's current level of growth and development

    c. Provide visual motor activities

    d. Assist parents in enrolling child in special programs for hearing impaired

    e. Provide contact information for community and national support groups

    f. Provide education and support to child/parents

4. Parent/child teaching
   a. Assess parents' current level of understanding
   b. Provide verbal and written information regarding:
      1) Ways to avoid risk factors for hearing impairment including not putting infant down to nap or sleep with bottle of juice or formula and not exposing child to secondhand smoke, loud noises, use of cotton-tipped applicators in ears, and ototoxic medications (if possible)
      2) Routine hearing evaluations for children
      3) Appropriate postoperative instructions including not allowing child to drink through a straw for at least two to three weeks; avoiding air travel for at least three weeks; avoiding rapid head movements, bending, jumping, or bouncing for three weeks; not coming in contact with people with respiratory infections; not washing child's hair or getting head wet for at least one week; not swimming for at least six weeks; blowing nose gently; sneezing with mouth open; reporting pain not controlled by medications, increased drainage, purulent drainage, or temperature > 37.5°C (101.2°F.)
      4) Care of hearing assistive devices including making sure batteries are functional; turning off unit when not in use (sleeping); keeping extra batteries available; not allowing child to wear device during ear infections; and teaching that if assistive device whistles, the ear mold is not inserted properly or a new mold is required
      5) Medication administration including importance of completing the prescribed medication regimen
      6) Signs and symptoms of adverse effects of medications
      7) Manifestations of worsening of condition
      8) Contact phone numbers for reporting signs and symptoms
      9) Importance of regular hand washing and appropriate technique
      10) Importance of follow-up with health care provider
   c. Provide adequate time for teaching and parents'/child's questions
   d. Document teaching and parents'/child's response

NIC

1. Communication Enhancement, Hearing Deficit
2. Communication Enhancement
3. Developmental Enhancement
4. Teaching: Illness Care, Treatment, Health Promotion

EVALUATION

1. Client uses and interprets speech cues.
2. Client uses communication aids as recommended.
3. Client engages in appropriate activities for level of development.
4. Client (if age-appropriate) and parents demonstrate understanding of prevention of hearing impairment, child's condition, treatment, and home care.

References

American Academy of Family Physicians. (2004). *Diagnosis and management of acute otitis media.* Retrieved May 17, 2007, from http://www.aafp.org/online/en/home/clinical/clinicalrecs/aom.html

Broyles, B. E. (2005). *Medical-surgical nursing clinical companion.* Durham, NC: Carolina Academic Press.

Centers for Disease Control and Prevention. (2004). *Hearing loss.* Retrieved May 17, 2007, from http://www.cdc.gov/ncbddd/dd/hi3.htm

Centers for Disease Control and Prevention. (2007). *Newborn hearing screening important for development.* Retrieved May 17, 2007, from http://www.cdc.gov/Features/NewbornHearing

National Institute on Deafness and Other Communication Disorders. (2007). *Testing in infants for prevention and diagnosis of hearing loss.* Retrieved May 17, 2007, from http://www.nidcd.nih.gov/research/stories/archives/06/04_02_07.htm

Potts, N. L., & Mandleco, B. L. (2007). *Pediatric nursing: Caring for children and their families* (2nd ed.). Clifton Park, NY: Delmar Cengage Learning.

Shah, R. K., & Lotke, M. (2007). *Hearing impairment.* Retrieved February 21, 2008, from http://www.emedicine.com/ped/topic931.htm

Spratto, G. R., & Woods, A. L. (2008). *2008 edition PDR Nurse's drug handbook.* Clifton Park, NY: Delmar Cengage Learning.

52

HEMOLYTIC UREMIC SYNDROME (HUS)

Definition

Hemolytic uremic syndrome (HUS) is an acute intravascular condition affecting the kidneys. HUS is most common in children and is the leading cause of acute renal failure in pediatric clients.

Pathophysiology

Although once relatively rare, HUS is increasing in children. It usually occurs following a gastrointestinal infection caused by a specific *Escherichia coli* (*E. coli* 0157:H7) bacterium found in contaminated meat. It has been termed "hamburger syndrome" (Potts & Mandleco, 2007). This microbe often is referred to by three other terms: (1) VTEC, or verotoxin-producing *E. coli*, (2) EHEC, or enterohemorrhagic *E. coli*, and (3) STEC, or Shiga toxin-producing *E. coli*. To a much lesser extent, HUS also has been associated with other enteric infections including *Shigella* and *Salmonella* and some nonenteric infections.

Two other sources for contamination by *E. coli* 0157:H7 were defined after two separate outbreaks in late 2006. The first one occurred in August and September from contaminated spinach. Of those diagnosed with the infection, "HUS occurred in approximately 18% of patients, on average, with the actual incidence ranging from 8%–35% in the different outbreaks" (Todd, 2007, p. 29). In December 2006, another outbreak in the northeastern part of the United States was traced to contaminated shredded lettuce, although this conclusion was based on a process of elimination comparing those individuals affected with those who ate with them but remained healthy (Stubenrauch, 2007).

This particular strain of *E. coli* attaches to the intestinal mucosa, secreting a Shiga toxin that destroys the endothelial cells of the capillary walls by binding to globotriaosylceramide (Gb3), a glycolipid receptor molecule on the surface of endothelial cells in the gastrointestinal tract, kidneys, and occasionally other organs (Beiga & Prauner, 2006). The toxin also destroys platelets and red blood cells. The resulting inflammatory process and the damaged red blood cells and platelets occlude the tiny renal capillaries or cause lesions in the kidneys. This results in occlusion of the capillaries in the renal glomeruli, decreasing filtration. These changes cause hemolytic anemia (from destruction of red blood cells); thrombocytopenia; inhibited fibrinolysis and microvascular thrombosis; nervous system manifestations; and in severe cases, renal failure (MedlinePlus, 2005). The linings of blood vessel walls also are damaged. This leads to elevated levels of blood urea nitrogen and creatinine, potassium, phosphorus, uric acid, bilirubin, liver enzymes, lactate dehydrogenase, and triglycerides. Bicarbonate and sodium concentrations are decreased, and protein and albumin levels are mildly decreased (Beiga & Prauner, 2006).

Initially, HUS is manifested as gastrointestinal symptoms including abdominal pain, vomiting, and bloody diarrhea usually lasting two to three days but sometimes persisting for up to two weeks. Even after the gastrointestinal manifestations subside, the child remains pale, tired, and irritable.

Complications

    Hemolytic anemia
    Thrombocytopenia
    Microvascular thrombosis

Nervous system manifestations

Acute renal failure

Risk for chronic renal failure

Incidence

HUS is most common in infants and children from 6 months to 4 years of age. According to Shapiro (2007), the average annual incidence is 2.65 cases per 100,000 in children under the age of 5 years. The incidence drops significantly in individuals aged 18 and younger, with the average annual incidence of 0.97 cases per 100,000. Incidence increases seasonally with the higher occurrence of *E. coli* 0157:H7 infections between June and September (Shapiro, 2007). "It is more prevalent in developing countries where sanitation and the undercooking of meats are a problem" (Potts & Mandleco, 2007, p. 647). "In Asia and Africa, it is often associated with Stx-producing *Shigella dysenteriae serotype 1*. Regarding Stx associated with *E. coli*, Stx-1 is almost identical to Stx associated with *S. dysenteriae type 1*, differing by a single amino acid. Stx-1 is 50% homologous with Stx-2. Stx-2 is associated with severe disease" (Parmar, 2006, Section 2).

Etiology

HUS is associated with a gastrointestinal infection caused by a specific *E. coli* (*E. coli* 0157:H7) bacterium. Seventy percent of the cases of HUS are secondary to this particular microorganism (Parmar, 2006). Several large outbreaks occurring in 1992 and 1993 attributed to undercooked hamburger contaminated with *E. coli* resulted in new supermarket labeling and new temperature guidelines for hamburger prepared at restaurants and fast-food chains (Centers for Disease Control and Prevention, 2006). In addition, HUS has been associated with other enteric infections, including those caused by *S. dysenteriae* and *Salmonella*, but not to the extent of *E. coli* 0157:H7. A few cases have occurred as the result of nonenteric conditions (MedlinePlus, 2008).

Clinical Manifestations

Bloody diarrhea

Abdominal pain

Vomiting

Pallor

Fatigue

Irritability

Anorexia

Decreased urinary output

Diagnostic Tests

Complete blood count

Serum chemistry levels

Urinalysis

Fecal culture

Electrocardiogram

Medical Management

According to the National Institutes of Health, the treatment (for HUS) is supportive, and about 60% of individuals receiving treatment will recover, and the outcome is better in children (MedlinePlus, 2008). The goals of management are early recognition of the disease, fluid volume control, reestablishment of electrolyte levels, reversal of acute renal failure, and effective treatment for hypertension and anemia.

In the presence of acute renal failure, close monitoring of fluid and electrolyte status is necessary. This may require frequent measurements of body weight, intake and output, vital signs, and serum electrolyte levels. The loop diuretic furosemide is the drug of choice for fluid overload (Broyles, Reiss, & Evans, 2007). Potassium should not be added to replacement fluids unless the child is hypokalemic. Dialysis usually is reserved for children who are anuric for 24 hours, experience seizures, or are extremely hypertensive (Potts & Mandleco, 2007). "Peritoneal dialysis is usually well tolerated and technically easier in small infants. Some data indicate that peritoneal dialysis may be preferred because it facilitates clearance of plasminogen activator inhibitor-1 (PAI-1) and promotes more rapid recovery of renal function. When dialysis is required, it is usually needed for 5–7 days" (Beiga & Prauner, 2006, Section 6). Severe hyperkalemia not controlled by dialysis may be treated with intravenous bicarbonate, glucose and insulin, and calcium (if cardiac rhythm changes are present). If chronic renal failure develops, renal transplantation is considered.

Hemolytic anemia may require transfusions of packed red blood cells if the child exhibits manifestations indicating decreased tissue perfusion, such as tachycardia or orthostatic changes in blood pressure or heart rate, or if the child's hematocrit falls rapidly. Because of the risk of fluid overload present with transfusions, administration of plasma products may be given to offset this occurrence. Platelet transfusions are recommended for symptomatic bleeding and before central line placement (for central venous pressure monitoring in the presence of central nervous system changes). The caution with platelet transfusions is the risk of platelet aggregation and further thrombus formation.

The agents of choice for the management of hypertension in children with HUS are hydralazine (vasodilator) and captopril (angiotensin-converting enzyme inhibitor) (Broyles et al., 2007). Total parenteral nutrition to maintain adequate energy intake may be required for children with severe vomiting and diarrhea.

In the presence of neurologic manifestations, treatment is supportive. Anticonvulsants are used to treat seizure activity; mannitol is the drug of choice for the treatment of increased intracranial pressure; manifestations resulting from metabolic acidosis are managed with intravenous sodium bicarbonate.

Nursing Management

ASSESSMENT

1. Obtain client history with focus on presence of a recent gastrointestinal infection
2. Obtain baseline height, weight, and vital signs including blood pressure
3. Complete a physical assessment
4. Assess parents for psychological impact of child's condition

NURSING DIAGNOSES (INCLUDING BUT NOT LIMITED TO)

1. Fluid volume excess R/T decreased renal function
2. Risk for injury, bleeding R/T decreased platelets and inhibited fibrinolysis
3. Ineffective tissue perfusion R/T decreased circulating erythrocytes
4. Parental anxiety R/T acuity of child's condition
5. Deficient knowledge R/T child's condition, treatment, risks of recurrence, and home care

PLANNING/GOALS

1. Client will regain and maintain fluid and electrolyte balance as evidenced by osmolality and electrolyte values within defined limits (WDL), absence of peripheral and pulmonary edema, and stable weight.
2. Client will not experience injury.

3. Client will regain and maintain adequate tissue perfusion as evidenced by level of consciousness, vital signs, and complete blood count WDL.
4. Parents will verbalize feelings and concerns and demonstrate use of positive coping strategies.
5. Parents will demonstrate understanding of condition, treatment, risks for recurrence, and home care.

NOC

1. Fluid Balance, Electrolyte and Acid/Base Balance
2. Risk Control
3. Circulation Status, Vital Signs
4. Anxiety
5. Knowledge: Illness Care, Treatment, Health Promotion

IMPLEMENTATION

1. Fluid and electrolyte balance
   a. Monitor intake and output
   b. Monitor weight
   c. Assess urine pH with each void
   d. Monitor serum electrolyte levels, reporting abnormal values to health care provider
   e. Auscultate breath sounds each shift and as needed
   f. Assess for peripheral edema and report findings to health care provider
   g. Turn child at least every 2 hours if peripheral edema is present
   h. Maintain dietary and fluid restrictions as prescribed, carefully monitoring for dehydration
   i. Administer total parenteral nutrition as prescribed
   j. Maintain intravenous access device, monitoring at least hourly
   k. Monitor blood pressure every 4 hours
   l. Administer diuretic agents as prescribed
   m. Administer antihypertensive agents as prescribed
   n. Prepare for dialysis as indicated, monitoring vital signs and indications of fluid deficit
2. Risk for bleeding
   a. Assess child for petechiae, bruising, epistaxis, and bleeding from other mucous membranes
   b. Monitor platelet counts and report abnormal findings to health care provider
   c. Test stools for blood
   d. Protect from falls
   e. Avoid intramuscular injections
   f. Initiate seizure precautions
   g. Assist with ambulation
   h. Maintain intravenous access, monitoring at least hourly
   i. Administer plasma products as prescribed
   j. Administer platelets as prescribed
3. Tissue perfusion
   a. Assess neurologic status
   b. Monitor vital signs with blood pressure

   c. Monitor intake and output

   d. Initiate and maintain hemodynamic monitoring as child's condition indicates

   e. Place on cardiorespiratory monitor if child has elevated potassium level

   f. Monitor complete blood count

   g. Maintain intravenous access, monitoring at least hourly

   h. Administer intravenous fluids as prescribed

   i. Administer blood products as prescribed, monitoring for transfusion reaction (Refer to Nursing Management in Chapter 35: Disseminated Intravascular Coagulation [DIC])

   j. Monitor intake and output

   k. Protect from injury and falls

   l. Monitor continuous pulse oximetry

   m. Administer oxygen, titrating to prescribed oxygen saturation

   n. Provide for adequate rest by clustering nursing care to provide undisturbed rest periods

   o. Maintain comfortable environmental temperature

   p. Encourage parents to spend as much time as possible with child

   q. Assess pain level hourly and medicate proactively to maintain pain control

4. Parental anxiety

   a. Assess parents for verbal and nonverbal indicators of anxiety

   b. Provide supportive environment

   c. Explain all equipment and procedures

   d. Encourage verbalization of feelings and concerns

   e. Encourage parents to participate actively in child's care

   f. Explain that child can sense parental anxiety

5. Parent teaching

   a. Assess parents' current level of knowledge

   b. Provide verbal and written information regarding:

      1) Risk factors for developing HUS and instructions as needed to avoid risk factors; for instance, importance of proper meat preparation

      2) Medication administration including importance of compliance with prescribed medication regimen

      3) Manifestations of adverse effects of medications

      4) Signs and symptoms of worsening of condition

      5) Contact phone numbers for reporting signs and symptoms and for making referral contacts

      6) Importance of hand washing and appropriate technique

      7) Importance of follow-up care with health care provider

   c. Provide adequate time for teaching

   d. Document teaching and parents' response

NIC

1. Fluid/Electrolyte Management, Fluid/Electrolyte Monitoring

2. Surveillance: Safety

3. Hemodynamic Regulation, Vital Signs Monitoring, Cerebral Perfusion Promotion, Neurologic Monitoring

4. Coping Enhancement
5. Teaching: Illness Care, Treatment, Health Promotion

EVALUATION

1. Client regains and maintains fluid and electrolyte balance as evidenced by osmolality and electrolyte values WDL, absence of peripheral and pulmonary edema, and stable weight.
2. Client does not experience injury.
3. Client regains and maintains adequate tissue perfusion as evidenced by level of consciousness, vital signs, and complete blood count WDL.
4. Parents verbalize feelings and concerns and demonstrate use of positive coping strategies.
5. Parents demonstrate understanding of condition, treatment, risks for recurrence, and home care.

References

Beiga, T., & Prauner, R. (2006). *Hemolytic-uremic syndrome.* Retrieved March 8, 2007, from http://www.emedicine.com/ped/topic960.htm

Broyles, B. E., Reiss, B. S., & Evans, M. E. (2007). *Pharmacological aspects of nursing care* (7th ed.). Clifton Park, NY: Delmar Cengage Learning.

Centers for Disease Control and Prevention. (2006). *Diarrheagenic* Escherichia coli. Retrieved March 5, 2007, from http://www.cdc.gov/ncidod/dbmd/diseaseinfo/diarrecoli_t.htm

MedlinePlus. (2005). *Hemolytic-uremic syndrome.* Retrieved May 17, 2007, from http://www.nlm.nih.gov/medlineplus/ency/article/000510.htm

Parmar, M. S. (2006). "*Hemolytic-uremic syndrome*". Retrieved May 17, 2007, from http://www.emedicine.com/med/topic980.htm

Potts, N. L., & Mandleco, B. L. (2007). *Pediatric nursing: Caring for children and their families* (2nd ed.). Clifton Park, NY: Delmar Cengage Learning.

Shapiro, W. (2007). *Hemolytic uremic syndrome.* Retrieved February 21, 2008, from http://www.emedicine.com/emerg/topic238.htm

Stubenrauch, J. M. (2007). Another 0157:H7 outbreak. *American Journal of Nursing, 107*(2).

Todd, B. (2007). Emerging infections: Outbreak: *E. coli* 0157:H7. *American Journal of Nursing, 107*(2).

53

HEMOPHILIA

Definition

Hemophilia is an X-linked hereditary bleeding disorder caused by deficiency of clotting factors VIII, IX, or XI (Potts & Mandleco, 2007).

Pathophysiology

Hemophilia is a lifelong disorder classified according to the clotting factor that is deficient. Clotting factors are proteins that are responsible for a part of the clotting cascade in the body (World Federation of Hemophilia, 2005). Hemophilia A, the most common type of hemophilia, accounting for 80–85% of hemophilia cases, reflects a deficiency of factor VIII. Hemophilia B, also known as Christmas disease, is about 5 times less common than hemophilia A and is the result of a deficiency of factor IX (Christmas factor) (National Heart Lung and Blood Institute, 2006). Finally, the least common form of hemophilia is hemophilia C, which is due to a lack of factor XI. Some children have a low level of one factor; for other children, the factor is completely missing.

Hemophilia is further classified depending on the severity of the disease: (1) mild, (2) moderate, or (3) severe. The severity is determined by the amount of clotting factor in the blood. Approximately 70% of individuals with hemophilia A have the severe form. In children and adults with normal factor VIII, the factor activity is 100%; individuals with severe hemophilia A have a factor VIII activity of less than 1% (National Heart Lung and Blood Institute, 2006).

Regardless of the type, hemophilia is a disturbance in the intrinsic pathway of the coagulation cascade. Factors VIII, IX, and XI are part of phase 1 of this pathway and are part of a sequence of enzymatic reactions needed to move to phase 2 of the common pathway, prothrombin activator complex. This complex facilitates the conversion of prothrombin to thrombin; and in phase 3, thrombin is necessary to convert fibrinogen to fibrin. This leads to prolonged bleeding even from small wounds. In traumatic injuries, hemorrhage, shock, and death from hypovolemia can occur (Potts & Mandleco, 2007).

In school-age children, hemarthrosis (bleeding into the joints) is a common complication because of the amount of running and other outdoor activities these children do. Hemarthrosis can be a recurrent complication and may lead to joint dysfunction, structural changes, contracture, pain, and deformity. Hemarthrosis most commonly occurs in the knees, elbows, shoulders, and ankles (Broyles, 2005).

Bleeding in the brain is a very serious complication of hemophilia that requires emergency treatment. This can occur as the result of a simple bump on the head or a more serious injury, such as what might occur in a motor vehicle or motor vehicle versus pedestrian accident. Common manifestations include long-lasting painful headaches, frequent vomiting, behavior changes, sleepiness, sudden extremity weakness, neck pain or stiffness, diplopia, unsteady gait, and seizures (National Heart Lung and Blood Institute, 2006).

Complications

Prolonged bleeding
Hemarthrosis
Hemorrhage

Neurologic devastation secondary to brain bleed
Shock
Death

Incidence

According to the National Hemophilia Foundation, hemophilia affects approximately 1 in 5,000 males born in the United States. It affects all races and economic groups equally (Potts & Mandleco, 2007; National Hemophilia Foundation, 2006). Each year about 400 babies are born with hemophilia (National Heart Lung and Blood Institute, 2006). Hemophilia A and B occur only in males; however, hemophilia C is equally distributed between males and females. In extremely rare cases, women who carry the gene for hemophilia A or B can experience hemophilia-like symptoms.

Etiology

Hemophilia is an X-linked recessive hereditary disorder. Hemophilia A is the result of a mutation in the F8 gene; hemophilia B is caused by a mutation in the F9 gene (Genetics Home Reference, 2007). In about 30% of cases, there is no family history of the disorder; the condition is the result of a spontaneous gene mutation. Refer to Figure 53-1.

(A) When the mother is a carrier for the disease, there is a 50% chance each child conceived will not have nor carry the disease. There is a 25% chance each child conceived will carry the disease and a 25% chance each child conceived will have the disease.

	Y	X
X	XY 25% Normal (Male)	XX 25% Normal (Female)
x	xY 25% Disease (Male)	Xx 25% Carrier (Female)

(B) When the father has the disease, there is a 50% chance each child conceived will not have the disease nor carry the disease and a 50% chance each child conceived will carry the disease.

	Y	x
X	XY 25% Normal (Male)	Xx 25% Carrier (Female)
X	XY 25% Normal (Male)	Xx 25% Carrier (Female)

Legend
x = Recessive disease gene
X or Y = Dominant normal gene
xx or xY = Disease state
Xx = Carrier state
YX or XX = Normal state

Figure 53-1: X-Linked Recessive Hereditary Etiology of Hemophilia.

Clinical Manifestations

Depends on the severity of the disease and the extent of the trauma

Bleeding following circumcision

Prolonged bleeding at umbilicus

Slow, persistent, prolonged bleeding

Stiffness and tenderness of joints in which bleeding occurs, progressing to swelling, warmth, and pain

Epistaxis

Ecchymosis

Hematoma formation

Hematuria

Severe bleeding including hemorrhage in the presence of moderate to severe injury

Diagnostic Tests

Platelet count

Ivy method (bleeding time)

Prothrombin time

Partial thromboplastin time

Quantitative immunoelectrophoretic assay

Factor assays

Medical Management

The goals of treatment are to prevent bleeding episodes and to limit complications of the disease. The standard of care for both prophylactic treatment and restorative treatment for children with hemophilia is factor replacement. The major issue with factor replacement is cost.

In the 1950s, fresh-frozen plasma as well as concentrates containing antihemophilic factors (AHFs) could be prepared; and "in 1958, Swedish clinicians began treating clients prophylactically with AHF to prevent joint damage. The success of their efforts supported the concept of prophylaxis, which remains the treatment of choice today. Innovations in prophylaxis have allowed outpatient and home treatment of hemophilia. As a result, the quality of life for those affected has dramatically improved. The life expectancy of people with hemophilia was 11 years of age in 1931; since 1980, the life expectancy has increased to 60 years with research continuing to improve this figure" (Broyles, 2005, p. 412).

For any kind of bleeding episode, treatment should not be postponed or deferred. For acute bleeds, rest and ice may be used; and in mild hemophilia, in addition to factor replacement, desmopressin acetate (DDAVP) may be used to stimulate the body's production of factor VIII. DDAVP acts on the endothelial cells, causing a release of von Willebrand factor (vWF) that binds with factor VIII, increasing the concentration of both factors. The most common problems associated with factor replacement are delaying replacement or discontinuing the therapy too early. Minor bleeding episodes should be treated for at least three days, and more severe injuries (surgery and trauma) may require ten days to two weeks of factor replacement therapy.

Home infusion replacement therapy is the norm for most families with children affected by hemophilia. Advantages to performing replacement therapy (both prophylactic and as-needed treatment) include treating the child quicker when a bleeding event occurs, experiencing fewer complications, making fewer health care provider or emergency department visits, incurring less cost, and helping the child accept treatment more readily.

Antifibrinolytic agents including tranexamic acid and aminocaproic acid are used with factor treatment. They prevent clots from breaking down and most often are used prior to dental work and for the treatment of epistaxis, bleeding of the oral mucous membranes, and mild intestinal bleeding (National Heart Lung and Blood Institute, 2006).

In children experiencing hemarthrosis, bed rest, ice, skin traction, and daily intravenous factor replacement are the standards of care. Pain management with acetaminophen (no aspirin or salicylate products) is usually sufficient because with no weight bearing or movement of the joint, pain is mild. However, if treatment is delayed, joint contracture can occur. This is treated with the use of a semiflexible splint or a desubluxation-type hinge cast (World Federation of Hemophilia, 2005) such as the Quingle cast, which allows for gradual reduction of the flexion contracture, usually over the course of approximately six weeks. For these children, pain management usually requires the use of opioid analgesics such as oxycodone or acetaminophen with codeine prior to each daily reduction session.

Nursing Management

ASSESSMENT
1. Obtain client history including history of injury
2. Assess for joint swelling, tenderness, and pain
3. Obtain height and weight (Factor replacement is based on kg/body weight)
4. Obtain vital signs

NURSING DIAGNOSES (INCLUDING BUT NOT LIMITED TO)
1. Ineffective tissue perfusion R/T bleeding episodes
2. Impaired physical mobility R/T treatment for hemarthrosis
3. Interrupted family processes R/T caring for a child with an inherited and potentially fatal disease
4. Deficient knowledge R/T child's condition, treatment, home care, and health promotion

PLANNING/GOALS
1. Client will be effectively treated by parents/caregivers who demonstrate ability to prevent bleeding episodes and to manage mild bleeding occurrences and mild hemarthrosis episodes.
2. Client will not experience complications associated with impaired mobility while on bed rest and in traction during hospitalization for moderate to severe hemarthrosis.
3. Parents/caregivers will verbalize feelings and concerns and use positive coping strategies and support systems.
4. Parents/caregivers will demonstrate understanding of child's condition, treatment, home care, and health promotion.

NOC
1. Circulation Status, Pain Control
2. Mobility
3. Coping
4. Knowledge: Illness Care, Treatment, Health Promotion

IMPLEMENTATION
1. Tissue perfusion
   a. Teach parents/caregivers about:
      1) Making the home environment as safe as possible
      2) Using padding on elbows and knees of toddlers
      3) Providing close observation of infants and toddlers
      4) Padding sides of crib and playpen

    5) Encouraging older children to participate in low-contact sports (swimming or tennis) or to assist with statistics or filming of other contact sports

    6) Using soft-bristled toothbrushes

    7) Preventing child from becoming overweight

    8) Obtaining a medical ID bracelet

    9) Applying pressure for 10–15 seconds to any bleed

    10) Immobilizing and elevating extremity and joint where bleeding is occurring

    11) Applying ice or cold to bleeding area

    12) Providing pain management for hemarthrosis (avoiding aspirin)

    13) Instituting active range-of-motion exercises after 48 hours of hemarthrosis treatment

    14) Administering replacement factor therapy and DDAVP as prescribed, handling factor carefully. *NOTE:* Each unit of factor costs more than one U.S. dollar, and many clients receive over 2,500 units/day during hospitalization for exacerbations.

2. Impaired physical mobility during hospitalization for hemarthrosis

   a. Assess skin at sites where traction is in contact with skin and over bony prominences

   b. Assess neurovascular status of extremity in skin traction

   c. Assess traction weights, ensuring that prescribed weight is maintained and weights hang free

   d. Assess traction pulleys to ensure that traction is functioning properly

   e. Assist with range-of-motion exercises to uninvolved joints using age-appropriate activities such as tossing paper wads into the trash receptacle

   f. Keep child's personal items within reach

   g. Encourage parents/caregivers to participate in child's care

   h. Medicate prior to reduction sessions if child is in a flexion contracture cast

   i. Provide age-appropriate diversionary activities (video games for school-age and adolescent boys)

   j. Explain all procedures, precautions, and equipment

   k. Assist client with use of trapeze

   l. Ensure that client does not slide to foot of bed

3. Family processes

   a. Assess parents/caregivers for verbal and nonverbal indicators of stress

   b. Encourage parents/caregivers to verbalize their feelings and concerns

   c. Listen actively

   d. Assist parents/caregivers in identifying positive coping strategies and support systems

   e. Encourage parents/caregivers to use these strategies and support systems

   f. Collaborate with social worker for possible family assistance

4. Parent/caregiver teaching
   a. Assess current level of understanding
   b. Provide verbal and written information regarding:
      1) Importance of maintaining a safe environment for the child, including reviewing risk factors for injuries and how to prevent injuries—for instance, using knee pads for young children, keeping sharp objects out of reach of children, avoiding use of razor blades for shaving (adolescents), performing daily mouth care carefully, and not participating in high-contact sports
      2) Measures to treat bleeding episodes and mild hemarthrosis
      3) Techniques for home infusion factor replacement therapy
      4) Importance of seeking medical attention immediately if more severe injury occurs
      5) Home health referral as needed to assist with medication administration including nasal administration of DDAVP and venipuncture and infusion techniques for self-administration of factor replacement
      6) Importance of compliance with medications
      7) Referral information and national and local support group information
      8) Manifestations of worsening of condition
      9) Contact phone numbers for reporting signs and symptoms
      10) Importance of follow-up with health care provider
   c. Provide adequate time for teaching and parent/caregiver interaction
   d. Document teaching and parent/caregiver response

NIC

1. Hemodynamic Regulation, Pain Management
2. Traction/Immobilization Care
3. Coping Enhancement
4. Teaching: Illness Care, Treatment, Health Promotion

EVALUATION

1. Client is effectively treated by parents/caregivers who demonstrate ability to prevent bleeding episodes and to manage mild bleeding occurrences and mild hemarthrosis episodes.
2. Client does not experience complications associated with impaired mobility while on bed rest and in traction during hospitalization for moderate to severe hemarthrosis.
3. Parents/caregivers verbalize feelings and concerns and use positive coping strategies and support systems.
4. Parents/caregivers demonstrate understanding of child's condition, treatment, home care, and health promotion.

References

Broyles, B. E. (2005). *Medical-surgical nursing clinical companion.* Durham, NC: Carolina Academic Press.

Genetics Home Reference. (2007). *What is hemophilia?* Retrieved March 8, 2007, from http://ghr.nlm.nih.gov/condition=hemophilia

National Heart Lung and Blood Institute. (2006). *Hemophilia.* Retrieved March 8, 2007, from http://www.nhlbi.nih.gov/health/dci/Diseases/hemophilia/hemophilia_what.html

National Hemophilia Foundation. (2006). *What is hemophilia?* Retrieved March 8, 2007, from
    http://www.hemophilia.org/NHFWeb/MainPgs/MainNHF.aspx?menuid=180&contentid=
    45&rptname=bleeding

Potts, N. L., & Mandleco, B. L. (2007). *Pediatric nursing: Caring for children and their families*
    (2nd ed.). Clifton Park, NY: Delmar Cengage Learning.

World Federation of Hemophilia. (2005). *Frequently asked questions about hemophilia.* Retrieved
    February 21, 2008, from http://www.wfh.org/index.asp?lang=EN&url=2/1/1_1_1_FAQ.htm

54

HEPATITIS

Definition

"Hepatitis is an acute or chronic inflammation of the liver" (Potts & Mandleco, 2007, p. 695).

Pathophysiology

As the major detoxifying organ in the body, the liver is exposed to all chemicals and microorganisms in the bloodstream. Following invasion by a hepatitis virus, inflammation occurs in the liver, causing it to become enlarged (hepatomegaly) and congested with phagocytes and fluid. As the disease progresses, hepatic necrosis and hepatic cell degeneration result. With hepatomegaly, portal vessel pressure increases interference with the blood supply to the liver lobules. In the presence of specific hepatic viruses, immune complex-mediated tissue damage occurs.

Hepatitis usually follows a well-defined course through three phases: (1) preicteric, (2) icteric, and (3) posticteric. The preicteric phase begins with exposure to the hepatitis virus and lasts until symptoms of jaundice and pain occur. The icteric phase is the active period characterized by jaundice that lasts four to six weeks. The posticteric phase is the recovery phase, which can last for months (Broyles, 2005).

Hepatitis A (HAV) occurs most frequently in children 5–14 years of age and is caused by oral intake of HAV that is found in the feces of infected individuals. Children in day care centers are at highest risk for contracting HAV because of the numbers of children in these centers and/or workers not observing proper hygiene habits (Potts & Mandleco, 2007). It can occur when a person ingests anything that is contaminated with HAV-infected stool—water, milk, food, and especially shellfish. HAV results only in acute hepatitis causing a short course of the disease or even an asymptomatic one.

Hepatitis B (HBV), also called serum hepatitis, is spread intravenously through direct contact with the blood or body fluids of an infected person. In children, most HBV infections are transmitted perinatally from an infected mother. Other methods of contracting HBV include coming in contact with infected body fluids (blood, saliva, semen, vaginal fluids, tears, and urine), engaging in sexual activity with a person infected with HBV, and sharing contaminated needles or syringes for injecting drugs. In the United States, contracting HBV from contaminated blood transfusions is rare.

Hepatitis C (HCV), commonly referred to as chronic hepatitis because of the percentage of individuals with HCV that develop chronic hepatitis, is transmitted by sharing drug needles, getting a tattoo or body piercing with unsterilized tools, being treated with blood transfusions prior to 1992, contracting it perinatally from an infected mother, and engaging in sexual contact (least common).

Hepatitis D (HDV) can occur only in the presence of HBV because HDV is an incomplete virus. It is rare in children in the United States because of the use of HBV immunizations. Hepatitis E is similar to HAV in terms of its transmission but also is rare in the pediatric population of the United States. Hepatitis G is the most recently identified strain of hepatitis viruses. Currently, no scientific evidence is available to support this virus as a cause of either acute or chronic hepatitis.

Complications

Transmission of disease

Liver failure

Incidence

The incidence of HAV is approximately 1 case per 100,000 children under the age of 5 years and 1.8 cases per 100,000 children aged 5–24. The incidence of HBV in children younger than 15 years of age is 0.03 cases per 100,000 children, and few cases of HCV were reported in children less than 15 years (Centers for Disease Control and Prevention, 2007b).

Etiology

The most common causes of hepatitis are the five hepatotropic viruses with corresponding names to the type of hepatitis that each virus causes—HAV, HBV, HCV, HDV, and HEV (Buggs & Lim, 2006). Hepatitis also can be a complication of other viral infections caused by cytomegalovirus (CMV), Epstein-Barr virus (EBV), herpes simplex virus (HSV), varicella zoster virus (VZV), enteroviruses (coxsackieviruses), echoviruses, rubella, (rubivirus), adenovirus, and parvovirus (referred to as fifth disease) (Children's Hospital Central California, 2006).

Clinical Manifestations

Flulike symptoms

Fever

Nausea and/or vomiting

Decreased appetite

Malaise

Abdominal pain or discomfort

Diarrhea

Joint and muscle pain

Itchy red hives on skin

Dark urine

Jaundice of eyes and skin

Diagnostic Tests

Liver function studies

Serum antibody studies

Complete blood count

Coagulation studies

Serum electrolytes

Ultrasonography

Abdominal computed tomography

Medical Management

The goals of management are preventing the disease, preventing its transmission, and maintaining optimal liver function. The primary method of preventing HAV is included in the new recommendations from the Centers for Disease Control and Prevention (CDC)—that the vaccine for HAV for children be given at age 1 and that high-risk children receive the HAV series between the ages of 2 and 18 years (CDC, 2007a). High-risk children include those living in areas of the country where the infection rate of HAV is above the national average. According to the American Academy of Pediatrics, these areas include Arizona, Alaska, Oregon, New Mexico, Utah, Washington, Oklahoma, South Dakota, Idaho, Nevada, and California. Other at-risk children are those living in areas where there has been a community outbreak, children with hemophilia, children attending child care centers that have had outbreaks of HAV, and children with chronic liver disease. To prevent HBV infections, a three-injection immunization series is recommended beginning with the first vaccination at birth, the second between 1 and 2 months of age, and the third between the ages of 6 and 18 months (Centers for Disease Control and Prevention, 2007a).

The best approach to preventing the spread of hepatitis is to educate the public about risk factors, that is, teaching children and those who care for them the importance of using appropriate hygiene measures. People should avoid crowded, unhealthy living conditions and take extra measures, particularly when drinking and swimming in areas of the world where sanitation is poor and water quality is uncertain. Shellfish that come from water sources that may be contaminated by sewage should be avoided; and using antiseptic cleansers to clean any toilet, sink, potty-chair, or bedpan used by someone in the family who develops hepatitis should be encouraged. Educating teens about the risks of drug use and unprotected sexual activities is an important component in any educational approach.

Children who have been exposed to a person with HAV should receive immune globulin within two weeks of the exposure. When administered within this time frame, immune globulin has demonstrated effectiveness in preventing the disease 80–90% of the time. Children exposed to HBV should receive the HBV immune globulin (HBIG) within two weeks of exposure. This agent has been shown to effectively prevent the child from developing HBV.

Treatment for hepatitis is primarily supportive. Physical rest is one of the most important components of care. This provides the liver time to heal by decreasing metabolic demands and increasing hepatic blood supply. Dietary modifications to include high-carbohydrate and high-calorie food containing moderate fat provides for healing and for growth and development needs. The use of pharmacological therapy may be indicated depending on the age of the child and the symptoms experienced. Antiemetic agents (lorazepam) may be prescribed to control nausea and vomiting. Biologic response modifiers have been approved by the FDA for use in treating HBV. These include interferon; and for children over 18 years of age, the newest agent, peginterferon alfa-2b, is available. In severe cases in children, antiviral agents such as ribavirin and lamivudine may be used in the treatment of HBV or HCV (Broyles, Reiss, & Evans, 2007).

Nursing Management

ASSESSMENT

1. Obtain client history
2. Assess parental knowledge of CDC's recommended immunization schedule
3. Assess child for manifestations of hepatitis
4. Obtain height, weight, and vital signs
5. Complete physical assessment
6. Assess psychosocial impact of disease on parents/child

NURSING DIAGNOSES (INCLUDING BUT NOT LIMITED TO)

1. Risk for infection R/T transmission of hepatitis viruses
2. Fatigue R/T disease process
3. Imbalanced nutrition: less than body requirements R/T decreased intake and increased metabolic demands
4. Deficient knowledge R/T prevention, causes, transmission, treatment, and home care

PLANNING/GOALS

1. Client will receive appropriate immunizations according to the CDC's recommended immunization schedule. Client will not become infected with the hepatitis virus.

2. Client will gradually increase activity level as fatigue decreases with rest.
3. Client will consume at least 90% of high-carbohydrate, high-calorie diet.
4. Parents and client (if age-appropriate) will demonstrate understanding of prevention strategies, child's condition, transmission, treatment, and home care.

NOC

1. Risk Control, Immune Status
2. Energy Conservation
3. Nutritional Status: Nutrient Intake
4. Knowledge: Infection Control, Illness Care, Treatment, Health Promotion

IMPLEMENTATION

1. Risk for infection
   a. Assess parents' knowledge about recommended immunizations
   b. Provide parents with CDC's recommended immunization schedule
   c. Assess for risk behaviors
   d. Instruct parents/adolescents about risk behaviors
   e. Encourage parents to discuss hygiene practices in any day care center they are considering for their child
   f. Use universal (standard) precautions and meticulous hand washing
   g. Instruct parents/children about proper hand washing technique with emphasis on washing hands after using the toilet or anytime they come in contact with fecal material
   h. Evaluate parents/children when performing hand washing
   i. Instruct health care workers to be immunized against HBV
   j. Administer immunizations according to CDC schedule
   k. Administer appropriate immune globulin to child exposed to hepatitis (needs to be administered within two weeks of exposure) as prescribed
2. Fatigue
   a. Assess child's level of fatigue
   b. Encourage rest
   c. Explain to parents/child importance of rest to the healing process
   d. Provide for several rest periods throughout the day if hospitalized
   e. Encourage parents to assist child with activities of daily living (ADL)
   f. Assist with providing and encouraging use of age-appropriate diversionary activities
   g. Administer antiviral agents as prescribed
3. Nutrition
   a. Monitor child's weight
   b. Assess child's food likes and dislikes
   c. Monitor intake and output
   d. Provide frequent small meals that are high in carbohydrates and calories

  e. Maintain an environment conducive to eating by eliminating noise and noxious odors

  f. Encourage parents to bring in favorite foods

  g. Provide supplemental vitamins and nutritional supplements as prescribed

  h. Administer antiemetic agents as prescribed and indicated

 4. Parent/child teaching

  a. Assess parents' current level of knowledge

  b. Provide verbal and written information regarding:

   1) CDC's recommended immunization schedule

   2) Risk factors for contracting and transmitting hepatitis

   3) Instructions about risk-taking behaviors and ways to avoid risk factors

   4) Dietary modifications to enhance healing

   5) Importance of frequent rest periods

   6) Medication administration including importance of completing prescribed medication regimen

   7) Signs and symptoms of adverse effects of medications

   8) Signs and symptoms of worsening of condition

   9) Contact phone numbers for reporting signs and symptoms

   10) Importance of regular hand washing and appropriate technique

   11) Importance of follow-up with health care provider

  c. Provide sufficient time for client and family questions, answering them honestly

  d. Document teaching and client's/family's response

NIC

 1. Immunization/Vaccination Management

 2. Energy Management

 3. Nutrition Management, Nutritional Monitoring

 4. Teaching: Infection Control, Illness Care, Treatment, Health Education

EVALUATION

 1. Client receives appropriate immunizations according to the CDC's recommended immunization schedule. Client does not become infected with the hepatitis virus.

 2. Client gradually increases activity level as fatigue decreases with rest.

 3. Client consumes at least 90% of high-carbohydrate, high-calorie diet.

 4. Parents and client (if age-appropriate) demonstrate understanding of prevention strategies, child's condition, transmission, treatment, and home care.

References

Broyles, B. E. (2005). *Medical-surgical nursing clinical companion.* Durham, NC: Carolina Academic Press.

Broyles, B. E., Reiss, B. S., & Evans, M. E. (2007). *Pharmacological aspects of nursing care* (7th ed.). Clifton Park, NY: Delmar Cengage Learning.

Buggs, A. M., & Lim, J. K. (2006). *Hepatitis.* Retrieved May 16, 2007, from http://www.emedicine.com/emerg/topic244.htm

Centers for Disease Control and Prevention. (2007a). *Recommended immunization schedules for persons aged 0–18 years—United States, 2007*. Retrieved May 10, 2007, from http://www.cdc.gov/mmwr/preview/mmwrhtml/mm5551a7.htm?s_cid=mm5551a7_e#fig1

Centers for Disease Control and Prevention. (2007b). *Surveillance for acute viral hepatitis—United States, 2005*. Retrieved May 16, 2007, from http://www.cdc.gov/ncidod/diseases/hepatitis/resource/PDFs/SS5603%20eBook.pdf

Children's Hospital Central California. (2006). *Hepatitis*. Retrieved March 10, 2007, from http://www.childrenscentralcal.org/content.asp?id=2219&parent=1&groupid=G0049

Potts, N. L., & Mandleco, B. L. (2007). *Pediatric nursing: Caring for children and their families* (2nd ed.). Clifton Park, NY: Delmar Cengage Learning.

HIRSCHSPRUNG DISEASE

Definition

Hirschsprung disease (Hirschsprung's disease), also termed *congenital aganglionic megacolon,* is an absence of parasympathetic ganglion cells in the large intestines (Potts & Mandleco, 2007).

Pathophysiology

During embryonic development, precursor ganglion cells derived from the neural crest of the developing brain normally migrate to the small intestine by the 7th week of gestation and reach the colon by the 12th week of gestation. These neuroblasts colonize in the gastrointestinal tract to provide innervation for peristalsis. Hirschsprung disease results from abnormal migration of these neuroblasts and impaired colonization of the distal portion of the gastrointestinal tract. In approximately 75% of cases, the lack of ganglion cells is limited to the rectosigmoid section of the bowel (Hockenberry, 2005). This lack of parasympathetic innervation interrupts the signal from the brain required for peristalsis. Lack of peristalsis and atonic contraction of the lumen causes a functional bowel obstruction because fecal contents cannot move forward normally. This results in the intestine becoming partially or completely obstructed and expanding to a larger-than-normal size as peristaltic movements occurring proximal to the aganglionic portion continue to move bowel contents up to the point of lack of innervation. Refer to Figure 55-1.

The problems a child experiences with Hirschsprung disease depend on how much of the intestine has normal nerve cells present and how much of the intestine is aganglionic. Most infants with Hirschsprung disease are missing nerve cells in only

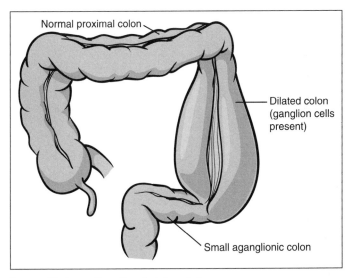

Figure 55-1: Hirschsprung Disease (Aganglionic Megacolon).

the last 1–2 feet of the large intestine; however, most infants have sufficient manifestations of bowel obstruction that 90% are diagnosed in the neonatal period (Lee & Puapong, 2006).

Eventually, a bacterial infection can develop in the digestive tract, causing serious problems. Severe worsening of the obstruction can lead to perforation and enterocolitis, which can carry a mortality rate as high as 30%. Untreated aganglionic megacolon in infancy may result in a mortality rate of as much as 80% compared to the very low mortality rate for the standard operative repairs for the disorder (Lee & Puapong, 2006). If a large segment lacks innervation, short gut syndrome occurs.

Complications

Perforation of the intestine
Enterocolitis
Short gut syndrome

Incidence

Hirschsprung disease occurs in 1 out of every 5,000 live births (Lucile Packard Children's Hospital at Stanford, 2007). The exact worldwide incidence is unknown. However, international studies have reported rates ranging from approximately 1 case per 1,500 newborns to 1 case per 7,000 newborns; it is rare in premature infants (Lee & Puapong, 2006). Hirschsprung disease is the cause for approximately 25% of all newborn intestinal obstruction and occurs 5 times more frequently in males than in females (MedlinePlus, 2007).

Etiology

The exact cause of Hirschsprung disease is not known; however, it is not considered a hereditary disorder even though inherited predisposition is relatively strong. "A family history can be obtained in about 7% of the cases, and the incidence in siblings is about 3.5%" (Potts & Mandleco, 2007, p. 674).

Clinical Manifestations

Failure to pass meconium stool within 24–48 hours after birth
Constipation
Abdominal distention
Vomiting
Watery diarrhea (in the newborn)
Poor weight gain
Slow growth in children 0–5 years of age
Malabsorption

Diagnostic Tests

Complete blood count
Chemistry panel
Abdominal radiography
Barium enema
Anal manometry
Rectal biopsy

Medical Management

All children with Hirschsprung disease require surgical treatment, so the goals of treatment are to surgically remove the aganglionic segment and return normal bowel function. The traditional repair is performed as a two-stage procedure. The first stage involves the creation of a colostomy during the neonatal period to relieve the obstruction and allow the megacolon to regain its tone. The second stage is performed when the infant is 6–15 months old or weighs 18–20 pounds. This procedure, called a pull-through, involves resecting or removing the aganglionic segment and anastomosing the normal bowel to the rectum and closing the colostomy.

Newer techniques are being used in some pediatric facilities. These include the one-stage pull-through procedure that resects the aganglionic portion and anatomoses the normal bowel to the rectum without the use of a temporary colostomy.

The newest procedure is the laparoscopic-assisted pull-through procedure that allows pediatric surgeons to enter the infant's body through the anus and pull the aganglionic segment of bowel through the opening without performing major abdominal surgery (Potts & Mandleco, 2007). This requires only one hospitalization and a much shorter hospital stay following the procedure. Both of the newer procedures show favorable results.

Nursing Management

ASSESSMENT

1. Obtain newborn history paying special attention to lack of passing meconium stool
2. Perform newborn assessment with focus on bowel assessment
3. Assess nutritional and hydration status
4. Obtain feeding history
5. Assess psychosocial impact on parents/family

NURSING DIAGNOSES (INCLUDING BUT NOT LIMITED TO)

1. Constipation R/T aganglionic colon obstruction
2. Risk for fluid volume deficit R/T malabsorption and surgical preparation
3. Impaired skin integrity R/T colostomy and surgical repair
4. Risk for infection R/T colostomy and surgical incision
5. Acute pain R/T surgical tissue trauma
6. Deficient knowledge R/T condition, treatment, and home and colostomy care

PLANNING/GOALS

1. Client will pass soft, formed stools without retention.
2. Client will experience fluid and electrolyte balance as evidenced by serum electrolyte levels within defined limits (WDL), urine output > 1–2 mL/kg/hr or six to eight wet diapers/day, and moist mucous membranes.
3. Client's skin will not experience breakdown and will regain and maintain integrity within six weeks following surgery.
4. Client will not experience infection around colostomy or surgical incision.
5. Client will demonstrate pain control as evidenced by ability to sleep and other behavioral indicators.
6. Parents will demonstrate understanding of condition, treatment, and colostomy and home care.

NOC

1. Bowel Elimination
2. Fluid Balance

3. Wound Healing: Primary Intention
4. Infection Control
5. Comfort Level
6. Knowledge: Illness Care, Treatment, Infant Care, Ostomy Care

IMPLEMENTATION

1. Bowel elimination
   a. Assess bowel sounds
   b. Assess characteristics of stools if present
   c. Assess for passage of meconium stool
   d. Measure abdominal girth
   e. Prepare infant/child for surgical repair and/or placement of colostomy
2. Fluid balance
   a. Maintain strict intake and output
   b. Monitor urine specific gravity
   c. Maintain nothing by mouth (npo) status preoperatively for age-appropriate time interval
   d. Initiate and maintain intravenous access, monitoring at least hourly
   e. Administer intravenous fluids as prescribed for hydration preoperatively and postoperatively until able to take fluids orally
   f. Begin oral fluids with electrolyte solution (Pedialyte or Infalyte)
3. Skin integrity
   a. Administer neomycin 1.0% solution preoperatively as prescribed
   b. Place a 4 x 4 gauze pad over colostomy, which may be sufficient initially to absorb colostomy drainage; hold in place with diaper
   c. Monitor vital signs every 4 hours; *do not take rectal temperature*
   d. Assess colostomy site immediately postoperatively and then every 2 hours
   e. Monitor colostomy for color and bleeding
   f. Assess skin surrounding colostomy for breakdown every two hours
   g. Assess anal area after pull-through for patency of any appliance that may be in place
   h. Collaborate with enterostomal therapist for colostomy and skin care
   i. Use appropriately sized hypoallergenic stoma supplies
   j. Provide meticulous skin care
4. Risk for infection
   a. Monitor infant's temperature every 4 hours during hospitalization
   b. Monitor vital signs
   c. Maintain patency of intravenous access, monitoring at least hourly
   d. Administer intravenous antimicrobials as prescribed
   e. Administer intravenous fluids as prescribed
   f. Weigh daily
   g. Monitor colostomy and surrounding skin for evidence of infection
   h. Monitor surgical incision for color, approximation, and drainage

5. Acute pain
    a. Assess pain level at least hourly using age-appropriate pain scale
    b. Administer analgesics proactively on scheduled basis as prescribed: intravenous analgesics are preferred; if using opiates, place infant on cardiorespiratory monitor
    c. Position for comfort
    d. Encourage parental involvement in care including holding, cuddling, and rocking
    e. Collaborate with health care provider if pain is not controlled
    f. Assess sleep pattern and avoid unnecessary interruptions of sleep
    g. Provide pacifier for infant
6. Parent teaching
    a. Assess parents' current level of knowledge
    b. Provide verbal and written instructions and demonstrations (as applicable) regarding:
        1) Surgical repair and recovery expectations
        2) Colostomy care and parental return demonstration prior to discharge
        3) Skin care
        4) Diet
        5) Infant care
        6) Medication administration (if prescribed)
        7) Referrals
        8) Symptoms to report to health care provider
        9) Contact number for health care provider and referral contacts
        10) Importance of follow-up care
    c. Provide adequate time for teaching, giving demonstrations, and observing return demonstrations; providing parental support; and encouraging verbalization of feelings and concerns
    d. Document teaching and parental response

NIC

1. Bowel Management
2. Fluid Management, Fluid Monitoring
3. Wound Care
4. Infection Precautions
5. Pain Management
6. Teaching: Illness Care, Treatment, Infant Care, Ostomy Care

EVALUATION

1. Client passes soft, formed stools without retention.
2. Client experiences fluid and electrolyte balance as evidenced by serum electrolyte levels WDL, urine output > 1–2 mL/kg/hr or six to eight wet diapers/day, and moist mucous membranes.
3. Client's skin does not experience breakdown and regains and maintains integrity within six weeks following surgery.
4. Client does not experience infection around colostomy or surgical incision.

5. Client demonstrates pain control as evidenced by ability to sleep and other behavioral indicators.

6. Parents demonstrate understanding of condition, treatment, and colostomy and home care.

References

Hockenberry, M. J. (2005). *Wong's essentials of pediatric nursing* (7th ed.). St. Louis, MO: Elsevier Mosby.

International Foundation for Functional Gastrointestinal Disorders. (2007). Retrieved March 31, 2008, from http://www.aboutconstipation.org/site/about-constipation/treatment/hirschsprungs-disease

Lee, S. L., & Puapong, D. (2006). *Hirschsprung disease*. Retrieved February 22, 2007, from http://www.emedicine.com/med/topic1016.htm

Lucile Packard Children's Hospital at Stanford. (2007). *Digestive and liver disorders: Hirschsprung's disease*. Retrieved February 20, 2007, from http://www.lpch.org/DiseaseHealthInfo/HealthLibrary/digest/hirschpr.html

MedlinePlus. (2007). *Hirschsprung's disease*. Retrieved February 21, 2008, from http://www.nlm.nih.gov/medlineplus/ency/article/001140.htm

Potts, N. L., & Mandleco, B. L. (2007). *Pediatric nursing: Caring for children and their families* (2nd ed.). Clifton Park, NY: Delmar Cengage Learning.

Hodgkin's Disease (Hodgkin's Lymphoma)

Definition

"Hodgkin's disease is a malignant neoplasm of lymphoid tissue first identified by Dr. Thomas Hodgkin in 1832" (Broyles, 2005, p. 434).

Pathophysiology

The lymphatic (lymph) system of the body is made up of lymph fluid containing lymphocyte cells, lymph vessels that carry lymph fluid throughout the body, and lymph nodes. Lymph nodes are located in the axilla, groin, neck, chest, and abdomen. They act as filters for the lymph fluid as it circulates through the body, and make and store lymphocytes. Also a part of the lymph system, the spleen is composed primarily of mature and immature lymphocytes and removes old cells and debris from the vascular system. The bone marrow and thymus also are parts of the lymph system. The thymus is a small organ in the chest that develops T cell lymphocytes, a major component of the immune system.

Due to how widespread the lymphatic tissue is in the body, Hodgkin's disease can initiate almost anywhere; however, it usually originates in the cervical lymph node before infiltrating into other parts of the lymph system. The cancer cells associated with Hodgkin's disease are called Reed-Sternberg cells, "distinctive giant cells with one or two large nuclei" (Rogers, 2005, p. 57).

The different types of Hodgkin's disease include (1) lymphocyte predominant, (2) nodular sclerosis, (3) mixed cellular, (4) lymphocyte depleting, (5) unclassified, and (6) nodular lymphocyte predominant. All of these forms are malignant, meaning that they grow, invade, compress, and destroy normal tissue and spread to other tissues (American Cancer Society, 2007).

To complete the diagnosis of Hodgkin's disease, the disease must be classified according to its stage. Stage I indicates that the disease is located in only one lymph node area or is localized. Stage II means that the disease is found in two or more lymph node areas on the same side of the diaphragm or that it has extended from the lymph node(s) to surrounding tissue. Stage III is characterized by the disease being found on both sides of the diaphragm or having extended into an adjacent organ or the spleen. Finally, stage IV (the most severe form of the disease) indicates that disease has metastasized to one or more organs outside the lymph system, most commonly the bone marrow or the liver (American Cancer Society, 2007).

Hodgkin's disease also can be progressive or recurrent. Progressive means that it spreads farther while the child is still being treated; recurrent means that the disease has returned weeks or years after the initial diagnosis. Refer to Figure 56-1.

Complications

Infection

Organ involvement

Organ failure

Incidence

Hodgkin disease is rare in children before 5 years of age. About 10–15% of cases are diagnosed in children 16 years of age and younger. However, the highest incidence is in adults in their mid to late twenties or after the age of 50 (Potts & Mandleco, 2007).

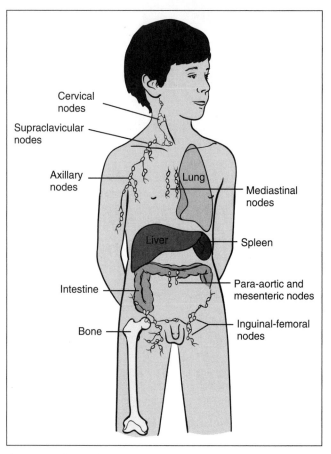

Figure 56-1: Lymph Nodes Affected by Hodgkin's Disease.

Etiology

The exact cause of Hodgkin's disease is unknown. However, preliminary research indicates that children who contract certain viruses (Epstein-Barr or HIV) or any condition that reduces the child's immune status have an increased incidence. The correlation has not been identified though (American Cancer Society, 2007).

Clinical Manifestations

Painless enlargement of the lymph nodes in neck, underarm, groin, and
   chest

Dyspnea secondary to enlarged nodes in the chest

Fever

Night sweats

Fatigue

Weight loss

Anorexia

Pruritus

Frequent viral infections

Diagnostic Tests

Excisional or incisional biopsy

Fine needle aspiration (FNA) biopsy

Diagnostic tests for the staging of Hodgkin's disease:

Chest radiography

Computed tomography

Magnetic resonance imaging

Gallium scan

Positron emission tomography (PET)

Lymphangiogram

Complete blood count

Bone biopsy and aspiration

Medical Management

The goal of treatment is to cure the condition while minimizing adverse or long-term effects of the disease or its treatment. The National Cancer Institute states that children and adolescents with any type of cancer should be treated in a children's cancer center. The approach to treatment is multidisciplinary and requires those professionals who are most familiar with the differences between children and adults, among them child psychologists, child life specialists, nutritionists, pediatric oncologists, and pediatric educators (National Cancer Institute, 2006).

Chemotherapy and radiation are the standards of care for the treatment of Hodgkin's disease. However, if the child has not reached physical maturity or has a smaller body size than an adult, chemotherapy is the treatment of choice. This is because radiation affects bone and muscle growth in children. Radiation must be administered in low doses for children, so the regimen for children must include chemotherapy.

The chemotherapy regimens usually are combinations of four drugs. The first of these is ABVD (adriamycin, bleomycin, vinblastine, and dacarbazine); the second is MOPP (mechlorethamine, oncovin, procarbazine, and prednisone) (Broyles, Reiss, & Evans, 2007). The success of this combined approach is excellent, demonstrating a cure rate of 85–100% in children with more advanced disease (American Cancer Society, 2007).

Bone marrow transplantation may be considered in the small number of cases in which the chemotherapy/low-dose radiation did not eradicate the disease. Two types of transplants are considered. The autologous bone marrow transplant involves harvesting the child's bone marrow and freezing it. Then the marrow is subjected to very high doses of chemotherapy (with or without radiation therapy) to destroy the cancer cells. Following the high-dose chemotherapy treatments, the bone marrow is thawed and administered back into the child intravenously.

Peripheral blood stem cell transplant also is autologous. However, with this procedure (leukapheresis), a phoresis machine collects small amounts of the child's blood, removes the stem cells, and returns the rest of the blood and blood products back to the child. Stem cell transplantation has been shown to be more effective when used earlier in treatment. This course is not recommended unless the first treatments do not eradicate the disease. On the other hand, if the disease relapses after a long-time remission, the first course of treatment still would be chemotherapy before a transplant would be recommended (American Cancer Society, 2007).

Nursing Management

Refer to Chapter 22: Chemotherapy and Chapter 87: Radiation Therapy.

References

American Cancer Society. (2007). *Hodgkin's disease in children.* Retrieved February 21, 2008, from http://www.cancer.org/docroot/CRI/content/CRI_2_2_1X_What_is_Hodgkins_disease_20.asp?sitearea=CRI

Broyles, B. E. (2005). *Medical-surgical nursing clinical companion.* Durham, NC: Carolina Academic Press.

Broyles, B. E., Reiss, B. S., & Evans, M. E. (2007). *Pharmacological aspects of nursing care* (7th ed.). Clifton Park, NY: Delmar Cengage Learning.

National Cancer Institute. (2006). *Childhood Hodgkin's lymphoma treatment (PDR).* Retrieved March 11, 2007, from http://www.cancer.gov/cancertopics/pdq/treatment/childhodgkins/healthprofessional/allpages

Potts, N. L., & Mandleco, B. L. (2007). *Pediatric nursing: Caring for children and their families* (2nd ed.). Clifton Park, NY: Delmar Cengage Learning.

Rogers, B. (2005). Looking at lymphoma and leukemia. *Nursing, 35*(7).

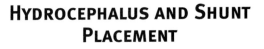

HYDROCEPHALUS AND SHUNT PLACEMENT

Definition

Hydrocephalus is an accumulation of cerebrospinal fluids (CSFs) in the brain's ventricular system resulting from increased production, impaired absorption, or blockage in the draining of CSF.

Pathophysiology

The cranial vault contains three components—the brain, intravascular blood, and CSF. The brain comprises 80% of the vault space, the intravascular volume is 10%, and CSF makes up the other 10%. According to the Monro-Kellie hypothesis, "When the volume of one component changes, there must be a compensatory change in another component in order to maintain constant volume" (Zomorodi, 2007, p. 3).

Normally, CSF circulates through the ventricles from the choroid plexus to the lateral ventricles. It then flows through the interventricular foramen of Monro to the third ventricle, the cerebral aqueduct of Sylvius, the fourth ventricle, the two lateral foramina of Luschka and one medial foramen of Magendie, the subarachnoid space surrounding the brain and spinal cord, the arachnoid granulations, and the dural sinus and finally into the venous drainage (Hord, 2006). With hydrocephalus, the CSF increases in volume, causing compression to the brain and its vascular supply. This can result in permanent damage to the neurons, resulting in damage to the cerebral and/or cerebellar structures and functions. Refer to Figure 57-1.

Hydrocephalus in children usually is congenital, occurring during the embryonic development of the cranial structures, and is classified as communicating or noncommunicating. In communicating hydrocephalus, an obstruction outside the ventricular system causes decreased absorption of CSF in the subarachnoid space at the subarachnoid villi (Potts & Mandleco, 2007).

Most fetal hydrocephalus is noncommunicating, resulting in an inability of the CSF to flow through the ventricles normally. This occurs due to a congenital malformation. Aqueductal stenosis, myelomeningocele, an obstruction in the foramina of Luschka and Magendie (Dandy-Walker syndrome), or Arnold-Chiari malformation/deformity (a defect in the posterior fossa allowing herniation of the cerebellum, medulla, pons, and fourth ventricle down into the cervical spine) predispose the child to hydrocephalus (Potts & Mandleco, 2007). Hydrocephalus in older children may be the result of injury, intracranial hemorrhage, or brain tumors.

With CSF unable to drain, the volume increases in the cranial vault, causing pressure against brain structures including compression of the cranial vasculature. As pressure (intracranial pressure, or ICP) increases, manifestations of the rising pressure and the resulting neuron damage emerge. Refer to Chapter 61: Increased Intracranial Pressure.

Complications

Intrauterine death
Motor dysfunction
Cognitive dysfunction
Sensory dysfunction
Vegetative state

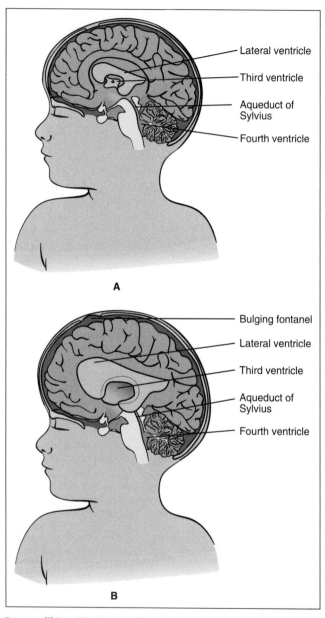

Lateral ventricle

Third ventricle

Aqueduct of Sylvius

Fourth ventricle

A

Bulging fontanel

Lateral ventricle

Third ventricle

Aqueduct of Sylvius

Fourth ventricle

B

Figure 57-1: **(A)** Normal Sized Ventricles, **(B)** Enlarged Ventricles Associated with Hydrocephalus.

Incidence

Incidence and prevalence data are difficult to establish as there is no existing national registry or database of people with hydrocephalus and closely associated disorders; however, hydrocephalus is believed to affect approximately 1 in every 500 children (National Institute of Neurological Disorders and Stroke, 2007). Most hydrocephalus is obstructive. An estimated 56,600 children and adolescents younger than 18 years have a ventriculoperitoneal (VP) shunt in place (Kramer & Azarow, 2007).

Etiology

The cause of hydrocephalus depends on the type of hydrocephalus the infant/child has. Communicating hydrocephalus most often is caused by defective absorption of CSF, although it also can result from overproduction of CSF (rare) or insufficient venous drainage of CSF. "An example of communicating hydrocephalus caused by CSF overproduction is the presence of choroid plexus papilloma in one of the ventricles. Examples of conditions with communicating hydrocephalus caused by impaired CSF absorption include IVH [intraventricular hemorrhage], meningitis, and head injury. Occasionally, obstructive and communicating hydrocephalus coexist and therefore cannot be differentiated" (Kramer & Azarow, 2007, Section 2).

Noncommunicating hydrocephalus occurs when CSF flow is obstructed within the ventricular system or in its outlets to the arachnoid space. Obstructive hydrocephalus is caused by obstruction of the flow of intraventricular or extraventricular CSF (Hord, 2006). Examples of conditions associated with obstructive hydrocephalus include congenital aqueductal stenosis, tumors of the ventricular system (colloid cyst of the third ventricle and astrocytoma of the third ventricle), and tumors of the posterior cranial fossa (cerebellar astrocytoma and medulloblastoma) (Kramer & Azarow, 2007, Section 2).

Clinical Manifestations

NEONATES/INFANTS: EARLY SIGNS

Bulging fontanels, most prominent in the anterior fontanel

Widely separated cranial sutures

Distended scalp veins

Increase head circumference

Thinning cranial bones

Poor feedings

Irritability

NEONATES/INFANTS: LATE SIGNS

Setting-sun sign—sclera visible above the iris

Frontal bone enlargement, or bossing

Vomiting

Altered respiratory pattern

Shrill, high-pitched cry

Sluggish and nonreactive pupils

Refer to Chapter 61: Increased Intracranial Pressure

CHILD: EARLY SIGNS

Strabismus

Frontal headache

Nausea and projectile vomiting

Diplopia

Restlessness and altered mental status

Personality changes

Ataxia

Papilledema

Sluggish and unequal papillary reaction to light

Neck pain indicating herniation

CHILD: LATE SIGNS

Elevated blood pressure

Bradycardia

Altered respirations

Seizures

Lethargy

Vomiting

Posturing (decerebrate)

Blindness

Diagnostic Tests

Prenatal ultrasonography

Radiography

Computed tomography

Magnetic resonance imaging

Pressure monitoring

Medical Management

The goals of treatment are to provide an alternative drainage path for the CSF and to prevent or reduce disability and death related to damage from increased ICP. To effectively achieve these goals, an alternative drainage path for the CSF needs to be established.

Surgical placement of a shunt system diverts the flow of CSF from a site within the central nervous system to an extracranial compartment where it can be absorbed into the circulatory system. Shunt placement is needed in at least 75% of hydrocephalus cases.

A shunt is a flexible but sturdy silastic tube that extends from the brain, lying under the skin, to the extracranial compartment. A shunt system is comprised of the shunt, a catheter, and a valve that maintains one-way movement of CSF and regulates its rate flow. When pressure in the brain increases above normal, the one-way valve opens, allowing the excess CSF to drain to the extracranial compartment, most commonly the peritoneum (VP shunt). Refer to Figure 57-2. After the shunt is inserted, the child should not be placed in an upright position to prevent overdrainage of CSF (Kramer & Azarow, 2007).

In children who experience recurrent failure of the VP shunt, the right atria of the heart can serve as the extracranial compartment (ventriculoatrial, VA, shunt) (National Institute of Neurological Disorders and Stroke, 2007). The VA shunt drains excess CSF from the cerebral ventricles through the jugular vein and superior vena cava into the right atrium. The disadvantages of this shunt include risk of cardiac dysrhythmias from the shunt moving and stimulating the myocardial muscle, risk of cardiac/pulmonary fluid overload, and repeated lengthening of the shunt to accommodate the child's growth.

The most frequent causes of shunt failure are infection (most common), kinking of the catheter, and the child's growth. To prevent the infant/child from outgrowing the shunt, pediatric neurosurgeons place a coiled shunt in the peritoneal cavity; the shunt uncoils as the child grows in height. Early detection of shunt failure (manifestations of increased ICP) and prompt medical attention is necessary. Hospitalization and administration of systemic antimicrobial agents are the first medical interventions used to treat shunt infections. If the therapy is not effective, intrathecal administration through a surgically placed external ventriculostomy system may be required. In addition, this system serves as a temporary drainage mechanism for the ventricles until the infection resolves and the VP shunt can be revised. Meticulous monitoring and maintenance of this system is needed because

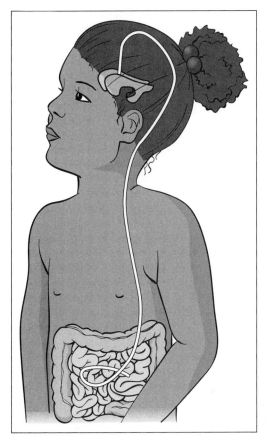

Figure 57-2: Ventriculoperitoneal Shunt.

its function is based on gravitational draining of the CFS from the ventricle. To prevent too much or too little CSF from draining through the ventriculostomy tube, the drainage system must be maintained at the level of the canthus of the ear (parallel to the ventricle).

Frequently, drugs are used to slow the production of CSF and temporarily reduce pressure in the brain until a shunt can be inserted. These agents include cetazolamide, furosemide, glycerol, digoxin, and isosorbide.

In a small number of infants/children with noncommunicating hydrocephalus (where there is a blockage of the passages that connect the ventricles), the surgical placement of a direct connection between one of the ventricles and the subarachnoid space can be inserted, allowing the fluid to drain without a shunt.

An alternative procedure called third ventriculostomy is used with a small number of children. In this procedure, a neuroendoscope is used to visualize the surface of the ventricle. The scope is guided into position so that a small hole can be bored in the floor of the third ventricle, allowing the CSF to bypass the obstruction and flow to the subarachnoid space for absorption.

The success in treating hydrocephalus depends on what its etiology is; how early in its course it was diagnosed and treated; and what, if any, coexisting conditions are present.

Close monitoring for shunt malfunction, rehabilitative therapies, and educational interventions are part of the multidisciplinary approach of the care of these children.

Nursing Management

Refer to Chapter 61: Increased Intracranial Pressure.

ASSESSMENT

1. Compare the head and chest circumference in the neonate
2. Palpate the anterior fontanel for size, bulging, and tenseness
3. Assess cranial suture separation
4. Assess for manifestations of increased ICP
5. Assess for level of consciousness (LOC), personality changes, interaction with the environment, sleep patterns, and developmental milestones in older child

NURSING DIAGNOSES (INCLUDING BUT NOT LIMITED TO)

1. Risk for ineffective cerebral tissue perfusion R/T inadequate circulation of CSF
2. Risk for infection R/T shunt placement
3. Acute pain R/T surgical shunt placement
4. Risk for delayed growth and development R/T neuron damage from increased ICP
5. Deficient parental knowledge R/T infant's/child's condition, treatment, and home care

PLANNING/GOALS

1. Client will maintain effective tissue perfusion as evidenced by presence and response of newborn reflexes, pediatric Glasgow Coma Scale and vital signs within defined limits (WDL), and age-appropriate behavior and thought processes.
2. Client will not experience shunt malfunction from infection as evidenced by temperature and central nervous system (CNS) function WDL.
3. Client will demonstrate effective pain management as evidenced by age-appropriate verbal and behavioral pain indicators.
4. Client will not experience delayed growth and development as evidenced by achieving developmental milestones.
5. Parents will demonstrate understanding of child's condition, treatment, and home care.

NOC

1. Neurologic Status
2. Risk Control
3. Pain Control
4. Child Development
5. Knowledge: Illness Care, Treatment, Health Promotion

IMPLEMENTATION

1. Cerebral tissue perfusion
   a. Establish neurologic baseline assessment including newborn reflexes, LOC, vital signs, and developmental milestones (child)
   b. Monitor anterior fontanel
   c. Monitor cranial sutures
   d. Monitor head circumference

    e. Place neonate in warming bed, monitoring continuous skin temperature

    f. Warm to prescribed body temperature (to decrease metabolic demands and ICP)

    g. Maintain head of crib/bed at 30–45 degrees

    h. Avoid prone position, neck flexion, and hip flexion

    i. Monitor neurologic status every hour and more often if condition indicates

    j. Assess for irritability and lethargy

    k. Place emergency equipment within easy access

    l. Monitor intake and output hourly

    m. Notify health care provider if urine output < 1 mL/kg/hr

    n. Establish and maintain intravenous access devices, monitoring at least hourly

    o. Administer medications as prescribed

    p. Monitor urine specific gravity each void

2. Risk for infection

    a. Assess temperature at least every 2 hours

    b. Monitor for heat, redness, and swelling along the shunt track under the skin

    c. Administer antipyretics as prescribed

    d. Perform neurologic assessments every 2 hours

    e. Assess head/abdominal dressings

    f. Position child off the shunt site for a minimum of the first two postoperative days

    g. Maintain intravenous access device, monitoring at least hourly

    h. Administer antimicrobial agents as prescribed. *NOTE:* Intravenous antimicrobial agents are particularly irritating to peripheral vessels and must be administered slowly through these accesses.

    i. Instruct parents about dressing changes (if needed) and signs of shunt infection and malfunction

3. Pain management

    a. Assess infant/child hourly for verbal and behavioral indicators of pain

    b. Administer pain medications on a regular schedule for 24–48 hours postoperatively. *NOTE:* Pain increases ICP.

    c. Place infant on cardiopulmonary monitor during time of opioid use for pain

    d. Hold, cuddle, and use diversionary therapy with child

    e. Encourage parental participation in care

    f. Provide calm, quiet environment that is conducive to low anxiety and encourages rest

    g. Reassure parents that infant/child will not become "addicted" to pain medication

4. Growth and development

    a. Assess neonate for presence and responsiveness of newborn reflexes

    b. Assess infant's/child's level of growth and development

    c. Instruct parents about age- and developmentally-appropriate play

    d. Collaborate with recreation therapists

    e. Encourage parental involvement in care

    f.   Assist parents to identify referrals they need to facilitate child's growth and development

5. Parent teaching

    a.   Assess parents' level of understanding

    b.   Provide verbal and written information regarding:

        1) Monitoring of child for indicators of increased ICP

        2) Medication administration if prescribed

        3) Monitoring of developmental milestones

        4) Age-appropriate play activities including avoidance of being overprotective and of allowing child to participate in contact sports

        5) Infant care

        6) Manifestations to report immediately to health care provider

        7) Contact number for health care provider and referral contact individuals

        8) Importance of lifelong follow-up care

    c.   Provide adequate time for teaching

    d.   Document teaching and parental response

NIC

1. Neurologic Monitoring
2. Infection Precautions
3. Pain Management
4. Infant Care, Developmental Enhancement: Child
5. Teaching: Illness Care, Treatment, Health Promotion

EVALUATION

1. Client maintains effective tissue perfusion as evidenced by presence and response of newborn reflexes, pediatric Glasgow Coma Scale and vital signs WDL, and age-appropriate behavior and thought processes.

2. Client does not experience shunt malfunction from infection as evidenced by temperature and CNS function WDL.

3. Client demonstrates effective pain management as evidenced by age-appropriate verbal and behavioral pain indicators.

4. Client does not experience delayed growth and development as evidenced by achieving developmental milestones.

5. Parents demonstrate understanding of child's condition, treatment, and home care.

References

Hord, E. (2006). *Hydrocephalus*. Retrieved March 11, 2007, from http://www.emedicine.com/NEURO/topic161.htm

Kramer, L. C., & Azarow, K. (2007). *Management of spina bifida, hydrocephalus and shunts*. Retrieved May 16, 2007, from http://www.emedicine.com/ped/topic2976.htm

National Institute of Neurological Disorders and Stroke. (2007). *Hydrocephalus fact sheet*. Retrieved March 11, 2007, from http://www.ninds.nih.gov/disorders/hydrocephalus/detail_hydrocephalus.htm#83433125

Potts, N. L., & Mandleco, B. L. (2007). *Pediatric nursing: Caring for children and their families* (2nd ed.). Clifton Park, NY: Delmar Cengage Learning.

Zomorodi, M. (2007, March). *ICP management*. Paper presented at the meeting of the University of North Carolina School of Nursing, Chapel Hill, NC.

58

Hypoplastic Left Heart Syndrome (HLHS)/Heart Transplantation

Definition

Hypoplastic left heart syndrome (HLHS) "encompasses a variety of deformities characterized by lack of the development of the left ventricle (during fetal development) secondary to mitral valve atresia or aortic atresia" (Potts & Mandleco, 2007, p. 787). Refer to Figure 58-1.

Pathophysiology

In HLHS, "the mitral and aortic valves are usually tiny or absent, as are the left ventricle and the first part of the aorta. Perhaps the most critical defect in HLHS is the small, underdeveloped left ventricle" (Congenital Heart Defects.com, 2006, p. 1). In a normal heart, the left ventricle is strong and muscular so it can pump blood to the body. When this chamber is small and poorly developed, it cannot pump effectively and cannot provide enough blood flow to meet tissue perfusion and metabolic needs of the body. For this reason, an infant with HLHS will not live long without surgical intervention.

Blood flow with HLHS is altered. Systemic venous return enters the right atria and flows through the tricuspid valve to the right ventricle, flows out the pulmonary artery

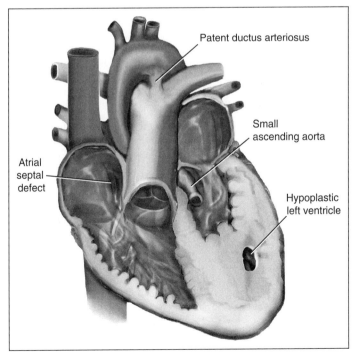

Patent ductus arteriosus

Small ascending aorta

Atrial septal defect

Hypoplastic left ventricle

Figure 58-1: Hypoplastic Left Heart Syndrome.

to the lungs, and then returns oxygenated blood to the left atria. At this point, because of atresia of the mitral valve and hypoplasia of the left ventricle, the blood cannot flow into the left ventricle. Consequently, it shunts from the left atria to the right atria through a patent foramen ovale. The only way blood can exit the heart via the aorta is by retrograde flow across a patent ductus arteriosus. As previously noted, cardiac output is insufficient to provide adequate tissue perfusion and an infant with this defect will not survive without surgical treatment.

Complications

Decreased cardiac output
Inadequate tissue perfusion
Death

Incidence

HLHS occurs in approximately 1–2% of all congenital heart defects (CHD). It is the leading cause of cardiac death in the infant less than 1 month old (Potts & Mandleco, 2007, p. 787). As many as 1.6–3.6 infants out of every 10,000 live births have HLHS (Rao & Turner, 2006). "It is one of the top three heart abnormalities to cause problems in the newborn. HLHS occurs slightly more often in boys than in girls" (Congenital Heart Defects.com, 2006, p. 1). According to the United Network for Organ Sharing, over 1,500 heart transplants have been performed on infants since 1988, with an average of 75 heart transplants per year in children under the age of 1 year. For all children 17 years of age and younger, over 4,300 heart transplants have been performed, with the lowest incidence in children 6–10 years old (OPTN: Organ Procurement and Transplantation Network, 2007).

Etiology

According to the American Heart Association, most of the time, the exact cause of congenital heart defects is unknown. Although the reason defects occur is presumed to be genetic, only a few genes have been discovered that have been linked to the presence of heart defects.

Heredity may play a role in HLHS as well as coexisting conditions such as Down syndrome or a mother contracting rubella during the first trimester of pregnancy. The mother's use of alcohol and illicit drugs during pregnancy increases the fetus's risk for developing HLHS (American Heart Association, 2007). "Hypoplastic left heart syndrome is the most common complex congenital heart defect for which a heart transplant is a potentially useful treatment" (American Heart Association, 2007, p. 1).

Clinical Manifestations

Cyanosis within hour of birth
Cardiovascular collapse
Hypotension
Tachycardia
Tachypnea

Diagnostic Tests

Chest radiography
Echocardiogram
Cardiac catheterization

Medical Management

For the neonate with HLHS to survive, surgical treatment is required. The most common procedure is "the Norwood"; it is a three-step procedure, the first stage being the

Norwood procedure. This is performed within the first few days of life. The second step is called the hemi-Fontan (which is frequently a bidirectional Glenn operation). It sends half the blood returning from the body to the lungs, reducing the workload on the heart. This second step is part of the preparation to transform the HLHS heart into a two-chamber pumping heart, which only functions to pump blood to the body. (After the third operation, all of the blood travels passively to the lungs.) The third operation, called the Fontan operation, is performed approximately 12 months after the hemi-Fontan procedure. "Completion of the Fontan procedure includes directing blood flow from the inferior vena cava to the pulmonary arteries by placing a tube within the right atrium. At the conclusion of the procedure, systemic venous blood returns to the lungs passively without passing through a ventricle" (Roa & Turner, 2006, Section 6).

Survival following a Norwood operation is approximately 80%, survival following a bidirectional Glenn operation is close to 100%, and survival following a Fontan operation is around 95%; the overall survival at 5 years of age is around 70–75% (Rao & Turner, 2006).

Another surgical procedure used to treat neonates/infants with HLHS is cardiac transplantation. Finally, the last surgical option is available only to a small percentage of HLHS children whose defect is reparable by a biventricular repair. Refer to Medical Management in Chapter 26: Congenital Heart Disease/Open Heart Surgery.

Cardiac transplantation involves the removal of the hypoplastic heart, which is replaced with a functioning donor heart. The infant's/child's major cardiac vessels (superior vena cava and aorta) are detached from the dysfunctional heart and connected to cardiopulmonary bypass. Following placement of the donor heart, the infant's major vessels are attached to the donor heart. The areas of connection are tested for leakage, and the open-heart surgery is completed. Because the donor heart is denervated and thus does not respond to autonomic stimulation, isoproterenol is needed to support the heart rate and cardiac output. Because of loss of vagal stimulation, the resting heart rate is faster than normal and takes longer to adapt to exercise and remains elevated longer after exercise ceases. The child receives immunosuppressant therapy for life including such medications as cyclosporine, tacrolimus, mycophenolate mofetil, prednisone, and azathioprine.

The transplant coordinator provides continuity for the child's outpatient care at the transplant center following heart transplantation. These professionals meet with families before, during, and after each transplant to educate and familiarize them with the hospital and outpatient settings.

Nursing Management

Refer to Nursing Management in Chapter 26: Congenital Heart Disease/Open Heart Surgery. Next is the Nursing Management of the Child Following Cardiac Transplantation (adapted from Broyles, 2005).

Nursing Management

ASSESSMENT

1. Obtain client history
2. Perform physical assessment
3. Assess preoperative laboratory values and diagnostic tests

NURSING DIAGNOSES (INCLUDING BUT NOT LIMITED TO)

1. Parental anxiety R/T complexity of heart transplantation, unknown future for child, and child being in the pediatric intensive care unit (PICU)
2. Decreased cardiac output R/T rejection, graft ischemia, and cardiac dysrhythmias
3. Ineffective protection R/T immunosuppressant therapy to prevent organ rejection

4. Risk for injury, complications R/T heart transplantation
5. Risk for ineffective health maintenance R/T lifelong immunosuppressant therapy, financial stressors of heart transplantation
6. Deficient parental knowledge R/T post transplantation hospital care, immunosuppressant therapy for life, infection protection, and home care

PLANNING/GOALS

1. Client's parents will demonstrate and verbalize a decrease in anxiety as evidenced by verbal and nonverbal cues.
2. Client will experience hemodynamic stability within 12–48 hours of transplant as evidenced by cardiac output, cardiac index, vital signs, oxygen saturation, and mixed venous oxygen saturation within defined limits (WDL).
3. Client will not experience infection as evidenced by body temperature WDL; however, if infection occurs, it will be treated promptly and effectively.
4. Client will not experience complications associated with cardiac transplantation and immunosuppressant therapy.
5. Parents will maintain immunosuppressant therapy and use resources available to them to maintain child's health.
6. Parents will demonstrate understanding of child's post transplantation hospital care, immunosuppressant therapy for life, infection protection, and home care.

NOC

1. Anxiety
2. Cardiac Pump Effectiveness
3. Immune Status
4. Risk Control
5. Knowledge: Health Promotion, Social Support
6. Knowledge: Infection Control, Medication, Health Promotion

IMPLEMENTATION

1. Parental pre- and post-transplant anxiety
   a. Encourage parents to verbalize fears and concerns
   b. Listen to their concerns
   c. Provide preoperative teaching to prepare parents for what to expect
   d. Refer questions appropriately
   e. Encourage parents to spend time with infant/child and participate in care
   f. Explain all medications, procedures, and equipment
2. Post-transplantation cardiac output
   a. Maintain continuous cardiorespiratory monitoring
   b. Maintain hemodynamic monitoring
   c. Maintain central venous access device, monitoring hourly
   d. Administer medications as prescribed, titrating to prescribed parameters
   e. Implement seizure precautions when administering high-dose steroids
   f. Wean intravenous medication infusions while maintaining hemodynamic parameters

    g. Administer intravenous volume expanders, monitoring closely for fluid overload

    h. Monitor laboratory results

    i. Auscultate heart sounds hourly during critical period

    j. Monitor peripheral pulses, capillary refill, and vital signs

    k. Monitor hourly urine output

    l. Maintain calm environment

    m. Keep parents informed of child's condition, encouraging them to visit PICU

    n. Administer immunosuppressant therapy as prescribed

3. Risk for infection

    a. Monitor continuous skin temperature during immediate postoperative period

    b. Monitor surgical incision for redness and drainage

    c. Maintain compromised host precautions following facility transplant protocols

    d. Limit visitors to child's healthy parents and grandparents; discourage children visitors

    e. Maintain meticulous asepsis during central venous access dressing changes

    f. Maintain meticulous hand washing

    g. Teach parents proper hand washing and compromised host precautions

    h. Report temperature elevations immediately to health care provider

4. Complications of cardiac transplantation

    a. Monitor for infection

    b. Monitor for hypertension and hypotension

    c. Monitor strict intake and output

    d. Monitor respiratory function

    e. Monitor renal function

    f. Monitor gastrointestinal function

    g. Monitor for cardiac changes secondary to loss of sympathetic and parasympathetic stimulation

    h. Provide information for parents concerning reasons for monitoring

5. Health maintenance

    a. Assess parental needs related to meeting child's health needs

    b. Collaborate with multidisciplinary team concerning identified needs

    c. Coordinate referrals to social worker, financial aid, dietician, occupational therapist, etc.

    d. Monitor parental feedback regarding services and needs being met

    e. Provide information regarding community and organ transplantation support services

    f. Encourage parental involvement in child's care, providing adequate time for providing information regarding child's care, medications, and infection protection

    g. Refer to "Parent discharge teaching"

6. Parent discharge teaching
   a. Assess parental level of understanding of home post transplantation care
   b. Provide verbal and written information regarding:
      1) Infant protection from infection
      2) Immunosuppressant medication administration
      3) Monitoring of infant's axillary temperature (avoiding rectal temperatures)
      4) Dressing changes as needed
      5) Manifestations of organ failure (increasing fatigue and decreased urine output)
      6) Adverse effects of immunosuppressant therapy
      7) Observations to report to health care provider immediately
      8) Referral information
      9) Contact numbers
      10) Importance of follow-up and long-term post transplant care
   c. Provide sufficient time for parental return demonstration of needed procedures and questions
   d. Document teaching and parental response

NIC

1. Anxiety Reduction
2. Cardiac Care, Hemodynamic Monitoring, Medication Administration, Vital Signs Monitoring
3. Infection Protection, Medication Administration, Risk Identification
4. Health Education, Risk Identification
5. Health Education, Risk Identification, Discharge Planning, Financial Resource Assistance
6. Health Education, Discharge Planning

EVALUATION

1. Client's parents demonstrate and verbalize a decrease in anxiety as evidenced by verbal and nonverbal cues.
2. Client experiences hemodynamic stability within 24 hours of transplant as evidenced by cardiac output, cardiac index, vital signs, oxygen saturation, and mixed venous oxygen saturation WDL.
3. Client does not experience infection as evidenced by body temperature WDL; however, if infection occurs, it is treated promptly and effectively.
4. Client does not experience complications associated with cardiac transplantation and immunosuppressant therapy.
5. Parents maintain immunosuppressant therapy and use resources available to them to maintain child's health.
6. Parents demonstrate understanding of child's post transplantation hospital care, immunosuppressant therapy for life, infection protection, and home care.

References

American Heart Association. (2007). *Heart transplants in infants and children.* Retrieved April 23, 2007, from http://www.americanheart.org/presenter.jhtml?identifier=4589

Broyles, B. E. (2005). *Medical-surgical nursing clinical companion.* Durham, NC: Carolina Academic Press.

Congenital Heart Defects.com. (2006). *Hypoplastic left heart syndrome.* Retrieved April 23, 2007, from http://www.congenitalheartdefects.com/typesofCHD.html#HLHS

OPTN: Organ Procurement and Transplantation Network. (2007). *Heart transplants in the U.S. by recipient age.* Retrieved February 25, 2008, from http://www.optn.org/latestData/rptData.asp

Potts, N. L., & Mandleco, B. L. (2007). *Pediatric nursing: Caring for children and their families* (2nd ed.). Clifton Park, NY: Delmar Cengage Learning.

Rao, P. S., & Turner, D. R. (2006). *Hypoplastic left heart syndrome.* Retrieved April 23, 2007, from http://www.emedicine.com/ped/topic1131.htm

59

IMMUNE (IDIOPATHIC) THROMBOCYTOPENIA PURPURA (ITP)

Definition

Idiopathic thrombocytopenia purpura (ITP) is a hematological bleeding disorder resulting from a deficiency in circulating platelets.

Pathophysiology

There are two classifications of thrombocytopenia purpura: intrinsic and immune. In children, the most common form is immune thrombocytopenia purpura, "formerly called idiopathic thrombocytopenia, but has since been found to be an autoimmune disorder. Consequently, the name was changed to reflect this discovery" (Potts & Mandleco, 2007, p. 844). Thrombocytopenia is the term meaning a deficiency in circulating platelets. Purpura is a condition characterized by small purple bruising occurring just beneath the skin or on the mucous membranes. Children with ITP also may have tiny hemorrhages that appear as tiny red or purple dots on the skin called petechiae (National Heart Lung and Blood Institute, 2007).

The function of platelets is to repair minute ruptures in the microcirculation. They adhere to each other and to the edges of the injured area, release chemical mediators at the site, and form a plug or clot. Minute ruptures in the microcirculation occur daily, and platelets are needed to make these repairs. In the presence of a deficiency in the numbers of platelets, these repairs cannot be made and purpura results.

In immune thrombocytopenia purpura, the deficiency of platelets results from an autoimmune response usually triggered by a viral infection. The autoimmune antibodies (proteins) "bind to the platelets causing them to become sequestered and destroyed prematurely in the spleen" (Potts & Mandleco, 2007, p. 844). This decreases the number of platelets and places the child at risk for bleeding that is difficult to control. This usually results in bleeding from mucous membranes, but it can lead to uncontrollable bleeding that requires platelet replacement. In adolescent girls, this can be a special problem because the blood loss associated with menses increases.

ITP can be acute or chronic. Acute ITP usually lasts less than six months and is the most common childhood ITP. Chronic ITP is "a long-lasting (6 months or longer) type of ITP that mostly affects adults. . . . Chronic ITP affects women two to three times more often than men" (National Heart Lung and Blood Institute, 2007, p. 1).

Complications

Epistaxis
Heavy menstrual flow
Uncontrolled bleeding

Incidence

An average estimate of the incidence in children is 50 cases per 1,000,000 annually in the United States. "Internationally: According to studies in Denmark and England, childhood ITP occurs in approximately 10–40 cases per 1,000,000 per year. A study in Kuwait reported a higher incidence of 125 cases per 1,000,000 per year. . . . Spontaneous remission occurs in more than 80% of cases in children. . . . Peak prevalence occurs in children aged 2–4 years. . . . Approximately 40% of all patients are younger than 10 years" (Silverman, 2007, Section 2).

Etiology

Most ITP in children is caused by an autoimmune response associated with a recent viral infection or live virus immunization. Viral infections associated with ITP include cytomegalovirus, Epstein-Barr virus, human immunodeficiency virus (HIV), and viral upper respiratory infections (National Heart Lung and Blood Institute, 2007).

Clinical Manifestations

Rapid onset

Ecchymosis

Purpura

Petechiae

Bleeding that is difficult to stop

Epistaxis

Bleeding oral mucous membranes

Heavy menstrual bleeding (menorrhagia)

Hepatosplenomegaly

Diagnostic Tests

Complete blood count

Platelet count

Blood smear

Stool for occult blood

Medical Management

The goal of treatment is supportive care until the ITP runs its course. The acute (temporary) type of ITP that occurs in children often goes away within a few weeks or months. The supportive care includes monitoring the child's platelet count. Treatment usually is not indicated in children with a platelet count greater than 50,000/mm^3 (Thiagarajan, 2006).

Although acute ITP is usually self-limiting, treatment is indicated if there is a risk of intracranial hemorrhage and in children whose platelet count is < 20,000/mm^3, especially if associated with extensive cutaneous (and especially mucosal) bleeding or if a protective environment cannot be assured. When treatment is needed, IV methylprednisolone at a dose of 30 mg/kg may be administered for 3 days. The corticosteroid prednisolone is used to decrease the activity in the immune system, resulting in an increase in the platelet count. The usual dose of a taper of prednisolone is 1–4 mg/kg/day for 21 days or until platelet count increases to > 20,000/mm^3 (Thiagarajan, 2006)

Corticosteroids produce adverse effects, however; and some children relapse when treatment is discontinued. Intravenous immune globulin (IVIG) and anti-(Rh)D immunoglobulin increase the platelet count. The usual dose of IVIG is 0.8–1.0 grams/kg/day for 1–2 days. Anti-D immunoglobulin usually is prescribed at a dose of 45–50 μg/kg (Thiagarajan, 2006). In 2006, the Food and Drug Administration and the pharmaceutical company that manufactures WinRho SDF (anti-D immunoglobulin intravenous) announced postmarketing safety surveillance showing rare but severe and sometimes fatal intravascular hemolysis and potentially serious complications, including disseminated intravascular coagulation in children with ITP being treated with WinRho SDF (Food and Drug Administration, 2006).

If bleeding continues to the point of being a life-threatening condition, the child may need to be treated with platelet transfusions or even a splenectomy. Although splenectomies are rare in children with ITP, they are used more frequently in adults who have not responded to steroid therapy.

Nursing Management

ASSESSMENT

1. Assess for manifestations of ITP
2. Obtain vital signs
3. Perform pediatric assessment
4. Assess neurologic status
5. Assess parents for psychosocial impact of child's illness

NURSING DIAGNOSES (INCLUDING BUT NOT LIMITED TO)

1. Risk for injury, bleeding R/T decreased circulating platelets
2. Deficient knowledge R/T child's condition, treatment, and home care
3. Risk for infection R/T corticosteroid therapy or splenectomy (if performed)

PLANNING/GOALS

1. Client will not experience bleeding that requires a splenectomy or platelet transfusion.
2. Parents will demonstrate understanding of child's condition, treatment, and home care.
3. Client will not experience infection.

NOC

1. Circulation Status
2. Knowledge: Illness Care, Treatment, Health Promotion
3. Risk Control, Immune Status

IMPLEMENTATION

1. Risk for bleeding
   a. Assess for purpura and petechiae
   b. Assess for epistaxis
   c. Assess neurologic status (rare, but risk for intracranial hemorrhage exists)
   d. Guaiac all stools
   e. Assess urine for blood
   f. Assess mucous membranes and nose for bleeding
   g. Initiate and maintain intravenous access device, monitoring at least hourly
   h. Administer intravenous or oral corticosteroids and IVIG
   i. Monitor platelet counts
   j. Assist in planning age-appropriate activities with low risk of being bruised or injured
   k. Do not use aspirin, ibuprofen, or rectal temperatures
   l. Closely monitor during invasive procedures
   m. Assist parent/child with use of soft-bristled toothbrush
   n. Collaborate with health care provider for treatment of heavy bleeding
   o. Administer medications as prescribed
2. Parent teaching
   a. Assess parents' current level of understanding
   b. Provide verbal and written information regarding:
      1) Medication administration and importance of compliance with medical regimen

      2) Assessment of nares and oral mucous membranes

      3) Types of age-appropriate activities

      4) Age-appropriate measures to make home environment safe

      5) Importance of weekly platelet counts

      6) Manifestations to report immediately to health care provider

      7) Importance of regular follow-up with health care provider

  c. Provide adequate time for teaching

  d. Document teaching and parental response

3. Risk for infection

  a. Assess for manifestations of infection

  b. Administer prophylactic antimicrobial agents as prescribed and emphasize importance of completing entire antimicrobial prescription

  c. Administer pneumococcus immunization

  d. Monitor white blood cell count

NIC

1. Vital Signs Monitoring

2. Teaching: Illness Care, Treatment, Health Promotion

3. Infection Precautions

EVALUATION

1. Client does not experience bleeding that requires a splenectomy or platelet transfusion.

2. Parents demonstrate understanding of child's condition, treatment, and home care.

3. Client does not experience infection.

References

Food and Drug Administration. (2006). *WinRhoSDF*. Retrieved February 21, 2008, from http://www.fda.gov/medwatch/safety/2006/WinRho_PI_%2005-DEC-2005.pdf

National Heart Lung and Blood Institute. (2007). *What is idiopathic thrombocytopenia purpura?* Retrieved March 13, 2007, from http://www.nhlbi.nih.gov/health/dci/Diseases/Itp/ITP_WhatIs.html

Potts, N. L., & Mandleco, B. L. (2007). *Pediatric nursing: Caring for children and their families* (2nd ed.). Clifton Park, NY: Delmar Cengage Learning.

Silverman, M. A. (2007). *Idiopathic thrombocytopenia purpura*. Retrieved March 13, 2007, from http://www.emedicine.com/emerg/topic282.htm

Thiagarajan, P. (2006). *Platelet disorders*. Retrieved February 21, 2008, from http://www.emedicine.com/med/topic987.htm

IMPERFORATE ANUS

Definition

Imperforate anus, also called anal atresia or anal agenesis, is the incomplete development of the distal end of the large intestines.

Pathophysiology

Imperforate anus occurs during the 4–16th week of embryonic development (Potts & Mandleco, 2007). "The embryogenesis of these malformations remains unclear. The rectum and anus are believed to develop from the dorsal portion of the hindgut or cloacal cavity when lateral ingrowth of the mesenchyme forms the urorectal septum in the midline. This septum separates the rectum and anal canal dorsally from the bladder and urethra. The cloacal duct is a small communication between the 2 portions of the hindgut. Downgrowth of the urorectal septum is believed to close this duct by 7 weeks' gestation. During this time, the ventral urogenital portion acquires an external opening; the dorsal anal membrane opens later. The anus develops by a fusion of the anal tubercles and an external invagination, known as the proctodeum, which deepens toward the rectum but is separated from it by the anal membrane. This separating membrane should disintegrate at 8 weeks' gestation. Interference with anorectal structure development at varying stages leads to various anomalies, ranging from anal stenosis, incomplete rupture of the anal membrane, or anal agenesis to complete failure of the upper portion of the cloaca to descend and failure of the proctodeum to invaginate. Continued communication between the urogenital tract and rectal portions of the cloacal plate causes rectourethral fistulas or rectovestibular fistulas" (Rosen & Beal, 2007, Section 2).

Anal stenosis is the narrowing or tightening of the anal sphincter. In this type of anal atresia, the anorectal structures are intact, but the narrowing of the sphincter interferes with the neonate's ability to eliminate the bowel. Incomplete rupture of the anal membrane occurs when the membrane that covers the anal opening during embryonic development remains as a covering over the anus. Like anal stenosis, all of the structures are present, but the membrane over the anus does not allow the bowel to empty. Low anal agenesis occurs when the anal portion of the large intestines ends in a pouch below the levator ani muscle that does not extend to the outside for elimination. High anal agenesis occurs when the anorectal portion of the large intestines ends in a blind pouch above the levator ani muscle. Refer to Figure 60-1.

Regardless of the type of imperforate anus, the neonate is unable to expel fecal matter. This results in constipation and intestinal obstruction.

Complications

Intestinal obstruction
Bowel incontinence
Constipation

Incidence

In the United States annually, anorectal anomalies occur at an incidence of 1 case per 5,000 live births (Rosen & Beal, 2007).

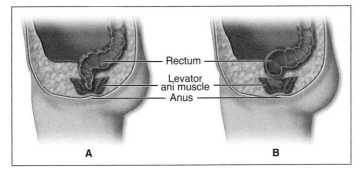

Figure 60-1: Imperforate Anus: **(A)** Low Anal Agenesis, **(B)** High Anal Agenesis.

Etiology

Imperforate anus is a congenital anomaly resulting from alterations in embryonic development of the intestines during the 4–16th week of gestation.

Clinical Manifestations

Absence of anal opening

Displaced anal opening

Anal opening very near the vaginal opening in the female

No passage of meconium stool within 24–48 hours after birth

Stool passed by way of vagina, base of penis or scrotum, or urethra

Abdominal distention (MedlinePlus, 2007)

Diagnostic Tests

Abdominal ultrasonography

Abdominal computed tomography

Abdominal radiography

Complete blood count

Serum electrolyte levels

Medical Management

The goal of treatment is to establish bowel elimination by medically or surgically repairing the anomaly. Anal stenosis usually is effectively treated by repeated anal dilatation. This begins in the hospital shortly after birth and extends to the home environment after parents are taught how to perform anal dilatation. Other forms of anal atresia are repaired surgically.

Surgery for a low-type imperforate anus involves creating an anal opening and sphincter and placing the rectal pouch in the anal opening (MedlinePlus, 2007). Complicated atresias and high atresias are repaired in a two-step surgical process. The first step involves creating a temporary colostomy. In the second step performed weeks or months later, the colostomy is closed and a pull-through procedure is performed that attaches the rectum to the anal sphincter.

Nursing Management:

Also refer to Chapter 100: Surgical Client.

ASSESSMENT

1. Perform neonatal assessment
2. Assess for passage of meconium stool within 24–36 hours following birth
3. Assess parents for psychosocial impact of child's illness

NURSING DIAGNOSES (INCLUDING BUT NOT LIMITED TO)

1. Risk for injury, intestinal obstruction R/T incomplete development of anorectal area
2. Impaired skin and tissue integrity R/T colostomy
3. Deficient knowledge R/T child's condition, treatment, and home care

PLANNING/GOALS

1. Client will not experience injury related to intestinal obstruction.
2. Client will not experience skin breakdown around the colostomy site, and ostomy tissue will show evidence of adequate tissue perfusion.
3. Parents will demonstrate understanding of child's condition, treatment, and home care.

NOC

1. Risk Control
2. Tissue Integrity: Skin
3. Knowledge: Illness Care, Treatment, Health Promotion

IMPLEMENTATION

1. Risk for intestinal obstruction
   a. Assess for anal opening
   b. Assess for abdominal distention
   c. Monitor for passage of meconium stool
   d. Perform anal dilatation for anal stenosis and instruct parents about correct technique
   e. Initiate and maintain intravenous access device for anal atresia requiring surgical repair, monitoring at least hourly
   f. Administer intravenous fluids as prescribed
   g. Monitor laboratory tests
   h. Prepare parents for surgical experience
   i. Begin teaching about colostomy
   j. Assess parents for manifestations of anxiety and fear
   k. Provide support to parents/neonate
   l. Administer medications as prescribed
2. Skin and tissue integrity (colostomy)
   a. Assess colostomy site postoperatively for evidence of adequate tissue perfusion and absence of bleeding
   b. Monitor colostomy site throughout hospitalization
   c. Collaborate with enterostomal therapist
   d. Provide hypoallergenic colostomy supplies to protect sensitive newborn skin
   e. Place a 4 x 4 gauze (secured by the diaper) while stools are liquid and occur in small amounts to provide sufficient protection without attaching ostomy bag

    f. Monitor skin closely for signs of breakdown

    g. Check at least hourly and change if soiled when using 4 x 4 gauze

    h. Empty colostomy bag when half full

    i. Teach colostomy care to parents

    j. Provide adequate time for teaching and for return demonstrations of skill by parents

3. Parent teaching

    a. Assess parents' current level of understanding

    b. Provide verbal and written information regarding:

        1) Infant care and feeding

        2) Reinforcement of instructions regarding colostomy care

        3) Contact information for enterostomal therapist

        4) Manifestations of altered tissue perfusion to colostomy

        5) Manifestations of infection at colostomy site

        6) Contact numbers for reporting manifestations

        7) Manifestations to report immediately to health care provider

        8) Importance of regular follow-up with health care provider

    c. Provide adequate time for teaching and return demonstration of colostomy care

    d. Document teaching and parental response

NIC

1. Risk Identification
2. Ostomy Care
3. Teaching: Illness Care, Treatment, Health Promotion

EVALUATION

1. Client does not experience injury related to intestinal obstruction.
2. Client does not experience skin breakdown around the colostomy site, and ostomy tissue shows evidence of adequate tissue perfusion.
3. Parents demonstrate understanding of child's condition, treatment, and home care.

References

MedlinePlus. (2007). *Imperforate anus*. Retrieved February 21, 2008, from http://www.nlm.nih.gov/medlineplus/ency/article/001147.htm

MedlinePlus. (2007). *Imperforate anus repair*. Retrieved February 21, 2008, from http://www.nlm.nih.gov/medlineplus/ency/article/002926.htm

Potts, N. L., & Mandleco, B. L. (2007). *Pediatric nursing: Caring for children and their families* (2nd ed.). Clifton Park, NY: Delmar Cengage Learning.

Rosen, N. G., & Beal, D. A. (2007). *Imperforate anus*. Retrieved May 16, 2007, from http://www.emedicine.com/ped/topic1171.htm

61

INCREASED INTRACRANIAL PRESSURE (ICP)

Definition

Increased intracranial pressure (ICP) occurs when the pressure within the cranial vault exceeds 20 mm Hg (the normal being 5–15 mm Hg). Increased ICP usually is the result of head trauma with traumatic brain injury (TBI).

Pathophysiology

The cranial vault contains three components—the brain (Refer to Figure 61-1), intravascular blood, and cerebrospinal fluid (CSF). The brain makes up 80% of the vault space, the intravascular volume is 10%, and CSF makes up the other 10%. According to the Monro-Kellie hypothesis, "When the volume of one component changes, there must be a compensatory change in another component in order to maintain constant volume" (Zomorodi, 2007, p. 3).

Normally, CSF circulates through the ventricles from the choroid plexus to the lateral ventricles. It then flows through the interventricular foramen of Monro to the third ventricle, the cerebral aqueduct of Sylvius, the fourth ventricle, the 2 lateral foramina of Luschka and 1 medial foramen of Magendie, the subarachnoid space surrounding the brain and spinal cord, the arachnoid granulations, and the dural sinus and then into the venous drainage (Hord, 2006).

With hydrocephalus, the CSF increases in volume, causing compression to the brain and its vascular supply. This can result in permanent damage to the neurons, resulting in damage to the cerebral and/or cerebellar structures and functions. Refer to Chapter 57: Hydrocephalus and Shunt Placement. The most common cause of increased ICP in a child is head trauma from motor vehicle accidents where the child is a pedestrian or a passenger. This results in an increase in blood volume in the cranial vault and interference in cerebral tissue perfusion from damage to blood vessels or compression of the blood vessels. Refer to Chapter 50: Head Trauma.

Regardless of the cause of increased ICP, the pathophysiology is similar. As the pressure in the cranial vault increases, the CSF compensates by decreasing production and circulation. Because CSF makes up only 10% of the vault volume, this compensation is limited. In infants, with the presence of fontanels and non-fused cranial sutures, the cranial vault can expand. However, after the sutures fuse and the anterior fontanel closes (by 14 months of age), the CSF must initiate compensation.

As the ICP continues to increase, brain mass is compressed against the cranium and blood vessels are compressed. With decreased vascular supply, neuron ischemia occurs, ultimately causing death to the cells. The sequence of complications of increased ICP depends on the areas of compression (lobes of the brain); but once the ICP reaches a pressure the cranium cannot accommodate, herniation of the medulla (vital center) and pons results because these structures are nearest the opening between the contents of the cranial vault and the cervical opening to the spine. Herniation frequently results in death.

"When a herniation occurs, it causes compression, destruction, and lacerations of the vascular system of the brain that further results in ischemia, cellular necrosis, and death. Among the more common herniation syndromes are cingulate herniation, uncal herniation, transtentorial (central) herniation, and transcranial (extracranial) herniation. Cingulate herniation compresses the cerebral artery and internal cerebral vein causing further increase in intracranial pressure. An uncal herniation is a life-threatening

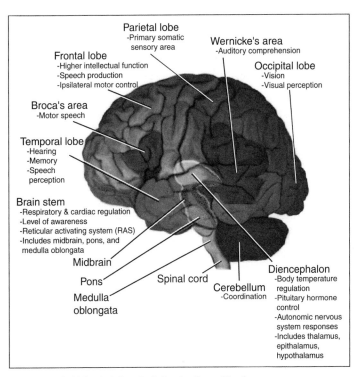

Figure 61-1: Cerebral Lobes, Brain Stem, Cerebellum: Locations and Functions.

situation occurring when the wound or lesion of the temporal fossa expands forcing the temporal lobe to the midline. Through its protrusion over the tentorium cerebelli, the oculomotor nerve and the posterior cerebral artery are compressed" (Broyles, 2005, p. 383). This causes physical damage to the nerve and vessel and a further increase in ICP. A transtentorial herniation may be an extension of a cingulated or uncal herniation that occurs when the tissue of the frontal, occipital, or parietal lobes expands causing the basal ganglia, diencephalons, thalamus, and hypothalamus to herniate through the tentorium cerebelli resulting in compression of the midbrain and posterior cerebral arteries. Finally, a transcranial herniation occurs when intracranial contents are forced through an opening in the cranial vault, such as a wound, skull fracture, or surgical incision (Broyles, 2005).

The frontal lobe receives the most damage because it frequently is the site of the original head trauma. The frontal lobes of the brain contain nerve tissue associated with impulse control, judgment, language, memory, motor function, problem solving, sexual behavior, socialization, and spontaneity. The frontal lobes also assist in planning, coordinating, controlling, and executing behavior. Because the occipital lobe (controls all aspects of vision) is opposite the frontal lobes, they frequently sustain collateral damage related to brain shifting. The temporal lobes are situated in pockets of the skull that allow more brain shifting.

Posturing indicates permanent brain damage. Decorticate posturing ("to the core" causing flexion) is associated with injuries that interrupt corticospinal pathways; decerebrate posturing (characterized by extension posture) usually indicates dysfunction of the brain stem.

Complications

Cognitive impairment

Motor impairment

Sensory impairment

Death

Incidence

Hydrocephalus is believed to affect approximately 1 in every 500 children (National Institute of Neurological Disorders and Stroke, 2007). According to the Centers for Disease Control and Prevention (CDC), among children under the age of 14 years, increased ICP from TBI results in an estimated 2,685 deaths, 37,000 hospitalizations, and 435,000 emergency department visits each year in the United States (Centers for Disease Control and Prevention, 2006). Over 1 million children experience brain injuries each year, and over 30,000 of these children have permanent disabilities as a result of the brain injury (National Dissemination Center for Children with Disabilities, 2006). The incidence of TBI is higher among children aged 0–4 years; and in motor vehicle-related accidents (including motor vehicle versus pedestrian) resulting in TBI, the death and hospitalization rates are highest among black children aged 0–9 years when compared with whites (Dawodu, 2007). Males are 2.5 times more likely to experience TBI than females (Su and Raghupathi, 2008).

Etiology

The most common cause of increased ICP in neonates is hydrocephalus. Refer to Chapter 57: Hydrocephalus and Shunt Placement. The most common cause of increased ICP in children over the age of 1 year is head trauma from motor vehicle accidents (as either a pedestrian or a passenger). Infections such as encephalitis can lead to increased ICP as well as conditions such as Reye syndrome and brain tumors.

Clinical Manifestations

NEONATES/INFANTS

Bulging fontanels, most prominent in the anterior fontanel

Widely separated cranial sutures

Distended scalp veins

Increased head circumference

Thinning cranial bones

Poor feedings

Irritability

Setting-sun sign (sclera visible above the iris)

Frontal bone enlargement, or bossing

Vomiting

Altered respiratory pattern

Shrill, high-pitched cry

Pupils sluggish and nonreactive

CHILDREN

Decreasing level of consciousness (LOC) (confusion, irritability, stupor, and coma)

Headache

Visual disturbances

Decreased coordination

Decreased muscle strength

Vomiting

Dizziness

Seizures

Papilledema

Decreased sensory perception

CHANGES IN VITAL SIGNS (LATE SIGN)

Irregular respirations

Increased blood pressure

Bradycardia

Pupil changes

Posturing (serious indication of brain damage)

Decorticate ("to the core"; arms, wrists, and fingers rigidly flexed; internal rotation of legs; and plantar flexion)

Decerebrate ("3 e's for extension," rigid extension of arms and legs, plantar flexion, pronation of arms, and opisthotonos)

Diagnostic Tests

Skull radiography

Computed tomography (CT)

Brain scan

Electroencephalogram

Cervical spine radiography

Magnetic resonance imaging (MRI)

Magnetic resonance arteriography (MRA)

Cerebral angiography

Evoked responses

Analysis of CSF

Complete blood count

Serum electrolytes and osmolality

Medical Management

The goals of management for increased ICP are to maintain a patent airway and gas exchange, reduce the ICP, and minimize complications secondary to brain tissue injury. Surgical intervention may be required to establish a patent airway (tracheostomy), however, initially oropharyngeal intubation is preferred. Mechanical ventilation usually is necessary depending on the child's ability to maintain adequate spontaneous ventilation. Surgical placement of a shunt is the standard of care for hydrocephalus.

Hypercapnia (elevated carbon dioxide levels) and hypoxia must be controlled because both of these conditions cause cerebral vasodilation and further increase ICP. During initial treatment "efforts should be made to maintain eucapnia at the low end of the reference range ($PaCO_2$ of 35–40 mm Hg) and prevent hypoxia ($PaO_2 < 100$ mm Hg) to prevent or to limit secondary brain injury" (Su and Raghupathi, 2008, Section 4). Drugs including etomidate, thiopental, and lidocaine are used to help prevent further increase of ICP during oropharyngeal intubation, and mechanical ventilation is used to prevent and/or treat hypercapnia and hypoxia. "Nasotracheal intubation should be avoided because of the risk of direct intracranial injury, especially in patients with basilar skull fractures" (Su and Raghupathi, 2008, Section 4).

Medical treatment is initiated to decrease ICP; surgical management includes evacuation of lesions, such as epidural, subdural, and intracranial hematomas, to decrease ICP secondary to head trauma and TBI. Other surgical management includes placement of an ICP monitoring system, debridement of wounds and brain tissue, repair of dural tears and lacerated cranial vessels, and removal of portions of the cranium to control ICP. Frontal lobectomies sometimes are performed to control severe increases in ICP.

Management of increased ICP is initially focused on monitoring the dynamics of the pressure. ICP should be maintained at < 20 mm Hg and cerebral perfusion pressure (CPP) > 40 mm Hg because higher mortality levels are seen if the ICP exceeds or CPP falls below these parameters.

Hemodynamic monitoring also is critical for these children. "Hypotension has been shown to significantly increase mortality rates in children with head injury, with or without the presence of hypoxia" (Su and Raghupathi, 2008, Section 4). Consequently, hypotension in children with TBIs must be avoided through "aggressive fluid resuscitation with isotonic fluids until euvolemia is achieved" (Su and Raghupathi, 2008, Section 4).

If ICP increases above 20 mm Hg, measures are taken to decrease it before brain cell damage occurs. ICP can be reduced through placement of an intraventricular or ventriculostomy system and drainage of CSF. To prevent herniation when these systems are used, the CSF drainage collection bag must be maintained at the level of the canthus of the ear. Positioning the child with the head elevated 30 degrees in the midline position remains the standard of care to help promote venous drainage and prevent obstruction.

A first-line therapy to decrease ICP is administration of the osmotic diuretic mannitol and the loop diuretic furosemide (Lasix). Furosemide should be administered at a dose of 1 mg/kg before and with mannitol doses (Gahart & Nazareno, 2008). These drugs are used to reduce cerebral edema by extracting fluid from the intracellular compartment of the brain. Because the fluid and electrolyte balance is so fragile in children, the increase in urine output from these two agents may place the child at risk for dehydration. In conjunction with the diuretics, dexamethasone, a steroidal anti-inflammatory agent, is used to decrease cerebral inflammation, thereby decreasing ICP.

Treatment with hypertonic saline "has been shown to be an effective therapy for intracranial hypertension following pediatric TBI. Hypertonic saline, typically 3% saline, has an osmolar mechanism of action similar to that of mannitol, without the diuretic effects" (Su and Raghupathi, 2008, Section 4). Renal insufficiency and rebound intracranial hypertension are two of the risks of this therapy. Adequate gas exchange must be maintained to ensure cerebral oxygenation. This is accomplished through oxygen administration via a delivery system appropriate for each client's condition—nasal cannula (for those children requiring < 40% oxygen) to mechanical ventilation (for those children requiring 100% oxygen and experiencing ineffective spontaneous ventilation). Mechanical ventilation frequently is used for children not only to provide for gas exchange but also to decrease the body's metabolic needs from the work of breathing.

Pain management is critical in the treatment of increased ICP. Pain increases ICP as well as metabolic demands (Su and Raghupathi, 2008). Unfortunately, treatment for pain in head trauma clients lacks adequacy in many cases because of an outdated philosophy that pain control will "mask symptoms" of neurologic damage. Currently, pain management is better in children than in adults with TBI. Usual medications include the benzodiazepine midazolam, opioid analgesics (fentanyl and morphine sulfate), and pancuronium that provide pain management and produce sedation to decrease demands so that cerebral blood supply can maintain cerebral function. A pediatric benefit of midazolam over other benzodiazepines is its short half-life (Broyles, Reiss, & Evans, 2007).

Other interventions focus on preventing complications associated with increased ICP including seizures, neurologic deficits, impaired physical mobility, disuse syndrome, nutritional deficits, gastrointestinal (GI) bleeding, and interferences with normal function associated with immobility and these are initiated in the pediatric intensive care unit. The anticonvulsant phenytoin is considered the first-line agent in the prevention and treatment of seizures (Olsen, 2006). Because of its toxicity to the veins if administered peripherally, intravenous phenytoin should always be administered through a central venous access device. The serum levels of phenytoin should be monitored closely because of "the narrow margin of error between therapeutic and toxic dose" (Gahart & Nazareno, 2008, p. 1056).

Muscle relaxants such as dantrolene may be used to prevent muscle spasms that can result in pain and contractures. Histamine-2 antagonists, proton pump inhibitors such as lansoprazole, and the GI stimulant metoclopramide are used to prevent the hyperacidity and gastric ulcer formation associated with enteral feedings and immobility. Increased nutritional requirements from the TBI and pediatric growth needs and the inability to take nutrition orally warrant the use of enteral feedings or total parenteral nutrition (TPN).

Children with head trauma require a multidisciplinary approach including physical therapy, occupational therapy, nutritional support, pharmacotherapeutics, psychosocial support for the child and family members, social services, rehabilitation, home health care, and community services. The initiation and coordination of these services is the combined responsibility of health care professionals.

Nursing Management (for children with increased ICP secondary to TBI)

Refer to Chapter 50: Head Trauma and Chapter 57: Hydrocephalus and Shunt Placement.

ASSESSMENT

1. Obtain client history immediately
2. Assess airway, breathing, and circulation
3. Perform rapid physical assessment
4. Perform continuous neurologic assessment (Glasgow Coma Scale, cranial nerves, motor status, sensory status, reflexes, and vital signs)
5. Assess psychosocial impact on parents/family

NURSING DIAGNOSES (INCLUDING BUT NOT LIMITED TO)

1. Impaired gas exchange R/T ineffective airway clearance, ineffective breathing pattern, and impaired spontaneous ventilation secondary to decreased ventilatory drive occurring from pressure on respiratory center, immobility, and possible neurogenic pulmonary edema
2. Ineffective cerebral tissue perfusion R/T increased ICP from compressed or bleeding intracranial vessels and rising increased ICP
3. Risk for injury, falls R/T decreased LOC
4. Risk for injury, seizures R/T lowered seizure threshold secondary to increased ICP and decreased cerebral tissue perfusion
5. Risk for infection R/T invasive treatment lines and procedures, surgical interventions
6. Risk for injury, complications R/T impaired physical mobility
7. Imbalanced nutrition: less than body requirements R/T increased demands and decreased intake
8. Parental anxiety R/T critical nature of child's condition
9. Risk for impaired home health maintenance R/T impaired cognitive functioning and extent of disability secondary to increased ICP resulting from TBI
10. Risk for caregiver role strain R/T deficient knowledge of care and available community services, fatigue, extent and complexity of client's care requirements, and social isolation
11. Deficient knowledge R/T child's condition, treatment, and home care

PLANNING/GOALS

1. Client will regain and maintain adequate gas exchange as evidenced by oxygen saturation > 94%/pulse oximetry, arterial blood gases (ABGs) within defined limits (WDL) airway patency, and respiratory rate and effort WDL.

2. Client will regain and maintain ICP < 20 mm Hg (normal 5–15 mm Hg), cerebral perfusion pressure (CPP) > 40 mm Hg, and systemic arterial pressure > 60 mm Hg (normal 60–150 mm Hg) as evidenced by pressure values and improvement of neurologic status.

3. Client will not experience injury from falls.

4. Client will not experience seizure activity or injury in the presence of a seizure.

5. Client will not experience infection as evidenced by temperature WDL; no redness, swelling, heat, or purulent drainage from wounds; complete blood count WDL; no evidence of leukocytes in CSF; and no clinical manifestations of encephalitis or meningitis.

6. Client will not experience complications from impaired physical mobility as evidenced by skin and tissue maintaining integrity and absence of contractures and disuse syndrome.

7. Client will regain and maintain adequate nutritional status as evidenced by nitrogen balance and stable weight within 24–48 hours prior to transfer from critical care unit.

8. Parents will verbalize feelings and concerns and use positive coping strategies and available support systems.

9. Client will rehabilitate to the highest level of growth, development, and wellness.

10. Parents/caregiver will utilize services, maintain adequate rest, and schedule activities outside of care environment to avoid social isolation.

11. Parents/caregiver will demonstrate understanding of child's condition, treatment modalities, home care, and community services available.

NOC

1. Respiratory Status: Gas Exchange
2. Neurologic Status
3. Risk Control
4. Risk Control
5. Infection Control
6. Risk Control
7. Nutritional Status: Nutrient Intake
8. Anxiety
9. Risk Control, Parenting Performance
10. Caregiver Emotional Health
11. Knowledge: Illness Care, Treatment, Health Promotion

IMPLEMENTATION

1. Gas exchange
   a. Assess respiratory rate, rhythm, and effort continuously during acute phase
   b. Auscultate lung sounds every 1–2 hours and report presence of adventitious breath sounds

    c. Initiate and maintain continuous pulse oximetry

    d. Administer oxygen as prescribed, titrating to maintain oxygen saturation > 94%/pulse oximetry and child's condition

    e. Monitor for manifestations of hypoxia including changes in LOC

    f. Maintain airway patency by proper positioning of neck and head of bed elevated 15–30 degrees

    g. Maintain mechanical ventilation

    h. Perform endotracheal or tracheostomy suctioning as indicated by increased respiratory rate, respiratory effort, or audible tracheal sounds. *NOTE:* Suctioning increases ICP, so avoid unnecessary suctioning.

    i. Perform tracheostomy care at least every 8 hours (per facility protocol)

    j. Collaborate with respiratory therapist for chest physiotherapy (CPT) as prescribed and in collaboration with physical therapist

    k. Monitor ABGs, maintaining patency of arterial line

2. Cerebral tissue perfusion

    a. Monitor systemic arterial pressure

    b. Monitor neurologic status

    c. Initiate and maintain indwelling urinary catheter

    d. Administer osmotic diuretic (mannitol), loop diuretic (furosemide), and steroidal anti-inflammatory agent (dexamethasone) as prescribed, monitoring for effectiveness (increased urinary output) and for adverse effects including dehydration and increased glucose levels (dexamethasone)

    e. Monitor ICP

    f. Administer anticonvulsant as prescribed

    g. Initiate seizure precautions

    h. Monitor for seizure activity

    i. Maintain client safety and assess seizure if one occurs

    j. Position with head of bed elevated 30 degrees as prescribed

    k. Administer oxygen as prescribed, titrating to oxygen saturation > 94% and child's response

    l. Assess for and correct factors that may increase ICP

    m. Adjust nursing care to limit activities that increase ICP > 5 mm Hg. Although many of these activities cannot be avoided (suctioning, positioning changes of neck, turning, bathing, providing sensory stimulation, and using wrist restraints), they need to be monitored to avoid sustained increases in ICP.

    n. Monitor ICP and CPP to insure they return to baseline or stay within acceptable parameters within 5 minutes of completion of tasks noted previously

    o. Maintain strict intake and output

    p. Assess for leakage of CSF (eyes, ears, and nose) by testing for presence of glucose if drainage presents

    q. Collaborate with health care provider to initiate bowel program to prevent constipation (Valsava's maneuver increases ICP), such as prophylactic stool softeners (docusate is drug of choice for children)

3. Risk for injury

    a. Maintain safe physical environment

    b. Assess neurologic status frequently

    c. Explain all procedures and equipment to child (if age-appropriate) and parents and repeat as frequently as needed

    d. Talk to child in calm manner

    e. Protect infusion lines, monitoring lines, and drainage tubes from being removed by child

    f. Follow facility's pediatric sedation protocol and health care provider's orders regarding TBI precautions

    g. Monitor balance and gait if ambulating

4. Risk for seizures

    a. Initiate and maintain seizure precautions

    b. Monitor neurologic status frequently

    c. Administer phenytoin according to intravenous precautions including dose not exceeding 25 mg/min and flushing before and after infusion with 0.9% normal saline or turning off continuous enteral feedings 1–2 hours (according to facility protocol) before and after phenytoin enteral administration if administering via enteral feeding tube (enteral feeding solutions alter the absorption of phenytoin)

    d. Monitor serum drug levels for therapeutic and toxic levels, reporting abnormal values to health care provider

    e. Monitor for gum hyperplasia

    f. Maintain patency of intravenous access, monitoring at least hourly

    g. Initiate and maintain continuous EEG monitoring if available

5. Risk for infection

    a. Monitor neurologic status frequently

    b. Monitor incisions and insertion sites (intravenous access, central venous access, and central venous pressure monitor; drainage tubes; enteral feeding tube; and monitoring sites) for redness, swelling, pain, heat, and purulent drainage

    c. Maintain strict asepsis during dressing changes, following facility protocols

    d. Administer antimicrobials as prescribed

    e. Culture wounds or insertion sites as indicated

    f. Instruct parents/family about hand washing and proper technique

    g. Maintain adequate nutritional intake

6. Risk for injury, complications

    a. Keep skin clean and dry

    b. Assess skin every 2 hours and as indicated for incontinence

    c. Avoid direct contact between skin and plastic protective pads by placing lift pad or draw sheet between client and protective pads

    d. Place on therapeutic mattress

    e. Monitor oral mucous membranes for breakdown from endotracheal tube (ET); change ET tube position (from one side of mouth to the other) according to facility protocol

    f. Administer prescribed medications to prevent GI ulcerations

    g. Assess baseline range of motion

    h. Perform passive range of motion to extremities 4 times a day, encouraging parental involvement in care

    i. Collaborate with physical therapist regarding ankle splints

    j. Maintain "on" and "off" schedule of use of ankle splints to prevent footdrop

    k. Maintain body alignment

    l. Collaborate with occupational therapist and physical therapist for other devices used

7. Nutrition

    a. Monitor daily weight

    b. Monitor skin integrity and turgor

    c. Provide nutrition via enteral feedings or TPN as prescribed

    d. Collaborate with dietician

    e. Monitor 24-hour urine nitrogen as prescribed

    f. Monitor strict intake and output

    g. Monitor serum electrolytes; if routine serum electrolyte levels are not prescribed, collaborate with health care provider as indicated

    h. Administer medications as prescribed to prevent GI complications

8. Parental anxiety

    a. Encourage parents to verbalize feelings and concerns

    b. Listen actively

    c. Explain all equipment and procedures

    d. Encourage parents to participate in child's care

    e. Assist parents in identifying positive coping strategies and activating support systems

    f. Provide for parental spiritual needs

9. Risk for impaired home maintenance

    a. Maintain multidisciplinary approach to care

    b. Assess parental ability to care for child at home following acute condition

    c. Assess child's neurologic status and collaborate with parents

    d. Assist parents in activating support systems

    e. Provide referral information including respite care

    f. Provide psychosocial support

    g. Make referrals in collaboration with health care provider

    h. Explain to parents the importance of seeking assistance as needed while maintaining as high a level of client independence as possible

10. Caregiver role strain

    a. Assess parent/caregiver for manifestations of caregiver role strain

    b. Assist parents in activating support systems

    c. Encourage verbalization of concerns

    d. Collaborate with health care provider for appropriate referrals

11. Parent teaching

    a. Assess parents' current level of knowledge and understanding of care required

    b. Provide verbal and written information regarding:

       1) Skin care

       2) Positioning

       3) Medication administration including importance of compliance with prescribed medication regime

       4) Alternative feeding methods

       5) Manifestations of adverse effects of medications and enteral feedings

       6) Manifestations of worsening condition

       7) Rehabilitation schedule and importance of compliance with schedule

       8) Importance of follow-up care with health care professionals

       9) Importance of parents getting enough rest and nutrition

       10) Referral information, contact person, and phone number

       11) Importance of using positive coping skills and support systems

       12) Importance of parents receiving time for personal business

  c. Demonstrate needed skills including hand washing, enteral feedings, dressing changes, tracheostomy care and suctioning, passive range of motion, and use of orthopedic devices required by caregiver, and provide adequate time for return demonstrations and questions

  d. Provide sufficient time for client (if age and cognitively appropriate) and family questions

  e. Document teaching and client and family response

NIC

1. Oxygen Therapy, Ventilation Assistance
2. Cerebral Perfusion Promotion, Intracranial Pressure Monitoring, Neurologic Monitoring
3. Risk Identification
4. Risk Identification
5. Infection Precautions
6. Risk Identification
7. Nutrition Management, Nutritional Monitoring
8. Coping Enhancement
9. Risk Identification, Home Maintenance Assistance
10. Caregiver Support, Coping Enhancement, Respite Care
11. Teaching: Illness Care, Treatment, Health Promotion

EVALUATION

1. Client regains and maintains adequate gas exchange as evidenced by oxygen saturation > 94%/pulse oximetry, ABGs WDL, airway patency, and respiratory rate and effort WDL.
2. Client regains and maintains ICP < 20 mm Hg (normal 5–15 mm Hg), cerebral perfusion pressure (CPP) > 40 mm Hg, and systemic arterial pressure > 60 mm Hg (normal 60–150 mm Hg) as evidenced by pressure values and improvement of neurologic status.
3. Client does not experience injury from falls.
4. Client does not experience seizure activity or injury in the presence of a seizure.
5. Client does not experience infection as evidenced by temperature WDL; no redness, swelling, heat, or purulent drainage from wounds; complete blood count WDL; no evidence of leukocytes in CSF; and no clinical manifestations of encephalitis or meningitis.

6. Client does not experience complications from impaired physical mobility as evidenced by skin and tissue maintaining integrity and absence of contractures and disuse syndrome.

7. Client regains and maintains adequate nutritional status as evidenced by nitrogen balance and stable weight within 24–48 hours prior to transfer from critical care unit.

8. Parents verbalize feelings and concerns and use positive coping strategies and available support systems.

9. Client rehabilitates to the highest level of growth, development, and wellness.

10. Parents/caregiver utilize services, maintain adequate rest, and schedule activities outside of care environment to avoid social isolation.

11. Parents/caregiver demonstrate understanding of child's condition, treatment modalities, home care, and community services available.

References

Broyles, B. E. (2005). *Medical-surgical nursing clinical companion*. Durham, NC: Carolina Academic Press.

Broyles, B. E., Reiss, B. S., & Evans, M. E. (2007). *Pharmacological aspects of nursing care* (7th ed.). Clifton Park, NY: Delmar Cengage Learning.

Centers for Disease Control and Prevention. (2006). *What is traumatic brain injury?* Retrieved March 2, 2007, from http://www.cdc.gov/ncipc/tbi/TBI.htm

Dawodu, S. T. (2007). *Traumatic brain injury: Definition, epidemiology, pathophysiology*. Retrieved March 4, 2008, from http://www.emedicine.com/pmr/topic212.htm

Gahart, B. L., & Nazareno, A. R. (2008). *2008 intravenous medications* (24th ed.). St. Louis, MO: Elsevier Mosby.

Hord, E. D. (2006). *Hydrocephalus*. Retrieved March 11, 2007, from http://www.emedicine.com/NEURO/topic161.htm

National Dissemination Center for Children with Disabilities. (2006). *Traumatic brain injury*. Retrieved March 1, 2007, from http://www.nichcy.org/pubs/factshe/fs18txt.htm

National Institute of Neurological Disorders and Stroke. (2007). *Hydrocephalus fact sheet*. Retrieved March 11, 2007, from http://www.ninds.nih.gov/disorders/hydrocephalus/detail_hydrocephalus.htm#83433125

Olsen, D. A. (2006). *Head injury*. Retrieved March 2, 2007, from http://www.emedicine.com/neuro/topic153.htm

Potts, N. L., & Mandleco, B. L. (2007). *Pediatric nursing: Caring for children and their families* (2nd ed.). Clifton Park, NY: Delmar Cengage Learning.

Su, F., & Raghupathi, R. (2008). *Neurointensive care for traumatic brain injury in children*. Retrieved March 4, 2008, from http://www.emedicine.com/ped/topic3082.htm

Zomorodi, M. (2007, March). *ICP management*. Paper presented at meeting of the University of North Carolina School of Nursing, Chapel Hill, NC.

62

INFLAMMATORY BOWEL DISEASE (IBD)

Definition

Inflammatory bowel disease (IBD) is a chronic inflammatory condition of the small and/or large intestines that includes two distinct disorders: (1) Crohn's disease and (2) ulcerative colitis (UC).

Pathophysiology

Crohn's disease is a chronic autoimmune condition that can occur at any point in the gastrointestinal (GI) tract and can affect all three levels of the intestinal mucosa. UC occurs basically in the colon and affects only the mucosal and submucosal layers of the colon wall.

Three main factors trigger an inflammatory response in the intestines: (1) viral, (2) allergic, and (3) immunologic. When one or more of these factors occur, the inflammatory response may be initiated, causing the perception that the tissues of the intestines have been injured or traumatized. Inflammation leads to capillary vasoconstriction and the stimulation for the release of cellular mediators, including histamine (Potts & Mandleco, 2007). Histamine causes vasodilation, which results in swelling and thickening of the mucosa, distorting the surface area of the villi. This leads to malabsorption in the intestines. Histamine also increases capillary permeability and further intestinal edema. This leads to cellular destruction and ulceration that progresses to fissures and fistulas that can result in bowel perforation. Adhesions and fibrous strictures can cause bowel obstruction. This manifests as severe abdominal pain, nausea, and vomiting. The increased cellular permeability and intestinal edema increase the amount of intestinal fluid, resulting in abdominal cramping and diarrhea (Broyles, 2005).

Crohn's disease is a chronic condition that involves all layers of the intestinal mucosa (transmural) and can occur at any point in the GI tract. However, the most common site is the ileum, the juncture of the small and large intestines. Crohn's disease can be rapidly fulminating; however, it usually manifests as recurrent exacerbations and remissions (Broyles, 2005).

Also a chronic condition, UC begins at the rectum and ascends, usually confining itself to the large intestine. However, it may extend as far up as the ileocecal valve. It causes intestinal congestion, abscess formation, and ulcerations. Over time, the intestinal mucosa becomes rigid and atrophied, affecting absorption of vitamins (especially vitamin B_{12}), electrolytes, and fluid. Secondary purulent bacterial dermatitis, termed *pyoderma gangrenosum,* with tissue wasting, particularly on the trunk, can occur.

Complications

   Bowel perforation
   Fistula formation
   Abscess formation
   Intestinal obstruction
   Fluid and electrolyte imbalance
   Impaired growth
   Complications of corticosteroid therapy
   Arthritis
   Colon cancer

Incidence

"Inflammatory bowel disease (IBD) is the most common chronic gastrointestinal (GI) disease of childhood and adolescence" (Colombo, Roberts, & Friessen, 2006, p. 1). Approximately 1 million people in the United States have either Crohn's disease or UC (Rowe, 2006). Crohn's disease affects approximately 7 out of every 100,000 people; UC occurs in 4–12 per 100,000 individuals. Twenty percent of these cases are children. Crohn's disease is seen in children as young as 7 years old, and males and females are affected equally. Crohn's disease appears to have a familial connection, with about 20% of individuals with Crohn's disease having a blood relative with IBD. For those people having a family history of Crohn's disease, the disease usually begins in the teens and twenties (Lucile Packard Children's Hospital at Stanford, 2007).

Etiology

The exact cause of IBD is not known; however, genetic, infectious, immunologic, and psychological factors have been implicated in influencing its development.

There is a genetic predisposition to the development of IBD. However, the triggering factor for activation of the body's immune system has yet to be identified. Factors that can turn on the body's immune system include an infectious agent (as yet unidentified), an immune response to an antigen (such as protein from cow's milk), or an autoimmune process. As the intestines are exposed to things that can cause immune reactions, more recent thinking is that there is a failure of the body to turn off normal immune responses (Rowe, 2006).

Clinical Manifestations

Abdominal pain, often in the lower right area

Abdominal distention

Diarrhea

Rectal bleeding

Obvious blood in the stools or black, tarlike stools

Fever

Weight loss

Anemia

Failure to grow

Diagnostic Tests

Complete blood count

Serum electrolyte levels

Erythrocyte sedimentation rate

Serum B_{12} levels

Stool for blood

Computed tomography

Upper endoscopy/esophagogastroduodenoscopy (EGD)

Colonoscopy

Small bowel enteroscopy

GI series (barium swallow/barium enema)

Biopsy

Medical Management

At this time, there is no cure for Crohn's disease; however, UC can be cured with surgical removal of the colon. The goals of treatment are to induce remission with medications to control inflammation, prevent relapse, correct nutritional and electrolyte deficiencies, and minimize adverse effects of treatment.

The first course of treatment for initial symptoms or exacerbations is the use of medications including anti-inflammatory agents, corticosteroids, and immunomodulators. Anti-inflammatory agents such as aminosalycilate, azulfidine, and 5-ASA compounds (sulfasalazine, olsalazine, and mesalamine) act directly on the bowel mucosa to treat inflammation and are usually the first line treatment. If the first course of treatment is not effective, it is followed by corticosteroids, infliximab, and methotrexate. Corticosteroids are anti-inflammatory agents used systemically for inflammatory disorders that require aggressive therapy for control. Infliximab is an immunosuppressant agent given to decrease immune-mediated inflammation, and methotrexate is an antineoplastic that also acts as an immunosuppressant (Broyles, Reiss, & Evans, 2007). In May 2006, the Food and Drug Administration (FDA) approved the use of Remicade for children with active Crohn's disease (Food and Drug Administration, 2006). Probiotics and antibiotics are used to manipulate "enteric microflora to improve the balance of aggressive and protective bacterial species in the patient with IBD . . . Last, biologic agents targeted against proinflammatory cytokines have shown promise as a therapy for IBD" (Colombo et al., 2006, p. 1).

Delayed growth and development is a major concern for children with IBD (Colombo et al., 2006). Children should receive dietary and vitamin supplements. Nutritional supplements for these children usually are in the form of high-calorie liquid supplements. Because some children avoid eating because of abdominal cramps and diarrhea, they need encouragement so that parenteral nutrition is not necessary. Ways to increase intake and decrease diarrhea include offering frequent small feedings; avoiding lactose products (milk and milk products); drinking liquids at room temperature and between meals instead of with meals; avoiding foods with sorbitol, xylitol, mannitol, and caffeine; and avoiding concentrated sweets (candy, cakes, and pies) and gas-producing foods (legumes, beans, peas, broccoli, onions, cauliflower, and cabbage). Children need to include sources of soluble fiber such as oatmeal, bananas, rice, applesauce, and tapioca.

Enteral feedings with polymeric or whole-protein formulas have been found not only to provide calories but also to reduce inflammation, "although optimal formulation of the enteral diet remains to be defined. Polymeric (whole-protein) formulas are as efficacious as elemental formulas (amino acid-based) in inducing remission, and are associated with greater weight gain. A polymeric formula rich in transforming growth factor β-2 has been developed as a Crohn's disease-specific formula (Modulen IBD). Although controlled trials have not been conducted, this formula has been associated with an anti-inflammatory effect in children with Crohn's disease, and induced complete remission in 79% of 29 children studied" (Colombo et al., 2006, p. 2). Usually, children on an enteral diet for Crohn's disease consume the formula exclusively for six to eight weeks although they also may have clear liquids. Food should be reintroduced gradually after that period (Colombo et al., 2006).

Surgical intervention is reserved for children with severe inflammation or life-threatening complications. However, surgical treatment of Crohn's disease cannot cure the disease. Because the recurrence or exacerbations of Crohn's tend to affect the same areas of the intestines, removal of these areas may provide short-term relief of symptoms. However, Crohn's disease will return and usually affects the area next to the one that was removed. Colostomy, ileostomy, or ileoanal reservoir may have to be placed surgically to provide an alternative outlet for feces. Repeated colon resections can lead to short bowel syndrome with resulting malabsorption syndrome. This usually requires total parenteral nutrition to provide adequate nutritional intake. Surgery also may be necessary to correct complications of the disease, including intestinal obstruction, perforation, abscess, or bleeding.

Medical treatment will be initiated to treat UC; however, surgical intervention may be required to relieve symptoms. Removal of the affected segment of colon usually cures UC.

Children with IBD need a multidisciplinary approach to care. Long-term effects of exacerbations and the manifestations, frequent medical care, and possibly hospitalization can cause psychosocial difficulties for these children and their parents/caregivers.

Nursing Management

ASSESSMENT

1. Obtain client and family history
2. Perform pediatric assessment
3. Assess for manifestations of IBD

NURSING DIAGNOSES (INCLUDING BUT NOT LIMITED TO)

1. Diarrhea R/T inflammation of the bowel
2. Acute pain R/T exacerbation of bowel inflammation and irritation
3. Impaired tissue integrity, GI R/T inflammation of bowel mucosa
4. Imbalanced nutrition: less than body requirements R/T increased metabolic rate, diarrhea, and decreased intake
5. Disturbed body image R/T body changes secondary to IBD and treatment of IBD
6. Deficient knowledge R/T condition, treatment, and home care

PLANNING/GOALS

1. Client will experience relief from diarrhea and return of normal bowel habits.
2. Client will experience pain control (as determined by client) to a level allowing for engagement in age-appropriate activities of daily living and activities of client's choice.
3. Client will experience decreased inflammation and injury to bowel mucosa.
4. Client will consume adequate nutrition for metabolic functions and growth and development as evidenced by gradual weight gain to within prescribed parameters.
5. Client will demonstrate improved body image as evidenced by verbal and nonverbal indicators using positive coping strategies to improve self-concept.
6. Parents/caregiver/client will demonstrate understanding of condition, chronicity of condition, treatment, and home care.

NOC

1. Bowel Elimination
2. Comfort Level
3. Tissue Integrity
4. Nutritional Status
5. Body Image
6. Knowledge: Illness Care, Diet, Medications, Procedures/Treatment, Health Promotion

IMPLEMENTATION

1. Diarrhea
   a. Monitor and document frequency and characteristics of bowel movements; for home treatment, have child/parent keep a journal
   b. Assess perineal and gluteal skin for breakdown

   c. Provide and teach skin care

   d. Measure abdominal girth every shift

   e. Auscultate bowel sounds every shift

   f. Administer medications as prescribed and teach parents/child about medications including why they are prescribed and what adverse effects may result

   g. Limit intake of food if diarrhea is acute, but encourage fluids

   h. Provide list of foods to avoid, especially during IBD exacerbations

   i. Monitor intake and output

   j. Initiate intravenous access, maintain patency, and monitor at least hourly if necessary

   k. Administer parenteral fluids as prescribed

   l. Monitor laboratory values

   m. Monitor vital signs every 4 hours

   n. Hemoccult stools

2. Pain

   a. Assess pain hourly

   b. Administer analgesics as prescribed. *NOTE:* Opiate analgesics help relax bowel and decrease bowel mobility.

   c. Administer anti-inflammatory and immunosuppressant agents as prescribed

   d. Provide nonpharmacological pain control methods, including age-appropriate diversionary activities

   e. Encourage verbalization of feelings and concerns

   f. Provide information and teaching to decrease anxiety, which can worsen pain perception

3. Tissue integrity

   a. Administer and teach about medications prescribed for IBD

   b. Monitor complete blood count

   c. Monitor stools and hemoccult test them

   d. Collaborate with health care provider regarding presence of blood in stools

4. Nutrition

   a. Weigh daily

   b. Monitor intake and output

   c. Collaborate with health care provider for caloric count and maintain count if prescribed

   d. Collaborate with child/parents regarding child's favorite fluids and foods

   e. Collaborate with dietician

   f. Monitor laboratory values, reporting abnormal values to health care provider

   g. Provide and teach about liquid nutritional supplements as needed

   h. Provide parenteral nutrition as prescribed. *NOTE:* If client is receiving TPN, review knowledge of care and maintenance of central venous access device.

   i. Administer vitamin supplements as prescribed

   j. Involve parents/child in dietary teaching, encouraging parents to bring favorite foods from home if not contraindicated

5. Body image
   a. Assess child for manifestations of concern about body changes
   b. Encourage child to verbalize feelings about body changes
   c. Encourage verbalization of physical changes and the consequences as perceived by child
   d. Encourage verbalization of effects of disease on school/peer relationships
   e. Encourage child participation in care and decision making
   f. Assist parents/child to identify positive coping strategies
   g. Discuss honestly possible effects of treatment options
   h. Instruct about other possible positive coping strategies (odor control, skin care, and dietary modifications)
6. Parent/caregiver and client teaching
   a. Assess current level of understanding
   b. Provide verbal and written information regarding:
      1) Importance of compliance with medication regimen (during remissions, child may not understand the importance of maintaining compliance.)
      2) Medication administration and possible adverse effects
      3) Risk factors for developing exacerbations of disease and instructions as needed to avoid risk factors (avoiding foods that worsen diarrhea and controlling emotional stress)
      4) Dietary modifications including adequate caloric, protein, and vitamin intake and foods high in vitamin B_{12}
      5) Skin care
      6) Manifestations of exacerbation
      7) Colostomy care as needed in collaboration with enterostomal therapist (including how to empty appliance, change appliance, care for skin, and control odor)
      8) Contact phone numbers for reporting signs and symptoms
      9) Importance of regular hand washing and appropriate technique
      10) Importance of long-term follow-up visits with health care provider
   c. Provide adequate time for teaching and feedback
   d. Document teaching and client/family response

NIC

1. Bowel Elimination Enhancement
2. Medication Management
3. Wound Care
4. Nutrition Monitoring, Nutrition Management
5. Body Image Enhancement
6. Teaching: Illness Care, Diet, Medications, Procedures/Treatment, Health Promotion

EVALUATION

1. Client experiences relief from diarrhea and return of normal bowel habits.
2. Client experiences pain control (as determined by client) to a level allowing for engagement in age-appropriate activities of daily living and activities of client's choice.

3. Client experiences decreased inflammation and injury to bowel mucosa.
4. Client consumes adequate nutrition for metabolic functions and growth and development as evidenced by gradual weight gain to within prescribed parameters.
5. Client demonstrates improved body image as evidenced by verbal and nonverbal indicators using positive coping strategies to improve self-concept.
6. Parents/caregiver/client demonstrate understanding of condition, chronicity of condition, treatment, and home care.

References

Broyles, B. E. (2005). *Medical-surgical nursing clinical companion.* Durham, NC: Carolina Academic Press.

Broyles, B. E., Reiss, B. S., & Evans, M. E. (2007). *Pharmacological aspects of nursing care* (7th ed.). Clifton Park, NY: Delmar Cengage Learning.

Colombo, J., Roberts, C., & Friessen, C. (2006). *Getting current on the treatment of inflammatory bowel disease.* Retrieved May 17, 2007, from http://www.modernmedicine.com/modernmedicine/article/articleDetail.jsp?id=378634

Food and Drug Administration. (2006). *FDA approves Remicade for children with Crohn's disease.* Retrieved May 17, 2007, from http://www.fda.gov/bbs/topics/NEWS/2006/NEW01376.html

Lucile Packard Children's Hospital at Stanford. (2007). *Digestive and liver disorders: Crohn's disease.* Retrieved March 15, 2007, from http://www.lpch.org/DiseaseHealthInfo/HealthLibrary/digest/crohns.html

Potts, N. L., & Mandleco, B. L. (2007). *Pediatric nursing: Caring for children and their families* (2nd ed.). Clifton Park, NY: Delmar Cengage Learning.

Rowe, W. A. (2006). *Inflammatory bowel disease.* Retrieved March 15, 2007, from http://www.emedicine.com/med/topic1169.htm

63

INTUSSUSCEPTION

Definition

Intussusception is the telescoping, or invagination, of one bowel segment into the lumen of an adjacent intestinal segment (Potts & Mandleco, 2007). Refer to Figure 63-1.

Pathophysiology

When one segment of the intestines telescopes into itself, obstruction occurs. The mesenteric vessels become trapped and compressed between the two bowel walls of the intussusception, resulting in ischemia to the tissues served by these vessels. The pressure of the bowel can cause bleeding and the currantlike stools that occur in 50% of children with intussusception. Mesenteric ischemia causes inflammation and edema that can lead to strangulation or infarction of the intestines. This can result in life-threatening

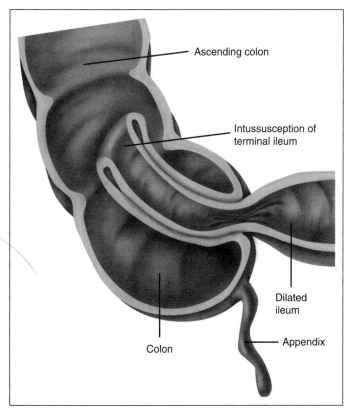

Figure 63-1: Intussusception of Terminal Ileum into the Ascending Colon.

complications, including bowel perforation or rupture, that further lead to peritonitis, sepsis, and death. Without treatment, death occurs within 2–5 days of onset (King, 2006).

Frequently, intussusception follows a viral infection (intestinal or respiratory). In response to the virus, the Peyer's patches (lymphatic components of the intestinal wall) experience significant enlargement. This causes the intestinal wall to thicken and predisposes the child to intussusception. Although most common in children under 3 years of age, when intussusception occurs in older children, it is usually the result of a pathologic lead point that is a recognizable anatomical abnormality such as Meckel's diverticulum or intestinal lymphoma that obstructs the bowel. This initiates the process of intussusception. Three types of intussusception have been identified: (1) ileocolic in which the small intestine invaginates into the colon, (2) ileoileal where the last segment of the small intestine telescopes into itself, and (3) colocolic with intussusception occurring between two segments of the large intestine. Ileocolic is the most common (Cincinnati Children's Hospital Medical Center, 2007).

Complications

Intestinal ischemia and necrosis
Bowel perforation
Sepsis
Shock
Recurrence

Incidence

Intussusception is the most common cause of intestinal obstruction in children between 3 months and 6 years of age; however, it is rare in infants younger than 3 months. The incidence is about 1–4 per 1,000 live births and affects males 3–4 times as often as females. As children get older, the gender difference is more pronounced, occurring 8 times as frequently in males compared to females after the age of 4 years. It is most common in infants aged 3–12 months and occurs at an average age of 7–8 months. With treatment, recurrence occurs in 3–11% of cases; and most of the recurrences involve children treated with contrast enemas (King, 2006). Intussusception appears to occur more often in the spring and fall months.

Etiology

Approximately 90% of cases are idiopathic in origin; if treated within 24 hours, most children recover. With treatment, the mortality rate is less than 4%. If left untreated, most children with intussusception die within 2–5 days. In neonates and children older than 3 years of age, mechanical lead points (addressed in "Pathophysiology") usually were present. Research also has shown a number of predisposing factors that increase the risk of intussusception. It often follows an intestinal virus (gastroenteritis) or another viral illness such as a respiratory infection. Some cases have been associated with infection, such as adenovirus, or with polyps or tumors (Centers for Disease Control and Prevention, 2006). Other factors include Henoch-Schönlein purpura, cystic fibrosis with accompanying dehydration, long-term indwelling gastrointestinal tubes (King, 2006), abdominal and intestinal tumors, and recent completion of chemotherapy for cancer.

A rotavirus vaccine approved by the Food and Drug Administration (FDA) in 1998 was discontinued in 1999 because of research indicating an association between the vaccine and an increased risk for intussusception in infants aged 1 year or younger. However, no research ever established a direct link to the vaccine as a cause of intussusception. The FDA approved a new rotavirus vaccine in 2006 that was evaluated in a clinical trial of over 70,000 children, and no increased risk of intussusception was found (Centers for Disease Control and Prevention, 1999). "DA is announcing the approval of RotaTeq, a new vaccine for the prevention of rotavirus gastroenteritis in infants. RotaTeq is the only US licensed vaccine that effectively prevents a viral infection, called rotavirus" (Food and Drug Administration, 2006, p. 1), with no history of association with the development of intussusception.

Clinical Manifestations

Usually healthy infant/child with sudden onset of paroxysmal
    abdominal pain
Triad of symptoms
    Nonbilious vomiting
    Intermittent abdominal pain
    Currant jelly stools (20%)
Other manifestations
    Diarrhea
    Abdominal tenderness
    Sausage-shaped mass in right upper quadrant of abdomen
    Grossly bloody stools 12–48 hours after onset of symptoms
    Inconsolable crying
    Fever
    Malaise
    Lethargy (progressive sign)

Diagnostic Tests

Stool testing for presence of blood and mucus
Abdominal radiography
Abdominal ultrasonography
Air or saline enema

Medical Management

The goals of treatment for intussusception are to relieve the intestinal obstruction and regain fluid and electrolyte balance. For all children with intussusception, intravenous fluid resuscitation and nasogastric decompression are initiated as soon as possible (Chahine, 2006).

Most cases (75%) can be reduced without surgery (King, 2006). The presence of peritonitis and any evidence of perforation revealed on plain abdominal X-rays are the only absolute contraindications for attempting nonoperative reduction with an enema. Reduction enemas may be hydrostatic, with either saline or water-soluble contrast, or pneumatic, with air insufflation. When a therapeutic enema is successful, the obstruction is relieved and the infant falls asleep almost immediately. This is followed by the resumption of a regular age-appropriate diet and a short period of overnight observation prior to discharge (Chahine, 2006).

If the intussusception is not resolved with a therapeutic enema or if the child is too ill for the procedure, surgical intervention is required. Under anesthesia, the surgeon makes an abdominal incision, locates the intussusception, and manually manipulates the telescoped sections back into place. The intestine is examined for tissue damage, perforation, lack of peristalsis, or other indicators of loss of function. If there is damage to a small intestinal segment, the section is removed and the two adjacent sections of healthy intestine are anastomosed together. If the injured section of intestine is large, requiring a significant amount of intestine to be removed, a colostomy may be done and peristalsis can resume. Depending on the amount of intestine removed, the colostomy may be temporary or permanent. Most colostomies are temporary with a pull-through procedure performed after a period of time for the healing of the traumatized intestinal tissue lapses. Intussusception recurs in 5–11% of children, and some children may have multiple recurrences. Surgery, even with resection, has a 1–4% incidence of recurrence (Cincinnati Children's Hospital Medical Center, 2007).

Nursing Management

ASSESSMENT

1. Obtain infant/child history with special attention to history of respiratory or gastrointestinal infection and clinical manifestations of intussusception
2. Perform assessment with focus on bowel assessment
3. Assess nutritional and hydration status
4. Obtain feeding history
5. Assess psychosocial impact on parents/family

NURSING DIAGNOSES (INCLUDING BUT NOT LIMITED TO)

1. Risk for injury, perforation R/T intestinal ischemia
2. Risk for fluid volume deficit R/T emesis, diarrhea, and nonsurgical reduction
3. Impaired skin integrity R/T colostomy and surgical repair
4. Risk for infection R/T colostomy and surgical incision
5. Acute pain R/T surgical tissue trauma
6. Deficient knowledge R/T condition, treatment, and home and colostomy care

PLANNING/GOALS

1. Client will not experience perforation.
2. Client will experience fluid and electrolyte balance as evidenced by serum electrolyte levels within defined limits (WDL), urine output > 1–2 mL/kg/hr or six to eight wet diapers/day, and moist mucous membranes.
3. Client's skin will not experience breakdown and will regain and maintain integrity within six weeks following surgery.
4. Client will not experience infection around colostomy or surgical incision.
5. Client will demonstrate pain control as evidenced by ability to sleep and other behavioral indicators.
6. Parents will demonstrate understanding of condition, treatment, and colostomy and home care.

NOC

1. Risk Control
2. Fluid Balance
3. Wound Healing: Primary Intention
4. Infection Control
5. Comfort Level
6. Knowledge: Illness Care, Treatment, Infant Care, Ostomy Care

IMPLEMENTATION

1. Risk for injury
   a. Assess bowel sounds
   b. Assess characteristics of stools

    c. Test stool for blood and mucus

    d. Measure abdominal girth

    e. Monitor vital signs

    f. Monitor intake and output

    g. Monitor electrolyte levels

    h. Monitor urine specific gravity

    i. Prepare infant/child for nonsurgical reduction, surgical repair, and/or placement of colostomy

2. Fluid balance

    a. Initiate and maintain intravenous access, monitoring at least hourly

    b. Administer intravenous fluids as prescribed for hydration pre-operatively and postoperatively until infant/child is able to take fluids orally

    c. Maintain strict intake and output

    d. Monitor urine specific gravity

    e. Maintain nothing by mouth status before procedure or before surgery for age-appropriate time interval

    f. Begin age-appropriate diet if nonsurgical reduction is successful

    g. Prepare infant/child for immediate surgery if nonsurgical reduction is not successful

3. Skin integrity

    a. Assess colostomy site immediately postoperatively and then every 2 hours

    b. Monitor colostomy for color and bleeding

    c. Monitor vital signs every 4 hours

    d. Assess skin surrounding colostomy for breakdown every 2 hours

    e. Collaborate with enterostomal therapist for colostomy and skin care

    f. Use appropriately sized hypoallergenic stoma supplies

    g. Try using a 4×4 gauze over colostomy to absorb colostomy drainage; hold in place with diaper

    h. Provide meticulous skin care

4. Risk for infection

    a. Monitor infant's temperature every 4 hours during hospitalization

    b. Monitor vital signs

    c. Maintain patency of intravenous access, monitoring at least hourly

    d. Administer intravenous antimicrobials as prescribed

    e. Administer intravenous fluids as prescribed

    f. Weigh daily

    g. Monitor colostomy and surrounding skin for evidence of infection

    h. Monitor surgical incision for color, approximation, and drainage

5. Acute pain

    a. Assess pain level at least hourly using age-appropriate pain scale

    b. Administer analgesics postoperatively and proactively on scheduled basis as prescribed: intravenous analgesics are preferred; if using opiates, place infant on cardiorespiratory monitor

    c. Position for comfort

d. Encourage parental involvement in care including holding, cuddling, and rocking

e. Collaborate with health care provider if pain is not controlled

f. Assess sleep pattern and avoid unnecessary interruptions of sleep

g. Provide pacifier for infant

6. Parent teaching

   a. Assess parents' current level of knowledge

   b. Provide verbal and written instructions and demonstrations (as applicable) regarding:

      1) Manifestations of recurrence to be reported to health care provider immediately

      2) Infant care and feeding

      3) Surgical repair and recovery expectations

      4) Colostomy care, encouraging parental return demonstration prior to infant's/child's discharge

      5) Skin care

      6) Diet

      7) Infant care

      8) Medication administration (if prescribed)

      9) Referrals

      10) Symptoms to report to health care provider

      11) Contact number for health care provider and referral contacts

      12) Importance of follow-up care

   c. Allow adequate time for teaching, demonstrations, and return demonstrations; parental support; and encouragement of verbalization of feelings and concerns

   d. Document teaching and parental response

NIC

1. Risk Identification
2. Fluid Management, Fluid Monitoring
3. Wound Care
4. Infection Precautions
5. Pain Management
6. Teaching: Illness Care, Treatment, Infant Care, Ostomy Care

EVALUATION

1. Client does not experience perforation.

2. Client experiences fluid and electrolyte balance as evidenced by serum electrolyte levels WDL, urine output > 1–2 mL/kg/hr or six to eight wet diapers/day, and moist mucous membranes.

3. Client's skin does not experience breakdown and will regain and maintain integrity within six weeks following surgery.

4. Client does not experience infection around colostomy or surgical incision.

5. Client demonstrates pain control as evidenced by ability to sleep and other behavioral indicators.

6. Parents demonstrate understanding of condition, treatment, and colostomy and home care.

References

Centers for Disease Control and Prevention. (1999). *Intussusception among recipients of rotavirus vaccine—United States, 1998–1999.* Retrieved May 17, 2007, from http://www.cdc.gov/ MMWR/preview/mmwrhtml/mm4827a1.htm

Centers for Disease Control and Prevention. (2006). *Intussusception—questions & answers.* Retrieved May 17, 2007, from http://www.cdc.gov/nip/diseases/rota/intussusception.htm

Chahine, A. A. (2006). *Intussusception.* Retrieved February 23, 2007, from http://www.emedicine .com/ped/topic1208.htm

Cincinnati Children's Hospital Medical Center. (2007). *Abdominal and digestive conditions/diagnoses: Intussusception.* Retrieved May 17, 2007, from http://www.cincinnatichildrens.org/health/info/ abdomen/diagnose/intussusception.htm

Food and Drug Administration. (2006). Product approval information—licensing action: RotaTeq™. Retrieved May 17, 2007, from http://www.fda.gov/CbER/products/rotamer020306qa.htm

King, L. (2006). *Pediatrics, intussusception.* Retrieved February 23, 2007, from http://www.emedicine .com/emerg/topic385.htm

Potts, N. L., & Mandleco, B. L. (2007). *Pediatric nursing: Caring for children and their families* (2nd ed.). Clifton Park, NY: Delmar Cengage Learning.

IRON DEFICIENCY ANEMIA (IDA)

Definition

Iron deficiency anemia (IDA) "is a hematologic condition characterized by decreased circulating erythrocytes related to the insufficient amounts of the mineral necessary for the manufacture of hemoglobin, poor absorption of the mineral, or loss of blood" (Broyles, 2005, p. 480).

Pathophysiology

Anemia occurs when there is insufficient hemoglobin to provide tissue perfusion to meet body needs. Iron is necessary for the manufacture of hemoglobin, the oxygen-carrying pigment of red blood cells. Hemoglobin is a crystallizable, conjugated protein that is responsible for carrying oxygen from the lungs to tissues (Potts and Mandleco, 2007). In the lungs, hemoglobin combines with oxygen to form oxyhemoglobin. In the tissues, the oxyhemoglobin exchanges its oxygen for carbon dioxide. If iron amounts are insufficient, hemoglobin cannot be manufactured at the normal rate and the tissues do not receive adequate oxygen due to increased peripheral resistance and increased cardiac workload. This results in the manifestations associated with anemia including dizziness, lightheadedness, vertigo, weakness, and even temporary loss of consciousness. In the presence of IDA, the normal body stores of iron have been depleted in the bone marrow. Iron-deficiency anemia in infants and toddlers can lead to long-term cognitive, motor, and behavioral impairment (Kazal, 2002).

The most common sources of iron are consumed in the diet and by recycling iron from old red blood cells. Foods high in iron include organ meat, dark green leafy vegetables, raisins, fish, egg yolks, and iron-fortified cereals.

Complications

Injury to tissues
Risk for falls

Incidence

The peak incidences of IDA in children are between 9 and 24 months of age and adolescence. In developed countries, approximately 7–12% of children and women have IDA; but in underdeveloped countries, the incidence is approximately 50% of the children and women (MedlinePlus, 2007). "Infants and toddlers 6–24 months of age need a lot of iron to grow and develop. The iron that full-term infants have stored in their bodies is used up in the first 4–6 months of life. After that, infants need to get iron from food or supplements. Premature and low-birth-weight babies are at even greater risk for iron-deficiency anemia because they don't have as much iron stored in their bodies" (National Heart Lung and Blood Institute, 2006, p. 1). In addition, approximately 50% of pregnant women have some level of IDA with the highest level among pregnant adolescents.

Etiology

IDA in children can result from insufficient dietary intake of iron through iron-rich foods, poor absorption of iron, or loss of blood. According to the National Institutes of Health, neonates have about 500 mg in iron stores when they are born; by adulthood, they need to have accumulated approximately 5,000 mg. To keep up with growth and development needs, children must absorb about 1 mg of iron per day. Since children absorb only approximately 10% of the iron they consume in their diets, they need an additional 8–10 mg per day. Because iron is absorbed more easily in breast milk, breast-fed infants require less dietary iron. Excess intake of cow's milk is a major cause of IDA in young children (MedlinePlus, 2005). Because of the menstrual cycle, adolescent girls are at risk for developing IDA; and as a result of increased vascular demands of pregnancy, pregnant adolescents and women are at highest risk. Poor absorption of iron can result from any chronic inflammatory bowel condition (Crohn's disease and celiac disease) that alters the duodenum's ability to absorb nutrients; decreased levels of folate, vitamin B_{12}, or vitamin C in the diet; or elevated lead in the body (National Heart Lung and Blood Institute, 2006).

Clinical Manifestations

- Pallor
- Fatigue
- Irritability
- Weakness
- Shortness of breath
- Sore tongue
- Brittle nails
- Anorexia
- Headache
- Dizziness
- Lightheadedness
- Blue-tinged or very pale sclerae

Diagnostic Tests

- Complete blood count
- Serum iron level
- Binding capacity of iron (total iron-binding capacity, or TIBC)
- Serum lead level
- Reticulocyte hemoglobin content analysis

Medical Management

The goals of treatment are to restore iron levels, identify the cause of the deficiency, and prevent further episodes. Especially in infants and toddlers, the focus is prevention of IDA because of the potential for long-term effects in the presence of severe or chronic iron deficiency sufficient to result in anemia. Unless an infant is at risk for IDA, risks (including GI distress, colic-like symptoms, diarrhea, constipation) from the use of iron-fortified formulas may outweigh the benefits of this supplementation because healthy neonates have a 4–6 month store of iron from birth. Infants 6–12 months of age may need iron supplementation in infant formulas, however, evidence is insufficient to recommend that those infants who are at low risk for IDA and asymptomatic need iron supplementation (Agency for Healthcare Research and Quality, 2006).

The standard of care for iron-deficiency anemia is oral iron supplementation. Ferrous sulfate and ferrous gluconate are the agents of choice because the ferrous form of iron is absorbed 3 times more readily than the ferric forms (Broyles, Reiss, & Evans, 2007). The iron preparations should be augmented by increased vitamin C because it facilitates the absorption of iron. The hematocrit should return to within defined limits (WDL) after 2 months of iron therapy, but health care providers recommend that iron supplements be continued for another 6–12 months for restoration of the body's iron stores in the bone marrow (MedlinePlus, 2005). Iron supplements should be taken on an empty stomach, but this results in gastrointestinal irritation; so for those children, the supplements can be taken with food.

Increasing dietary iron and taking iron supplements is necessary during pregnancy and lactation. Dietary modification to include red meats (especially liver), whole grain bread, poultry, fish, egg yolks, raisins, and legumes will increase dietary iron intake. In severe cases of IDA, which are very rare, hospitalization and intravenous infusions of packed red blood cells may be required.

Nursing Management

ASSESSMENT
1. Obtain client history
2. Obtain client's height and weight for comparison to standardized chart
3. Perform pediatric assessment

NURSING DIAGNOSES (INCLUDING BUT NOT LIMITED TO)
1. Ineffective cerebral tissue perfusion R/T decreased hemoglobin secondary to depleted iron stores
2. Imbalanced nutrition: less than body requirement R/T inadequate intake/absorption of iron
3. Deficient knowledge R/T condition, treatment, and home care

PLANNING/GOALS
1. Client will experience adequate tissue perfusion as evidenced by resolution of symptoms, oxygen saturation > 94%, and hemoglobin/ hematocrit levels WDL.
2. Parents/client will comply with medication therapy and dietary modifications to increase intake of iron-rich foods as evidenced by verbal confirmation and hemoglobin/hematocrit levels WDL.
3. Parents/caregiver and client (if age-appropriate) will demonstrate understanding of risks, condition, treatment, and home care.

NOC
1. Circulation Status, Neurologic Status
2. Nutritional Status
3. Knowledge: Medications, Diet, Health Promotion

IMPLEMENTATION (FOR HOSPITALIZED CHILD)
1. Tissue perfusion
   a. Assess for manifestations of ineffective tissue perfusion
   b. Monitor oxygen saturation continuously using pulse oximetry
   c. Administer oxygen as prescribed to maintain oxygen saturation within prescribed limits
   d. Monitor laboratory values
   e. Encourage parents to participate in care
   f. Assist with ambulation as needed
   g. Administer iron supplements and vitamin C as prescribed and reinforce teaching
   h. Establish intravenous access with an intravenous catheter of sufficient gauge to infuse blood products if transfusion of packed red blood cells is needed

    i. Transfuse blood following facility protocol including these universal protocols:

        1) Type and cross-match client's blood

        2) Obtain client's vital signs before transfusion begins and upon completion of transfusion

        3) Check red blood cell unit with another licensed person for typing, expiration date, and child's identification

        4) Administer blood with normal saline *only*. *NOTE:* For infants and toddlers, use $\frac{1}{2}$ units and begin transfusion at half the rate required to complete transfusion within 4 hours. Increase rate in small increments over the first hour to achieve needed hourly rate to complete transfusion within 4 hours.

        5) Remain at bedside, monitoring client for a minimum of 15–30 minutes after initiation of transfusion to assess for signs of transfusion reaction. If reaction occurs, immediately stop the transfusion, maintain patency of the intravenous access, and notify health care provider.

        6) Closely monitor transfusion to ensure that it is completed within 4 hours of initiation

2. Nutrition

    a. Perform nutritional assessment in collaboration with dietician

    b. Obtain baseline weight

    c. Instruct parents and child (if age-appropriate) about foods rich in iron

    d. Instruct parents of infant not to allow infant to consume cow's milk

    e. Instruct parents of toddler to decrease child's milk intake and substitute iron-fortified liquid supplement (PediaSure)

3. Parent/caregiver and client (if age-appropriate) teaching

    a. Assess parents' and/or child's current level of understanding

    b. Provide verbal and written instructions regarding:

        1) Medications prescribed and importance of compliance with therapy

        2) The fact that most iron preparations are necessary only on a temporary basis

        3) Iron preparations that cause gastric distress can be given to child with food

        4) Dietary modifications to include foods rich in iron (raisins, whole grains, fish, iron-fortified cereals, liquid supplements, egg yolks, dark green leafy vegetables, pastas, and peanut butter)

        5) Importance of refraining from giving infants cow's milk

        6) Importance of decreasing toddler's milk intake, substituting liquid supplementation (PediaSure)

        7) Importance of follow-up lab work

        8) Importance of follow-up visits with health care provider

        9) Contact numbers of health care provider and referrals (if necessary)

    c. Provide adequate time for teaching

    d. Document teaching and parent/child response

NIC

1. Cerebral Perfusion Promotion
2. Nutrition Management
3. Teaching, Medications, Diet, Health Promotion

EVALUATION

1. Client exhibits adequate tissue perfusion as evidenced by resolution of symptoms, oxygen saturation > 94%, and hemoglobin/hematocrit levels WDL.
2. Parents/client comply with medication therapy and dietary modifications to increase intake of iron-rich foods as evidenced by verbal confirmation and hemoglobin/hematocrit levels WDL.
3. Parents/caregiver and client (if age-appropriate) demonstrate understanding of risks, condition, treatment, and home care.

References

Agency for Healthcare Research and Quality. (2006). *Screening and supplementation for iron-deficiency anemia.* Retrieved March 4, 2008, from http://www.ahrq.gov/clinic/uspstf/uspsiron.htm

Broyles, B. E. (2005). *Medical-surgical nursing clinical companion.* Durham, NC: Carolina Academic Press.

Broyles, B. E., Reiss, B. S., & Evans, M. E. (2007). *Pharmacological aspects of nursing care* (7th ed.). Clifton Park, NY: Delmar Cengage Learning.

Kazal, L. A. (2002). *Prevention of iron deficiency in infants and toddlers.* Retrieved May, 17, 2007, from http://www.aafp.org/afp/20021001/1217.html

MedlinePlus. (2007). *Iron deficiency anemia—children.* Retrieved March 4, 2008, from http://www.nlm.nih.gov/medlineplus/ency/article/000584.htm

National Heart Lung and Blood Institute. (2006). *Iron-deficiency anemia: Who is at risk for iron-deficiency anemia?* Retrieved March 4, 2008, from http://www.nhlbi.nih.gov/health/dci/Diseases/ida/ida_whoisatrisk.html

Potts, N. L., & Mandleco, B. L. (2007). *Pediatric nursing: Caring for children and their families* (2nd ed.). Clifton Park, NY: Delmar Cengage Learning.

65

Juvenile Rheumatoid Arthritis (JRA)

Definition

Juvenile rheumatoid arthritis (JRA) or juvenile idiopathic arthritis (JIA) is a group of systemic chronic inflammatory disorders of the joints and connective tissues (Potts & Mandleco, 2007).

Pathophysiology

JRA/JIA generally progresses through four stages. The onset of the first stage is gradual and involves immune complexes in the blood and synovial tissue initiating an inflammatory response by activating the plasma protein complement causing the release of prostaglandins and kinin. This leads to increased permeability of the vessels in the synovial membranes that attracts leukocytes and lymphocytes to the synovial membranes. Neutrophils and macrophages ingest the immune complexes, resulting in the release of enzymes that inflame the synovium by damaging the articular surfaces of the joints. Stage two is characterized by increased fluid production in the joint. However, unlike synovial fluid that lubricates and nourishes the joint cartilage, this fluid causes the synovium to swell and the villi to thicken. This leads to nodules called pannas formations that protrude into the joint cavity over the articular cartilage, causing it to deteriorate. During the third stage, tough, fibrous connective tissue replaces the granulation, causing occlusion of the joint space (or fibrous ankylosis) and leading to malalignment, joint stiffness, altered angle of tendon pull, instability, and decreased range of motion of the joints involved. The joint capsules and ligaments become restricted, resulting in tendonitis. The fourth stage is characterized by scar tissue calcification resulting in contractures because of the adhesions that form between the joint surfaces and the ankylosis that occurs (Broyles, 2005).

There are three main categories of JRA in this group of disorders: pauciarticular, polyarticular, and systemic. Pauciarticular JRA, which involves fewer than five joints, is the most common type affecting about 50% of all children with arthritis and predominantly affecting girls. Frequently, a single knee joint is affected. Children who develop this form of JRA before the age of 7 years have the best chance of having their joint disease subside with time. However, they are at increased risk of developing iritis or uveitis that may persist independently of the arthritis. These children are more likely to have a positive antinuclear antibody titer. Children older than 7 years of age who develop pauciarticular JRA may experience multiple joint involvement that persists into adulthood. Polyarticular JRA involves five or more joints during the first six months of the illness. This type can develop into the adult form of rheumatoid arthritis that begins at an earlier-than-usual age. Systemic onset JRA begins with a recurrent fever that can be 39.5°C (103°F) or higher, frequently accompanied by an intermittent pink rash. This type of JRA can cause inflammation of the internal organs as well as the joints. Joint swelling may not appear initially but may develop months or even years after the onset of recurring fever. Anemia and leucocytosis also are typical manifestations of this type (American College of Rheumatology, 2007).

Complications of JRA/JIA include pain, contractures, and impaired mobility. The chronicity of this condition can lead to psychosocial issues and delayed growth and development.

Complications

   Pain
   Contractures
   Impaired mobility
   Iritis
   Uveitis
   Delayed growth and development
   Psychosocial issues
   Adult rheumatoid arthritis

Incidence

JRA/JIA occurs in approximately 1 out of every 1,000 children. Systemic onset JRA affects about 10% of children with arthritis, and pauciarticular JRA occurs in approximately 50% of all children with arthritis. Native American children have the highest incidence, and African-Americans and Asian-American children have the lowest incidence. Girls are at higher risk than boys (Potts & Mandleco, 2007; American College of Rheumatology, 2007).

Etiology

The cause of JRA is unknown; as a result, it also is termed *juvenile idiopathic arthritis.* "Research suggests that some children have a genetic predisposition to JRA, but develop the condition only after exposure to an infectious trigger—as yet unknown. Dietary and emotional factors do not appear to play a role in the development of JRA" (American College of Rheumatology, 2007, p. 1).

Clinical Manifestations

   Joint swelling
   Joint pain
   Joint stiffness
   Fever
   Decreased physical mobility
   Decreased range of motion
   Malaise
   Fatigue
   Anorexia
   Weight loss
   Lethargy

Diagnostic Tests

   Erythrocyte sedimentation rate
   Complete blood count
   C-reactive protein
   Serum antinuclear antibody titer
   Serum rheumatoid factor
   Radiography
   Magnetic resonance imaging

Medical Management

The goals of treatment are to decrease joint inflammation, maintain joint function, and prevent psychosocial complications. This is best provided through a multidisciplinary approach including a health care provider, nurses, social worker, occupational therapist, physical therapist, and recreational or child-care specialist.

The standard of care for JRA is the use of nonsteroidal anti-inflammatory drugs (NSAIDs). These may include ibuprofen, naproxen, indomethcin, tolmetin, and salicylates. Because of the gastric irritation associated with these medications, the use of the COX-2 selective inhibitor celecoxib was approved for use in children 2 years and older in the treatment of JRA. This approval by the Food and Drug Administrations (FDA) was published in 2007 and "was based on the serious nature of JRA, the lack of adequate available therapies, and the data . . . which supports the efficacy and safety profile" (Food and Drug Administration, 2007, p. 1). The risk of developing heart complications associated with the use of celecoxib will need long-term study in children. Immunomodulators such as sulfasalazine, methotrexate, and etanercept also are used frequently in the treatment of JRA.

Sulfasalazine is an antimicrobial anti-inflammatory agent, and methotrexate is a folic acid antagonist and cytotoxic agent. Etanercept (also classified as a biologic response modifier), which was developed for the treatment of moderate to severe rheumatoid arthritis in adults, is approved for use in children 4 years and older. Etanercept binds with the tumor necrosis factor (TNF) and blocks TNF interaction with the cell surface of TNF receptors, resulting in the deactivation of TNF, a critical cytokine for normal inflammatory and immune responses (Broyles, Reiss, & Evans, 2007). Etanercept may be used in combination with methotrexate therapy (Spratto & Woods, 2008). Other medications used in the treatment include hydroxychloroquine (an antimalarial agent) and corticosteroids.

Children treated with methotrexate or corticosteroids need to be monitored for increased risk of infection associated with the use of these agents. Child-life specialists are important members of the multidisciplinary team because of their expertise in facilitating growth and development while therapeutically assisting the child with coping strategies related to pain and chronic illness.

Nursing Management

ASSESSMENT

1. Obtain client history
2. Perform physical assessment
3. Obtain pain assessment
4. Assess family's response to disease process

NURSING DIAGNOSES (INCLUDING BUT NOT LIMITED TO)

1. Chronic pain and fatigue R/T swollen or inflamed joints and chronic disease state
2. Impaired physical mobility R/T joint stiffness and restricted movement
3. Delayed growth and development R/T activity intolerance and joint immobility
4. Disturbed body image R/T joint disfiguration and delayed growth and development
5. Risk for injury R/T joint stiffness and restricted movement
6. Deficient knowledge R/T condition, treatment, and home care

PLANNING/GOALS

1. Client's pain will be effectively managed (as determined by client).
2. Client will regain and maintain optimal mobility within constraints of disease process.
3. Client will regain and maintain optimal level of growth and development.

4. Client will demonstrate improved body image and use of positive coping strategies.
5. Client will not experience injury.
6. Parent/client will demonstrate understanding of condition, treatment, and home care.

NOC

1. Pain Control, Energy Conservation
2. Mobility, Joint Movement
3. Child Development
4. Body Image
5. Risk Control
6. Knowledge: Illness Care, Disease Process, Treatment, Health Promotion

IMPLEMENTATION

1. Pain/fatigue
   a. Assess pain level using age-appropriate assessment scale
   b. Administer analgesics proactively as prescribed
   c. Administer anti-inflammatory agents and other antirheumatic agents as prescribed
   d. Position for comfort
   e. Administer heat and cold therapy
   f. Encourage participation in low-impact age-appropriate activities until fatigue subsides
   g. Collaborate with child-life, occupational, and physical therapists
   h. Maintain body alignment
   i. Encourage parental participation in child's care
2. Physical mobility
   a. Assess for joint stiffness, decrease in range of motion, and joint immobility
   b. Assist with and teach range-of-motion exercises
   c. Collaborate with physical therapist for continuity of exercises
   d. Collaborate with health care provider and physical therapist for home exercises
   e. Provide needed reinforcement of instructions given by other members of multidisciplinary team
   f. Provide periods of rest
   g. Encourage age-appropriate activities
   h. Encourage parents to participate in age-appropriate and physical exercise activities
   i. Monitor bowel function
   j. Monitor respiratory function
   k. Monitor serum creatine and serum creatine kinase (CPK) levels
   l. Maintain age-appropriate hydration and nutrition
3. Growth and development
   a. Assess level of growth and development
   b. Recognize child's need to regress in response to illness
   c. Collaborate with child-life specialist for activities to facilitate growth and development
   d. Encourage parents to actively participate in child's care
   e. Collaborate with social worker and occupational therapist

4. Body image
   a. Encourage verbalization of fears, concerns, and feelings about body changes
   b. Listen actively
   c. Assist parents and child in identifying positive coping strategies
   d. Collaborate with social worker for community services
   e. Explain all equipment and procedures
   f. Provide age-appropriate play within child's energy, physical ability, and interest
   g. Promote positive body image by assisting with hairstyle and selection of clothes and age-appropriate jewelry
5. Risk for injury
   a. Assess mobility
   b. Assess gait when ambulating
   c. Assist with ambulation in a nonintrusive manner
   d. Note changes in joint pain, swelling, tenderness, and range of motion after exercise/ambulation
   e. Administer antirheumatoid medications as prescribed
   f. Use splints, applications of heat or cold, and positioning with support during periods of inflammation
   g. Assess for manifestations of infection in children receiving methotrexate, corticosteroids, or biologic response modifier
   h. Assess for visual complications (iritis or uveitis)
6. Parent/client teaching
   a. Assess parent's/child's level of understanding
   b. Provide verbal and written information regarding:
      1) Activity level limits
      2) Home physical activity exercises (for example, benefits of swimming)
      3) Medication administration and importance of compliance with therapy
      4) Referral information and contact information
      5) Child developmental needs and age-appropriate activities
      6) Diet and hydration needs
      7) Coordination of health care provider appointments, referrals, and physical therapy appointments
      8) Importance of long-term follow-up with health care provider
      9) Importance of annual eye exams with an ophthalmologist
      10) Manifestations of worsening condition and contact information
   c. Provide adequate time for teaching in collaboration with multidisciplinary team members
   d. Document teaching and parent's/child's response

NIC

1. Analgesic Administration, Environment Comfort, Calming Techniques, Energy Management
2. Exercise Therapy: Joint Mobility
3. Developmental Enhancement

4. Body Image Enhancement
5. Surveillance: Safety
6. Teaching: Illness Care, Disease Process, Treatment, Health Promotion

EVALUATION

1. Client's pain is effectively managed (as determined by client).
2. Client regains and maintains optimal mobility within constraints of disease process.
3. Client regains and maintains optimal level of growth and development.
4. Client demonstrates improved body image and use of positive coping strategies.
5. Client does not experience injury.
6. Parent/client demonstrate understanding of condition, treatment, and home care.

References

American College of Rheumatology. (2007). *Arthritis in children.* Retrieved March 17, 2007, from http://www.rheumatology.org/public/factsheets/arth_in_children.asp?aud=pat

Broyles, B. E. (2005). *Medical-surgical nursing clinical companion.* Durham, NC: Carolina Academic Press.

Broyles, B. E., Reiss, B. S., & Evans, M. E. (2007). *Pharmacological aspects of nursing care* (7th ed.). Clifton Park, NY: Delmar Cengage Learning.

Food and Drug Administration. (2007). *Summary of clinical review of studies submitted in response to the pediatric written request for NDA 20-998, supplement 021.* Retrieved March 17, 2007, from http://www.fda.gov/cder/foi/esum/2006/020998s021_Celecoxib_Clinical_BPCA.pdf

Potts, N. L., & Mandleco, B. L. (2007). *Pediatric nursing: Caring for children and their families* (2nd ed.). Clifton Park, NY: Delmar Cengage Learning.

Spratto, G. R., & Woods, A. L. (2008). *2008 edition: PDR Nurse's drug handbook.* Clifton Park, NY: Delmar Cengage Learning.

66

KAWASAKI DISEASE (KD)

Definition

Kawasaki disease (KD) is a multisystem immune complex disorder characterized by generalized vasculitis including inflammation of the coronary vessels.

Pathophysiology

Also termed *mucocutaneous lymph node syndrome,* KD was first identified by Dr. Tomisaku Kawasaki, a Japanese pediatrician, in 1967. KD is a pediatric disorder characterized by fever; rash; edema of the hands and feet; redness and irritation of the sclera; lymphedema in the neck; and inflammation of the mouth, lips, and throat. The acute manifestations of KD usually are not serious; however, chronic complications, especially in the coronary vessels, can be observed as early as 14 days following the onset of the disease (American Heart Association, 2008a).

During the acute phase of KD (usually the first 10 days), T-helper cells are more abundant than T-suppressor cells. Increased numbers of B cells spontaneously secrete immunoglobulin G (IgG) and immunoglobulin M (IgM), forming antibody complexes that bind with the vascular endothelium. The inflammation and hypertrophy of the vessels cause them to enlarge rather than to form aneurysms (although aneurysms may develop in the future). This enlargement is termed *ectasia,* meaning "larger than normal for age." This results in pancarditis, or inflammation of the entire heart structure, and can lead to pericardial effusion. Other vessels affected may include the iliac, femoral, axillary, and renal arteries with the same pathological changes.

Following the acute period, inflammation decreases, including desquamation of the skin on the hands and feet. The pronounced changes in the proximal segments and distal branching segments of the coronary arteries decrease. However, in children who developed aneurysms during the acute phase, the aneurysms can become stenotic, decreasing the vessel lumen. This can lead to congestive heart failure, aneurysm rupture, or myocardial infarction. In severe cases, this can result in death.

Complications

Coronary heart disease
Aneurysms
Myocardial infarction

Incidence

The incidence of KD is highest in Japan (approximately 1 case in 1,000 children) although it occurs throughout the world. In the United States, it affects approximately 1 in 10,000 children and is more frequent among Asian-American children although it can occur in any racial or ethnic group. Approximately 80% of cases are found in children under 5 years of age, with its peak incidence in children 2 years of age and younger (Potts & Mandleco, 2007). KD is considered a self-limiting condition usually lasting about 12 days. However, in the United States, as many as 25% of children with KD develop cardiac-related complications including coronary artery aneurysms. KD is a major cause of heart disease in children and results in 4,200 hospitalizations for KD-related heart conditions each year (Metules & Bauer, 2006). Recently, KD has occurred most often in localized outbreaks during the late winter or spring, but is seen year-round. KD affects boys almost twice as often as girls (American Heart Association, 2008a).

Etiology

The exact cause of KD is unknown; however, because it frequently occurs in outbreaks, viral origin is most likely. It is not contagious or hereditary, rarely affecting more than one child in a family. KD is believed to be an antibody-mediated immune complex injury.

Clinical Manifestations

ACUTE

Fever for five days or longer
Erythema of palms and soles
Edema of hands and feet
Erythema and fissures of the lips
Strawberry tongue
Irritability
Bilateral conjunctivitis without exudate
Polymorphous erythematous rash
Enlarged cervical lymph nodes
Desquamation of hands and feet (after acute period)
Leucocytes in the urine

SECONDARY

Arthritis
Arthralgia
Diarrhea
Photophobia
Erythema and fissures of the lips
Inflamed throat
Difficulty eating

Diagnostic Tests

Presence of fever and four of the Clinical Diagnostic Criteria for KD:

1. "Fever persisting for at least 5 days
2. Changes in extremities:
   Acute: Erythema and edema of hands and feet
   Convalescent: Membranous desquamation of fingertips
3. Polymorphous exanthem
4. Bilateral, painless bulbar conjunctival infection without exudate
5. Changes in lips and oral cavity: Erythema and cracking of lips, strawberry tongue, diffuse infection of oral and pharyngeal mucosae
6. Cervical lymphadenopathy ($\geq$ 1.5 cm in diameter), usually unilateral"
   (American Heart Association, 2008b, p. 1; Newburger et al., 2004)

Urinalysis
Complete blood count
Erythrocyte sedimentation rate
C-reactive protein

Electrocardiogram

Echocardiogram (Newburger et al., 2004)

Magnetic resonance imaging

Medical Management

The goals of treatment are to prevent cardiac complications, control the fever, and provide supportive care of the clinical manifestation of KD. The standards of care for these children are intravenous immune globulin (IVIG) and aspirin therapy to reduce formation of coronary aneurysm and to control the fever. The treatment is most beneficial when administered within 10 days of the onset of symptoms. Two preparations of IVIG are used to treat KD. Gamimune N is administered 1 gram/kg as a single dose or 400 mg/kg for four consecutive days; Iveegam EN or Venoglobulin-S is administered as a single dose of 2 grams/kg infused over 10–12 hours. If manifestations continue, another 2 grams/kg dose may be given over 10–12 hours. IVIG is used concomitantly with 80–100 mg/kg/day of aspirin (Gahart & Nazareno, 2008). Most health care providers decrease the dose of aspirin to 3–5 mg/kg/day after the fever subsides; however, aspirin therapy should continue for six to eight weeks (Potts & Mandleco, 2007).

Because of the risk of Reye syndrome in children who have recently experienced a varicella or influenza infection, children taking aspirin (salicylates) long term should receive an annual influenza vaccine (Newburger et al., 2004).

Anticoagulant therapy with warfarin may be required for children with large aneurysms to prevent thrombus formation in the coronary arteries. For a child experiencing coronary artery occlusion, tissue plasminogen is an effective thrombolytic. The prognosis is good with KD having a 1% mortality rate.

Nursing Management

ASSESSMENT

1. Obtain client history
2. Assess for presence of recent varicella or influenza infection
3. Assess for manifestations of KD
4. Obtain vital signs
5. Perform pediatric assessment

NURSING DIAGNOSES (INCLUDING BUT NOT LIMITED TO)

1. Risk for decreased cardiac output R/T inflammation of the coronary arteries
2. Risk for deficient fluid volume R/T fever
3. Acute pain R/T skin desquamation of hands and feet and inflammation of the joints
4. Anxiety R/T child's hospitalization, condition, and uncertain prognosis
5. Deficient knowledge R/T child's condition, treatment, prognosis, and home care

PLANNING/GOALS

1. Client will maintain cardiac output within defined limits (WDL).
2. Client will maintain fluid balance as evidenced by urine output of 1–2 mL/kg/hr and urine specific gravity and vital signs WDL.
3. Client will demonstrate pain management as evidenced by verbal and behavioral indicators and engagement in age-appropriate activities.

4. Parents/caregiver/child will exhibit decreased manifestations of anxiety as evidenced by verbal and behavioral indicators and will use positive coping strategies.

5. Parents/caregiver will demonstrate understanding of child's condition, treatment, prognosis, and home care.

NOC

1. Risk Control, Cardiac Pump Effectiveness
2. Risk Control, Fluid Balance
3. Pain Control
4. Anxiety
5. Knowledge: Disease Process, Medications, Treatment, Health Promotion

IMPLEMENTATION

1. Cardiac output
   a. Assess vital signs frequently at least every 4 hours
   b. Assess heart sounds every 4 hours
   c. Position with head of bed/crib elevated
   d. Initiate and maintain patency of intravenous access, monitoring at least hourly
   e. Administer premedications of diphenhydramine and acetaminophen as prescribed prior to IVIG infusion
   f. Have epinephrine available in the event of an anaphylactic response to IVIG
   g. Administer IVIG as prescribed
   h. Monitor for adverse effects of IVIG (facial flushing, chest tightness, chills, dizziness, nausea, vomiting, diaphoresis, or hypotension)
   i. Administer aspirin as prescribed, collaborating with health care provider if child has history of recent varicella or influenza infection
   j. Encourage fluid intake by providing child's favorite beverages
   k. Assess temperature 30–45 minutes following aspirin administration

2. Fluid balance
   a. Monitor intake and output
   b. Monitor urine specific gravity
   c. Assess skin turgor
   d. Maintain integrity of intravenous access, monitoring at least hourly
   e. Encourage fluid intake by providing child's favorite beverages
   f. Maintain pain control at a level of 1 on the 1–5 faces scale

3. Pain
   a. Assess pain level hourly
   b. Administer pain medication proactively as prescribed
   c. Administer IVIG and aspirin as prescribed
   d. Administer soothing sponge bath
   e. Keep skin clean and dry
   f. Offer cool or frozen liquids by mouth
   g. Apply local throat anesthetics 15–60 minutes prior to meals
   h. Provide mouth care including topical medications for lips
   i. Cluster activities that require touching child and use palms of hands when lifting child

     j. Line bed with soft blankets from home if possible

     k. Encourage child to participate in age-appropriate diversionary activities

     l. Encourage parents to participate in care and play

4. Anxiety

     a. Encourage parents to verbalize feelings and concerns

     b. Listen actively

     c. Explain all equipment and procedures

     d. Reinforce information about child's condition provided by health care provider

     e. Encourage parents to participate in child's care

     f. Assist parents to identify positive coping strategies and activate support systems

     g. Involve child in age-appropriate diversionary activities

     h. Provide for parental spiritual needs

5. Parent/caregiver teaching

     a. Assess parents'/caregiver's current level of understanding

     b. Provide verbal and written information regarding:

          1) Skin care, avoiding soaps and gently rinsing child's skin with water only

          2) Care of oral mucous membranes

          3) Pain management

          4) Medication administration including importance of compliance with aspirin therapy

          5) Importance of child's drinking fluids

          6) Dietary modifications including low-cholesterol diet, low-acid liquids that are high in calories, bland foods offered first, and child's favorite foods made available

          7) Procedure to monitor morning and evening temperature and to record on chart

          8) Importance of follow-up care with health care provider including bringing temperature chart to visits

          9) Manifestations of disease complications

          10) Contact information for reporting manifestations to health care provider

          11) Referral information if needed

NIC

1. Risk Identification, Medication Administration, Vital Signs Monitoring, Cardiac Precautions
2. Fluid Management, Fluid Monitoring
3. Medication Administration
4. Coping Enhancement
5. Teaching: Disease Process, Medications, Treatment, Health Promotion

EVALUATION

1. Client maintains cardiac output WDL.
2. Client maintains fluid balance as evidenced by urine output of 1–2 mL/kg/hr and urine specific gravity and vital signs WDL.

3. Client demonstrates pain management as evidenced by verbal and behavioral indicators and engagement in age-appropriate activities.

4. Parents/caregiver/child exhibit decreased manifestations of anxiety as evidenced by verbal and behavioral indicators and use positive coping strategies.

5. Parents/caregiver demonstrate understanding of child's condition, treatment, prognosis, and home care.

References

American Heart Association. (2008a). *Diagnostic guidelines for Kawasaki disease.* Retrieved March 4, 2008, from http://www.americanheart.org/presenter.jhtml?identifier=11163

American Heart Association. (2008b). *Kawasaki disease.* Retrieved March 4, 2008, from http://www.americanheart.org/presenter.jhtml?identifier=162

Gahart, B. L., & Nazareno, A. R. (2008). *2008 intravenous medications* (24th ed.). St. Louis, MO: Elsevier Mosby.

Metules, T., & Bauer, J. (2006). Be on the lookout for this seasonal ailment. *RN, 69*(2).

Newburger, J. W., Takahashi, M., Gerber, M. A., Gewitz, M. H., Tani, L. Y., Burns, J. C., Shulman, S. T., Bolger, A. F., Ferrieri, P., Baltimore, R. S., Wilson, W. R., Baddour, L. M., Levison, M. E., Pallasch, T. J., Falace, D. A., & Taubert, K. A. (2004, October 26). Diagnosis, treatment, and long-term management of Kawasaki disease: A statement for health professionals from the Committee on Rheumatic Fever, Endocarditis and Kawasaki Disease, Council on Cardiovascular Disease in the Young, American Heart Association. *Circulation, 110*(17), 2747–2771. Retrieved May 17, 2007, from http://www.guideline.gov/summary/summary.aspx?ss=15&doc_id=6180&nbr=3979#s23

Potts, N. L., & Mandleco, B. L. (2007). *Pediatric nursing: Caring for children and their families* (2nd ed.). Clifton Park, NY: Delmar Cengage Learning.

67

LEUKEMIA/STEM CELL TRANSPLANTATION

Definition

Leukemia is a neoplasm of the blood-forming cells that occurs when "cells arising from stem cells lose the ability to differentiate into white blood cells, red blood cells, and platelets" (Rogers, 2005, p. 61). Hematopoietic stem cell transplantation, also known as bone marrow transplantation or bone marrow transplant (BMT) or hematopoietic stem cell transplant (HSCT), is the replacement of a child's stem cells after the child's "own bone marrow has been destroyed by disease or by the treatment of a malignant disease" (Potts & Mandleco, 2007, p. 933).

Pathophysiology

Leukemia is characterized by the proliferation of immature white blood cells within the bone marrow that disseminates systemically to other organs (Broyles, 2005). It is divided into four types: (1) acute lymphocytic leukemia (ALL), also called acute lymphoblastic leukemia, (2) acute myelogenous leukemia (AML), also called acute myeloid leukemia, (3) chronic lymphocytic leukemia (CLL), and (4) chronic myelogenous leukemia. The chronic forms of leukemia are extremely rare in children, most often affecting adults. Juvenile myelomonocytic leukemia is a rare type of leukemia that is neither chronic nor acute. It originates from myeloid cells but does not grow as fast as AML or as slow as chronic myeloid leukemia. Some types of leukemia have features of both ALL and AML and are termed *hybrid* or *mixed lineage leukemias*. They often are treated like ALL and respond to treatment like ALL (American Cancer Society, 2007). This discussion will focus on ALL and AML. Stem cell transplants (SCTs) will be discussed under "Medical Management" in this chapter.

ALL develops from lymphocyte-forming cells in the bone marrow and is further classified according to the type of cell involved. Most ALL cases are of B-cell origin; the rest are of T-cell origin. AML develops from the bone marrow cells that form granulocytes, monocytes, erythrocytes, or platelets. Both types most likely occur from a fundamental genetic mutation in the stem cell, so all cells derived from this stem cell also have the defect.

ALL is the most common leukemia in children and is characterized by malignant growth of immature blast cells called lymphoblasts (B cell or T cell) that normally make lymphocytes in the bone marrow. These lymphocytes mature to help the body defend itself from infection. In ALL, the immature lymphoblasts proliferate in the bone marrow until most of the marrow is almost completely saturated with them. These undifferentiated and immature lymphoblasts are not capable of preventing infection. They proliferate rapidly and have a prolonged life span, not responding to the body's biofeedback mechanism that normally controls cellular growth. In the bone marrow, they crowd out the mature lymphocytes, the erythrocytes, and platelet-producing cells by depriving them of oxygen and nutrients. This leads to leukopenia, anemia, and thrombocytopenia. This places the child at risk for infection, ineffective tissue perfusion, and bleeding. As the immature blast cells continue to proliferate, they enter systemic circulation, crossing the blood-brain barrier and infiltrating the central nervous system, reticuloendothelial system (lymph nodes, liver, and spleen), and other body tissues and systems. In these systems, they compete with normal functioning cells for nutrients and metabolites, causing premature death to these normal cells.

The spleen and liver are saturated by these cells resulting in splenomegaly and hepatomegaly, respectively (Broyles, 2005).

In AML the bone marrow produces large numbers of blast cells called myeloblasts instead of all three types of mature white blood cells (neutrophils, lymphocytes, and monocytes). These myeloblasts then enter the systemic circulation, also crossing the blood-brain barrier. In addition to the brain, they can invade the skin, the ovaries and testes, and other organs, competing with normal cells and causing their premature death. AML cells occasionally form a solid tumor called an isolated granulocytic sarcoma or chloroma (National Cancer Institute, 2007).

Complications

Life-threatening infection
Anemia
Thrombocytopenia
Bleeding/Hemorrhage
Organ failure

Incidence

ALL represents 23% of cancer diagnoses among children younger than 15 years of age (National Cancer Institute, 2007) and 75–80% of all leukemia cases in children. Approximately 3, 930 new cases of ALL are diagnosed annually in the United States in children and adolescents under the age of 19 (Leukemia & Lymphoma Society, 2007). ALL occurs at a rate of 30–40 children per million annually in the United States. The peak incidence of ALL is in children aged 2–3 years (> 80/million/year), with rates declining to 20 per million for children aged 8–10 years. The incidence of ALL in Caucasian children is 3 times higher than in African-American children; however, the highest incidence (43 per million) is in Hispanic children (National Cancer Institute, 2007). Approximately 85% of cases of ALL are B-cell type; the other 13–15% are T-cell-originated and occur more often in older children. "The American Cancer Society estimates that about 2,790 new cases of ALL leukemia will be found in children in 2007" (American Cancer Society, 2007, p. 1). AML is more common in the first two years of life. It affects 0.9 per 100,000 children under 4 years of age and 0.8 per 100,000 children 15–19 years of age (National Cancer Institute, 2007).

Etiology

Lifestyle risk factors that affect the incidence of cancers in adults (diet, exercise, and use of tobacco) are not linked to childhood cancers. Although the exact cause of ALL and AML is unknown, certain genetic conditions including Down syndrome, Klinefelter's syndrome, and Li-Fraumeni syndrome are risk factors for ALL (American Cancer Society, 2006) and for familial monosomy 7 syndrome, Fanconi anemia, congenital dyskeratosis, Bloom's syndrome, neurofibromatosis type 1, and Noonan's syndrome. These conditions result in altered immune systems and increase the risk of the child developing leukemia. Alcohol intake in a pregnant woman may increase the risk that her child will develop AML. An identical twin of a child who develops leukemia before the age of 6 years has a 20–25% higher risk than other children. Other risk factors for developing leukemia include exposure to high doses of radiation and immunosuppression therapy used to treat posttransplant children (American Cancer Society, 2007).

Scientific research concerning how certain changes in DNA can cause bone marrow stem cells to develop into leukemia is progressing rapidly. Research has determined that DNA changes linked to leukemia occur after birth rather than having been inherited, and these changes occur for no apparent reason(s). DNA is housed in 23 pairs of chromosomes, and translocations of DNA (one chromosome attaches to the wrong chromosome) can lead to cancer (American Cancer Society, 2007).

Clinical Manifestations

Fatigue

Pallor

Fever

Neutropenia

Infection

Easy bleeding or bruising

Petechiae

Purpura

Bone pain

Abdominal distention

Lymphadenopathy

Coughing

Dyspnea

Facial edema

Headache

Visual disturbances

Vomiting

Rashes

Weakness

Seizure activity

Diagnostic Tests

Complete blood count

Bone marrow biopsy

Serum electrolytes

Lumbar puncture

Lymph node biopsy

Chest radiography

Computed tomography

Ultrasonography

Magnetic resonance imaging

Bone scan

Gallium scans

Medical Management

The goals of treatment for leukemia are to eradicate the cancer cells with minimal complications and to provide the child with a cancer-free future. A multidisciplinary approach is important to best meet the physical and psychosocial needs of the child and family. The multidisciplinary team approach incorporates the skills of the primary health care provider, pediatric surgical subspecialists, radiation oncologists, pediatric medical oncologists/hematologists, rehabilitation specialists, pediatric nurse specialists, and social workers. Many people are not aware of the 90–95% remission rate with ALL. As a result of this deficient knowledge, people continue to view leukemia as a "fatal disease," which increases the psychosocial impact of the diagnosis. Education is a critical part of the care of this family.

Chemotherapy is the standard of care for the treatment of leukemia. Although other routes of administration (oral and intrathecal) may be used, intravenous administration is most common. Because of the toxic nature of intravenous antineoplastic agents, these agents are infused through a surgically placed central venous access device (CVAD) (tunneled catheter or implanted port). Chemotherapy for leukemia involves combination therapy or regimens. Refer to Chapter 22: Chemotherapy.

Current chemotherapy regimens for the treatment of ALL usually involve three phases. The first phase is induction, in which 95% of children achieve remission (meaning that 99% of the cancer cells have been destroyed) after one month of treatment. This phase focuses on eradicating the immature lymphoblasts in the bone marrow. During induction, the child spends some or much of the time in the hospital. All children need to have lumbar punctures to inject chemotherapy intrathecally (into the cerebrospinal fluid) to prevent central nervous system involvement. The second phase, consolidation, is directed at destroying the leukemic cells in other areas of the body where they "hide." This phase lasts for a minimum of four to eight months. Finally, the maintenance phase begins after the induction and consolidation phases have substantially reduced the number of leukemia cells. The entire chemotherapy regimen lasts two to three years for most children with ALL (American Cancer Society, 2007). Prognosticating factors for chemotherapy in children include age (best prognosis in children diagnosed between 2 and 10 years of age), gender (girls have a better prognosis than boys), type of leukemia (ALL has a better prognosis than AML), and white blood cell count at diagnosis (a normal or slightly low count has a better prognosis than a high white cell count).

Antineoplastic agents used to treat ALL include asparaginase (enzyme), corticosteroids, cyclophosphamide (alkylating agent), cytarabine (antimetabolite), daunorubicin (antibiotic), doxorubicin (antibiotic), etoposide (plant alkaloid), idarubicin (antibiotic), ifosfamide (alkylating agent), mercaptopurine (antimetabolite), methotrexate (antimetabolite), PEG-L-asparaginase (enzyme), teniposide (plant alkaloid), thioguanine (antimetabolite), and vincristine (plant alkaloid). Combination chemotherapeutic regimens include OAP (Oncovin (vincristine), Ara-C (cytarabine), and prednisone), COAP (cyclophosphamide, Oncovin, Ara-C, and prednisone), Ad-OAP (Adriamycin, Oncovin, Ara-C, and prednisone), and DAT (daunorubicin, Ara-C, and thioguanine) (Broyles, Reiss, & Evans, 2007).

Treatment for children with AML has two phases: induction and intensification. During induction, the combinations of antineoplastic agents used to treat AML differ from those used in the treatment of ALL. Chemotherapy agents used to treat AML include azacitidine (antimetabolite) with premedication of ondansetron, cytarabine (antimetabolite), doxorubicin (antibiotic), etoposide (plant alkaloid), fludarabine (antimetabolite), hydroxyurea (antimetabolite), idarubicin (antibiotic), mercaptopurine (antimetabolite), and thioguanine (antimetabolite) (Gahart & Nazareno, 2008; Potts & Mandleco, 2007).

Therapy is administered in cycles usually extending over several days, and these cycles are repeated every four weeks until the bone marrow appears to be free of leukemic cells (remission). Remission occurs in 75–85% of these children following induction therapy. Intrathecal chemotherapy is often administered as an adjunct to treatment given intravenously. The intensification phase begins after remission and usually involves the administration of one or two rounds of chemotherapy. Most children treated for AML do not require maintenance chemotherapy (American Cancer Society, 2007).

Because AML recurs more often than ALL, some pediatric oncologists recommend SCT for some children with AML immediately after they have gone into remission if they have a brother or sister who can donate cells. If the cancer returns following the first round of chemotherapy, most health care providers will suggest SCT as soon as the child goes into remission again.

Although 75–85% of children with AML achieve remission following induction chemotherapy, the cure rate for AML with standard treatment is 40–50%. Treatment with SCT from a sibling with a good tissue match results in a 55–60% cure rate (American Cancer Society, 2007).

BONE MARROW TRANSPLANT (BMT) OR PERIPHERAL BLOOD/ HEMATOPOIETIC STEM CELL TRANSPLANT (SCT)

SCT is used for children who have a poor prognosis with standard or intensive chemotherapy. SCT is more frequently used with children with AML than with ALL. This treatment can be used for children whose chances of survival are very poor with standard or even intensive chemotherapy.

SCTs are typed according to the source of the donor: (1) allogeneic (bone marrow used is from another person who is genetically similar), (2) autologous (stem cells come from the child), and (3) syngeneic (cells are donated from an identical twin). The most common type of SCT used is allogeneic. Syngeneic is least commonly used, especially with leukemia. Identical twins have an increased risk of leukemia if one twin has it, and there is the risk that the donor cells may possess the genetic mutation for leukemia. Autologous SCT is rarely used to treat leukemia because (1) there may be a risk that some of the stem cells have cancer and (2) leukemia has a higher chance of recurrence. The donor for allogeneic SCT usually is a sibling of the child; but if this is not possible, health care providers must search for a human leukocyte antigen (cell marker)-matched donor. Allogeneic transplants require the child to receive long-term immunosuppressant therapy to prevent rejection of the donor cells (American Cancer Society, 2007).

Prior to the transplant, stem cells are harvested from the posterior iliac crest of the donor or from the bloodstream in a process called apheresis. Both of these donor sites contain stem cells from which all blood cells are formed. Umbilical cord blood is another source of stem cells that can be donated for SCT. The harvested stem cells are frozen and stored. The child is then given high doses of chemotherapy with busulfan and cyclophosphamide (and sometimes radiation) to destroy existing bone marrow and malignant cells. After treatment, the stored stem cells are thawed and transfused intravenously into the child. The stem cells travel to the sites that produce bone marrow and establish themselves. It takes approximately two to four weeks for the graft to "take," which is called engraftment, at which time the bone marrow becomes functional and produces erythrocytes, leukocytes, and platelets. Until engraftment occurs, the child is at high risk for potentially life-threatening infection and bleeding. Antimicrobial agents are used to help prevent and treat opportunistic infections until engraftment occurs. Blood transfusions of packed red blood cells and platelets may help increase tissue perfusion and prevent bleeding until engraftment occurs. Complete recovery of immune function can take up to one to two years for allogeneic SCT (National Cancer Institute, 2007).

Immunosuppressant agents (cyclosporine, methotrexate, FK 506, OKT3, antithymocyte globulin, azathioprine, and sandimmune) and corticosteroids (prednisone and methylprednisolone) are used to prevent graft-versus-host disease (GVHD), a complication of allogeneic SCT. GVHD or stem cell rejection occurs during engraftment by the donor lymphocytes when they activate donor T cells against the recipient's histocompatibility complex antigens. This causes cell death from cell-mediated cytotoxic effects. GVHD occurs only in the presence of three factors: (1) when the graft contains immunocompetent cells, (2) when the recipient is immunocompromised (all transplant recipients are treated with immunosuppressants), and (3) when there are histocompatibility differences between the graft and the host. GVHD can be acute or chronic. Acute GVHD occurs within the first 100 days posttransplant and is characterized by ear, palm, sole, and trunk erythema as well as enteritis, cholestatic hepatitis, and recurring malignancy. Chronic GVHD occurs after the first 100 days posttransplant and manifests as systemic lupus erythematosus (SLE) and primary biliary cirrhosis.

Stem cell transplantation is very expensive (more than $100,000) and requires a lengthy hospital stay. Because it is so costly, parents should be sure to get a written approval from their insurer if their child is to have this treatment (National Cancer Institute, 2007).

Nursing Management (Leukemia and SCT)

Also refer to Chapter 22: Chemotherapy and Chapter 87: Radiation Therapy.

ASSESSMENT

1. Obtain client history
2. Assess for manifestations of leukemia
3. Perform pediatric physical assessment
4. Assess for psychosocial impact of diagnosis for family

NURSING DIAGNOSES (INCLUDING BUT NOT LIMITED TO)

LEUKEMIA (AND LEUKEMIA BEING TREATED WITH CHEMOTHERAPY)

1. Risk for infection R/T lack of mature leukocytes
2. Risk for bleeding R/T depleted platelets
3. Risk for ineffective tissue perfusion R/T depleted erythrocytes
4. Anxiety R/T diagnosis, procedures, treatment, and prognosis
5. Deficient knowledge R/T condition, treatment, and home care

POSTSTEM CELL TRANSPLANTATION

6. High risk for infection R/T immunocompromised state pre- and posttransplant
7. Risk for bleeding R/T bone marrow and platelet destruction prior to transplant
8. Risk for altered tissue perfusion R/T red blood cell destruction
9. Acute pain R/T to cellular destruction secondary to chemotherapy/irradiation
10. Imbalanced nutrition: less than body requirements R/T anorexia, stomatitis/esophagitis, nausea, and vomiting
11. Risk for injury, complications associated with pretransplant chemotherapy/irradiation
12. Risk for injury, GVHD R/T allogeneic transplant
13. Deficient knowledge R/T stem cell transplantation, complications, and home care

PLANNING/GOALS

LEUKEMIA (AND LEUKEMIA BEING TREATED WITH CHEMOTHERAPY)

1. Client will not experience infection; but if infection occurs, it will be promptly detected and treated.
2. Client will not experience bleeding episodes; but if bleeding occurs, it will be promptly detected and treated.
3. Client will not experience impaired tissue perfusion; but if anemia occurs, it will be promptly detected and treated.
4. Client/family will express feelings and concerns and use positive coping strategies.
5. Client/family will demonstrate understanding of condition, treatment, and home care, maintaining compliance with therapeutic regimen.

POSTSTEM CELL TRANSPLANT

6. Client will not contract infection; but if infection occurs, it will be effectively treated.
7. Client will not experience bleeding complications; but if bleeding occurs, it will be effectively treated.
8. Client will maintain adequate tissue perfusion as evidenced by capillary refill, oxygen saturation, and vital signs within defined limits (WDL).

9. Client will maintain pain control as determined by client using age-appropriate pain scale as evidenced by verbal and behavioral indicators.
10. Client will consume adequate nutrition to maintain and support growth.
11. Client will not experience complications associated with pretransplant chemotherapy/irradiation.
12. Client will not experience GVHD; but if GVHD occurs, it will be promptly and effectively treated.
13. Client (if age-appropriate) and family will demonstrate understanding of stem cell transplantation and necessary home care.

NOC

LEUKEMIA (AND LEUKEMIA BEING TREATED WITH CHEMOTHERAPY)

1. Risk Control, Immune Status
2. Risk Control, Circulation Status
3. Risk Control, Tissue Perfusion
4. Anxiety
5. Knowledge: Disease Process, Treatment, Medications

POSTSTEM CELL TRANSPLANT

6. Risk Control, Immune Status
7. Risk Control, Circulation Status
8. Risk Control, Tissue Perfusion
9. Pain Level
10. Nutrition Status
11. Risk Control, Immune Status
12. Risk Control, Immune Status
13. Knowledge: Treatment, Health Promotion

IMPLEMENTATION

LEUKEMIA (AND LEUKEMIA BEING TREATED WITH CHEMOTHERAPY)

1. Risk for infection
   a. Monitor temperature at least every 4 hours during hospitalization
   b. Provide environment to protect against infection
   c. Ensure that all people coming in contact with client maintain meticulous hand washing
   d. Restrict visitors with upper respiratory infections and communicable diseases
   e. Maintain and assist with thorough hygiene care
   f. Instruct parents/child regarding how to perform oral hygiene after each meal and assist as needed
   g. Avoid invasive procedures
   h. Monitor white blood cell count and differential
   i. Perform CVAD care using strict asepsis
   j. Restrict presence of fresh flowers, fruits, and vegetables if neutropenic and place on neutropenic precautions according to facility protocol
   k. Administer prescribed antibiotics
2. Risk for bleeding
   a. Assess all mucous membranes for bleeding
   b. Monitor vital signs
   c. Monitor platelet count

    d. Use soft toothbrush or toothettes for oral hygiene

    e. Avoid foods that may damage oral mucous membranes

    f. Avoid invasive procedures including rectal temperatures, urinary catheterization, and intramuscular injections. Do not perform biopsies and lumbar punctures if platelet count < 50,000 cells/mm^3.

    g. Apply pressure to puncture sites (lumbar puncture and discontinued intravenous access) for 3–5 minutes and to arterial blood gas sites for 20 minutes

    h. Administer medications as prescribed

    i. Administer platelets as prescribed

    j. Assess for epistaxis

    k. Instruct to avoid picking nose, blowing nose, coughing or sneezing forcefully, and straining to have bowel movement

    l. Engage child in low-impact age-appropriate activities

    m. Collaborate with health care provider for prescription for stool softener

    n. Inform older children to avoid safety razors and use only electric razors

3. Risk for ineffective tissue perfusion

    a. Assess for manifestations of ineffective tissue perfusion with focus on neurologic assessment

    b. Monitor erythrocyte count, hemoglobin, and hematocrit

    c. Instruct child to seek assistance when ambulating

    d. Administer packed red blood cells as prescribed and follow facility protocol for blood administration

    e. Administer epoetin alfa recombinant (Procrit)

    f. Monitor continuous pulse oximetry

    g. Administer oxygen as prescribed, titrating to pulse oximetry to maintain oxygen saturation > 94%

    h. Monitor frequent vital signs

    i. Provide periods of undisturbed rest

4. Anxiety

    a. Try to be with child and family when diagnosis of leukemia is verbalized to them

    b. Maintain calm and empathetic affect

    c. Encourage expression of feelings and concerns

    d. Listen actively

    e. Anticipate grieving process and assist with progression through the stages

    f. Provide information concerning treatment and facts about how research has provided improved prognosis for children with leukemia in collaboration with health care provider

    g. Contact pastoral care or client's minister according to wishes of client/family

    h. Assist child (if age-appropriate) and family in identifying positive coping strategies

    i. Engage child in age-appropriate activities

    j. Collaborate with child-life specialist for pediatric relaxation techniques, diversionary activities, and guided imagery

     k.   Collaborate with health care provider for prescription for anxiolytics as indicated by client, depending on child's age. *NOTE:* This might be necessary for school-age or adolescent child.

5. Parent/caregiver/client teaching

     a.   Assess child's (if age-appropriate) and family's level of understanding

     b.   Provide demonstration of CVAD care if client is being discharge with access; provide adequate time for return demonstration

     c.   Provide verbal and written information regarding:

         1) Accurate data concerning prognosticating statistics in collaboration with health care provider

         2) Risk factors for developing infection, bleeding, and anemia and instructions as needed to avoid risk factors and signs and symptoms to report immediately

         3) Medication administration including importance of compliance with the prescribed medication regime

         4) Chemotherapy schedule

         5) Manifestation of adverse effects of chemotherapy (infection, bleeding, and anemia)

         6) Care of central venous access

         7) Manifestations of worsening of condition

         8) Contact phone numbers for reporting signs and symptoms

         9) Importance of regular hand washing and appropriate technique

         10) Importance of follow-up lab tests with health care provider

     d.   Provide adequate time for teaching, demonstrations, and return demonstrations

     e.   Document teaching and child's/family's response including evaluation of return demonstrations

POSTSTEM CELL TRANSPLANT

6. High risk for infection

     a.   Monitor temperature at least every 4 hours

     b.   Maintain protective isolation precautions

     c.   Monitor leukocyte counts and differential

     d.   Instruct visitors to carefully wash hands prior to entering child's room

     e.   Assess CVAD site hourly and maintain sterile technique during dressing changes and lab draws from CVAD

     f.   Obtain blood cultures as prescribed if temperature elevates

     g.   Note any reddened areas on skin as this can be a sign of infection in the compromised client

     h.   Infuse marrow/stem cells according to facility protocol

     i.   Administer antibiotics and/or lymphocyte transfusion as prescribed

7. Risk for bleeding

     a.   Assess for bleeding from nose and oral mucous membranes

     b.   Assess urine every void for blood

     c.   Hemoccult test each stool

     d.   Monitor child receiving oxygen via nasal cannula closely for bleeding

     e.   Report any bleeding to health care provider and institute bleeding precautions

   f. Use mouth swab or soft tooth brush for oral hygiene
   g. Do not administer intramuscular or subcutaneous injections
   h. Do not assess temperature rectally
   i. Monitor platelet count
   j. Maintain patency of intravenous access, monitoring hourly
   k. Infuse marrow/stem cells as prescribed and per facility protocol
   l. Administer platelets as prescribed

8. Risk for ineffective tissue perfusion
   a. Assess vital signs every 4 hours
   b. Assess continuous oxygen saturation using pulse oximetry
   c. Administer oxygen as prescribed, titrating to maintain oxygen saturation > 94%
   d. Monitor erythrocyte count, hemoglobin, and hematocrit values
   e. Infuse marrow/stem cells according to facility protocol
   f. Administer blood products (packed red blood cells) as prescribed and per facility blood transfusion protocol
   g. Monitor capillary refill with shift assessment as indicated by client manifestations
   h. Assess child's ability to perform activities of daily living (ADL) and assist as needed
   i. Assist with ambulation to maintain safety

9. Pain
   a. Assess pain level hourly using age-appropriate pain assessment tool
   b. Assess mucous membranes for signs of stomatitis
   c. Assess for painful swallowing or other indications of esophagitis
   d. Administer intravenous opioid analgesics (morphine sulfate and hydromorphone) as indicated by client's assessment of pain level. *NOTE:* Pain is what the client says it is.
   e. Collaborate with health care provider for moderate to severe client pain to provide for continuous infusion and patient-controlled analgesia (PCA) dosing until pain is controlled
   f. Provide age-appropriate diversionary activities
   g. Position for comfort
   h. Encourage parents/caregiver to participate in child's care and to provide comfort to child

10. Nutrition
   a. Assess for presence of mucositis
   b. Assess for nausea and vomiting
   c. Administer medications as prescribed
   d. Assess child's food and fluid preferences
   e. Provide Popsicles, cold juice, and other drinks
   f. Collaborate with dietician to provide child's favorite foods
   g. Maintain environment conducive to nutritional intake
   h. Encourage parents/family to join child at mealtime

11. Risk for complications of stem cell transplant
   a. Premedicate for chemotherapy as prescribed, which usually involves using serotonin-blocking agents (ondansetron (Zofran), granisetron (Kytril), and dolasetron (Anzanet))
   b. Monitor intake and output
   c. Assess for diarrhea and resulting dehydration

    d. Maintain patency of CVAD, monitoring at least hourly

    e. Administer intravenous hydration as prescribed

    f. Monitor vital signs every 4 hours for indications of thyroid deficiency from irradiation

    g. Assess for skin breakdown from radiation

    h. Monitor pulmonary, cardiac, liver, and metabolic function to note chronic effects of SCT

12. Risk for GVHD

    a. Administer immunosuppressant agents as prescribed

    b. Instruct parents/family about immunosuppressant therapy and importance of compliance with this regimen

    c. Monitor for adverse effects associated with immunosuppressant and corticosteroid therapy

    d. Instruct parents/family about manifestations of acute and chronic GVHD to monitor for at home

    e. Monitor for manifestations of acute GVHD

13. Parent/client teaching

    a. Assess client's (if age-appropriate) and parent's current level of understanding

    b. Provide verbal and written instructions regarding:

       1) Reinforcement of CVAD care

       2) Use of pain medication

       3) Contact phone number for health care provider

       4) Manifestations to report immediately to health care provider including elevated temperature, bleeding, dizziness, acute GVHD, and chronic GVHD

       5) Importance of avoiding crowds and exposure to individuals with a communicable disease until child's leukocyte count is WDL

       6) Use of age-appropriate activities with low risk for injury

       7) Importance of compliance with immunosuppressant therapy

       8) Referral information and contact phone numbers

       9) Importance of follow-up lab work (blood drawing through CVAD) and monitoring by health care provider

    c. Provide adequate time for teaching, client and parental questions, and return demonstrations

    d. Document teaching and child/parental response including evaluation of return demonstration of skills required at home

NIC

LEUKEMIA (AND LEUKEMIA BEING TREATED WITH CHEMOTHERAPY)

1. Risk Identification, Infection Precautions

2. Risk Identification, Bleeding Precautions

3. Risk Identification, Vital Signs Monitoring, Oxygen Therapy

4. Coping Enhancement

5. Teaching: Disease Process, Treatment, Medications

POSTSTEM CELL TRANSPLANT

6. Risk Identification, Infection Precautions

7. Risk Identification, Bleeding Precautions

8. Risk Identification, Vital Signs Monitoring, Oxygen Therapy

9. Analgesia Administration
10. Nutrition Management, Nutrition Monitoring
11. Risk Identification
12. Risk Identification
13. Teaching: Treatment, Health Promotion

EVALUATION

LEUKEMIA (AND LEUKEMIA BEING TREATED WITH CHEMOTHERAPY)

1. Client did experience infection, but it was promptly detected and treated.
2. Client did experience bleeding episodes, but they were promptly detected and treated.
3. Client did experience impaired tissue perfusion, but it was promptly detected and treated.
4. Client/family express feelings and concerns and use positive coping strategies.
5. Client/family demonstrate understanding of condition, treatment, and home care, maintaining compliance with therapeutic regimen.

POSTSTEM CELL TRANSPLANT

6. Client did contract infection, but it was effectively treated.
7. Client did experience bleeding complications, but they were effectively treated.
8. Client maintains adequate tissue perfusion as evidenced by capillary refill, oxygen saturation, and vital signs WDL.
9. Client maintains pain control as determined by client using age-appropriate pain scale as evidenced by verbal and behavioral indicators.
10. Client consumes adequate nutrition to maintain and support growth.
11. Client does not experience complications associated with pretransplant chemotherapy/irradiation.
12. Client experiences GVHD, but it is promptly and effectively treated.
13. Client (if age-appropriate) and family demonstrate understanding of stem cell transplantation and necessary home care.

References

American Cancer Society. (2007). *Overview: Leukemia—children's.* Retrieved March 4, 2008, from http://www.cancer.org/docroot/CRI/CRI_2_1x.asp?dt=24

Broyles, B. E. (2005). *Medical-surgical nursing clinical companion.* Durham, NC: Carolina Academic Press.

Broyles, B. E., Reiss, B. S., & Evans, M. E. (2007). *Pharmacological aspects of nursing care* (7th ed.). Clifton Park, NY: Delmar Cengage Learning.

Gahart, B. L., & Nazareno, A. R. (2008). *2008 intravenous medications* (24th ed.). St. Louis, MO: Elsevier Mosby.

Leukemia & Lymphoma Society. (2007). *Acute lymphocytic leukemia.* Retrieved May 17, 2007, from http://www.leukemia-lymphoma.org/all_page?item_id=7049

National Cancer Institute. (2007). *Childhood acute lymphoblastic leukemia treatment (PDQ).* Retrieved May 17, 2007, from http://www.cancer.gov/cancertopics/pdq/treatment/childALL/healthprofessional

Potts, N. L., & Mandleco, B. L. (2007). *Pediatric nursing: Caring for children and their families* (2nd ed.). Clifton Park, NY: Delmar Cengage Learning.

Rogers, B. (2005). Looking at lymphoma & leukemia. *Nursing, 35*(7).

68

LYME DISEASE

Definition

Lyme disease is an infection transmitted to humans by the bite of an infected long-legged tick species *Ixodes scapularis* and *Ixodes pacificus*.

Pathophysiology

Lyme disease was discovered in 1977 near Lyme, Connecticut, when a number of children in the community were diagnosed with arthritis (Bachur & Harper, 2006). Once the bacterium was identified, scientists determined that it was transmitted to humans by the bite of infected deer ticks (vectors). The bacterium was named in 1982 even though European health care providers in the early 1900s observed similar manifestations that they termed *erythema migrans* (Broyles, 2005).

Lyme disease presents in three stages: early disease, early disseminated disease, and late disease. Early disease occurs approximately 7–14 days following the bite by an infected tick. The manifestations of this stage are the characteristic erythema migrans rash (Figure 68-1), flulike symptoms, and tenderness at the site of bite (Bachur & Harper, 2006). Without treatment, the early disseminated disease stage (affecting approximately 25% of those infected) occurs from 3–10 weeks after the tick bite. Erythemic oval-shaped macules develop as well as fever, myalgias, arthralgias, malaise, and headache. "Aseptic meningitis may develop at this stage. Cranioneuropathies, especially peripheral seventh nerve (Bell palsy), are common (3% of Lyme disease)" (Bachur & Harper, 2006, Section 3). Finally, the late disease stage develops weeks to months following the bite. Arthritis is the classic manifestation of this stage (Bachur & Harper, 2006).

The clinical manifestations of the disease will subside without treatment. However, if aggressive treatment is not initiated in the early stages of the disease, chronic problems can develop including arthritis, cardiac abnormalities, and neurologic complications. When Lyme disease is not treated until later in the course of the illness, the clinical manifestations appear more neuropsychiatric and the response to treatment is less effective. In a large group of children with Lyme disease referred to a pediatric neurologist, headaches were the most commonly reported manifestation of neurologic involvement. Other manifestations included disturbances of behavior and mood. Magnetic imaging resonance testing showed abnormalities in the deep white matter of the brain. The most commonly noted neurocognitive manifestations included behavioral changes,

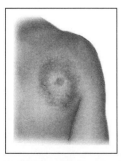

Figure 68-1: Erythema Migrans.

forgetfulness, declining school performance, headache, and fatigue (Lyme Disease Research Studies, 2007).

Complications

Arthritis

Neurologic manifestations (cognitive and psychiatric)

Lyme carditis

Skin disorders

Visual disturbances

Severe fatigue

Weakness

Difficulty with coordination

Incidence

Lyme disease is the most frequently reported vector-borne infection in both North America and Europe. In the United States, Lyme disease tends to be endemic in several regions, particularly areas of the northeastern states, upper midwestern states, and California, although cases are increasing in the mid-Atlantic states as far south as South Carolina. According to the Centers for Disease Control and Prevention (CDC), Lyme disease continues to be a rapidly emerging infectious disease although fewer than 20,000 people are infected each year. The majority of cases (95%) are reported in Connecticut, Rhode Island, New York, Pennsylvania, Delaware, New Jersey, Maryland, Massachusetts, Maine, Minnesota, New Hampshire, and Wisconsin (Centers for Disease Control and Prevention, 2007). The incidence is highest in children aged 5–10 years. The highest international incidence is in the Scandinavian countries, Germany, Switzerland, and Austria (Bachur & Harper, 2006). In addition, cases have been reported in Asia, Europe, and parts of Canada. Most outbreaks occur between April and October, particularly in June and July. Depending on the location, anywhere from less than 1% to more than 50% of the ticks are infected with the spirochetes (Lucile Packard Children's Hospital at Stanford, 2007).

Etiology

Lyme disease is caused by the spirochete *Borrelia burgdorferi,* which is transmitted by the bite of the long-legged tick species *Ixodes scapularis* and *Ixodes pacificus* (Centers for Disease Control and Prevention,).

Clinical Manifestations

(Refer to "Pathophysiology")

Presence of tick embedded in skin

Fever

Erythema migrans (present in approximately 80% of cases and resembling a bull's-eye and usually appearing 7–14 days after the tick has been removed) Refer to Figure 68-1.

LATE SIGNS

Fatigue

Weakness

Headache

Arthritis

Personality disturbances

Mood disturbances

Changes in cardiac rhythm

Difficulty with coordination

Diagnostic Tests

Erythema migrans: the only manifestation of Lyme disease in the United States that is sufficiently distinctive to allow clinical diagnosis in the absence of laboratory confirmation (Wormser et al., 2006)

ELISA antibody/antigen test

Immunofluorescence antibody/antigen test

Immunoglobulin M (IgM) and immunoglobulin G (IgG) immunoblots

Medical Management

The goals for treatment of Lyme disease are prevention of tick bites through health education, prevention of Lyme disease after a recognized tick bite, and early aggressive treatment once Lyme disease has been diagnosed. Refer to "Parent/child teaching" under "Nursing Management" for instructions on how to prevent tick bites.

The following are the Clinical Practice Guidelines by the Infectious Diseases Society of America published by Wormser et al. in 2006:

Although routine use of antimicrobial prophylaxis is not recommended, a single dose of doxycycline may be offered to children 8 years of age and older of 4 mg/kg up to a maximum dose of 200 mg if *all* of the following circumstances exist: (a) the attached tick can be reliably identified as an adult or nymph form of *I. scapularis* tick that is estimated to have been attached for 36 hours or more on the basis of the degree of engorgement of the tick with blood or if child/parent is certain about the time of exposure to the tick, (b) prophylaxis can be started within 72 h of the time that the tick was removed, (c) ecologic information indicates that the local rate of infection of these ticks with *B. burgdorferi* is greater than 20%, and (d) doxycycline treatment is not contraindicated.

The recommended treatment for children with diagnosed Lyme disease is doxycycline [4 mg/kg per day in 2 divided doses (maximum of 100 mg per dose)], amoxicillin [50 mg/kg per day in 3 divided doses (maximum of 500 mg per dose)], cefuroxime axetil [30 mg/kg per day in 2 divided doses (maximum of 500 mg per dose)]. Doxycycline is contraindicated during pregnancy or lactation and in children less than 8 years of age.

Macrolide antibiotics are not recommended as first-line therapy for early Lyme disease, because they have been found to be less effective than those noted above. However, in children who cannot tolerate the recommended agents of treatment, the recommended agents and dosages of macrolides are: azithromycin, 10 mg/kg per day (maximum of 500 mg per day); clarithromycin, 7.5 mg/kg twice per day (maximum of 500 mg per dose); or erythromycin, 12.5 mg/kg 4 times per day (maximum of 500 mg per dose). Children who are treated with macrolides need to be closely monitored to ensure their effectiveness in resolving the clinical manifestations.

For children with Lyme meningitis or other neurologic manifestations, ceftriaxone (50–75 mg/kg per day) in a single daily intravenous dose (maximum, 2 grams) is recommended. If necessary, an alternative dose for cefotaxime is 150–200 mg/kg per day divided into 3 or 4 intravenous doses per day, not to exceed 6 grams per day. Penicillin G is an alternative agent with dosing of 200,000–400,000 units/kg per day, not to exceed 18–24 million U per day. These doses should be divided into 6 intravenous infusions per day. For symptomatic children with Lyme carditis, hospitalization with continuous monitoring and pharmacotherapy with either oral or parenteral antibiotic therapy for 14–21 days is the recommended treatment (Wormser et al., 2006).

Nursing Management

ASSESSMENT

1. Obtain client history with focus on potential or actual tick bite exposure
2. Perform physical assessment

3. Note presence of erythema migrans
4. Assess psychosocial impact of child's condition

Nursing Diagnoses (including but not limited to)

1. Altered protection R/T living in high-risk environment
2. Risk for injury R/T chronic Lyme disease complications
3. Deficient knowledge R/T prevention, child's condition, treatment, and home care

Planning/Goals

1. Client will not experience infection however, if infection occurs, parents will seek treatment for client early in the disease process.
2. Client will not experience complications of the disease.
3. Parents/caregiver and child (if age-appropriate) will demonstrate understanding of prevention of Lyme disease, child's condition, treatment, and home care.

NOC

1. Risk Control, Immune Status
2. Risk Control
3. Knowledge: Infection Prevention, Illness Care, Treatment, Health Promotion

Implementation

1. Protection
   a. Refer to "Parent/caregiver/child teaching" regarding prevention techniques
   b. Begin treatment as soon as possible for child who develops erythema migrans
2. Risk for long-term complications
   a. Refer to "Parent/caregiver/child teaching" regarding prevention techniques
   b. Monitor child with history of Lyme disease during well-child follow-up visits for manifestations of complications
   c. Notify health care provider of any assessment data that may indicate chronic complications
3. Parent/caregiver/child teaching
   a. Assess parent's/child's current level of understanding
   b. Provide verbal and written information regarding:
      1) Medication administration and importance of compliance with antimicrobial therapy
      2) Importance of avoiding direct sunlight on skin because of the adverse effect of photosensitivity for child on doxycycline (Broyles, Reiss, & Evans, 2007)
      3) Use of protective clothing (long-sleeved shirt tucked into pants and long pants tucked into socks)
      4) Use of light-colored clothing
      5) Use of tick and insect repellents that contain N,N-Diethyl-3-methylbenzamide (DEET) applied to the skin or clothing. (Use an insect repellent for children checked with child's health care provider before using DEET.)

6) Importance of using soap and water to wash skin treated with DEET after returning indoors

7) Necessity of checking children often for ticks, especially behind knees, between fingers and toes, under arms, in the groin, in the umbilicus, in and behind ears, on the neck and hairline, and on top of the head. In addition, check children where elastic waistband of underwear touches the skin, where bands from pants or skirts touch the skin, and anywhere else clothing presses on the skin.

8) Importance of showering or bathing children at the end of all outdoor activities for the day

9) Importance of walking on cleared paths and pavement through wooded areas and fields when possible

c. Provide time for questions

d. Document teaching and client/parent response

NIC

1. Risk Identification, Safety Surveillance
2. Risk Identification
3. Teaching: Infection Precautions, Illness Care, Treatment, Health Promotion

EVALUATION

1. Client did experience Lyme disease, but it was detected early and treated effectively.
2. Client does not experience complications of the disease.
3. Parents/caregiver and child (if age-appropriate) demonstrate understanding of prevention of Lyme disease, child's condition, treatment, and home care.

References

Bachur, R. G., & Harper, M. (2006). *Lyme disease.* Retrieved May 12, 2007, from http://www.emedicine.com/ped/topic1331.htm

Broyles, B. E. (2005). *Medical-surgical nursing clinical companion.* Durham, NC: Carolina Academic Press.

Broyles, B. E., Reiss, B. S., & Evans, M. E. (2007). *Pharmacological aspects of nursing care* (7th ed.). Clifton Park, NY: Delmar Cengage Learning.

Centers for Disease Control and Prevention. (2007). *Lyme disease.* Retrieved March 4, 2008, from http://www.cdc.gov/ncidod/dvbid/lyme/index.htm

Lucile Packard Children's Hospital at Stanford. (2007). *Common childhood injuries and poisonings: Lyme disease.* Retrieved March 19, 2007, from http://www.lpch.org/DiseaseHealthInfo/HealthLibrary/poison/lyme.html

Lyme Disease Research Studies. (2007). *Overview of neuropsychiatric Lyme disease.* Retrieved May 17, 2007, from http://www.columbia-lyme.org/flatp/lymeoverview.html#timecourse

Potts, N. L., & Mandleco, B. L. (2007). *Pediatric nursing: Caring for children and their families* (2nd ed.). Clifton Park, NY: Delmar Cengage Learning.

Wormser, G. P., Dattwyler, R. J., Shapiro, E. D., Halperin, J. J., Steere, A. C., Klempner, M. S., Krause, P. J., Bakken, J. S., Strle, F., Stanek, G., Bockenstedt, L., Fish, D., Dumler, J. S., & Nadelman, R. B. (2006). *The clinical assessment, treatment, and prevention of Lyme disease, human granulocytic anaplasmosis, and babesiosis: Clinical practice guidelines by the Infectious Diseases Society of America.* Retrieved March 4, 2008, from http://www.journals.uchicago.edu/doi/full/10.1086/508667?cookieSet=1

69

MENINGITIS

Definition

Meningitis is an inflammation of the membranes covering the structures of the central nervous system (CNS) as a result of an infection.

Pathophysiology

When infectious agents (bacteria, virus, or fungus) infiltrate the three layers of the meninges membranes (pia, arachnoid, and dura), meningitis can occur. Especially in children, it usually results secondary to upper respiratory infections such as pneumonia, otitis media, sinusitis, mastoiditis, pharyngitis, or osteomyelitis. These infections disperse by way of vascular dissemination throughout the body and into the meninges where the organisms can rapidly multiply, especially in the arachnoid space. They disseminate through the brain and spinal cord via cerebral spinal fluid. The microorganisms and their exudates accumulate and can lead to increased intracranial pressure (ICP). Meningitis is classified according to the causative organism and includes cryptococcal, syphilitic, aseptic, *Haemophilus influenzae*, meningococcal (*Neisseria meningitidis*), pneumococcal, staphylococcal, tuberculous, aseptic, gram-negative, and carcinomatous (Broyles, 2005).

Acute bacterial meningitis is a medical emergency because of the rapid infiltration of the bacteria in the CNS and the neurologically devastating effects they can cause, including death. Acute bacterial meningitis requires hospitalization and early aggressive treatment to prevent the child from dying. Regardless of the type of meningitis, the clinical manifestations vary only in severity and most complications are secondary to increased ICP originating with the inflammatory process.

Complications

Increased ICP
Neurologic complications including auditory dysfunction
Neurologic devastation
Death

Incidence

Two peaks in the incidence of invasive meningococcal disease (IMD) occur in pediatric patients: infants younger than 1 year and adolescents 15–18 years of age with the highest fatality rate among adolescents (Centers for Disease Control and Prevention, 2005). "Prior to the routine use of the pneumococcal conjugate vaccine, the incidence of bacterial meningitis in the United States was about 6000 cases per year; roughly half of these were in pediatric patients ($\leq$ 18 y). *N. meningitidis* caused about 4 cases per 100,000 children (aged 1–23 mo). The rate of *S. pneumoniae* meningitis was 6.5 cases per 100,000 children (aged 1–23 mo). This number has since declined given the routine use of conjugate pneumococcal vaccine in children. The recent introduction of conjugate meningococcal vaccine in the United States is expected to reduce the incidence of bacterial meningitis even further. Incidence of neonatal bacterial meningitis is 0.25–1 case per 1000 live births. In addition, incidence is 0.15 case per 1000 full-term births and 2.5 cases per 1000 premature births. Approximately 30% of newborns with clinical sepsis have associated bacterial meningitis" (Miller, Gaur, & Kumar, 2008, Section 2).

"Prior to the availability of the Hib vaccine, *H. influenzae* was the leading cause of bacterial meningitis in children under 5 years of age. It occurred most frequently in children from 1 month up to 4 years, with a peak at 6 to 9 months. Since the introduction of the vaccine in the U.S., *H. influenzae* now occurs in less than 2 in 100,000 children" (MedlinePlus, 2006, p. 1).

In a 2002 investigational study published in *The Journal of Pediatrics,* researchers found that children with cochlear implants experienced over 30 times the incidence of pneumococcal meningitis compared to children in the general population of the United States (Biernath et al., 2006). The Food and Drug Administration (FDA) in conjunction with the Centers for Disease Control and Prevention (CDC) further confirmed this risk.

Etiology

Meningitis can be caused by a variety of microorganisms. As a result, it is classified according to the causative organism. These types include cryptococcal, syphilitic, aseptic, *H. influenzae,* meningococcal (*N. meningitidis*), pneumococcal, staphylococcal, tuberculous, aseptic, gram-negative, and carcinomatous. In addition, the causative organism is often age-related. "Neonates develop meningitis as a result of *Escherichia coli, Haemophilus influenzae,* type B: Group B *Streptococcus, Neisseria meningitides, Streptococcus pneumoniae, and herpes.* Infants and children are susceptible to *Haemophilus influenzae,* type B *Neisseria meningitidis, Streptococcus pneumoniae* . . . adolescents are at risk from exposure to *Neisseria meningitidis, Streptococcus pneumoniae, herpes,* adenovirus, and arbovirus" (Potts & Mandleco, 2007, p. 1079).

Clinical Manifestations

High fever
Headache
Nucal rigidity
Positive Kernig's sign
Positive Brudzinski's sign
Opisthotonos (lying with the back arched and head, back, and chin up)
  Refer to Figure 69-1.
Nausea
Vomiting

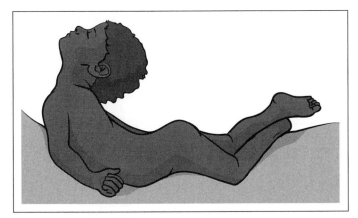

Figure 69-1: Opisthotonic Position.

Photophobia

Confusion

Lethargy

In newborns and small infants, the classic symptoms of fever, headache, and neck stiffness may be absent or difficult to detect. The infant may have bulging fontanels; may be inactive or irritable; may only appear to be slow or inactive; or may be irritable, vomiting, or feeding poorly. As the disease progresses, clients of any age may have seizures (Centers for Disease Control and Prevention, 2005).

Diagnostic Tests

Xpert EV test. *NOTE:* The FDA approved this test on March 16, 2007, for distinguishing viral and bacterial meningitis. The test takes only $2\frac{1}{2}$ hours and predicts with over 95% accuracy (Food and Drug Administration, 2007b).

Lumbar puncture

Cerebrospinal fluid for culture and sensitivity

Gram stain and culture of cerebral spinal fluid

Chest radiography

Head computed tomography (CT)

Medical Management

The goals of treatment are to prevent meningitis through immunization and to treat cases of meningitis effectively to prevent neurologic complications or death. A tetravalent meningococcal polysaccharide-protein conjugate vaccine (MCV4) is recommended for all children at their routine preadolescent (11–12 years of age) health care provider maintenance visit. For those who have not received MCV4 previously, a dose is recommended at high school or college entry. The vaccine also is available to other adolescents who want to decrease their risk of contracting meningitis. The CDC further recommends that individuals at increased risk for meningitis—including college freshmen living in dormitories, U.S. military recruits, anyone who has a damaged spleen or whose spleen has been removed, anyone who is immunosuppressed, anyone who is traveling to countries that have an outbreak of meningococcal disease, and those individuals who might have been exposed to meningitis during an outbreak—should be vaccinated. MCV4 is the preferred vaccine for people 11–55 years of age in these risk groups, but MPSV4 can be used if MCV4 is not available. MPSV4 should be used for children 2–10 years old and adults over 55 who are at risk. A newly approved vaccine (pneumococcol conjugate) appears to be effective in infants and is recommended for all children over 2 years of age (American Academy of Pediatrics, 2005; Centers for Disease Control and Prevention, 2005).

Because of the increased risk of meningitis in children with cochlear implants, the Food and Drug Administration in conjunction with the CDC provide guidelines for prophylaxis in children with cochlear implants. These recommendations are:

1. "Children with cochlear implants aged 2 years and older who have completed the pneumococcal conjugate vaccine (Prevnar) series should receive one dose of the pneumococcal polysaccharide vaccine (Pneumovax 23). If they have just received pneumococcal conjugate vaccine, they should wait at least two months before receiving pneumococcal polysaccharide vaccine.

2. Children with cochlear implants between 24 and 59 months of age who have never received either pneumococcal conjugate vaccine or pneumococcal polysaccharide vaccine should receive two doses of pneumococcal conjugate vaccine two or more months apart and

then receive one dose of pneumococcal polysaccharide vaccine at least two months later.

3. Persons aged 5 years and older with cochlear implants should receive one dose of pneumococcal polysaccharide vaccine." (Food and Drug Administration, 2007a, p. 1).

Most children with viral meningitis recover without treatment. In the event that a child develops bacterial meningitis, intravenous antimicrobial therapy should be initiated immediately because this type is considered a medical emergency. Third-generation cephalosporins are the agents of choice for meningococcal meningitis. In infants younger than 4 weeks, the use of ampicillin and cefotaxime or an aminoglycoside is the standard of care. In infants aged 4–12 weeks, the treatment is ampicillin and a third-generation cephalosporin. In children aged 12 weeks to 18 years, a third-generation cephalosporin or ampicillin in addition to chloramphenicol is the preferred therapy. In the event that the sensitivity testing reveals that the causative microbe is resistant to penicillin, therapy should be changed to ceftriaxone or cefotaxime as monotherapy (Gondim & Singh, 2007). Vancomycin and ceftazidime (fourth-generation cephalosporin) are used to treat staphylococcal meningitis; and third-generation cephalosporins, rifampin, and vancomycin are prescribed to treat streptococcal meningitis. For fungal-originated meningitis, amphotericin B and fluconazole are the agents of choice.

Dexamethasone is used as an adjunct to decrease ICP in children and to prevent auditory loss, a common complication. "Dexamethasone can reduce the subarachnoid space inflammatory response—a major factor in morbidity and mortality caused by bacterial meningitis—and may therefore alleviate many of the pathologic consequences of bacterial meningitis (e.g., cerebral edema, cerebral vasculitis, change in cerebral blood flow, increase in intracranial pressure, neuronal injury). There is some concern that adjunctive dexamethasone therapy may inhibit the efficacy of cerebrospinal fluid (CSF) vancomycin and would therefore be harmful to patients with penicillin- or cephalosporin-resistant strains" (American Academy of Family Physicians, 2005, p. 1). Mannitol and anticonvulsant agents may be required to treat or prevent complications of increased ICP. Surgical treatment for meningitis is used only for the treatment of the accompanying increased ICP including shunt placement. Refer to Chapter 61: Increased Intracranial Pressure (ICP).

Nursing Management

Refer to Chapter 61: Increased Intracranial Pressure (ICP).

ASSESSMENT

1. Obtain client history
2. Assess for recent history of upper respiratory infection
3. Perform pediatric physical assessment
4. Note any manifestations of meningitis and report them to health care provider immediately

NURSING DIAGNOSES (INCLUDING BUT NOT LIMITED TO)

1. Ineffective protection R/T infection process in CNS
2. Risk for imbalanced fluid volume R/T cerebral edema, osmotic diuretics, and increased metabolic needs secondary to meningitis
3. Deficient knowledge R/T prevention, child's condition, treatment, and home care

PLANNING/GOALS

1. Client will not experience injury or complications associated with meningitis as evidenced by complete recovery without neurologic deficits.
2. Client will regain and maintain appropriate fluid balance as evidenced by urine output > 1–2 mL/hr for young children

and > 30 mL/hr for adolescents, show an increase in response to measures for decreasing ICP, show mucous membranes and skin within defined limits (WDL), and show a return of body temperature to WDL.

3. Parents and child (if age-appropriate) will demonstrate understanding of prevention, child's condition, treatment, and home care.

NOC

1. Immune Status
2. Fluid Balance
3. Knowledge: Infection Prevention, Illness Care, Treatment, Health Promotion

IMPLEMENTATION

1. Ineffective protection
   a. Place child on continuous cardiorespiratory monitoring and pulse oximetry
   b. Administer oxygen, titrating to oxygen saturation to within prescribed limits
   c. Assess neurologic status every 4 hours
   d. Report immediately any changes in level of consciousness to health care provider
   e. Position with head of bed elevated 30–45 degrees
   f. Initiate and maintain patency of intravenous access, monitoring at least hourly
   g. Administer antimicrobial agents as prescribed. *NOTE:* Intravenous antimicrobials are irritating to peripheral veins; so they should be infused slowly or, more appropriately, infused through a peripherally inserted central catheter (PICC).
   h. Institute seizure precautions
   i. Instruct parents and visitors on importance of hand washing and appropriate technique
   j. Assist child with hand washing as needed

2. Fluid balance
   a. Monitor hourly urine output
   b. Monitor strict intake and output
   c. Weigh daily
   d. Assess skin turgor and mucous membranes for indications of dehydration
   e. Monitor urine specific gravity each void
   f. Monitor blood urea nitrogen (BUN) and creatinine ratio
   g. Assess temperature every 4 hours
   h. Maintain intravenous access, monitoring at least hourly
   i. Administer intravenous fluids as prescribed

3. Parent/child teaching
   a. Assess current level of understanding
   b. Provide verbal and written information regarding:
      1) Recommended immunization schedule
      2) Risk groups that also should received immunization
      3) Medication administration including importance of compliance with the prescribed medication regime

    4) Manifestations of adverse effects of medications

    5) Manifestations of worsening of condition

    6) Contact phone numbers for reporting signs and symptoms

    7) Importance of regular hand washing and appropriate technique

    8) Importance of follow-up with health care provider

    9) Importance of audiological exam on discharge

c. Provide adequate time for teaching and questions

d. Document teaching and parent/child response

NIC

1. Infection Protection, Immunization/Vaccination Management

2. Fluid Management, Fluid Monitoring

3. Teaching: Infection Precautions, Illness Care, Treatment, Health Promotion

EVALUATION

1. Client does not experience injury or complications associated with meningitis as evidenced by complete recovery without neurologic deficits.

2. Client regains and maintains appropriate fluid balance as evidenced by urine output > 1–2 mL/hr for young children and > 30 mL/hr for adolescents, show an increase in response to measures for decreasing ICP, show mucous membranes and skin WDL, and show a return of body temperature to WDL.

3. Parents and child (if age-appropriate) demonstrate understanding of prevention, child's condition, treatment, and home care.

References

American Academy of Family Physicians. (2005). *Practice guidelines: Management of bacterial meningitis: New guidelines from the IDSA.* Retrieved May 18, 2007, from http://www.aafp.org/afp/20050515/practice.html

American Academy of Pediatrics. (2005). *Prevention and control of meningococcal disease: Recommendations for use of meningococcal vaccines in pediatric patients.* Retrieved March 20, 2007, from http://aappolicy.aappublications.org/cgi/content/abstract/pediatrics;116/2/496

Biernath, K. R., Reefhuis, J., Whitney, C. G., Mann, E. A., Costa, P., Eichwald, J., & Boyle, C. (2006). Bacterial meningitis among children with cochlear implants beyond 24 months after implantation. *Pediatrics, 117*(2).

Broyles, B. E. (2005). *Medical-surgical nursing clinical companion.* Durham, NC: Carolina Academic Press.

Centers for Disease Control and Prevention. (2005). *Meningococcal disease.* Retrieved March 4, 2008, from http://www.cdc.gov/ncidod/dbmd/diseaseinfo/meningococcal_g.htm

Food and Drug Administration. (2007a). *Use of meningitis vaccine in persons with cochlear implants.* Retrieved March 4, 2008, from http://www.cdc.gov/vaccines/vpd-vac/mening/cochlear/dis-cochlear-gen.htm

Food and Drug Administration. (2007b). *FDA clears rapid test for meningitis.* Retrieved June 6, 2007, from http://www.fda.gov/bbs/topics/NEWS/2007/NEW01588.html

Gondim, A. A., & Singh, M. K. (2007). *Meningococcal meningitis.* Retrieved March 20, 2007, from http://www.emedicine.com/NEURO/topic210.htm

Miller, M. L., Gaur, A. H., & Kumar, A. (2008). *Meningitis, bacterial.* Retrieved March 4, 2008, from http://www.emedicine.com/PED/topic198.htm

MedlinePlus. (2006). *Meningitis—H. influenzae.* Retrieved March 20, 2007, from http://www.nlm.nih.gov/medlineplus/ency/article/000612.htm

Potts, N. L., & Mandleco, B. L. (2007). *Pediatric nursing: Caring for children and their families* (2nd ed.). Clifton Park, NY: Delmar Cengage Learning.

70

MENINGOCELE/MYELOMENINGOCELE

Definition

Meningocele and myelomeningocele are congenital neural tube defects where there is incomplete closure of the vertebrae and the neural tube. These two types of spina bifida defects are referred to as spina bifida manifesta. The other types of spina bifida are occulta and closed neural tube defect (National Institute of Neurological Disorders and Stroke, 2007).

Pathophysiology

During the first 28 days of gestation, the vertebral column closes around the spinal cord enclosed in the neural tube of the spine. Meningoceles and myelomeningoceles occur during this initial month of embryonic development. Other neural tube anomalies are anencephaly (absence of the cranial vault), cranioschisis (cranial defect), exancephaly (defect characterized by exposure of the brain or evidence of the brain herniated through a skull defect), encephalocele (protrusion of the brain and meninges through a defect in the cranium), and rachischisis (fissure in the vertebral column causing exposure of the spinal cord and meninges) (Potts & Mandleco, 2007).

A meningocele is a "sac-like herniation through the bony malformation containing the meninges and cerebrospinal fluid. The sac covering may be thin and translucent or membranous" (Potts & Mandleco, 2007, p. 1072). Refer to Figure 70-1.

A myelomeningocele (sometimes referred to as meningomyelocele) is a "sac-like extrusion through the bony defect containing the meninges, cerebrospinal fluid, and a portion of the spinal cord or nerve roots" (Potts & Mandleco, 2007, p. 1072). This protrusion may be poorly covered, so some cerebrospinal fluid may be leaking at the site. The most common sites for myelomeningoceles are the lumbar and lumbar-sacral regions of the spine. Refer to Figure 70-2.

Myelomeningocele is the most common, comprising 96% of the cases of spina bifida manifesta anomalies. It also is the more severe of the two. The complications of myelomeningocele depend on a number of factors including the location of the defect on the spinal column and the extent of damage to the spinal cord or nerve roots. The higher the myelomeningocele is located on the vertebral column, the more severe the complications, including the increased risk of fetal demise. All nerves located below the level of the defect are affected. The severity of damage incurred by the nerve cells determines the amount of motor and/or sensory loss. Complications can range from minor physical alterations to severe physical and mental disabilities; however, most children with spina bifida have normal intelligence (National Institute of Neurological Disorders and Stroke, 2007). In some children, learning difficulties can occur, including attention-deficit hyperactivity disorder (ADHD) and problems with language, comprehension, and math. Because the innervation to the bowel and bladder is located at S_3 to S_5, neurogenic bowel and bladder are common with the accompanying problem of latex allergies resulting from intermittent catheterization to empty the urinary bladder.

Because the fetus develops in a cephalocaudal manner, a defect in one area of the system is often accompanied by defects in other areas of the system. In addition to loss of sensation and paralysis, another neurologic complication associated with myelomeningocele is

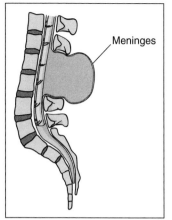

Figure 70-1: Meningocele.

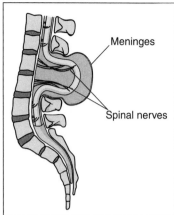

Figure 70-2: Myelomeningocele.

a Chiari II malformation, in which the brainstem and the cerebellum have herniated into the spinal canal. This can result in compression of the spinal cord, leading to difficulties with feeding and swallowing and breathing. It also can cause a blockage of cerebrospinal fluid, resulting in hydrocephalus. Refer to Chapter 57: Hydrocephalus and Shunt Placement. Because of the exposure of the spinal cord or nerve roots to the environment, some neonates develop meningitis. Refer to Chapter 69: Meningitis. Further, many children with myelomeningocele develop progressive tethering of the spinal cord (tethered cord syndrome), resulting in loss of muscle function to the lower extremities and neurogenic bowel and bladder (National Institute of Neurological Disorders and Stroke, 2007). Refer to Chapter 102: Tethered Cord Syndrome.

Complications

Physical impairment
Neurogenic bowel and bladder
Sensory impairment
Cognitive impairment
Chiari II malformation
Hydrocephalus
Tethered cord syndrome
Fetal demise

Incidence

Spina bifida is the most common neural tube defect in the United States—affecting 1,500 to 2,000 of the more than 4 million neonates born each year (National Institute of Neurological Disorders and Strokes, 2007). Meningoceles and myelomeningoceles occur in approximately 7 out of every 10,000 births annually in the United States (Spina Bifida Association, 2006). Of these infants born with "spina bifida manifesta," about 4% have the meningocele form and approximately 96% have the myelomeningocele form. Neural tube anomalies are more common in Caucasian children than in African Americans, and there is a higher incidence in Hispanic children than in non-Hispanics.

Research studies have consistently shown that if all women of childbearing age took a multivitamin with folic acid (400 mcg or 4000 mcg/day in women who have a history of neural tube defect pregnancy), the risk of neural tube defects could be reduced by up to 70% (Spina Bifida Association, 2006; National Institute of Neurological Disorders and Stroke, 2007; March of Dimes, 2006).

Etiology

In the United States, there are 60 million women of childbearing age and each one is potentially at risk of having a pregnancy affected by a neural tube anomaly. In fact, 95% of neural tube defects occur in women with no personal or family history of the defect (March of Dimes, 2006). Some risk factors have been identified that increase a woman's potential for having a child with a neural tube defect. A woman who experienced a previous neural tube defect pregnancy is 20 times more likely to have another affected pregnancy than a woman without such a history. Other factors include maternal insulin-dependent diabetes; use of certain anticonvulsant agents (valproic acid and carbamazapine); medically diagnosed obesity; elevated temperatures early in pregnancy, such as prolonged febrile conditions or hot tub use; and folic acid deficiency (National Institute of Neurological Disorders and Stroke, 2007).

Clinical Manifestations

Fluid-filled sac protruding from the spinal cord

Meningocele—sac covered by thin layer of skin

Myelomeningocele—spinal cord tissue

Manifestations of hydrocephalus

Diagnostic Tests

Prenatal ultrasonography

Second trimester maternal serum alpha fetoprotein (MSAFP)

Amniocentesis

Transillumination (shining a light through the sac)

Computed tomography

Magnetic resonance imaging

Medical Management

The goals of treatment are to prevent infection from developing through the exposed nerves and tissue and to protect the exposed nerves and structures from additional trauma. Usually, a neonate with meningocele/myelomeningocele will have surgery within the first few days of life to close the defect. If the newborn also is diagnosed with hydrocephalus, a shunt is placed. Care of the neonate with a neural tube defect should be provided by a multidisciplinary team including pediatric neurosurgery personnel, physical therapists, nurses, urology specialists, social workers, and child-life therapists. The child with spina bifida has lifelong needs requiring support for both child and parents as the child grows and matures.

Recently, pediatric neurosurgeons have begun performing fetal surgery for treatment of myelomeningocele because of the belief that the earlier the defect is corrected, the better the prognosis for the child by preventing further loss of physical and sensory function. This surgery cannot restore neurological function that has already been lost due to exposure of spinal tissue to amniotic fluid, which is considered toxic to internal tissues of the fetus.

Fetal repair surgery involves making an incision into the mother's uterus, a laparotomy, and suturing the opening over the developing fetus's spinal cord. Surgeons have discovered an additional benefit of this surgery as it appears the procedure affects the way the brain develops in utero, allowing Chiari II with associated hydrocephalus to correct itself and reducing or even eliminating the need for shunt placement. This surgical procedure does pose risks to both the mother and the fetus, however, so it is still considered experimental. The major risks to the fetus include organ immaturity, cerebral hemorrhage, and death because the surgery may stimulate premature labor and birth. Risks to the mother include infection, hemorrhage, gestational diabetes, and weight gain due to bed rest (National Institute of Neurological Disorders and Stroke, 2007).

Early surgery on the spinal cord to repair the tethered cord may allow the child to regain a normal level of functioning and prevent further neurologic deterioration. Some children with myelomeningocele will need subsequent surgeries to manage structural problems with the feet, hips, or spine. Infants with hydrocephalus may need shunt placement and may require additional surgeries to replace the shunt if it malfunctions.

Physical therapy is a critical component in the treatment of children with neural tube defects. An early exercise program will help preserve muscle function and strength. Some children may need to use assistive devices to improve physical mobility, including braces, crutches, or wheelchairs (in cases of a high defect on the spine). However, with special physical therapy, these children may be able to ambulate unaided. Intermittent urinary catheterization is required for most children with myelomeningoceles; however, bladder training can reduce the number of times this must be performed daily. Surgical bladder augmentation may be performed to improve urinary function during the child's preschool or school-age years.

The following is from the National Institute of Neurological Disorders and Stroke (NINDS), a component of the National Institutes of Health and part of the U.S. federal government, concerning current research in neural tube defects:

1) A study supported by NINDS involves researchers looking at the hereditary basis of neural tube defects. The goal of this research is to find the genetic factors that make some children more susceptible to neural tube defects than others with the focus of using this knowledge to prevent these defects. In addition, the study looks at gene expression during the process of neural tube closure, which will provide information on the human nervous system during development.

2) NINDS-supported scientists are working to identify, characterize, and evaluate genes for neural tube defects. The goal is to understand the genetics of neural tube closure, and to develop information that will translate into improved clinical care, treatment, and genetic counseling.

3) Other research focuses on studying genetic risk factors for spina bifida, especially those that decrease folic acid function in the mother during pregnancy, possibly leading to spina bifida in the fetus. This study hopes to show how folic acid prevents spina bifida and may lead to improved forms of folate supplements.

4) The National Institute of Child Health and Human Development (NICHD) is conducting the Management of Myelomeningocele Study (MOMS), a large 5-year study to determine if fetal surgery to correct spina bifida in utero is safer and more effective than the post-natal surgery. NICHD also is a part of the National Institutes of Health (National Institute of Neurological Disorders and Stroke, 2007).

Nursing Management

ASSESSMENT

1. Obtain maternal obstetrical history
2. Assess neonate for presence of neural tube defect
3. Perform neonatal assessment
4. Assess psychosocial impact of the defect on parents/family

NURSING DIAGNOSES (INCLUDING BUT NOT LIMITED TO)

1. Risk for infection R/T impaired skin integrity and exposed spinal tissue and nerves
2. Risk for injury, complications R/T neural tube defect
3. Impaired urinary elimination R/T altered sensorimotor innervation to urinary bladder
4. Parental anxiety R/T child's condition, surgery, and prognosis
5. Impaired bowel elimination R/T altered sensorimotor innervation to the bowel
6. Deficient knowledge (parental) R/T child's condition, treatment, prognosis, and home care

PLANNING/GOALS

1. Client will not experience infection or further damage to exposed spinal tissue and nerves.
2. Client will be effectively treated for any associated complications of neural tube defect.
3. Client will not experience further impaired urinary elimination, and parents will demonstrate ability to perform urinary catheterization.
4. Parents will verbalize feelings and concerns and use positive coping strategies.
5. Client will experience effective bowel elimination, and parents will demonstrate understanding of and compliance with child's bowel training program.
6. Parents will demonstrate understanding of child's condition, treatment, prognosis, and home care.

NOC

1. Risk Control, Infection Severity: Newborn
2. Risk Control, Health Screening and Treatment
3. Urinary Continence
4. Anxiety
5. Bowel Continence
6. Knowledge: Illness Care, Treatment, Health Promotion

IMPLEMENTATION

1. Risk for infection
   a. Maintain sterile saline-soaked gauze preoperatively over myelomeningocele as prescribed
   b. Position neonate prone with head of crib elevated
   c. Place on continuous cardiopulmonary monitoring
   d. Monitor hourly temperature
   e. Monitor frequent vital signs
   f. Monitor for manifestations of meningitis

   2. Complications
     a. Perform neurologic assessment
     b. Monitor for manifestations of hydrocephalus
        1) Assess fontanels for bulging every 2–4 hours
        2) Assess head circumference daily
        3) Assess cranial sutures every 2–4 hours
        4) Monitor for changes in neonatal behavior every 2–4 hours
     c. Assess for manifestations of meningitis
     d. Assess for extremity movement
     e. Monitor urinary pattern, noting dribbling of urine
     f. Perform intermittent catheterization as prescribed
     g. Monitor for bowel function
     h. Monitor feeding patterns
     i. Provide tactile stimulation (touching and stroking)
     j. Avoid use of latex products

   3. Urinary function
     a. Assess urinary stream, noting dribbling of urine
     b. Monitor intake and output
     c. Perform intermittent catheterization as prescribed
     d. Demonstrate intermittent urinary catheterization to parents and provide for return demonstration
     e. Evaluate parental ability to perform catheterization
     f. Monitor urine for clarity, noting manifestations of urinary tract infection

   4. Parental anxiety
     a. Assess parents for manifestations of anxiety
     b. Encourage parents to express feelings and concerns
     c. Listen actively
     d. Facilitate parental bonding with neonate, providing support
     e. Assist parents in identifying support systems and positive coping strategies
     f. Encourage parental involvement in infant's care
     g. Collaborate with health care provider for as-needed referrals

   5. Bowel function
     a. Assess bowel function, noting continuous oozing of feces or constipation
     b. Assess for abdominal distention, emesis, poor feeding, or behavior indicators of pain
     c. Collaborate with health care provider regarding bowel training program

   6. Parent teaching
     a. Assess parents' current level of knowledge
     b. Provide verbal and written information (and skill demonstrations) regarding:
        1) Infant care including psychosocial development
        2) Infant feeding
        3) Manifestations of infection at surgical site
        4) Manifestations of shunt obstruction or malfunction (symptoms of increased intracranial pressure)

5) Urinary catheterization
6) Bladder training
7) Reinforcement of postoperative instructions
8) Reinforcement of physical therapy exercise program
9) Importance of treating child according to cognitive rather than physical abilities
10) Referrals including contact numbers
11) Local and national support groups
12) Importance of follow-up care
13) Contact number for report concerns or questions

c. Provide adequate time for teaching, skills demonstrations, and parental return demonstrations

d. Document teaching and parental response

NIC

1. Infection Precautions
2. Risk Identification, Latex Precautions
3. Bladder Training, Infection Precautions
4. Anxiety Reduction, Coping Enhancement
5. Bowel Training
6. Teaching: Illness Care, Treatment, Health Promotion

EVALUATION

1. Client does not experience infection or further damage to exposed spinal tissue and nerves.
2. Client is effectively treated for any associated complications of neural tube defect.
3. Client does not experience further impaired urinary elimination, and parents demonstrate ability to perform urinary catheterization.
4. Parents verbalize feelings and concerns and use positive coping strategies.
5. Client experiences effective bowel elimination, and parents demonstrate understanding of and compliance with child's bowel training program.
6. Parents demonstrate understanding of child's condition, treatment, prognosis, and home care.

References

March of Dimes. (2006). *Spina bifida*. Retrieved March 25, 2007, from http://www.marchofdimes.com/pnhec/4439_1224.asp

National Institute of Neurological Disorders and Stroke. (2007). *Spina bifida fact sheet*. Retrieved March 25, 2007, from http://www.ninds.nih.gov/disorders/spina_bifida/detail_spina_bifida.htm

Potts, N. L., & Mandleco, B. L. (2007). *Pediatric nursing: Caring for children and their families* (2nd ed.). Clifton Park, NY: Delmar Cengage Learning.

Spina Bifida Association. (2006). *Frequently asked questions about spina bifida*. Retrieved March 25, 2007, from http://www.spinabifidaassociation.org/site/c.liKWL7PLLrF/b.2642327/k.5899/FAQ_About_Spina_Bifida.htm

71

MIGRAINE HEADACHES

Definition

A migraine headache (vascular headache) is an episodic disorder characterized by throbbing unilateral, frontotemporal pain and vomiting in children.

Pathophysiology

Although the exact mechanism of migraine headaches is not clear, the most accepted theory is that the large intracranial blood vessels dilate as a result of decreased serotonin levels. This causes irritation of the nerve fibers that line the vessels and results in throbbing vascular pain so intense that it causes vomiting in children (American Academy of Family Physicians, 2006). "This theory is supported by the auras associated with migraine headaches and the success of medications that alter 5-hydoxytryptamine (serotonin)" (Broyles, 2005, p. 551). The throbbing pain usually lasts an hour or more and then dulls. The dull pain may continue for 4–12 hours. Current therapy with medications has resulted in a more rapid recovery from each migraine episode.

Complications

Debilitating pain
Risk for aspiration from vomiting
Psychosocial implications from the chronicity of migraine headaches

Incidence

Migraine headaches affect approximately 2.5% of children under the age of 7 years (Potts & Mandleco, 2007). Approximately 5% of school-age children and 20% of adolescents experience migraine headaches. These headaches affect girls more often than boys; and boys who get migraines have them more often when they are about 10–12 years old, experiencing as many as two or three a week (American Academy of Family Physicians, 2006). At least 90% of children and adolescents who experience migraines have other family members who also battle with migraines. When both parents have a history of migraines, there is a 70% chance that the child will develop migraines; if only one parent has a history of migraines, the risk drops to 25–50%.

Etiology

As noted in the Pathophysiology section, the exact mechanism of migraine headache is not confirmed; however, a number of "triggers" have been identified. All of the triggers are associated with lowered serotonin levels and include strong or unusual odors; bright lights or loud noises; changes in weather or altitude; fatigue; stress; depression; changes in sleeping patterns or sleeping time; menstrual periods or hormones; intense physical activity; missing meals or fasting; and consuming certain foods especially those than contain tyramine, sodium nitrate, or phenylalanine. Trigger foods include canned or processed bologna, game, ham, herring, hot dogs, pepperoni, and sausage; aged cheese; aspartame (artificial sweetener); avocados; beans (pole, lima, Italian, navy, pinto, and garbanzo); caffeine; canned soup or bouillon cubes; chocolate; buttermilk and sour cream; figs; lentils; meat tenderizer; monosodium glutamate (MSG); nuts and peanut butter; onions; pea pods; pickles; raisins; red plums; sauerkraut; seasoned salt; and soy sauce (American Academy of Family Physicians, 2006). This is not an exhaustive list because many food triggers are idiosyncratic to certain individuals. In addition, considering 90% of children with migraine headaches have family members with the same condition, heredity appears to play a significant role in whether a child will experience migraine headaches.

Clinical Manifestations

  Throbbing frontotemporal headaches
  Nausea
  Abdominal pain
  Visual changes
  Photophobia
  Phonophobia
  Vomiting (occurs in 90% of children with migraines)
  Relief with sleep

Diagnostic Tests

  Complete blood count
  Computed tomography of head
  Magnetic resonance imaging of brain

Medical Management

The goals of treatment focus primarily on pain management and prevention. Currently, the standard of care is the administration of ibuprofen and acetaminophen, having the child lie down in a cool, dark room with a cool, wet cloth over the eyes and forehead (Lewis et al., 2004). Among the drugs researched, pediatric dosages for children 8 years and older have been identified as sumatriptan: 12.5–25 mg orally (not to exceed 100 mg daily), sumatriptan nasal spray: 5 mg intranasally as needed, sumatriptan subcutaneous injection: 0.02 mg/kg as needed, zolmitriptan: 2.5 mg orally (not to exceed 10 mg daily), naratriptan: 1 mg orally (not to exceed 5 mg daily, and rizatriptan: 5 mg orally (not to exceed 30 mg daily). The sumatriptan nasal spray has been studied extensively in adolescents, with positive results (Lenaerts & Gay, 2006; Lewis et al., 2004). "As of now, use of these drugs for migraine relief in children has not been formally approved. However, evidence has accumulated regarding efficacy and safety in this population by several clinical studies, and many pediatric neurologists are beginning to use them in children. The decision to choose these drugs might be reserved best for consultation" (Lenaerts & Gay, 2006, Section 7).

The most effective means for preventing migraine headaches is through parent/child education. Assistance in identifying triggering factors through biofeedback (children are very receptive to this) will help parent/child avoid the migraines. Lifestyle changes such as regular sleep and eating habits are mandatory. In addition, children need an adequate fluid intake. Limiting caffeine and sugar intake, learning relaxation techniques, and decreasing stress and fatigue are very helpful in preventing migraines in children. Narcotic analgesics should be avoided because some opioid analgesics actually intensify vasodilation, making the headaches more severe. Health care providers and parents must collaborate with the child's school to ensure that treatment is available and provided at the onset of a headache. Preventative medication usually is limited to children who experience migraines more than once a month or have particularly distressing headaches (National Headache Foundation, 2005). As the child grows older and into adolescence, depression related to the temporary debilitating effects of migraine headaches may become an issue requiring treatment.

Nursing Management

ASSESSMENT

1. Obtain client history
2. Assess quality of headache (location, quality, severity, frequency, and triggers)
3. Assess vital signs including blood pressure
4. Assess height and weight
5. Perform pediatric physical examination including neurologic exam with exam of optic fundi
6. Assess psychosocial impact of headaches on child/parents

NURSING DIAGNOSES (INCLUDING BUT NOT LIMITED TO)

1. Acute pain R/T nerve irritation secondary to cerebral vessel vasodilation
2. Deficient knowledge R/T condition, prophylactic and therapeutic treatment, and home care

PLANNING/GOALS

1. Client will achieve pain control at a level of 0–2/10 as determined by client using age-appropriate pain assessment tool, verbalizations, and behaviors.
2. Parents/client/family will demonstrate understanding of condition, prophylaxis, therapy, and home care.

NOC

1. Comfort Level
2. Knowledge: Illness Care, Treatment, Medication, Health Promotion

IMPLEMENTATION

1. Acute pain
   a. Assess pain level
   b. Administer medications as prescribed
   c. Place in cool room with cool, wet cloth over eyes and forehead
   d. Encourage child to sleep after medication administration
   e. Assist parents/child in identifying migraine triggers
   f. Collaborate with child-life therapist for relaxation techniques
2. Parent/child teaching
   a. Assess parent's and child's (if age-appropriate) current level of understanding
   b. Provide verbal and written information regarding:
      1) Manifestations of migraine headache versus other types of headaches that may require further diagnostics and treatment
      2) Medication administration
      3) Cool room with cool, wet cloth over eyes and forehead to relieve pain
      4) Biofeedback techniques
      5) Regular mealtimes with no skipping of meals
      6) Regular sleep schedule and exercise
      7) Triggers for migraine headaches (certain foods, stress, too much exercise or physical activity, certain activities, or stress)
      8) Reinforcement of biofeedback and relaxation techniques

      9) Importance of preventing interruption in school

     10) Importance of follow-up care with health care provider

     11) Contact number for health care provider

  c. Provide adequate time for teaching

  d. Document teaching and parent/child response

NIC

1. Medication Management, Biofeedback
2. Teaching: Illness Care, Medication, Treatment, Health Education

EVALUATION

1. Client achieves pain control at a level of 0–2/10 as determined by client using age-appropriate pain assessment tool, verbalizations, and behaviors.
2. Parents/client/family demonstrate understanding of condition, prophylaxis, therapy, and home care.

References

American Academy of Family Physicians. (2006). *Migraine headache in children and adolescents.* Retrieved March 26, 2007, from http://familydoctor.org/757.xml

American Academy of Neurology. (2007). *Treatment of migraine headache in children and adolescents.* Retrieved March 26, 2007, from http://www.aan.com/professionals/practice/pdfs/Headache_Peds_Patients.pdf

Broyles, B. E. (2005). *Medical-surgical nursing clinical companion.* Durham, NC: Carolina Academic Press.

Lenaerts, M. E., & Gay, C. (2006). *Headache, children.* Retrieved March 26, 2007, from http://www.emedicine.com/oph/topic334.htm

Lewis, D., Ashwal, S., Hershey, A., Hirtz, D., Yonker, M., & Silberstein, S. (2004). *Practice parameter: Pharmacological treatment of migraine headache in children and adolescents.* Retrieved May 18, 2007, from http://www.neurology.org/cgi/content/full/63/12/2215

National Headache Foundation. (2005). *Headache in children.* Retrieved March 26, 2007, from http://www.headaches.org/consumer/topicsheets/children.html

Potts, N. L., & Mandleco, B. L. (2007). *Pediatric nursing: Caring for children and their families* (2nd ed.). Clifton Park, NY: Delmar Cengage Learning.

72

MUSCULAR DYSTROPHY (DUCHENNE)

Definition

Muscular dystrophy (MD) is a rare, inherited, progressive degenerative disease of the muscle fibers, primarily affecting voluntary muscles (Muscular Dystrophy Association, 2006; Potts & Mandleco, 2007).

Pathophysiology

Duchenne muscular dystrophy (DMD), one of more than 20 types of MD, is the most common type of childhood MD and the most common of all other types of MD. It is named after a French neurologist Guillaume Duchenne de Boulogne who worked in Paris in the mid-nineteenth century and described DMD in the 1860s after writing a comprehensive account of 13 boys with the condition. "A milder form of the disease is known as Becker muscular dystrophy (BMD). The combined spectrum of these diseases is referred to as Duchenne/Becker muscular dystrophy (DBMD)" (Centers for Disease Control and Prevention, 2006, p. 1). Both Duchenne and Becker MD are X-linked defects carried by the mother and affecting male offspring.

DMD is caused by a genetic mutation. Dystrophin is the largest known human gene, and it provides blueprints for making a protein called dystrophin. The gene makes many different versions of dystrophin, which is located chiefly in skeletal muscles used for movement and in the myocardium. Small amounts of the protein are present in nerve cells in the brain. Dystrophin is part of a protein complex (dystrophin-glycoprotein complex) that strengthens muscle fibers and forms a protective membrane to protect the fibers from injury as they contract and relax. The dystrophin complex acts as an anchor or glue, connecting each muscle cell's structural framework (cytoskeleton) with the lattice of proteins and other molecules outside the cell (extracellular matrix). The dystrophin-glycoprotein complex also may play a role in cell signaling by interacting with proteins that send and receive chemical signals. Little is known about the function of dystrophin in nerve cells. Research suggests that the protein is important for the normal structure and function of synapses where cell-to-cell communication occurs (Genetics Home Reference, 2007).

When the protective membrane is damaged, muscle fibers begin to leak the protein creatine kinase necessary for the chemical reactions that produce energy for muscle contractions and take on excess calcium, further damaging the muscle fibers. As a result, the affected muscle fibers branch and split and eventually are phagocytosized and die, leading to progressive muscle degeneration as muscle tissue is replaced by connective tissue and fat. This also can result in chronic or permanent shortening of tendons and muscles and loss of tendon reflexes (Muscular Dystrophy Association, 2006).

The disease follows a well-documented course. Most affected boys develop the first signs of difficulty in ambulation between the ages of 1 and 3 years when they are unable to run or jump like other toddlers and preschoolers, often struggling to get up off the floor or to climb stairs (Broyles, 2005). Refer to Figure 72-1.

This progresses in early childhood to a child's inability to walk as far or as fast as the child's friends. Usually, this is the age that learning and behavioral difficulties begin. (Approximately one third of boys with DMD have cognitive disabilities.) Between the ages of 8 and 11 years, the boys lose the ability to ambulate. Around the age of 10 years, respiratory muscle function may begin to decline due to the weakening of the diaphragm from scar tissue formation secondary to muscle degeneration. In addition, the muscles responsible

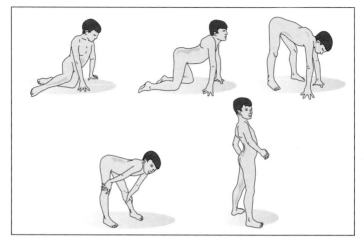

Figure 72-1: Gower's Sign: A Series of Maneuvers that a Child with MD Must Use to Rise from a Sitting or Lying Position.

for coughing weaken and are unable to support the diaphragm. At this point, breathing can become compromised and the child becomes susceptible to respiratory infections. With these children, a non-complex viral infection can progress rapidly to viral and then secondary bacterial pneumonia (National Institute of Neurological Disorders and Stroke, 2007). Joint and tendon cord contractures resulting from fibrosis can occur as well as eating and language difficulties because of weakening of the facial muscles. Scoliosis affects these children in early adolescence. Without medical management, these children die by the age of 20 due to cardiorespiratory failure. However, with many forms of treatment available now, these young men can live productive lives into young adulthood.

Complications

Muscle weakness
Contractures
Lordosis
Scoliosis
Physical immobility
Learning disabilities
Cardiorespiratory failure

Incidence

DMD affects approximately 1 out of every 3,500 male births (National Institute of Neurological Disorders and Stroke, 2007). The annual incidence is approximately 400 to 600 boys born with DMD. A female with one copy of the DMD genetic mutation can pass the disease to her male offspring without being affected herself. This means that a female who is a carrier of the defective gene can be born into any family at any time (Centers for Disease Control and Prevention, 2006). The incidence in other developed countries is the same as the United States (Muscular Dystrophy Campaign, 2007).

Etiology

As discussed in the Pathophysiology section, MD is caused by an X-linked gene, meaning that only boys are affected but that their mothers may be carriers. Actually, almost 50% of boys affected may have developed the defective or mutated gene rather than having genetically inherited it. After a mother gives birth to a son affected by DMD, each subsequent son of a carrier has a 50-50 chance of being affected and each daughter has a 50-50 chance of being a carrier. A small number of female carriers of the gene have a mild degree of muscle weakness themselves and are known as "manifesting carriers" (Muscular Dystrophy Campaign, 2007).

Clinical Manifestations

Generalized muscle weakness
Difficulty running, climbing stairs, or getting up off the floor
Pseudohypertrophy of the calves
Gowers' sign
Learning disabilities
Language difficulties
Loss of ambulation
Lordosis
Tendon cord and joint contractures
Scoliosis

Diagnostic Tests

Serum creatine kinase
Electromyography
Nerve conduction testing
Muscle biopsy

Medical Management

Currently, no cure exists for MD. However, research spearheaded by the Muscular Dystrophy Association continues its focus on gene therapy and treatments to help the child with MD lead a productive life into young adulthood. Experimental treatment called myoblast transfer therapy presently is being supported by the Food and Drug Administration. This involves injecting the patient with healthy donor myoblasts with the intent that these cells will fuse to each other in the unhealthy cells of the recipient.

The focus of medical management is to slow the progression of the disease through exercise and pharmacotherapeutics. At one time, it was believed that exercise hastened the degenerative process. This theory has changed, and physical and occupational therapy are used to maximize the function of muscle and to maintain independence for as long as possible. Exercises can maintain range of motion, prevent contractures of the joints, and delay curvature of the spine.

Anti-inflammatory agents and corticosteroid therapy are used to help slow the progression. Stool softeners and laxatives prevent constipation and fecal impactions that can occur after loss of mobility and bowel control. Because of the risk of respiratory infections so common in later stages of the disease, vaccinations against pneumonia and influenza should be kept up to date. Eventually, mechanical ventilation may become necessary as the muscles of the respiratory system weaken.

Children should stay in school as long as possible to prepare them for employment. Of course, they will not be able to do a job requiring any muscle strength; their leisure activities also will be restricted. From the earliest days at school, education is extremely important to foster the children's talents so that they can be fully developed. Computers offer a genuine opportunity to help these children develop skills within the constraints of their abilities. With more online education programs becoming available, pursuing higher education is a real possibility for them.

Nursing Management

ASSESSMENT

1. Obtain client history
2. Perform pediatric physical assessment focusing on motor and respiratory function
3. Assess vital signs
4. Perform psychosocial assessment (to determine presence of coping strategies and possible developmental delays and to aid in genetic counseling)

NURSING DIAGNOSES (INCLUDING BUT NOT LIMITED TO)

1. Delayed growth and development R/T muscle weakness and possible learning disabilities
2. Impaired physical mobility/impaired mobility: wheelchair R/T muscle weakness and wasting
3. Ineffective breathing pattern R/T progressive weakness of respiratory muscles
4. Ineffective individual/family coping R/T increasing demands of care, financial responsibilities, and client needs
5. Anticipatory grieving R/T to poor prognosis in children with DMD
6. Deficient knowledge R/T MD, treatment, prognosis, and home care

PLANNING/GOALS

1. Client will develop to highest level of growth and development.
2. Client will maintain independence for as long as possible and perform activities of daily living (ADL) on his own and with family assistance as needed.
3. Client will maintain respiratory function even when mechanical assistance is required.
4. Client/parents/family will demonstrate positive coping mechanisms and use community support.
5. Client/parents/family will effectively work through anticipatory grieving process.
6. Family will demonstrate understanding of child's condition, treatment options, prognosis, and home care including use of community resources.

NOC

1. Child Development
2. Mobility
3. Respiratory Status: Ventilation
4. Coping
5. Coping
6. Knowledge: Disease Process, Illness Care, Medications, Exercise, Treatment, Health Promotion

IMPLEMENTATION

1. Growth and development
   a. Assess child's current level of growth and development every 24 hours during acute care and every visit to health care provider during outpatient care
   b. Enhance growth and development by beginning at the point where the child is

   c. Collaborate with child-life specialist for assistance as needed

   d. Encourage age-appropriate activities, altering them to accommodate muscle weakness

   e. Reinforce physical therapy exercises

   f. Reinforce occupational therapy interventions

   g. Encourage parents to communicate with child's school to ensure accommodations for child as condition progresses

   h. Encourage parents to actively participate in child's activities

   i. Monitor development through clinic/health care provider visits

2. Physical mobility

   a. Assess physical mobility and ability to perform self-care activities every 8 hours during acute care and every visit to health care provider during outpatient care

   b. Encourage activities such as swimming and walking to promote range of motion while able

   c. Encourage quiet activities with family and friends as disease progresses

   d. Reinforce physical therapy exercises and assistive and adaptive equipment

   e. Maintain adequate nutritional intake

   f. Maintain adequate fluid intake to prevent urinary stasis

   g. Administer medications as prescribed

   h. Perform and teach client/family urinary catheterization as indicated

3. Breathing pattern

   a. Assess respiratory function including breath sounds every 4 hours during hospitalization

   b. Document and report changes in respiratory status

   c. Protect child from exposure to individuals with communicable or infectious diseases

   d. Maintain vaccination schedule

   e. Maintain patency of intravenous access during hospitalization, monitoring at least hourly

   f. Administer antimicrobials as prescribed, taking care to administer on time to maintain blood level, avoiding infusing these medications too rapidly when using a peripheral venous access

   g. Maintain mechanical support as indicated

4. Coping

   a. Encourage verbalization of feelings and concerns and promote environment for expression

   b. Listen actively and provide honest answers and refer questions to health care provider as needed

   c. Collaborate with health care provider regarding referrals to social services, physical and occupation therapy, child-life specialist, and community support groups

   d. Perform ongoing assessment of client/family affect and emotional status

   e. Encourage visitation of friends and family according to client's wishes

   f. Involve child in age-appropriate activities adapted to physical limitations

    g. Provide information concerning MD support groups

    h. Provide parents/family with information about growth and development needs and ways these can be met

5. Anticipatory grieving

    a. Assess child's/family's anticipatory grieving state

    b. Listen to concerns and feelings

    c. Use therapeutic silence when appropriate

    d. Spend time with client/family as indicated by their responses

    e. Encourage client/family to discuss feelings with each other

    f. Assist client/family to discuss death issues

    g. Consult pastoral care or encourage family minister to visit and provide support if client desires

6. Parent/client teaching

    a. Assess client's (if age-appropriate) and family's current level of knowledge about MD

    b. Provide verbal and written information regarding:

       1) Medication administration

       2) Modification of home to make it wheelchair-accessible and modification of bathroom to facilitate bathing and toileting

       3) Methods of providing clothing that allows for ease of dressing and maintenance of independence

       4) Importance of protecting child from respiratory infections

       5) Vaccination schedule and importance of compliance with it

       6) Use of pulmonary hygiene and respiratory exercises as indicated

       7) Urinary catheterization including return demonstration

       8) Suggestions on how to modify diet to provide for adequate nutrition, prevent obesity, and promote independence

       9) Referrals and community resources available and the services they offer

      10) Importance of follow-up with health care provider

      11) Contact information for health care provider

    c. Coordinate regular monitoring by multidisciplinary team

    d. Provide adequate time for teaching and demonstrations

    e. Evaluate family learning through return demonstrations of skills

    f. Document teaching and client/family response

NIC

1. Developmental Enhancement: Child
2. Exercise Therapy, Exercise Promotion, Self-Care Assistance
3. Respiratory Monitoring, Vital Signs Monitoring
4. Coping Enhancement
5. Coping Enhancement, Grief Work Facilitation
6. Teaching: Disease Process, Illness Care, Medications, Exercise, Treatment, Health Education

EVALUATION

1. Client develops to highest level of growth and development.
2. Client maintains independence for as long as possible and performs ADL on his own and with family assistance as needed.

3. Client maintains respiratory function even when mechanical assistance is required.

4. Client/parents/family demonstrate positive coping mechanisms and use community support.

5. Client/parents/family effectively work through anticipatory grieving process.

6. Family demonstrates understanding of child's condition, treatment options, prognosis, and home care including use of community resources.

References

Broyles, B. E. (2005). *Medical-surgical nursing clinical companion.* Durham, NC: Carolina Academic Press.

Centers for Disease Control and Prevention. (2006). *Single gene disorders and disability (SGDD).* Retrieved July 7, 2007, from http://www.cdc.gov/ncbddd/duchenne/who.htm

Genetics Home Reference. (2007). *DMD.* Retrieved March 27, 2007, from http://ghr.nlm.nih .gov/gene=dmd;jsessionid=F72979C724568932AD06F4CB5BF48134

Muscular Dystrophy Association. (2006). *Facts about muscular dystrophy (MD).* Retrieved March 27, 2007, from http://www.mda.org/publications/fa-md-qa.html

Muscular Dystrophy Campaign. (2007). *Duchenne muscular dystrophy factsheet.* Retrieved March 27, 2007, from http://www.muscular-dystrophy.org/information_resources/factsheets/ medical_conditions_factsheets/duchenne.html

National Institute of Neurological Disorders and Stroke. (2007). *Muscular dystrophy: Hope through research.* Retrieved March 27, 2007, from http://www.ninds.nih.gov/disorders/md/detail_md.htm

Potts, N. L., & Mandleco, B. L. (2007). *Pediatric nursing: Caring for children and their families* (2nd ed.). Clifton Park, NY: Delmar Cengage Learning.

73

NEAR DROWNING/DROWNING (IMMERSION SYNDROME/ SUBMERSION SYNDROME)

Definition

Drowning is a process in which immersion or submersion in water or another fluid medium prevents an individual from breathing, resulting in respiratory compromise (Ross, 2005; Shepherd et al., 2008; American Heart Association, 2008).

Pathophysiology

Drowning often is referred to as death within 24 hours following an immersion or submersion episode (Shepherd, et al, 2008); it is differentiated from near-drowning, defined as when a person initially survives suffocation after being immersed in water or another fluid medium, requiring medical attention and leading to morbidity and mortality (Potts & Mandleco, 2007). The International Liaison Committee on Resuscitation (ILCOR), a group formed in 1992 to improve communication among the primary resuscitation organizations in the world, recommends the use of the term *drowning* to incorporate both terms by providing a broader definition of drowning. This has been endorsed by the American Heart Association and published in its journal (Idris et al., 2003). The ILCOR definition will be the term used in this discussion.

Drowning is a medical emergency. When a child is submerged in water, he attempts to breathe and either aspirates (wet drowning) or experiences laryngospasm without aspiration (dry drowning). Most children with submersion injury have aspirated a small amount of water or gastric contents into their lungs; however, approximately 10–15% of them become asphyxiated without evidence of aspiration. Fluid aspiration alters surfactant function, resulting in the inability of the alveoli to exchange oxygen and carbon dioxide. Pulmonary edema also interferes with gas exchange. Release of inflammatory mediators causes vasoconstriction, further increasing the hypoxia. The hypoxemic state interferes with cardiac function, leading to potentially life-threatening dysrhythmias (ventricular tachycardia, fibrillation, and asystole). This leads to initiation of the shock process and a downward spiral in the child's condition. Hypoxia results in neurologic damage, devastation, and even death. At least one third of victims of drowning episodes experience moderate to severe neurologic damage (Verive, Heidemann, & Fiore, 2007).

"If immersion occurs in extremely cold water, a protective mechanism known as the dive reflex slows the heart rate, constricts peripheral vessels, shunts blood to the heart and brain, and dramatically lowers metabolism. This mechanism can prolong tissue life and prevent permanent damage beyond the 10-minute time frame usually associated with brain death. An individual that is conscious when admitted to the emergency department has a good prognosis of survival. In the presence of neurological damage, the prognosis is less favorable" (Broyles, 2005, p. 285).

Complications

Asphyxia
Aspiration
Pulmonary edema
Hypoxemia

Neurologic damage
Cardiorespiratory failure
Death

Incidence

Approximately 2,000 children die in the United States each year from drowning injuries. Boys are 3 times more likely to experience near-drowning or drowning than girls; however, bathtub drowning accidents occur more often in girls. The peak incidence of 3.22 per 100,000 occurs in children under the age of 4 years; most of these injuries occur in swimming pools, with 90% occurring in residential pools (Potts & Mandleco, 2007; Verive et al., 2007). African-American children die from drowning at 2.5 times the rate of Caucasian children between the ages of 5 through 19 years. Alcohol is a factor in 25–50% of adolescent and adult drowning deaths. Immersion accidents are the second leading cause of accidental death in children between the ages of 1 and 14 years and are second only to motor vehicle accidents (Potts & Mandleco, 2007).

Etiology

The leading cause of near-drowning injuries and drowning deaths is inadequate adult supervision of children around residential swimming pools. In most instances, a gate entering the pool has been left opened. "Although no individual characteristics have been found to predict survivability, the Orlowski score has been found to identify the likelihood of neurologically intact survival. In using the Orlowski score, 1 point is given for each item; scores of 2 or less are associated with a 90% likelihood of complete recovery, and submersion-injury patients with scores of 3 or more have only a 5% chance of survival. The items in the Orlowski score are as follows: age 3 years or older, submersion time of more than 5 minutes, no resuscitative efforts for more than 10 minutes after rescue, comatose on admission to the emergency department, and arterial pH of less than 7.10" (Verive et al., 2007, Section 2).

Clinical Manifestations

Altered level of consciousness
Restlessness
Apprehension
Dyspnea
Cough
Wheezing
Vomiting
Apnea
Tachypnea
Pink, frothy sputum
Tachycardia
Cardiac dysrhythmias
Hypotension

Diagnostic Tests

Carboxyhemoglobin levels
Arterial blood gases
Chest X-ray
Serum electrolyte levels
Bronchoscopy
Pulse oximetry
Complete blood cell count
Prothrombin time with international normalized ratio (INR)

Partial thromboplastin time, fibrinogen, D-dimer

Liver enzymes, especially aspartate aminotransferase and alanine aminotransferase

Renal function tests (blood urea nitrogen [BUN] and creatinine)

Cardiac troponin I testing

Brain scan

Medical Management

The goals of management are to promote client survival and limit the long-term complications of the drowning episode. The initial treatment for the victim is cardiopulmonary resuscitation to promote gas exchange and tissue perfusion to the heart and brain and, it is hoped, to restore respirations. Chest compressions are more effective at removing aspirated water than the Heimlich maneuver. Endotracheal intubation and mechanical ventilation may be required to maintain a patent airway and provide adequate alveolar ventilation. All near-drowning victims require 100% supplemental oxygen to be administered as soon as possible. Endotracheal suctioning helps remove excess secretions and fluid. An intravenous access device should be initiated as soon as possible for the administration of intravenous volume expanders (lactated Ringer's solution) to treat intravascular volume depletion. A central venous access device may need to be placed depending on the child's response to treatment. Inotropic support for hypotension and cardiac dysrhythmias may be required using dopamine and/or dobutamine.

The respiratory acidosis resulting from hypercapnea usually is reversed after correction of volume depletion and oxygenation. In the event of severe acidosis, sodium bicarbonate may be administered. To prevent neurologic damage, health care providers may induce hypothermia or a barbiturate-induced coma. Corticosteroids and osmotic diuretics (mannitol) may be needed to decreased intracranial pressure (ICP) if the drowning is accompanied by head trauma and increased ICP (Broyles, Reiss, & Evans, 2007). A nasogastric tube is placed for removal of swallowed water and debris, urinary catheter placement is needed for assessment of urine output, and placement of an arterial line is necessary for monitoring blood gases. In the event the child does not respond to conventional mechanical ventilation or high-frequency ventilation, extracorporeal membrane oxygenation (ECMO) may be required (Verive et al., 2007). Rehabilitation is based on the presence and extent of persistent neurologic damage.

Nursing Management

ASSESSMENT

1. Obtain client history of submersion including length of submersion and temperature and type of water
2. Perform rapid initial cardiopulmonary assessment
3. Assess neurologic status
4. Obtain vital signs, height, and weight

NURSING DIAGNOSES (INCLUDING BUT NOT LIMITED TO)

1. Ineffective airway clearance R/T aspiration of fluid
2. Impaired gas exchange R/T presence of fluid in alveoli and washing away of surfactant
3. Ineffective cerebral tissue perfusion R/T decreased oxygen and ineffective airway clearance
4. Impaired spontaneous ventilation R/T asphyxia
5. Parental anxiety R/T potential for intubation, mechanical ventilation, critical care, and death
6. Deficient knowledge R/T prevention, treatment, home care, or potential life-threatening condition

PLANNING/GOALS

1. Client will regain and maintain patent airway as evidenced by effective respiratory rate and effort.
2. Client will regain and maintain adequate gas exchange as evidenced by arterial blood gases and oxygen saturation within defined limits (WDL).
3. Client will regain and maintain cerebral tissue perfusion as evidenced by neurologic status WDL.
4. Client will regain and maintain spontaneous ventilation.
5. Parents will exhibit a decrease in anxiety as evidenced by verbal and nonverbal indicators.
6. Parents will demonstrate understanding of condition, prevention, treatment, and home care.

NOC

1. Respiratory Status: Airway Patency
2. Respiratory Status: Gas Exchange
3. Circulation Status
4. Respiratory Status: Ventilation
5. Anxiety
6. Knowledge: Child Physical Safety, Disease Process, Illness Care, Health Promotion

IMPLEMENTATION

1. Airway
   a. Assess respiratory status frequently according to assessment findings
   b. Place on continuous cardiorespiratory monitor
   c. Assess amount, color, and consistency of sputum
   d. Assist with coughing and deep breathing for child not on mechanical ventilation
   e. Position with head of bed (HOB) elevated to facilitate breathing
   f. Perform the following if child is on mechanical ventilation:
      1) Assess endotracheal tube to ensure proper placement
      2) Stabilize endotracheal tube to prevent displacement
      3) Reposition from one side of the mouth to the other according to facility protocol to prevent oral mucous membrane breakdown
      4) Assess breath sounds
      5) Maintain ventilator settings as prescribed
      6) Suction endotracheal tube as indicated by child's need
      7) Administer bronchodilators as prescribed
      8) Perform chest physiotherapy to loosen secretions for suctioning
      9) Maintain sedation as prescribed to conserve client energy and prevent "fighting the ventilator"
2. Gas exchange
   a. Monitor continuous pulse oximetry
   b. Monitor serial arterial blood gases
   c. Administer supplemental oxygen, titrating rate to pulse oximetry and child's response

    d. Administer sodium bicarbonate as prescribed

    e. Position with HOB elevated to facilitate alveolar ventilation

    f. Assess neurologic status every 2–4 hours and as needed

    g. Assess skin and nail bed color for changes and presence of cyanosis

    h. Monitor pulmonary artery pressure

    i. Provide frequent mouth care

    j. Maintain mechanical ventilation (if present)

    k. Collaborate with respiratory therapist to regain and maintain effective gas exchange

    l. Collaborate with health care provider regarding changes in child's status

3. Cerebral tissue perfusion

    a. Assess neurologic status frequently

    b. Monitor ICP for signs of increasing levels

    c. Monitor vital signs as a part of each neurologic assessment

    d. Position with HOB elevated

    e. Maintain head in neutral position

    f. Maintain effective ventilation and oxygenation

    g. Maintain patency of intravenous access, monitoring at least hourly

    h. Provide care for intravenous access according to facility protocol

    i. Administer corticosteroids and osmotic diuretics as prescribed

    j. Administer inotropic support as prescribed

    k. Administer sodium bicarbonate as prescribed

    l. Monitor urinary output as objective indicator of effectiveness of osmotic diuretics

4. Spontaneous ventilation

    a. Refer to "Implementation for Airway and Gas Exchange"

    b. Wean from mechanical ventilation as prescribed and according to facility protocol

5. Anxiety

    a. Assess child/parents for indications of anxiety

    b. Support parents experiencing feelings of guilt

    c. Explain all procedures and equipment, assessing parents for indications of understanding

    d. Be available to child and parents. *NOTE:* With endotracheal tube in place, child is unable to communicate verbally.

    e. Keep parents informed of client's condition

    f. Encourage parents to visit as often as possible

    g. Encourage verbalization of feelings and concerns

    h. Listen actively

    i. Answer questions honestly, referring questions to appropriate health care personnel as indicated

    j. Maintain calm affect and environment

6. Parent teaching

    a. Assess parent's and child's (if age-appropriate) current level of knowledge

    b. Provide verbal and written information regarding:

1) Risk factors for drowning accidents, avoidance of these factors, and rules of water safety:

    a) Supervise children closely while they are swimming, watching them constantly

    b) Teach children never to go near the water unless an adult is present

    c) Do not allow children around pools unless pools have self-latching gates

    d) Ensure that pools are gated and locked when adults are not in attendance

    e) Comply with water speed limits when boating

    f) Never consume alcohol while swimming or boating

    g) Wear life jackets (vests) at all times while boating

    h) Never allow child to swim alone

    i) Swim only in designated swimming areas

    j) Have child wait at least 30 minutes after consuming a meal before swimming

    k) Have children take swimming classes

    l) Learn cardiopulmonary resuscitation

    m) Check the water depth before allowing children to swim

    n) Do not allow children to chew gum or eat while swimming, diving, or playing in water, thus preventing choking

    o) Do not leave standing buckets of water unattended

2) Medication administration if appropriate, including importance of completing the prescribed medication regime

3) Signs and symptoms of adverse effects of medications

4) Contact phone numbers for reporting signs and symptoms

5) Importance of follow-up with health care provider

6) Referrals as indicated for children with neurologic deficits

c. Provide adequate time for teaching

d. Document teaching and client/family response

NIC

1. Airway Management, Airway Suctioning
2. Oxygen Therapy, Acid/Base Management, Ventilation Assistance
3. Cerebral Perfusion Promotion
4. Airway Management, Respiratory Monitoring, Ventilation Assistance
5. Anxiety Reduction
6. Teaching: Child Safety, Disease Process, Illness Care, Health Education

EVALUATION

1. Client regains and maintains patent airway as evidenced by effective respiratory rate and effort.
2. Client regains and maintains adequate gas exchange as evidenced by arterial blood gases and oxygen saturation WDL.
3. Client regains and maintains cerebral tissue perfusion as evidenced by neurologic status WDL.
4. Client regains and maintains spontaneous ventilation.

5. Parents exhibit a decrease in anxiety as evidenced by verbal and non-verbal indicators.

6. Parents demonstrate understanding of condition, prevention, treatment, and home care.

References

American Heart Association. (2008). *International Liaison Committee on Resuscitation (ILCOR) guideline recommendations.* Retrieved March 10, 2008, from http://circ.ahajournals .org/cgi/reprint/CIRCULATIONAHA.107.186228

Broyles, B. E. (2005). *Medical-surgical nursing clinical companion.* Durham, NC: Carolina Academic Press.

Broyles, B. E., Reiss, B. S., & Evans, M. E. (2007). *Pharmacological aspects of nursing care* (7th ed.). Clifton Park, NY: Delmar Cengage Learning.

Idris, A. H., Berg, R. A., Bierens, J., Bossaert, L., Branche, C. M., Gabrielli, A., Graves, S. A., Handley, A. J., Hoelle, R., Morley, P. T., Papa, L., Pepe, P. E., Quan, L., Szpilman, D., Wigginton, J. G., Modell, J. H., Atkins, D., Gay, M., Kloeck, W., & Timerman, S. (2003). *Recommended guidelines for uniform reporting of data from drowning: The "Utstein style."* Retrieved July 7, 2007, from http://circ.ahajournals.org/cgi/content/full/108/20/ 2565?maxtoshow=&HITS=10&hits=10&RESULTFORMAT=&fulltext=drowning& searchid=1&FIRSTINDEX=0&resourcetype=HWCIT

Potts, N. L., & Mandleco, B. L. (2007). *Pediatric nursing: Caring for children and their families* (2nd ed.). Clifton Park, NY: Delmar Cengage Learning.

Ross, J. L. (2005). Summer injuries: Near drowning. *RN, 68*(7).

Shepherd, S. M., Martin, J., & Shoff, W. H. (2008). *Drowning.* Retrieved March 10, 2008, from http://www.emedicine.com/emerg/topic744.htm

Verive, M., Heidemann, S., & Fiore, M. (2007). *Near drowning.* Retrieved July 7, 2007, from http://www.emedicine.com/ped/topic2570.htm

74

NECROTIZING ENTEROCOLITIS (NEC)

Definition

Necrotizing enterocolitis (NEC) is a potentially life-threatening acquired disease of the gastrointestinal tract of the neonate resulting in ischemia and death of intestinal tissue (MedlinePlus, 2007). It can vary in intensity from a mild self-limiting disease to a severe inflammatory complex resulting in diffuse or patchy necrosis in the intestinal mucosal and submucosal layers.

Pathophysiology

NEC is most prevalent in preterm infants with some type of intestinal injury. The immune systems of these infants are very immature, and this injury can cause vascular compromise and decreased blood supply to the intestines. Ischemia of the intestinal mucosa leads to the risk of perforation, allowing intestinal contents to enter the peritoneal cavity. Normal intestinal bacteria hydrolyze formula in the intestine, "forming gas or air in the bowel wall called pneumatosis intestinalis. The bowel becomes edematous and distended. Progressive infiltration of the bowel wall with bacteria leads to more extensive tissue inflammation, destruction, and necrosis" (Potts & Mandleco, 2007, p. 690). Paralytic ileus occurs.

During this process, sodium levels decrease (hyponatremia) and blood components are impacted resulting in thrombocytopenia, leukopenia or leukocytosis, and neutropenia. The thrombocytopenia, prolonged prothrombin time (PT) and activated partial thromboplastin time (aPTT), decreasing fibrinogen, and rising fibrin split products increase the infant's risk for bleeding. In advanced stages, metabolic acidosis, shock response, and cardiovascular collapse can result in infant death.

Complications

Paralytic ileus
Hyponatremia
Metabolic acidosis
Thrombocytopenia
Leukopenia or leukocytosis with left shift
Neutropenia
Prolonged PT and aPTT, decreasing fibrinogen, and rising fibrin split products (in cases of consumption coagulopathy)
Perforation
Sepsis
Shock
Death

Incidence

The incidence of NEC has occurred at a stable prevalence over the past 25 years at 0.3–2.4 cases per 1,000 live births. The disease is most prevalent in preterm infants with an inverse ratio of weight versus occurrence. The smaller the preterm neonate, the more likely the infant will develop NEC. The condition, however, has been reported among term infants who have experienced perinatal asphyxia or congenital heart disease

(Springer & Annibale, 2006). "[T]he incidence is increasing because of the improved survival rate in the high-risk group of infants born prematurely" (Woods, 2005, Section 2).

Etiology

The exact cause of NEC is unknown; however, several factors have been identified as predisposing the neonate to this disease. Among these factors are intestinal ischemia, intestinal infectious process, and presence of hypertonic solutions in the intestines usually from concentrated formulas (Potts & Mandleco, 2007). Other factors that can predispose the preterm neonate include exchange blood transfusions, perinatal asphyxia, respiratory distress syndrome, abnormal mesenteric artery, and placement of umbilical catheters (Woods, 2005; Potts & Mandleco, 2007).

Clinical Manifestations

Feeding intolerance
Abdominal pain/tenderness
Abdominal distention
Bloody stools
Decreased bowel sounds
Increased gastric residuals
Bradycardia
Temperature instability
Lethargy
Apnea
Cyanosis in extremities
Abnormal clotting
Decreased urinary output
Shock

Diagnostic Tests

Complete blood count
Serum electrolytes
Arterial blood gases (ABGs)
Abdominal radiography
Abdominal ultrasonography
Rectal biopsy

Medical Management

The goal of treatment is to preserve the infant's life through early detection and treatment or surgical intervention (required in 40–50% of cases) to resect the necrotic bowel. If the disease is detected early, medical management includes withholding enteral feedings; placing a nasogastric tube for continuous gastric decompression; maintaining adequate oxygenation; and inserting an intravenous access for fluid resuscitation, reestablishment of acid-base balance, and administration of broad-spectrum antimicrobials. Intravenous sodium bicarbonate is used to treat the metabolic acidosis. Vancomycin, cefotaxime (third-generation cephalosporin), clindamycin, and metrodiazole (antifungal) are the antimicrobials of choice for NEC (Springer & Annibale, 2006).

In the event of manifestations of shock, crystalloid intravenous volume expanders are needed. Lactated Ringer's usually is the fluid of choice because it expands vascular volume; in addition, the lactate ions convert to bicarbonate to buffer the metabolic acidosis. Colloids including 5% albumin may be used to expand plasma volume (Broyles, Reiss, & Evans, 2007). A central venous pressure (CVP) line is inserted to monitor the infant's response and to identify subtle changes that would indicate the presence of cardiovascular overload and pulmonary edema. Vasopressors dopamine and dobutamine are used to treat NEC infants experiencing decreased tissue perfusion and compromised cardiac output (CO). These infants must be closely monitored for fluid overload and the risk of increased intracranial pressure. Inotropic agents (digoxin) may be used to increase CO; oxygen therapy also is a first-line therapy for shock. Mechanical ventilation to support respiratory function frequently is needed to decrease energy consumption used for the work of breathing so that the brain and heart can maintain adequate oxygen perfusion. Hemodynamic monitoring is imperative in the treatment of NEC to provide critical information about the infant's condition, response to therapy, and overall prognosis. Cardiac enzymes are monitored and replacement therapy for clotting factors and platelets is initiated in the presence of coagulation irregularities.

When surgical intervention is required, a resection of the necrotic portion of the bowel is performed. In some cases, removal of extensive amounts of the bowel may necessitate the creation of a temporary ileostomy, jejunostomy, or colostomy (Potts & Mandleco, 2007).

Nursing Management

ASSESSMENT

1. Obtain client history
2. Perform pediatric assessment
3. Monitor cardiorespiratory status
4. Obtain frequent assessments of abdominal girth in preterm infant
5. Assess gastric residuals and bowel sounds

NURSING DIAGNOSES (INCLUDING BUT NOT LIMITED TO)

1. Risk for injury, NEC R/T intestinal injury in preterm infants
2. Ineffective tissue perfusion R/T disease process and shock response
3. Decreased CO R/T decreased blood volume
4. Deficient fluid volume R/T body fluid shift
5. Ineffective thermoregulation R/T prematurity and disease process
6. Ineffective protection R/T prematurity and disease process
7. Imbalanced nutrition: less than body requirements R/T lack of oral intake and energy expenditure
8. Parental anxiety R/T critical condition of infant and potential death
9. Deficient knowledge (parental) R/T infant's condition, treatment, and home care

PLANNING/GOALS

1. Client's NEC will be detected early and treated effectively.
2. Client will regain and maintain adequate tissue perfusion as evidenced by maintenance of vital signs, oxygen saturation, and urine output within defined limits (WDL) and alertness within 48–72 hours of diagnosis.
3. Client will regain and maintain CO WDL to maintain tissue perfusion.
4. Client will regain and maintain adequate fluid volume as evidenced by urinary output > 30 mL/hr, stable vital signs WDL, CO WDL, and peripheral pulses > 2+; client will be awake and alert consistent with age.
5. Client will regain and maintain temperature stability WDL.
6. Client will regain and maintain stabilization of preterm condition as evidenced by resolved edema, clear breath sounds, resolution of adventitious heart sounds, and CO WDL.

7. Client will have adequate nutrition as evidenced by nitrogen balance and stable weight within 24–48 hours prior to transfer from critical care unit.

8. Parents will express concerns and use positive coping mechanisms and support systems.

9. Parents will demonstrate understanding of condition, treatment, and home care.

NOC

1. Risk Control
2. Circulation Status
3. Circulation Status
4. Fluid Balance
5. Thermoregulation
6. Immune Status
7. Nutritional Status
8. Anxiety
9. Knowledge: Disease Process, Illness Care, Treatment, Medications, Health Promotion: Infant

IMPLEMENTATION

1. Risk for injury
   a. Assess abdominal girth frequently
   b. Assess for abdominal distention or bowel loops
   c. Measure gastric residual prior to each feeding
   d. Monitor bowel sounds
   e. Monitor laboratory test results
   f. Test all stools for blood
   g. Monitor vital signs (no rectal temperatures)

2. Tissue perfusion
   a. Maintain on continuous cardiorespiratory monitoring and pulse oximetry
   b. Assess for adequate tissue perfusion
   c. Monitor capillary refill and color of extremities
   d. Maintain patency of central venous access device (CVAD), monitoring at least hourly
   e. Administer intravenous fluids as prescribed, monitoring effectiveness
   f. Administer antimicrobial agents as prescribed, monitoring effectiveness
   g. Administer vasopressor agents as prescribed, monitoring effectiveness
   h. Monitor intake and output
   i. Administer oxygen as prescribed, titrating to oxygen saturation
   j. Place on mechanical ventilation as prescribed

3. Cardiac output
   a. Refer to interventions used to support tissue perfusion
   b. Monitor mean arterial pressure (MAP), blood pressure, pulmonary artery pressure (PAP), ABGs, and heart rate and rhythm continuously
   c. Assess CO every 1–4 hours and after administration of vasopressor agents

    d. Maintain patency of CVAD, monitoring at least hourly

    e. Auscultate breath sounds every 1–2 hours and report any adventitious sounds that may indicate a need for increase in dosage or change in diuretic

    f. Monitor urine output continuously and report if urine output does not respond to diuretic therapy

    g. Monitor renal function tests including BUN and creatinine

    h. Administer oxygen, titrating to maintain oxygen saturation/pulse oximetry

    i. Monitor for dysrhythmias and report to health care provider

4. Fluid balance

    a. Monitor daily weight

    b. Maintain strict intake and output

    c. Maintain nothing by mouth

    d. Monitor hourly urine output

    e. Maintain patency of CVAD, monitoring at least hourly

    f. Administer intravenous fluids, monitoring vital signs and urine output to determine effectiveness

    g. Administer medications as prescribed, monitoring for effectiveness and adverse effects

    h. Monitor vital signs continuously

    i. Monitor cardiac telemetry continuously for dysrhythmias

    j. Monitor lungs sounds for crackles and rhonchi that may indicate fluid overload

    k. Monitor serum laboratory values

    l. Reestablish oral/enteral feedings once paralytic ileus and NEC have been resolved

5. Thermoregulation

    a. Monitor continuous skin temperature

    b. Place on warming bed as needed to maintain prescribed temperature

    c. Administer acetaminophen as prescribed for temperature elevations

    d. Monitor skin and respiratory status

    e. Place in temperature-controlled isolette as indicted by infant's condition

6. Altered protection

    a. Refer to Thermoregulation for interventions

    b. Monitor for manifestations of worsening NEC

    c. Protect skin from injury

    d. Monitor coagulation studies

    e. Assess for bleeding from skin, mucous membranes, stool, gastric secretions, and urine

    f. Provide tactile stimulation and use a soft, soothing voice

    g. Encourage parents to visit and interact with infant within the constraints of the infant's condition

    h. Maintain on continuous hemodynamic monitoring

    i. Institute infection precautions

    j. Assess incision site for redness, swelling, heat, and purulent drainage

k. Maintain strict asepsis during dressing changes (CVAD, wound, A-line, etc.)

l. Culture any suspicious drainage or secretions

m. Maintain sterile integrity of intravenous accesses, tubing and intravenous fluids, and medications

n. Change intravenous tubing every 72 hours or per facility protocol

o. Administer therapeutic or prophylactic antimicrobials as prescribed

p. Perform indwelling urinary catheter care per facility protocol including maintaining catheter integrity

q. Maintain mechanical ventilation, ET suction as indicated by increased respiratory rate, effort, and audible tracheal mucous sounds

r. Protect from injury

s. Provide nutritional support to maintain nitrogen balance

7. Nutrition

a. Monitor daily weight

b. Monitor skin integrity and turgor

c. Provide nutrition via enteral feedings as prescribed or total parenteral nutrition (TPN)

d. Collaborate with dietician

e. Coordinate multidisciplinary team approach

f. Monitor strict intake and output

g. Monitor serum electrolytes

8. Anxiety

a. Encourage parents to express feelings and concerns

b. Listen actively

c. Encourage parents to visit infant in critical care unit

d. Explain all procedures and equipment to parents

e. Keep parents informed of infant's condition when they are not permitted to visit due to infant's condition or critical care unit protocols

f. Serve as liaison between family and health care provider

g. Make referrals to chaplain and other parent support services in collaboration with health care provider as needed

9. Parent teaching

a. Assess parents' current level of knowledge

b. Explain all equipment and procedures to parents—in particular, the extensive equipment involved in the critical care environment, which can be quite overwhelming

c. Provide parents with information regarding visitation schedule for critical care unit (neonatal intensive care unit or pediatric intensive care unit)

d. Encourage parent/family visitation and questions

e. Provide honest and truthful answers to parents' questions

f. Refer questions to health care provider as necessary

g. Provide preoperative teaching if indicated

h. Provide written and verbal instructions regarding home care, including infant care and feedings, medication administration, signs and symptoms to report to health care provider, and importance of follow-up medical visits

i. Provide adequate time for teaching

j. Document teaching and parental response

NIC

1. Risk Identification, Surveillance: Safety

2. Hemodynamic Monitoring

3. Hemodynamic Monitoring

4. Fluid and Electrolyte Monitoring/Management, Acid/Base Monitoring/Management

5. Temperature Regulation

6. Infection Protection, Bleeding Precautions

7. Nutrition Monitoring, Nutrition Management

8. Anxiety Reduction, Coping Enhancement

9. Teaching (Parent): Disease Process, Illness Care, Treatment, Medications, Health Education

EVALUATION

1. Client's NEC is detected early and treated effectively.

2. Client regains and maintains adequate tissue perfusion as evidenced by maintenance of vital signs, oxygen saturation, and urine output WDL and alertness within 48–72 hours of diagnosis.

3. Client regains and maintains CO WDL to maintain tissue perfusion.

4. Client regains and maintains adequate fluid volume as evidenced by urinary output > 30 mL/hr, stable vital signs WDL, CO WDL, and peripheral pulses > 2+; client is awake and alert consistent with age.

5. Client regains and maintains temperature stability WDL.

6. Client regains and maintains stabilization of preterm condition as evidenced by resolved edema, clear breath sounds, resolution of adventitious heart sounds, and CO WDL.

7. Client has adequate nutrition as evidenced by nitrogen balance and stable weight within 24–48 hours prior to transfer from critical care unit.

8. Parents express concerns and use positive coping mechanisms and support systems.

9. Parents demonstrate understanding of condition, treatment, and home care.

References

Broyles, B. E., Reiss, B. A., & Evans, M. A. (2007). *Pharmacological aspects of nursing care* (7th ed.). Clifton Park, NY: Delmar Cengage Learning.

MedlinePlus. (2007). *Necrotizing enterocolitis.* Retrieved July 7, 2007, from http://www.nlm.nih .gov/medlineplus/ency/article/001148.htm

Potts, N. L., & Mandleco, B. L. (2007). *Pediatric nursing: Caring for children and their families* (2nd ed.). Clifton Park, NY: Delmar Cengage Learning.

Springer, S. C., & Annibale, D. J. (2006). *Necrotizing enterocolitis.* Retrieved July 7, 2007, from http://www.emedicine.com/ped/topic2601.htm

Wood, B. P. (2005). *Necrotizing enterocolitis.* Retrieved July 7, 2007, from http://www.emedicine .com/radio/topic469.htm

75

NEPHROTIC SYNDROME

Definition

Nephrotic syndrome is a kidney disorder characterized by proteinuria, hypoproteinemia (hypoalbuminemia), and edema (Broyles, 2005). The most common type of nephrotic syndrome in children is termed *minimal change disease* (National Kidney and Urologic Diseases Information Clearinghouse (NKUDIC), 2005).

Pathophysiology

The event that initiates nephrotic syndrome is unknown; however, it causes the glomerular capillaries in the kidneys to selectively increase their permeability to protein (albumin). Refer to Figure 75-1. This increased filtering of albumin is greater than the ability of the tubules to reabsorb protein, resulting in proteinuria. The protein being excreted is drawn from the vascular system, leading to hypoproteinemia or hypoalbuminemia. Albumin is a critical component of plasma proteins that help maintain vascular oncotic pressure. Decreased serum albumin reduces oncotic pressure causing extravasation of plasma water from the vascular compartment to the interstitial space. This results in edema. In addition, with the decrease in plasma volume, renal perfusion decreases resulting in stimulation of the renin-angiotensin complex leading to an increase in secretion of the antidiuretic hormone causing the renal tubules to increase the reabsorption of sodium and water. The result is an increase in the severity of the edema (Travis, 2005).

Edema usually begins in the extremities, but it can third-space to the lungs and brain, resulting in increased intracranial pressure. Peripheral edema poses a risk for impaired skin integrity due to pressure decreasing tissue perfusion as well as increased stress to the skin with an increased risk of skin breakdown. "The loss of antithrombin III and plasminogen via urine and the simultaneous increase in clotting factors, especially factors I, VII, VIII, and X, increases the risk for arterial thrombosis, venous thrombosis, and pulmonary embolism, which occurs in 5% of children with nephrotic syndrome" (Agraharkar & Gala, 2007, Section 2).

In approximately 20% of children with nephrotic syndrome, scarring or deposits in the glomeruli have been revealed through renal biopsy. This can cause permanent damage to the glomeruli that may lead to nephron damage and the onset of renal failure. The positive aspect of nephrotic syndrome is that most children outgrow it by their late teens with no permanent damage to their kidneys.

Very rarely, a neonate may be born with congenital nephropathy, a condition that causes primary congenital nephrotic syndrome. "The classifications of primary congenital nephrotic syndrome include infantile microcystic disease (Finnish type—most commonly seen in infants of Finnish descent), infantile microcystic disease (non-Finnish type), diffuse mesangial sclerosis, minimal-lesion nephrotic syndrome, and [focal segmental glomerulosclerosis] FSGS. The classifications of secondary congenital nephrotic syndrome include intrauterine infections (eg, toxoplasmosis, cytomegalovirus)" (Agraharkar & Gala, 2007, Section 2).

Complications

Decreased renal perfusion
Edema
Skin breakdown
Renal failure

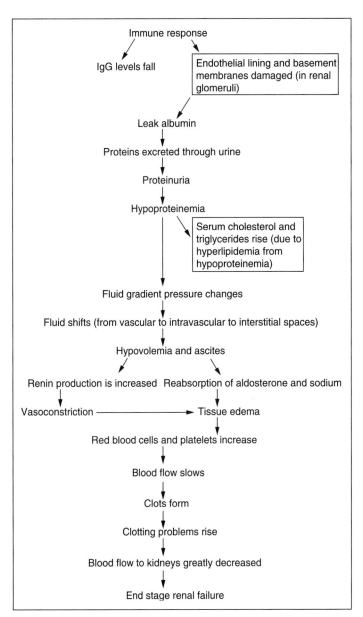

Figure 75-1: Pathophysiology of Nephrotic Syndrome.

Incidence

Pediatric nephrotic syndrome can occur at any age but is most prevalent between the ages of 1½ and 5 years with a peak incidence at 2 years of age. Over 75% of children under 16 years of age who develop nephrotic syndrome do so before the age of 6. It seems to affect boys more often than girls (National Kidney and Urologic Diseases Information Clearinghouse [NKUDIC], 2005). The overall incidence of nephrotic syndrome in childhood is approximately two to seven cases per 100,000 children (Agraharkar & Gala, 2007).

Etiology

The exact cause of nephrotic syndrome is unknown; primary nephrotic syndrome (PNS) is believed to be caused by an immune response triggered by either glomerular disease or a systemic infection (Potts & Mandleco, 2007). Other primary causes include systemic lupus erythematosus (SLE); rheumatoid arthritis; polyarteritis nodosa; Henoch-Schönlein purpura; hereditary nephritis; sickle cell disease (SCD); diabetes mellitus (DM); amyloidosis; malignancies including leukemia, lymphoma, Wilms' tumor, and pheochromocytoma; toxins from bee sting, poison ivy and oak, and snake venom; medications including probenecid, fenoprofen, captopril, lithium, warfarin, penicillamine, mercury, gold, trimethadione, and paramethadione; and heroin use (Agraharkar & Gala, 2007). Secondary causes in children are related to postinfectious diseases including tuberculosis, varicella, hepatitis B, human immunodeficiency virus (HIV) type 1, infectious mononucleosis, and group A beta-hemolytic streptococci (Agraharkar & Gala, 2007).

Clinical Manifestations

Edema
Anorexia
Abdominal pain
Fatigue
Increased weight

Diagnostic Tests

Urinalysis
Renal ultrasonography
Kidney biopsy

Medical Management

The goals of treatment are to decrease protein loss, control edema, and prevent infection. The standard of care is the administration of corticosteroids, prednisone, and prednisolone. These agents decrease inflammation and loss of proteins, resulting in the return of vascular oncotic pressure and a decrease in edema. This treatment usually is continued for 4–8 weeks. Depending on the severity of the child's condition, the corticosteroids initially may be administered intravenously, but the majority of the treatment is oral with a tapering of prednisone over the course of several weeks. Also, if the edema is severe, the loop diuretic furosemide may be prescribed until the edema is under control. Furosemide acts by inhibiting the reabsorption of sodium and chloride in the ascending loop of Henle, thus decreasing the kidneys' ability to concentrate urine, resulting in increased water excretion (Broyles, Reiss, & Evans, 2007).

The relapse rate for nephrotic syndrome is 50–60%; if relapse occurs, high-dose steroid therapy is initiated but is continued for a much shorter period of time and discontinued when the child is free of proteinuria for three days. For nephrotic syndrome that does not respond to steroid therapy, immunosuppressant agents including cyclophosphamide, chlorambucil, and alternate treatments with cyclosporine are used for 8–12 weeks. Recent experience with angiotensin-converting enzyme (ACE) inhibitors indicates that these agents are useful in preventing proteinuria and preventing kidney damage in children with nephrotic syndrome.

Since pharmacological agents have little effect on congenital nephropathy, transplantation usually is required by the second or third year of life. Until that point, health care providers may recommend infusions of albumin to replace protein lost in urine and prescribe a diuretic to facilitate removal of excess fluid from edema. If the child's immune system is weakened, antimicrobial agents are prescribed at the first sign of infection. Congenital nephropathy can alter thyroid function, so the child may need thyroid replacement with thyroxine to promote growth and strengthen bones. The anticoagulant warfarin sodium may be prescribed to prevent thrombus formation. In addition, enteral feedings may be necessary to ensure proper nutrition. In the event the proteinuria and hypoalbuminemia cannot be controlled, the diseased kidney may need to be removed to eliminate proteinuria. Dialysis then will be necessary until the child can receive a renal transplant. Peritoneal dialysis is preferable to hemodialysis for young children because of the risk of hypotension related to the hemodialysis process and the fact that peritoneal dialysis provides better control in children. In peritoneal dialysis, a catheter (usually called a Tenckhoff peritoneal catheter) that is surgically placed in the child's peritoneal cavity is used to introduce diasylate solution into the abdominal cavity (peritoneum). The solution draws wastes and excess fluid from the child's bloodstream; and after a specified "dwell time," the solution is drained by gravity into a urine receptacle. Cycles of introducing diasylate solution, dwell time, and drainage are performed according to what a nephrologist prescribes (usually four or five times per day).

Nursing Management

ASSESSMENT

1. Obtain client history (in children, focus on recent history of upper respiratory infection)
2. Assess urine for protein
3. Perform pediatric assessment noting presence of edema, skin integrity, and breath sounds
4. Assess vital signs
5. Obtain weight and height
6. Monitor laboratory values

NURSING DIAGNOSES (INCLUDING BUT NOT LIMITED TO)

1. Excess fluid volume R/T edema
2. Risk for impaired skin integrity R/T edema
3. Ineffective protection R/T immunosuppression and hypercoagulability
4. Fatigue R/T anemia, loss of plasma proteins, and anorexia
5. Parental anxiety R/T child's condition and potential loss of renal function
6. Deficient knowledge R/T child's condition, treatment, prognosis, and home care

PLANNING/GOALS

1. Client will regain and maintain appropriate fluid volume as evidenced by resolution of hypoproteinemia, edema, and proteinuria.
2. Client will maintain skin integrity as evidenced by intact skin.
3. Client will not experience infection or thromboemboli.
4. Client will gradually regain energy level to resume activities of daily living (ADL) as evidenced by verbalization and increased involvement in age-appropriate activities.

5. Parents will verbalize feelings and concerns and use positive coping strategies.
6. Parents will demonstrate understanding of condition, treatment, prognosis, and home care.

NOC

1. Fluid Balance
2. Risk Control, Tissue Integrity: Skin
3. Immune Status
4. Fatigue
5. Anxiety
6. Knowledge: Illness Care, Disease Process, Treatment, Medications, Health Promotion

IMPLEMENTATION

1. Excess fluid volume
   a. Assess skin integrity every 2 hours when repositioned
   b. Monitor vital signs every 4 hours and as needed
   c. Assess breath sounds every 4 hours
   d. Administer medications as prescribed, monitoring effectiveness and adverse effects
   e. Maintain strict intake and output
   f. Monitor urine specific gravity
   g. Monitor urine for protein
   h. Weigh daily
   i. Assess and document presence of edema
   j. Monitor serum electrolytes, hemoglobin, and creatinine
   k. Collaborate with health care provider for dietary referral if needed
   l. Maintain dietary modifications as prescribed
   m. Initiate and maintain patency of intravenous access if prescribed, monitoring at least hourly
2. Skin integrity
   a. Assess for degree of edema
   b. Assess skin integrity every 1–2 hours
   c. Reposition every 1–2 hours
   d. Elevate edematous extremities
   e. Administer medications as prescribed, monitoring for effectiveness and adverse effects
   f. Provide skin protection as indicated
3. Ineffective protection
   a. Assess vital signs every 4 hours
   b. Monitor complete blood count
   c. Assess for other signs of infection, such as wound drainage and urine cloudiness
   d. Use meticulous hand washing and teach appropriate technique to child/parents
   e. Avoid or minimize invasive procedures
   f. Administer medications as prescribed
   g. Maintain diet with complete proteins
   h. Monitor for manifestations of thrombus formation

4. Fatigue
    a. Assess energy level
    b. Encourage low-energy, age-appropriate activities
    c. Assist with ADL as needed and encourage parent participation in care
    d. Provide for adequate rest by clustering activities when possible
    e. Collaborate with dietician and health care provider for frequent small meals and diet with complete proteins, iron, and adequate calories
    f. Support child and parents with understanding and active listening
5. Anxiety
    a. Encourage verbalization of feelings and concerns
    b. Support with understanding and active listening
    c. Assist parents in identifying positive coping strategies that were effectively used previously
    d. Encourage participation in child's care
    e. Answer questions honestly, referring those requiring health care provider input
6. Parent teaching
    a. Assess parents' current level of knowledge
    b. Provide verbal and written information regarding:
        1) Medication administration and importance of compliance with regime
        2) Infection protection (avoiding crowds, avoiding people with contagious diseases, and washing hands using appropriate technique)
        3) Manifestations of adverse effects of medications
        4) Skin protection and care
        5) Manifestations of worsening of condition or relapse (dyspnea, edema, and decreased urine output)
        6) Contact phone numbers for reporting signs and symptoms
        7) Importance of follow-up with health care provider
    c. Provide adequate time for teaching
    d. Document teaching and parental response

NIC

1. Fluid Management, Fluid Monitoring
2. Skin Surveillance, Positioning
3. Infection Protection
4. Energy Enhancement
5. Anxiety Reduction, Coping Enhancement
6. Teaching: Illness Care, Disease Process, Treatment, Medications, Health Education

EVALUATION

1. Client regains and maintains appropriate fluid volume as evidenced by resolution of hypoproteinemia, edema, and proteinuria.
2. Client maintains skin integrity as evidenced by intact skin.
3. Client does not experience infection or thromboemboli.
4. Client gradually regains energy level to resume ADL as evidenced by verbalization and increased involvement in age-appropriate activities.

5. Parents verbalize feelings and concerns and use positive coping strategies.
6. Parents demonstrate understanding of condition, treatment, prognosis, and home care.

References

Agraharkar, M., & Gala, G. (2007). *Nephrotic syndrome.* Retrieved March 10, 2008, from http://www.emedicine.com/MED/topic1612.htm

Broyles, B. E. (2005). *Medical-surgical nursing clinical companion.* Durham, NC: Carolina Academic Press.

Broyles, B. E., Reiss, B. S., & Evans, M. E. (2007). *Pharmacological aspects of nursing care* (7th ed.). Clifton Park, NY: Delmar Cengage Learning.

National Kidney and Urologic Diseases Information Clearinghouse (NKUDIC). (2005). *Childhood nephrotic syndrome.* Retrieved March 29, 2007, from http://kidney.niddk.nih.gov/kudiseases/pubs/childkidneydiseases/nephrotic_syndrom/index.htm

Potts, N. L., & Mandleco, B. L. (2007). *Pediatric nursing: Caring for children and their families* (2nd ed.). Clifton Park, NY: Delmar Cengage Learning.

Travis, L. (2005). *Nephrotic syndrome.* Retrieved July 7, 2007, from http://www.emedicine.com/ped/topic1564.htm

76

NEUROBLASTOMA

Definition

Neuroblastoma is a tumor originating from the primordial neural crest cells that are embryonic precursors of the adrenal medulla and sympathetic nervous system (Potts & Mandleco, 2007).

Pathophysiology

Neuroblastoma originates in the adrenal medulla or the paraspinal sites where sympathetic nervous system tissue is present. The adrenal glands, positioned on top of the kidneys, secrete hormones and other substances. The abnormal cells, present in the fetus, later develop into a detectable tumor. These cells compete with the normal cells for oxygen, nutrients, and metabolites; and because they do not have the same homeostatic checks and balances of the normal cells, they proliferate without restriction, metastasizing to bone, the retrobulbar region, the liver, and other areas of the sympathetic nervous system. This can lead to organ failure and death if not diagnosed and treated early, usually within the first year of life. For children with high-risk neuroblastoma, long-term survival ranges from 10–40% (National Cancer Institute, 2007).

The most common presentation of neuroblastoma is an abdominal mass. The most common symptoms in high-risk children are due to a tumor mass or bone pain from metastases. Ptosis and periorbital ecchymosis may occur, resulting from retrobulbar metastasis. Extensive bone marrow metastasis may cause pancytopenia. Abdominal distention with respiratory compromise due to massive liver metastases may occur in infants. Because they originate in paraspinal ganglia, neuroblastomas may invade through neural foramina and compress the spinal cord extradurally, causing paralysis. On rare occasions, children may have severe, watery diarrhea due to the secretion of vasoactive intestinal peptide by the tumor or may have protein-losing enteropathy with intestinal lymphangiectasia (Schneider Children's Hospital, 2007).

Neuroblastomas are divided into low-, intermediate-, and high-risk groups and are based on biologic factors they have been divided into three biological groups. One type, the hyperdiploid, expresses the TrkA neurotrophin receptor. This type tends to spontaneously diminish. Another type that expresses the TrkB neurotrophin receptor has an additional chromosome, 17q, and has loss of heterozygosity of 14q or 11q. The third type is characterized by the addition of 17q, the loss of chromosome 1p, and the amplification of the oncogene called the MYCN gene (National Cancer Institute, 2007).

Complications

Metastasis
Respiratory compromise
Bone pain
Organ failure
Death

Incidence

Neuroblastoma is the most common tumor of the sympathetic nervous system, accounting for 97% of tumors in this system. Neuroblastoma affects approximately 500–1,000 children annually in the United States (Neuroblastoma Children's Cancer Society, 2007).

The incidence is approximately 9.4 cases per 100,000 live births. In children under the age of 1 year, the incidence is 64 cases per 1 million infants; during the second year, it is 29 per million. It accounts for about 7.7% of all childhood tumors occurring in children under the age of 15 years. The survival rate from diagnosis in infants is 83%; and in children 5 years and older, the rate is 40% (National Cancer Institute, 2007). Because neuroblastoma derives from embryonic cells, approximately 40% of cases are diagnosed before the age of 1 year; 89% are diagnosed before the age of 5 years (Potts & Mandleco, 2007).

Etiology

The cause of neuroblastoma is currently unknown; however, it occurs more often in children born with fetal hydantoin syndrome, neurofibromatosis, and Beckwith-Wiedeman syndrome. The exact relationship between these conditions and the disease are not known (National Cancer Institute, 2007).

Clinical Manifestations

Abdominal mass
Thoracic mass
Peripheral edema
Altered urinary elimination
Bone marrow involvement (pain, limping, paralysis, or weakness)
Diarrhea
Ecchymosis of the eyelid
Ptosis

Diagnostic Tests

Complete blood count
Urinalysis
Magnetic resonance imaging
Electron microscopy
Serum catecholamines
Urine catecholamine metabolites
Bone marrow aspirate
Trephine biopsy

Medical Management

The goals of treatment are early detection, complete resection through surgery, and/or establishment of remission. Treatment can be accomplished by surgery, radiation therapy, chemotherapy, and/or stem cell transplantation. The treatment depends on the stage of the disease, prognostic markers, and the child's age. For the child who presents with a stage 1 or stage 2 neuroblastoma, complete surgical resection usually provides a cure for the disease.

The determination of high-risk neuroblastoma is established by the International Neuroblastoma Staging System (INSS) stage and tumor biology (MYCN gene amplification, Shimada classification, and DNA ploidy). According to the National Cancer Institute, the following children are identified as high-risk, requiring combination therapy including multidrug chemotherapy (with commonly used agents such as cyclophosphamide, ifosfamide, cisplatin, carboplatin, vincristine, doxorubicin, and etoposide) and stem cell transplantation:

1. INSS stage 2A/2B tumors in children older than 1 year and in whom the tumor has both unfavorable Shimada classification and MYCN gene amplification
2. INSS stage 3 tumors in infants younger than 1 year and in whom the tumor demonstrates MYCN gene amplification

3. INSS stage 3 tumors in children older than 1 year and in whom the tumor demonstrates either MYCN gene amplification or unfavorable Shimada classification

4. INSS stage 4 tumors in infants younger than 18 months at diagnosis and in whom the tumor demonstrates MYCN gene amplification

5. INSS stage 4 tumors in children older than 18 months with or without MYCN gene amplification

6. INSS stage 4S tumors in infants younger than 1 year at diagnosis and in whom the tumor demonstrates MYCN gene amplification

In advanced disease, multidrug chemotherapy brings about a high degree (83%) of success; however, recurrence rates are high as well (National Cancer Institute, 2007). Radiation therapy is not used as a monotherapy, but rather in conjunction with chemotherapy and stem cell transplantation. End-of-life care is an important part of the multidisciplinary approach for children in the end stage of the disease (Broyles, Reiss, & Evans, 2007). Refer to Chapter 22: Chemotherapy, Chapter 67: Leukemia/Stem Cell Transplantation, Chapter 87: Radiation Therapy, and Chapter 100: Surgical Client.

Nursing Management

Refer to Chapter 22: Chemotherapy, Chapter 67: Leukemia/Stem Cell Transplantation, Chapter 87: Radiation Therapy, and Chapter 100: Surgical Client. Refer to the chapters listed previously for the nursing management of a child with neuroblastoma.

References

Broyles, B. E., Reiss, B. S., & Evans, M. E. (2007). *Pharmacological aspects of nursing care* (7th ed.). Clifton Park, NY: Delmar Cengage Learning.

National Cancer Institute. (2007). *Sympathetic nervous system tumors.* Retrieved April 4, 2007, from http://seer.cancer.gov/publications/childhood/sympathetic.pdf

Neuroblastoma Children's Cancer Society. (2007). *What is neuroblastoma?* Retrieved July 9, 2007, from http://www.neuroblastomacancer.org/scripts/content.cgi?template=default&args=main, education

Potts, N. L., & Mandleco, B. L. (2007). *Pediatric nursing: Caring for children and their families* (2nd ed.). Clifton Park, NY: Delmar Cengage Learning.

Schneider Children's Hospital. (2007). *Oncology: Neuroblastoma.* Retrieved April 4, 2007, from http://www.schneiderchildrenshospital.org/peds_html_fixed/peds/oncology/nbt.htm

Non-Hodgkin's Lymphoma (NHL)

Definition

Non-Hodgkin's lymphoma (also called NHL or lymphoma) is cancer that originates in lymphoid tissue (American Cancer Society, 2006b).

Pathophysiology

Lymphoid tissue, which includes the lymph nodes and other organs that are part of the body's immune system, forms blood and protects against infection. Lymphoid tissue is found throughout the body including the spleen, thymus, bone marrow, tonsils, adenoids, stomach, and intestinal tract. The primary cells found in the lymphoid tissue are lymphocytes: B cells and T cells. Approximately 85% of lymphomas originate in the B cells (Broyles, 2005). Lymph nodes become enlarged in the presence of infection; however, large lymph nodes are the cardinal manifestation of lymphoma. The spleen manufactures lymphocytes, the thymus gland is critical in the development of T cells, and lymphocytes also are produced in the bone marrow along with erythrocytes and platelets (American Cancer Society, 2006b). Because of the diffuse nature of lymphoid tissue, NHL has a rapid onset and usually presents with widespread involvement (Stages III and IV) (Potts & Mandleco, 2007).

There are about 30 types of NHLs including (1) diffuse large B-cell lymphoma, (2) follicular lymphoma, (3) Burkitt's lymphoma, (4) lymphoblastic lymphoma, (5) nonlymphoblastic lymphoma, and (6) anaplastic large cell lymphoma. Diffuse large B-cell lymphomas make up about 30% of lymphoma cases and occur most frequently in older adults. Follicular lymphomas make up about 14% of cases of lymphoma, and the cells tend to grow in a circular pattern in the lymph nodes. This is a slow-growing cancer. It is found most often in the elderly and is rare in very young children. Burkitt's lymphoma, lymphoblastic lymphoma, and anaplastic large cell lymphoma are the most common types found in children. With current treatments, about 80% of children and adolescents with NHL survive at least five years.

In addition to the type of NHL, another of the prognostic factors is the stage of the disease when it is diagnosed. The higher the stage, the more difficult it is to treat successfully. Children with Stage I disease (a single extra-abdominal/extrathoracic tumor) have an excellent prognosis and a five-year survival rate of approximately 90% regardless of histology. Children with NHL arising in the bone have an excellent prognosis regardless of histology. Children and adolescents with nonlymphoblastic NHL involving the mediastinum have a poorer prognosis compared with other sites of the disease. In Stage II, the disease is limited to a single tumor with regional node involvement, two or more tumors or nodal areas involved on one side of the diaphragm, or a primary completely resected gastrointestinal tumor with or without regional node involvement.

Stage III childhood NHL describes tumors or involved lymph node areas that occur on both sides of the diaphragm, primary intrathoracic (mediastinal, pleural, or thymic) disease, extensive primary intra-abdominal disease, or any paraspinal or epidural tumors. With Stage IV NHL, the tumors involve bone marrow and/or central nervous system (CNS) disease regardless of other sites of involvement (National Cancer Institute, 2007).

Complications

Mediastinal involvement
Intra-abdominal disease

CNS tumors

Bone marrow tumors

Tumor lysis syndrome (related to multidrug chemotherapy treatment)

Death

Incidence

Lymphoma (Hodgkin's and non-Hodgkin's) is the third most common childhood malignancy, and NHL accounts for approximately 7% of cancers in children under the age of 20. The annual incidence in the United States is about 800 new cases of NHL affecting approximately 10 per 1,000,000 children. NHL occurs most commonly in children between the ages of 11 and 19 years. The incidence of NHL is higher in Caucasians than in African Americans, and NHL is more common in males than in females (National Cancer Institute, 2007).

Etiology

The exact cause of NHL in children is unknown although viral, genetic, immunologic, and environmental factors have been implicated in the search for a cause. Immunodeficiency, both congenital and acquired (human immunodeficiency virus [HIV] infection or post-transplant), increases the risk of NHL. Epstein-Barr virus (EBV) is associated with most cases of NHL seen in the immunodeficient population (National Cancer Institute, 2007).

Clinical Manifestations

Lymph node pain and swelling

Mediastinal mass, pleural effusion, and lymphadenopathy (lymphoblastic NHL)

Abdominal mass and CNS involvement (Burkitt's lymphoma)

Infection

Headache

Nausea

Vomiting

Petechiae

Ecchymosis

Bone pain

Diagnostic Tests

Biopsy

Computed tomography

Lumbar puncture

Bone scan

Gallium scan

Complete blood count

Serum electrolytes

Medical Management

The goals of treatment are to arrest neoplastic growth and to achieve remission and a cure. Because of the widespread involvement usually present at diagnosis, multidrug chemotherapy is the treatment of choice. Chemotherapy may be used alone or in conjunction with radiation therapy (American Cancer Society, 2006a). Agents used in combination chemotherapeutic regimens include CHOP (cytoxan, hydroxydaunorubicin, Oncovin, and prednisone), COP (cytoxan, Oncovin, and prednisone), and BACOP (bleomycin, doxorubicin, cyclophosphamide, vincristine, and prednisone) (Broyles, Reiss, & Evans, 2007). Children with limited disease (Stage I or II) have an excellent prognosis, achieving a 90–100% cure rate. Children with more extensive disease experience a 70–90% cure rate (Potts & Mandleco, 2007). Refer to Chapter 22: Chemotherapy and Chapter 87: Radiation Therapy.

Nursing Management

Refer to Chapter 22: Chemotherapy and Chapter 87: Radiation Therapy.

References

American Cancer Society (ACS). (2006a). *Detailed guide: Lymphoma, non-Hodgkin type: Chemotherapy.* Retrieved April 9, 2007, from http://www.cancer.org/docroot/CRI/content/CRI_2_4_4X_Chemotherapy_32.asp?rnav=cri

American Cancer Society (ACS). (2006b). *Overview: Lymphoma, non-Hodgkin type: What is non-Hodgkin lymphoma?* Retrieved April 5, 2007, from http://www.cancer.org/docroot/CRI/content/CRI_2_2_1x_What_is_Non-Hodgkin_Lymphoma.asp?sitearea=

Broyles, B. E. (2005). *Medical-surgical nursing clinical companion.* Durham, NC: Carolina Academic Press.

Broyles, B. E., Reiss, B. S., & Evans, M. E. (2007). *Pharmacological aspects of nursing care* (7th ed.). Clifton Park, NY: Delmar Cengage Learning.

National Cancer Institute. (2007). *Childhood non-Hodgkin lymphoma treatment (PDQ).* Retrieved April 4, 2007, from http://www.cancer.gov/cancerinfo/pdq/treatment/child-non-hodgkins/healthprofessional

Potts, N. L., & Mandleco, B. L. (2007). *Pediatric nursing: Caring for children and their families* (2nd ed.). Clifton Park, NY: Delmar Cengage Learning.

78

OMPHALOCELE

Definition

Omphalocele is a congenital anomaly of the gastrointestinal tract where a defect in the abdominal wall at the umbilicus allows abdominal contents covered by a thin layer of parietal peritoneum to herniate through the abdominal wall. The abdominal contents covered by this peritoneal sac are in contrast to gastroschisis, where the herniated contents lie openly on the abdomen (MedlinePlus, 2006a; Khan & Thomas, 2005). Refer to Figure 78-1.

Pathophysiology

Omphalocele results from the failure of the intestines to reenter the abdominal cavity at approximately seven weeks' gestation (Potts & Mandleco, 2007). Omphaloceles are classified as small or large, and they are more serious than gastroschisis because infants with the defect are more likely to have other birth defects including chromosomal abnormalities, congenital heart defects, and congenital diaphragmatic hernia. Approximately 25–40% of neonates with an omphalocele have other birth defects (MedlinePlus, 2006b).

According to Khan and Thomas, chromosomal anomalies including trisomies 13, 18, and 21, Turner's syndrome, and Klinefelter's syndrome occur in 40–60% of infants with omphalocele. Coexisting cardiac defects present in 16–47% of these children and

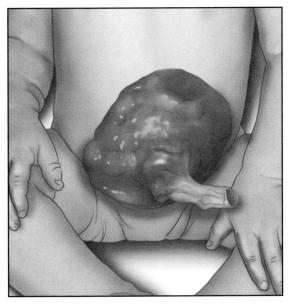

Figure 78-1: Omphalocele.

include "ventricular and atrial septal defects, tetralogy of Fallot, pulmonary stenosis, pulmonary hypoplasia, a double-outlet right ventricle, bicuspid aortic valve syndrome, transposition of the great vessels, coarctation of the aorta, ectopia cordis, and an absent inferior vena cava" (Khan & Thomas, 2005, Section 2).

Khan and Thomas include additional gastrointestinal defects such as cleft lip, diaphragmatic hernia, malrotation, intestinal duplications, atresias, ascites, absent gallbladder, abnormal fixation of the liver, tracheoesophageal fistula, and imperforate anus as being present in 40% of omphalocele cases. Also occurring in 40% of these cases are genitourinary anomalies such as exstrophy of the bladder, obstruction of the ureteropelvic junction, renal malpositioning (cephalic renal displacement), and cloacal exstrophy. Musculoskeletal anomalies occur in 10–30% of infants with omphalocele and include scoliosis, dwarfism, clubfeet, syndactyly, and other anomalies of the digits. Neural tube defects, cerebral hypoplasia, and encephalocele are additional coexisting anomalies (Khan & Thomas, 2005).

Neonates with omphaloceles commonly experience intrauterine growth retardation (IUGR), immaturity at birth, prematurity, and a single umbilical artery. Polyhydramnios frequently is seen in the antepartal mother and warrants further evaluation because it is a common indictor of congenital anomalies.

Complications

Presence of potentially life-threatening coexisting congenital anomalies
Intestinal infection
IUGR

Incidence

The incidence of small omphaloceles is 1 case per 5,000 live births, whereas large omphaloceles occur in 1 per 10,000 live births in the United States. The morbidity/mortality rate depends on the existence of coexisting anomalies. However, in the presence of chromosomal alterations and heart defects, the rate is 100%. More boys than girls are affected (Khan & Thomas, 2005; Lucile Packard Children's Hospital at Stanford, 2007).

Etiology

The exact cause of omphalocele is unknown.

Clinical Manifestations

Protrusion of the sac containing abdominal organs outside the abdominal wall
Small for age

Diagnostic Tests

Prenatal alfa-fetoprotein levels
Prenatal ultrasonography (usually diagnosed during second trimester)
Prenatal magnetic resonance imaging

Medical Management

The goals of treatment are the prevention of hypothermia, maintenance of homeostasis in the presence of other congenital anomalies, surgical closure of the abdominal wall, and prevention of complications of the anomaly and low birth weight. If omphalocele is diagnosed prenatally, a cesarean section delivery is recommended to avoid damage to the abdominal contents that can occur during vaginal delivery. Delivery, however, is not performed prior to term unless fetal distress occurs.

Immediately following delivery, the exposed abdominal sac is covered with warm, sterile saline-soaked gauze. Usually, a nasogastric (NG) tube is inserted to provide gastric decompression to prevent aspiration of gastric contents. Omphaloceles are repaired with surgery, although not always immediately. Because a sac provides some protection for the abdominal contents, other more serious anomalies, such as heart defects, can be managed first if necessary.

As soon as the neonate is stable, surgery is performed. During surgery, the sac is covered with a synthetic material and the covering is sutured in place. Over time, as the abdomen grows, the abdominal contents are pushed into the abdomen. Once the abdominal wall allows the omphalocele to fit inside, the synthetic material is removed and the abdomen is closed (MedlinePlus, 2006b).

Following surgery, the neonate is transferred to the neonatal intensive care unit (NICU); thermoregulation, intravenous fluids, antimicrobial agents, pain management, and oxygen are standards of care. Mechanical ventilation frequently is required for these neonates to maintain gas exchange following general anesthesia during the surgical repair. Gastric decompression continues until bowel function resumes; then feedings are started very slowly. If the infant does not tolerate oral feedings, enteral feedings are used. For all infants receiving enteral feedings, a pacifier should be used to stimulate and maintain the suck reflex.

Nursing Management

ASSESSMENT

1. Assess neonate's airway, breathing, and circulation
2. Perform rapid neonatal assessment
3. Assess exposed abdominal contents
4. Assess parental response to neonate's condition

NURSING DIAGNOSES (INCLUDING BUT NOT LIMITED TO)

1. Ineffective thermoregulation R/T environmental adjustment of the neonate
2. Risk for injury R/T presence of additional congenital anomalies
3. Risk for infection R/T exposed sac-covered abdominal contents
4. Ineffective breathing pattern R/T high intra-abdominal pressure secondary to return of intestinal contents to a closed abdominal cavity
5. Risk for deficient fluid volume R/T gastric decompression and inadequate intake
6. Risk for imbalanced nutrition: less than body requirements R/T gastric decompression and inadequate intake
7. Parental anxiety R/T critical nature of neonate's condition and surgery
8. Deficient knowledge R/T neonate's condition, treatment, and home care

PLANNING/GOALS

1. Client will maintain thermoregulation as evidenced by body temperature within defined limits (WDL).
2. Client will be stabilized, and other congenital anomalies will be identified and treated effectively if possible.
3. Client will not experience infection.
4. Client will regain/maintain respiratory status WDL.
5. Client will maintain adequate hydration as evidenced by urine output > 1–2 mL/kg/hr.
6. Client will regain and maintain adequate nutrition for growth according to standardized growth chart.

7. Parents will verbalize concerns and feelings and use positive coping strategies.
8. Parents will demonstrate understanding of neonate's condition, treatment, and home care.

NOC

1. Thermoregulation: Newborn
2. Risk Control
3. Risk Control
4. Respiratory Status: Ventilation, Vital Signs
5. Fluid Status
6. Nutritional Status
7. Anxiety
8. Knowledge: Illness Care, Treatment, Health Promotion

IMPLEMENTATION

1. Thermoregulation
   a. Place neonate in infant warmer
   b. Monitor continuous skin temperature
   c. Avoid drafts in deliver room and nursery
   d. Assess skin for mottling
   e. Assess continuous respiratory status
2. Risk for presence of additional congenital anomalies
   a. Monitor prenatal diagnostics
   b. Provide hemodynamic monitoring as required
   c. Maintain hemodynamic status according to presenting condition
   d. Provide care for infants with additional anomalies according to presenting condition
   e. Keep parents informed of infant's condition
   f. Encourage parental visitation
   g. Provide support for parents, especially in the event of fetal or neonatal demise
3. Risk for infection
   a. Use sterile technique for care of exposed sac
   b. Cover exposed sac immediately in delivery room with sterile saline-soaked gauze
   c. Monitor continuous skin temperature. *NOTE:* Temperature elevation may be masked by neonate's lowered body temperature immediately after birth
   d. Minimize manipulation of exposed sac
   e. Use sterile technique for maintenance of central venous access device
   f. Use sterile technique for surgical dressing changes following surgery
   g. Monitor complete blood count
4. Breathing pattern
   a. Place on continuous cardiorespiratory monitoring
   b. Place on continuous pulse oximetry
   c. Administer oxygen, titrating to neonate's oxygen saturation as prescribed

   d. Monitor vital signs at least hourly

   e. Position to maximize ventilatory efforts

   f. Monitor temperature, peripheral pulses, capillary refill, and skin color

   g. Monitor for increased respiratory rate, nasal flaring, and sternal retractions

   h. Support ventilatory efforts with mechanical ventilation as prescribed

5. Fluid balance

   a. Assess oral mucous membranes

   b. Monitor strict intake and output

   c. Weigh diapers for accurate urine output

   d. Weigh daily

   e. Assess fontanels

   f. Monitor serum electrolyte levels

   g. Maintain central venous access, monitoring at least hourly

   h. Administer intravenous fluids as prescribed

   i. Maintain NG tube for gastric decompression

   j. Replace gastric output with intravenous boluses as prescribed

   k. Offer pacifier (holding pacifier in neonate's mouth for sucking, as normal movement of tongue pushes pacifier out of mouth)

6. Nutrition

   a. Monitor daily weight

   b. Monitor for return of bowel sounds

   c. Monitor strict intake and output

   d. Maintain intravenous access, monitoring at least hourly

   e. Monitor and maintain parenteral nutrition therapy

   f. Offer oral or NG fluids slowly after return of bowel function

   g. Offer nipple feeding and then whatever prescribed amount of feeding is not consumed orally, administer enteral feeding

7. Parental anxiety

   a. Assess parents for manifestations of anxiety

   b. Encourage parents to verbalize feelings and concerns

   c. Listen actively

   d. Assist parents in identifying positive coping strategies and support systems

   e. Collaborate with members of health care team to provide answers to parental questions

   f. Assist with parent-infant bonding

   g. Encourage parents to visit infant in NICU

   h. Explain all equipment and procedures

   i. Provide for parental spiritual needs

8. Parent teaching

   a. Assess parents' current level of knowledge

   b. Provide verbal and written information regarding:

      1) Wound care

      2) Infant feedings

      3) Infant care

      4) Infant's developmental needs

       5) Importance of holding, cuddling, and bonding with neonate

       6) Infection precautions

       7) Medication administration if needed

       8) Manifestations of complications (bowel obstruction, infection, or feeding intolerance)

       9) Contact information for reporting manifestations to health care provider

       10) Contact information for nutrition support if applicable

       11) Importance of follow-up care

       12) Referral information and contact numbers as needed

   c. Provide adequate time for teaching, demonstrations, and return demonstrations

   d. Document teaching and parental response

NIC

1. Temperature Regulation, Newborn Care
2. Surveillance: Safety
3. Infection Control, Infection Precautions
4. Ventilation Assistance, Respiratory Monitoring, Vital Signs Monitoring
5. Fluid Management, Fluid Monitoring
6. Nutrition Management, Nutrition Monitoring
7. Anxiety Reduction, Coping Enhancement
8. Teaching: Illness Care, Treatment, Health Promotion

EVALUATION

1. Client maintains thermoregulation as evidenced by body temperature WDL.
2. Client is stabilized, and other congenital anomalies are identified and treated effectively if possible.
3. Client does not experience infection.
4. Client regains/maintains respiratory status WDL.
5. Client maintains adequate hydration as evidenced by urine output > 1–2 mL/kg/hr.
6. Client regains and maintains adequate nutrition for growth according to standardized growth chart.
7. Parents verbalize concerns and feelings and use positive coping strategies.
8. Parents demonstrate understanding of neonate's condition, treatment, and home care.

References

Khan, A. N., & Thomas, N. (2005). *Omphalocele.* Retrieved March 1, 2007, from http://www.emedicine.com/radio/topic483.htm

Lucile Packard Children's Hospital at Stanford. (2007). *High-risk newborn: Omphalocele.* Retrieved July 9, 2007, from http://www.lpch.org/diseasehealthinfo/healthlibrary/hrnewborn/omphaloc.html

MedlinePlus. (2006a). *Gastroschisis.* Retrieved March 1, 2007, from http://www.nlm.nih.gov/medlineplus/ency/article/000992.htm

MedlinePlus. (2006b). *Omphalocele.* Retrieved March 1, 2007, from http://www.nlm.nih.gov/medlineplus/ency/article/000994.htm

Potts, N. L., & Mandleco, B. L. (2007). *Pediatric nursing: Caring for children and their families* (2nd ed.). Clifton Park, NY: Delmar Cengage Learning.

79

Osteogenesis Imperfecta (OI)

Definition

Osteogenesis imperfecta (OI) is a genetic connective tissue disorder characterized by bones that fracture easily, often from little or no apparent cause (Osteogenesis Imperfecta Foundation, 2007).

Pathophysiology

OI results from a genetic defect that affects the body's production of type I collagen. Collagen is the major fibrous insoluble protein of the body's connective tissue representing approximately 30% of the body's protein. It provides a meshwork to help strengthen the bones and ligaments. In children with OI the "type I collagen fibers are composed of a left-handed helix formed by intertwining of pro-alpha 1 and pro-alpha 2 chains. Mutations in the loci encoding these chains (*COL1A1* on band 17q21 and *COL1A2* on band 7q22.1, respectively)" (Plotkin & Pattekar, 2006, p. 2). The mutations may cause the collagen to be less in amount than normal or weaker in structure than normal. This leads to disturbed periosteal bone formation, which causes the bones to be weak and fracture easily, including the cranium. For instance, an infant with OI can receive a tibial-fibula fracture just by using the lower legs to lift the buttocks off the changing table when being diapered (Potts & Mandleco, 2007). Bumps that normally would not result in any more than a reddened mark on the head can result in a skull fracture for an infant with OI.

According to the Osteogenesis Imperfecta Foundation, there are six identified types of OI, which vary in severity and presentations. Type I, the most common, is the mildest form of OI. Type II is the most severe form frequently resulting in death before or shortly after birth from respiratory dysfunction or cerebral trauma. Type III is a moderate form of OI characterized by fractures at birth and evidence of fractures in utero. Types IV and V are similar in severity, with levels from mild to severe; and Type VI is a severe form. Refer to Clinical Manifestations, adapted from the Osteogenic Imperfecta Foundation.

Complications

Fractures
Abnormal dentition
Spinal curvatures
Respiratory compromise
Death

Incidence

OI affects 1 in 20,000 live births; but the mild form may be underdiagnosed, so the number may be higher. It affects children with no gender or race discrimination (Plotkin & Pattekar, 2006). It is estimated that a minimum of 20,000 and possibly as many as 50,000 individuals are affected in the United States (Osteogenesis Imperfecta Foundation, 2007). It is estimated that 6 or 7 per 100,000 individuals worldwide are affected by OI. Types I and IV are the most common forms of OI, occurring in 4 or 5 per 100,000 people. Approximately 1 or 2 per 100,000 people are affected by types II and III (Genetics Home Reference, 2006).

Etiology

In 85–90% of children with OI, the cause is an autosomal dominant inherited mutation of type 1 collagen; however, 10–15% of cases do not have a type I collagen defect. In some cases, the cause is spontaneous mutation. In 2007, a recessive form of the disease was identified characterized by a defective CRTAP (cartilage-associated protein) gene that results in death (Osteogenesis Imperfecta Foundation, 2007). Some families are scanned for possible child abuse before OI is diagnosed.

Clinical Manifestations

Type I

- Tendency for bones to fracture easily with most fractures occurring before puberty
- Normal or near-normal stature
- Loose joints and muscle weakness
- Blue, purple, or gray tint to the sclera
- Triangular face
- Tendency toward spinal curvature
- Absent or minimal bone deformity
- Possibility of brittle teeth
- Hearing loss often beginning in early adulthood
- Normal collagen structure, but less-than-normal amount

Type II

- Likelihood of death at or shortly after birth, often due to respiratory problems
- Numerous fractures and severe bone deformity
- Small stature with underdeveloped lungs
- Improperly structured collagen

Type III

- Tendency for bones to fracture easily
- Fractures often present at birth, and x-rays may reveal healed fractures that occurred before birth
- Short stature
- Blue, purple, or gray tinted sclera
- Loose joints and poor muscle development in arms and legs
- Barrel-shaped rib cage
- Triangular face
- Spinal curvature
- Respiratory difficulties
- Severe bone deformity
- Brittle teeth
- Hearing loss
- Collagen of altered structure

Type IV

- Between type I and type III in severity
- Tendency for bones to fracture easily, occurring most often before puberty
- Shorter-than-average stature
- Normal white sclera
- Mild to moderate bone deformity
- Tendency toward spinal curvature

      Barrel-shaped rib cage

      Triangular face

      Possibility of brittle teeth

      Possibility of hearing loss

      Improperly formed collagen

Type V

      Clinically similar to type IV

      Dense band seen on X-rays adjacent to growth plate of long bones

      Unusually large calluses, called hypertrophic calluses, at sites of fractures
        or surgical procedures

      Calcification of membrane between radius and ulna leading to
        restriction of forearm rotation

      White sclera

      Normal teeth

      Meshlike appearance of bone when viewed under a microscope

Type VI

      Moderately to severely affected

      Normal white sclera

      Slightly elevated alkaline phosphatase

      "Fish-scale" appearance of bone when viewed under a microscope

(Adapted from Osteogenesis Imperfecta Foundation, 2007)

Diagnostic Tests

      Collagen synthesis analysis

      Prenatal DNA mutation analysis

      Prenatal ultrasonography (at 14–18 weeks)

      Bone density analysis

      Type I collagen study

      Radiography

      Bone biopsy

Medical Management

The goals of treatment for the child with OI are preventing or controlling the symptoms, maximizing independent mobility, and developing optimal bone mass and muscle strength. This involves care of fractures, extensive surgical and dental procedures, and physical therapy. Refer to Chapter 46: Fractures, Casts, and Traction.

The use of wheelchairs, braces, and other mobility aids is common, particularly among children with more severe types of OI, although these aids may be required in less severe types. A surgical procedure called "rodding" often is considered a useful treatment for OI. This treatment involves inserting metal rods through the length of the long bones to strengthen them and prevent and/or correct deformities. Exercise is encouraged, especially swimming and water therapy. For those who are able, walking is excellent exercise. Nutrition is an important part of the treatment for OI. Maintaining a healthy weight by eating a nutritious diet and exercising under the guidance of the health care provider and physical therapist are beneficial practices. Vitamin supplements such as calcium, magnesium, and vitamins can strengthen bone material. Although a cure for OI is not available at this time, gene targeting is being tested as a potential treatment or cure for OI (Osteogenesis Imperfecta Foundation, 2007).

Nursing Management

Refer to Chapter 46: Fractures, Casts, and Traction.

ASSESSMENT

1. Obtain client history and family history
2. Perform pediatric assessment
3. Assess for manifestations of OI

NURSING DIAGNOSES (INCLUDING BUT NOT LIMITED TO)

1. Risk for injury, fractures R/T fragility of bones
2. Risk for impaired gas exchange R/T structural changes in the thorax
3. Delayed growth and development R/T severity and chronicity of disease
4. Acute pain R/T fractures
5. Ineffective coping (parental) R/T severity and chronicity of child's disease
6. Deficient knowledge R/T child's condition, treatment, safety precautions, and home care

PLANNING/GOALS

1. Client will experience a reduction in fracture episodes, and fractures will be detected and treated in a timely manner.
2. Client will experience breathing pattern within defined limits (WDL).
3. Client will reach his/her highest level of growth and development within the constraints of the disease.
4. Client will demonstrate effective pain management as determined by client.
5. Parents will verbalize feelings and concerns and use positive coping strategies.
6. Parents will demonstrate understanding of child's condition, treatment, safety precautions, and home care.

NOC

1. Risk Control
2. Risk Control
3. Growth and Development: Child
4. Pain Level
5. Coping
6. Teaching: Illness Care, Treatment, Health Promotion

IMPLEMENTATION

1. Risk for fractures
   a. Discuss safety measures with parents to prevent injury
   b. Monitor diagnostic studies
   c. Coordinate referrals to physical therapy, dietary services, and social services
   d. Reinforce exercise instructions from physical therapy
   e. Reinforce dietary modifications
2. Gas exchange
   a. Monitor respiratory status
   b. Encourage positioning to enhance respiratory effort
   c. Collaborate with health care provider for kyphosis and scoliosis screening

3. Growth and development
   a. Assess child's current level of growth and development
   b. Assist with developmentally appropriate activities within safety constraints to prevent fractures
   c. Encourage parents to participate in child's care during hospitalization

4. Pain
   a. Assess pain hourly
   b. Use age-appropriate pain assessment tool
   c. Position for comfort
   d. Assess cast borders for skin irritation
   e. Assess skin around pins (if external fixator is present)
   f. Administer analgesics and anti-inflammatory agents proactively as prescribed
   g. Administer pain medications at equal intervals during first 24 hours after fracture/surgery
   h. Encourage parents and child (if age-appropriate) to be proactive with pain management
   i. Collaborate with health care provider for patient-controlled analgesia if pain control is not adequate

5. Ineffective coping
   a. Encourage parents to verbalize feelings and concerns
   b. Listen actively
   c. Assist parents in identifying positive coping strategies and support systems
   d. Provide information about community resources in collaboration with social services
   e. Provide information about the Osteogenesis Imperfecta Foundation

6. Parent teaching
   a. Assess current level of understanding
   b. Provide verbal and written information regarding:
      1) Safety precautions to use at home to prevent injury
      2) Fracture care
      3) Cast care
      4) Dietary modifications
      5) Medications if prescribed
      6) Physical therapy exercises
      7) Manifestations of fractures
      8) Contact information to report fractures to health care provider or to report immediately to emergency department of local acute care facility
      9) Importance of follow-up with health care provider, physical therapy, and social services
      10) Contact information for local and national support groups
   c. Provide adequate time for teaching
   d. Document teaching and parental response

NIC

1. Risk Identification, Surveillance: Safety
2. Risk Identification, Respiratory Monitoring

3. Developmental Enhancement: Child
4. Analgesia Administration
5. Coping Enhancement
6. Teaching: Illness Care, Treatment, Health Education

EVALUATION

1. Client experiences a reduction in fracture episodes, and fractures are detected and treated in a timely manner.
2. Client experiences breathing pattern WDL.
3. Client reaches his/her highest level of growth and development within the constraints of the disease.
4. Client demonstrates effective pain management as determined by client.
5. Parents verbalize feelings and concerns and use positive coping strategies.
6. Parents demonstrate understanding of child's condition, treatment, safety precautions, and home care.

References

Genetics Home Reference. (2006). *Osteogenesis imperfecta.* Retrieved July 9, 2007, from http://ghr.nlm.nih.gov/condition=osteogenesisimperfecta

Osteogenesis Imperfecta Foundation. (2007). *Fast facts on osteogenesis imperfecta.* Retrieved April 9, 2007 from http://www.oif.org/site/PageServer?pagename=FastFacts

Plotkin, H., & Pattekar, M. A. (2006). *Osteogenesis imperfecta.* Retrieved April 9, 2007, from http://www.emedicine.com/PED/topic1674.htm

Potts, N. L., & Mandleco, B. L. (2007). *Pediatric nursing: Caring for children and their families* (2nd ed.). Clifton Park, NY: Delmar Cengage Learning.

80

OSTEOGENIC SARCOMA (OS)

Definition

Osteogenic sarcoma (OS), or osteosarcoma, is a tumor of the bone usually occurring in the end of the long bones or growth metaphysis (Potts & Mandleco, 2007).

Pathophysiology

OS arises from the primitive bone-forming cells, similar to osteoblasts (cells that make up the bone matrix). The neoplastic growth of the bone-producing cells invades the medullary canal of the bone with nonfunctional cells, crowding out normal functioning cells, and rapidly spreads to the surrounding soft tissue. This causes pain over the tumor site and may or may not manifest as a mass. Movement or weight bearing on the limb usually increases the pain, and trauma or injury to the limb serves as a catalyst for treatment and subsequent diagnosis of OS. The most common site of the tumor is the distal femur, proximal humerus, or proximal tibia; and about 10–20% of all children have metastases when they present for diagnosis of OS. The most common sites for metastases are the lungs. Other sites include the kidneys, the adrenal glands, the lining of the lungs, other bones, and the myocardium. Manifestations may be present for as long as six months before the tumor is diagnosed (Children's Healthcare of Atlanta, 2007). Long-term survival is about 70% without metastasis; however, less than 30% of children with localized resectable primary tumors that are treated with surgery alone survive free of relapse (National Cancer Institute, 2007).

Complications

Pain
Impaired mobility
Metastasis
Surgery
Death

Incidence

OS is the most common bone cancer in children, accounting for 5% of all childhood tumors. More than 50% of tumors arise from the bones around the knee (National Cancer Institute, 2007). There are approximately 400 new cases of OS in the United States annually with the average age at diagnosis being 15, possibly because of the rapid growth rate at this age. This cancer is more prevalent in males than in females during adolescence. Prior to adolescence, the percentage of affected males and females is equal (Lucile Packard Children's Hospital at Stanford, 2007).

Etiology

As with all cancer, there is no known cause for OS. Research has shown some families with a higher incidence. In addition, children with a history of retinoblastoma (cancer of the retina of the eye) have an increased risk of OS. Genetics may play a significant role in the development of OS. Children and adults with other hereditary abnormalities, including exostoses (bony growths), osteogenesis imperfecta, polyostotic fibrous dysplasia, and Paget's disease, have an increased risk of developing OS. Finally, OS has been linked to exposure to ionizing irradiation associated with radiation therapy for other types of cancer including Hodgkin's and non-Hodgkin's lymphomas (Lucile Packard Children's Hospital at Stanford, 2007).

Clinical Manifestations

Bone pain (sharp or dull) at site of tumor
Edema and/or redness at site of tumor
Increased pain with activity or lifting
Limping
Decreased movement of affected limb

Diagnostic Tests

Radiography
Bone scan
Magnetic resonance imaging
Ultrasonography
Complete blood count
Serum chemistry
Tumor biopsy

Medical Management

The goals of treatment are to remove the tumor and prevent metastasis. The standard of care is surgical resection of the tumor. This usually involves limb salvage, bone/skin grafts, and bone reconstruction; however, in rare cases, amputation is required. Limb salvage procedure is the surgical resection of the tumor while "sparing" the rest of the limb and is preferred over amputation. The resected area of bone is replaced by cadaver bone and grafted into place (Potts & Mandleco, 2007). Multidrug chemotherapy including agents such as doxorubicin, cisplatin, carboplatin, cyclophosphamide, ifosfamide, methotrexate, and dactinomycin is used in conjunction with surgery (Broyles, Reiss, & Evans, 2007). Also, radiation therapy is used to destroy any microscopic disease that could lead to metastasis. In addition, if amputation is necessary, rehabilitation including physical and occupational therapy and psychosocial adapting as well as prosthesis fitting and training is needed.

Nursing Management

Refer to Chapter 22: Chemotherapy, Chapter 87: Radiation Therapy, and Chapter 100: Surgical Client.

ASSESSMENT

1. Obtain client history
2. Perform pediatric assessment
3. Assess for manifestations of OS
4. Assess for psychosocial impact of diagnosis on parents/child

NURSING DIAGNOSES (INCLUDING BUT NOT LIMITED TO)

1. Acute pain R/T tumor growth, surgical resection of tumor, chemotherapy, and radiation therapy
2. Fear and anxiety R/T diagnosis and potential loss of limb
3. Disturbed body image R/T loss or impairment of limb
4. Impaired physical mobility R/T pain and loss or impairment of limb
5. Deficient knowledge R/T condition, treatment, rehabilitation, and home care

Planning/Goals

1. Client will demonstrate effective pain management at a level of 2–3/10 as determined by client.
2. Parents/child will verbalize feelings of fear and anxiety and use positive coping strategies.
3. Client will return to appropriate growth and development activities and use positive coping strategies.
4. Client will regain mobility to acceptable level for client.
5. Parents/child will demonstrate understanding of condition, treatment, rehabilitation, and home care.

NOC

1. Pain Level
2. Fear, Anxiety
3. Child Development: Adolescence
4. Mobility
5. Knowledge: Illness Care, Treatment, Rehabilitation, Health Promotion

Implementation

1. Pain
   a. Assess pain level hourly during hospitalization, using age-appropriate pain assessment tool
   b. Administer analgesics proactively
   c. Collaborate with health care provider to increase the dose or change the medication if pain is not managed. *NOTE:* Postoperatively, patient-controlled analgesia (PCA) should be prescribed. If not prescribed, collaboration with the prescribing health care provider should be initiated by the nurse.
   d. Involve child in age-appropriate activities
   e. Encourage adolescent friends to visit in hospital
   f. Position for comfort
   g. Monitor vital signs
2. Fear and anxiety
   a. Assess for verbal and nonverbal cues indicating fear and anxiety
   b. Encourage verbalization of feelings and concerns
   c. Listen actively
   d. Collaborate with recreation therapist or child-life specialist
   e. Introduce to another adolescent with similar diagnosis for peer interaction
   f. Involve in age-appropriate activities
   g. Provide preoperative teaching
   h. Reinforce or explain health care provider's instructions
   i. Assist client/parents with identifying positive coping strategies
3. Body image
   a. Assess for verbal and nonverbal cues indicating body image disturbance
   b. Encourage verbalization of feelings and concerns
   c. Listen actively
   d. Collaborate with recreation therapist or child-life specialist

   e. Introduce to another adolescent with similar diagnosis for peer interaction

   f. Involve in age-appropriate activities

   g. Assist client/parents with identifying positive coping strategies

4. Physical mobility

   a. Assess physical limitations

   b. Collaborate with physical therapist for continuity

   c. Encourage involvement in self-care activities

   d. Encourage early ambulation with crutches, reinforcing crutch-walking techniques from physical therapy

   e. Prepare for extensive exercise and the need to be compliant with rehabilitation

   f. Coordinate with professional in charge of prosthetics if amputation was required and assess for correct fit when client uses prosthetic

   g. Encourage prescribed physical activity

5. Parent/child teaching

   a. Assess parents'/child's current level of understanding

   b. Provide verbal and written information and demonstration regarding:

      1) Postoperative care

      2) Chemotherapy

      3) Radiation therapy

      4) Medication administration

      5) Physical therapy exercises

      6) Assessment of stump skin before and after using prosthesis if applicable

      7) Community services available

      8) Contact numbers for referrals and health care provider

      9) Importance of follow-up care with physical therapist and health care provider

   c. Provide adequate time for teaching, demonstrations (as needed), and return demonstrations

   d. Document teaching and parents'/child's response

NIC

1. Pain Management
2. Coping Enhancement
3. Developmental Enhancement, Adolescent
4. Exercise Therapy: Ambulation
5. Teaching: Illness Care, Treatment, Rehabilitation, Health Education

EVALUATION

1. Client demonstrates effective pain management at a level of 2–3/10 as determined by client.
2. Parents/child verbalize feelings of fear and anxiety and use positive coping strategies.
3. Client returns to appropriate growth and development activities and uses positive coping strategies.
4. Client regains mobility to acceptable level for client.
5. Parents/child demonstrate understanding of condition, treatment, rehabilitation, and home care.

References

Broyles, B. E., Reiss, B. S., & Evans, M. E. (2007). *Pharmacological aspects of nursing care* (7th ed.). Clifton Park, NY: Delmar Cengage Learning.

Children's Healthcare of Atlanta. (2007). *Osteogenic sarcoma.* Retrieved April 10, 2007, from http://www.choa.org/default.aspx?id=419

Lucile Packard Children's Hospital at Stanford. (2007). *Oncology: Osteogenic sarcoma.* Retrieved April 10, 2007, from http://www.lpch.org/DiseaseHealthInfo/HealthLibrary/oncology/ostsar.html

National Cancer Institute. (2007). *Osteosarcoma/malignant fibrous histiocytoma of bone treatment (PDQ).* Retrieved July 9, 2007, from http://www.cancer.gov/cancertopics/pdq/treatment/osteosarcoma/healthprofessional

Potts, N. L., & Mandleco, B. L. (2007). *Pediatric nursing: Caring for children and their families* (2nd ed.). Clifton Park, NY: Delmar Cengage Learning.

81

OTITIS MEDIA (OM)

Definition

Otitis media (OM) is an infection or blockage of the structures in the middle ear (Broyles, 2005). Refer to Figure 81-1.

Pathophysiology

OM usually is a complication of an upper respiratory infection in children. Most often upper respiratory infections originate with viral invasion; then as the self-limiting virus follows its course, the immune system is stressed sufficiently to allow normal bacterial flora in the respiratory tract to multiply and become pathogenic. Most often OM is related to dysfunctional eustachian tube drainage; and because of the continuous nature of the mucous membranes, the middle ear and the air cells of the mastoid become involved in the infection process. In children, the eustachian tube is short and provides easy access to the structures in the middle ear. Mucosal edema that accompanies upper respiratory infections causes a "vacuum," or negative pressure, in the middle ear and leads to increased fluid pressure. This causes pain as the fluid presses against middle ear structures. As fluid accumulates, it becomes an excellent medium for bacterial growth. If OM is left untreated, the eardrum can perforate or rupture as a result of the pressure and the toxins emitted by the bacteria (Broyles, 2005). Ear pain is the most common manifestation of OM, although 90% of infants and toddlers with OM have associated rhinitis symptoms (National Guidelines Clearinghouse, 2007). Infants and nonverbal children pull down on the pinna of the ear, which in small children, results in opening the ear canal and temporarily relieving pressure and pain.

There are two types of OM in children: acute otitis media (AOM) and OM with effusion. AOM, the most common form of middle ear infection, is caused by the presence of excessive fluids in the ear. Its symptoms are pain, possibly a light fever, as

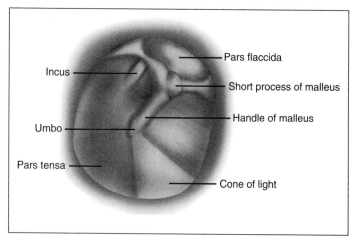

Figure 81-1: Middle Ear Structures.

well as the change of the color of the eardrum (usually becomes red). OM with effusion results when fluids in the middle ear persist for more than six weeks.

Complications

Pain
Perforation or rupture of the tympanic membrane
OM with effusion
Conductive hearing loss

Incidence

Almost every child experiences some form of ear infection before 6 years of age. Before they are 3 years old, more than 75% of children have experienced some form of OM. It is estimated that 30 million cases of OM are reported in the United States annually, accounting for 20–40% of pediatric office visits for children under the age of 5 (Potts & Mandleco, 2007).

Etiology

As previously noted, OM usually follows an upper respiratory infection caused by *Streptococcus pneumoniae, Haemophilus influenzae*, and *Moraxella catarrhalis* (Potts & Mandleco, 2007). The infection moves up the very narrow and quickly obstructed eustachian tubes of young children. Other factors that increase a child's risk of developing OM include first- or secondhand cigarette smoke, allergies that manifest in the respiratory system, tonsillitis, water entering the ear when a child is bathing or swimming, placement of an infant in a community child care facility, and placement of an infant supine in bed with a bottle. Cigarette smoking dries the cilia in the ear that are necessary to keep fluids moving out of the ear; placing a baby in a crib with a bottle allows food overflow to the eustachian tube, leading to infection. Community child care facilities expose infants and small children to close encounters with multiple children.

Clinical Manifestations

Ear pain (indicated in preverbal children by fussiness and tendency to
    pull down on the pinna of the ear)
Drainage from the ear
Red (rather than the normal pearly gray color) tympanic membrane
Conductive hearing loss
Fever
Chills
Irritability
Nausea and vomiting
Difficulties with balance
"Popping" sound in the ear

Diagnostic Tests

Otoscopic examination
Inspection of ear structures
Cultures of ear drainage
Sinus radiography
Computed tomography (CT)
Magnetic resonance imaging (MRI)

Medical Management

The goals of treatment are to eliminate the infection and prevent hearing loss. The first-line antibiotic for the treatment of AOM is amoxicillin. The second-line agent is amoxicillin/potassium clavulanate (Augmentin) (Broyles, Reiss, & Evans, 2007). After 2–3 days of antimicrobial therapy, the pain usually is relieved completely; and after a week, the purulent drainage changes to serous drainage and then is referred to as OM with effusion. Antimicrobials are prescribed for 10 days although the effusion may take weeks or months to resolve. Pain and fever management usually is achieved with the use of acetaminophen or ibuprofen.

If complications occur, surgical intervention may be indicated. A myringotomy is an incision into the tympanic membrane to release ear pressure and may include the placement of myringotomy tubes for continuous drainage of fluid in the middle ear. A tympanoplasty is performed to repair a perforated or ruptured tympanic membrane (eardrum).

Nursing Management

ASSESSMENT

1. Obtain client history including recent history of upper respiratory infection
2. Assess for presence of clinical manifestations of OM
3. Assess pain level
4. Assess vital signs, height, and weight

NURSING DIAGNOSES (INCLUDING BUT NOT LIMITED TO)

1. Acute pain R/T middle ear inflammation and infection and pressure on the tympanic membrane
2. Ineffective protection R/T presence of infectious organisms
3. Risk for delayed growth and development R/T hearing impairment
4. Risk for deficient fluid volume R/T decreased fluid intake and fever
5. Deficient knowledge (parental) R/T child's condition, treatment, and home care

PLANNING/GOALS

1. Client will experience effective pain control (0 or 1 on a scale of 0 to 5) as evidenced by verbal and nonverbal indicators.
2. Client will become afebrile, and infection will be effectively eradicated.
3. Client will maintain hearing function.
4. Client will maintain balanced fluid volume as indicated by urinary output within defined limits (WDL), moist mucous membranes, and elastic skin turgor.
5. Parents will demonstrate understanding of child's condition, treatment, and home care.

NOC

1. Pain Level
2. Immune Status
3. Sensory Function: Hearing
4. Fluid Balance
5. Knowledge: Illness Care, Treatment, Health Promotion

IMPLEMENTATION

1. Pain
   a. Assess pain level
   b. Instruct parents to administer acetaminophen every 4 hours or pediatric ibuprofen every 6 hours or alternate the two for fever and pain management

    c. Instruct parents on proper administration of antibiotic therapy at equal intervals for at least the first 24 hours of therapy

    d. Stress the importance of completing full course of antibiotic therapy

2. Infection

    a. Assess temperature

    b. Instruct parents to administer acetaminophen every 4 hours or pediatric ibuprofen every 6 hours or alternate the two for fever and pain management

    c. Instruct parents to provide fluids every 2–3 hours, including fruit juices, Pedialyte, and Pedialyte frozen pops

    d. Instruct parents on proper administration of antibiotic therapy including administering antibiotic at equal intervals for the first 24 hours

    e. Stress with parents the importance of completing full course of antibiotic therapy

    f. Instruct concerning factors to avoid in order to prevent further episodes of OM

3. Sensory perception

    a. Assess for age-appropriate hearing acuity

    b. Encourage hearing screening if parents note that child does not babble by 7 months of age or does not respond to name

4. Fluid balance

    a. Instruct parents to provide fluids every 2–3 hours, including fruit juices, Pedialyte, and Pedialyte frozen pops

    b. Instruct parents on proper administration of antibiotic therapy including administering antibiotics at equal intervals for at least the first 24 hours of therapy

    c. Stress the importance of completing full course of antibiotic therapy

    d. Monitor temperature

    e. Monitor intake and output

    f. Instruct parents that infant should have six to ten wet diapers each 24-hour period

    g. Instruct parents concerning manifestations of dehydration

5. Parent teaching

    a. Assess parents' current level of understanding

    b. Provide verbal and written information regarding:

        1) Risk factors for developing OM, including first- and secondhand smoke, community child care facilities, horizontal positioning of infant for feeding, and infant going to bed with a bottle

        2) Breast feeding to provide immune factors that can help prevent OM

        3) Antimicrobial administration including the importance of completing the entire prescription

        4) Medication administration for fever and pain

        5) Manifestations of worsening of condition

        6) Contact numbers for reporting worsening of condition

        7) Importance of four-week follow-up with child's health care provider

    c. Provide adequate time for teaching

    d. Document teaching and parental response

1. Analgesic Administration
2. Infection Protection
3. Communication Enhancement, Infection Protection
4. Fluid Management, Fluid Monitoring
5. Teaching: Illness Care, Treatment, Health Education

EVALUATION

1. Client experiences effective pain control (0 or 1 on a scale of 0 to 5) as evidenced by verbal and nonverbal indicators.
2. Client is afebrile, and infection is effectively eradicated.
3. Client maintains hearing function.
4. Client maintains balanced fluid volume as indicated by urinary output WDL, moist mucous membranes, and elastic skin turgor.
5. Parents demonstrate understanding of child's condition, treatment, and home care.

References

Broyles, B. E. (2005). *Medical-surgical nursing clinical companion*. Durham, NC: Carolina Academic Press.

Broyles, B. E., Reiss, B. S., & Evans, M. E. (2007). *Pharmacological aspects of nursing care* (7th ed.). Clifton Park, NY: Delmar Cengage Learning.

National Guidelines Clearinghouse. (2007). *Diagnosis and treatment of otitis media in children*. Retrieved April 10, 2007, from http://www.guideline.gov/summary/summary.aspx?doc_id=5450

Potts, N. L., & Mandleco, B. L. (2007). *Pediatric nursing: Caring for children and their families* (2nd ed.). Clifton Park, NY: Delmar Cengage Learning.

PATENT DUCTUS ARTERIOSUS (PDA)

Definition

Patent ductus arteriosus (PDA) occurs when the connective structure between the aorta and the pulmonary artery does not close spontaneously within a few hours to three weeks after birth.

Pathophysiology

During fetal development, the ductus arteriosus acts as a fetal shunt that directs oxygenated maternal blood into fetal systemic circulation since the fetal lungs do not function to oxygenate fetal blood. When the fetus is born, pressure changes within the cardiopulmonary system, cause the ductus to close off as the neonate breathes on his/her own, and the lungs perform the function of oxygenating the neonate's blood. In PDA, the ductus arteriosus remains open; and depending on the size of the PDA and the condition of the lungs, the neonate may be asymptomatic or may experience moderate to severe decreases in cardiac output as a result of increased pulmonary blood flow and eventually pulmonary congestion and right-sided heart failure (Potts & Mandleco, 2007). Refer to Figure 82-1. The hemodynamics of PDA are similar to any other left to right shunt but this shunt occurs because of the increased pressure in the aorta shunting blood into the lower pressure pulmonary artery (fluid moves from an area of greater pressure to that of lesser pressure). Shunted oxygenated blood from the aorta to the pulmonary artery is then recirculated through the lungs increasing pulmonary resistance. This in turn increases the resistance against which the right ventricle must pump increasing the workload on the right ventricle.

The hemodynamics of a patent ductus arteriosus is similar to other left to right shunts. Oxygenated blood in the higher pressure aorta is shunted into the lower pressure of the pulmonary artery through the PDA causing this blood to be recirculated through the lungs. This increases the volume and thus the pressure within the lungs resulting in increased pulmonary resistance causing the right ventricle to work harder to pump blood into the lungs against this resistance. This increased workload eventually will take its toll on the effectiveness of right ventricular function.

Complications

Pulmonary congestion
Heart failure

Incidence

"The incidence of PDA in a nonpremature infant is approximately 5–10% of all CHD [congenital heart disease/defects]" (Potts & Mandleco, 2007, p. 775). The incidence in the premature infant is 5 to 8 times greater, with infants weighing less than 1000 grams having the higher risk. "Patent ductus arteriosus is the sixth most common congenital heart defect . . . [and] occurs twice as often in girls as in boys" (CongenitalHeartDefects .com, 2007, p. 1).

Etiology

"Most of the time we do not know [what causes congenital heart defects]. Although the reason defects occur is presumed to be genetic, only a few genes have been discovered

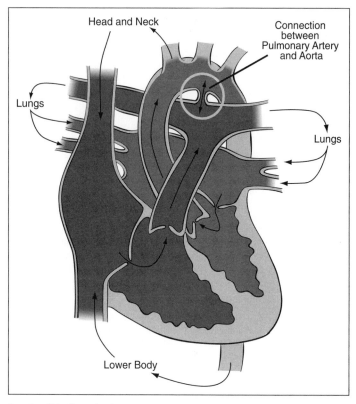

Figure 82-1: Patent Ductus Arteriosus.

that have been linked to the presence of heart defects. Rarely the ingestion of some drugs and the occurrence of some infections during pregnancy can cause defects" (American Heart Association, 2007, p. 1).

Clinical Manifestations

Most infants are asymptomatic except for the presence of a systolic
    murmur
Larger PDAs
Tachycardia
Tachypnea
Moist breath sounds
Systemic edema

Diagnostic Tests

Chest radiography
Echocardiogram
Cardiac catheterization

Medical Management

No medical/surgical treatment is required in children with asymptomatic PDA. If clinical manifestations of altered cardiac output occur, the most common treatment for closure of the PDA is the nonsurgical placement of coils, which may be all that is required to occlude a PDA. "These coils sit in the PDA and expand to the point where they block all the blood flow" (CongenitalHeartDefects.com, 2007, p. 1). If the PDA is too complex, open-heart surgical repair is required.

Refer to Medical Management in Chapter 26: Congenital Heart Disease/Open Heart Surgery.

Nursing Management

Refer to Nursing Management in Chapter 26: Congenital Heart Disease/Open Heart Surgery.

References

American Heart Association. (2007). *Patent ductus arteriosus (PDA).* Retrieved July 9, 2007, from http://www.americanheart.org/presenter.jhtml?identifier=1672

CongenitalHeartDefects.com. (2007). *Patent ductus arteriosus (PDA).* Retrieved July 9, 2007, from http://www.congenitalheartdefects.com/typesofCHD.html#PDA

Potts, N. L., & Mandleco, B. L. (2007). *Pediatric nursing: Caring for children and their families* (2nd ed.). Clifton Park, NY: Delmar Cengage Learning.

83

PNEUMONIA

Definition

"Pneumonia is an acute inflammation of the pulmonary parenchyma associated with alveolar consolidation" (Potts & Mandleco, 2007, p. 721).

Pathophysiology

Normally, the defense mechanisms for the respiratory tract protect individuals from inhaled pathogens. These mechanisms include the cough reflex, the immune system, the inflammatory response, mucociliary activity, and phagocytosis by alveolar macrophages (Potts & Mandleco, 2007). When pathogens such as bacteria, viruses, fungi, and parasites invade the lungs, they release toxins that combine with by-products of the body's defense mechanisms. These substances damage the pulmonary parenchyma and pulmonary mucous membranes, resulting in accumulation of exudates and debris. The immune system cascade triggers the leakage of plasma and the loss of surfactant, causing consolidation in the alveoli, resulting in air loss. The lungs may fill with fluid, causing pulmonary edema resulting from pathogenic invasion. This causes the lungs to become stiff and less distensible, leading to a decrease in tidal volume (Bennett, Domachowske, & Virella-Lowell, 2007). The infection can spread rapidly through vascular dissemination and invade the entire body, resulting in sepsis, septic shock, and death.

The incubation period for pneumonia varies according to the type of virus or bacteria causing the infection. For instance, the incubation period for respiratory syncytial virus (RSV) is four to six days; for influenza, 18–72 hours. With effective treatment, most types of bacterial pneumonia can be cured within 1–2 weeks. Viral pneumonia may last longer. Mycoplasmal pneumonia may take 4–6 weeks to resolve completely.

Viral pneumonia is characterized by a slow onset with the accumulation of mononuclear cells in the submucosa and perivascular space, causing partial obstruction of the airway. This leads to wheezing and crackles. As the disease progresses, the alveolar type II cells become structurally damaged and surfactant production is decreased. This leads to the development of pulmonary edema, resulting in further impaired gas exchange.

Bacterial pneumonia is characterized by a rapid onset and high fever caused by the alveoli filling with proteinaceous fluid that causes an influx of red blood cells and polymorphonuclear cells (red hepatization) followed by the deposition of fibrin and the degradation of inflammatory cells (gray hepatization). During resolution, intra-alveolar debris is ingested and removed by the alveolar macrophages. This consolidation leads to decreased air entry and dullness to percussion. Inflammation in the small airways leads to crackles. Wheezing is less common in bacterial pneumonia than it is in viral infections (Bennett et al., 2007).

Complications

  Empyema
  Pulmonary edema
  Impaired gas exchange
  Sepsis
  Death

Incidence

"Pneumonia accounts for 13% of all infectious illnesses in the first 2 years of life. In a large community-based study conducted by Denny and Clyde, the annual attack rates of pneumonia were 4 cases per 100 children in the preschool age group, 2 cases per 100 children in the 5- to 9-year age group, and 1 case per 100 children in the 9- to 15-year age group. The United Nations Children's Fund (UNICEF) estimates that 3 million children die worldwide from pneumonia each year. Although most of these fatalities occur in developing countries, pneumonia remains a significant cause of morbidity in industrialized nations" (Bennett et al., 2007, Section 2).

Etiology

Respiratory viruses are the most common causes of pneumonia in young children, peaking between the ages of 2 and 3. These viruses include adenoviruses, rhinovirus, influenza virus, RSV, and parainfluenza virus. By the time children become school age, the bacterium *Mycoplasma pneumoniae* becomes more common (The Children's Hospital, 2006). The organism *Streptococcus pneumoniae* is the most common cause of bacterial pneumonia (American Lung Association, 2006). Risk factors for developing pneumonia include chronic respiratory disease (cystic fibrosis) and immunosuppression either from disease (human immunodeficiency virus, HIV) or from medical treatment for conditions such as neoplasms and organ transplantation.

Clinical Manifestations

Tachypnea
Fever
Chills
Cough
Adventitious breath sounds
Wheezing
Grunting
Sternal or rib retractions
Nasal flaring (in infants)
Diarrhea
Vomiting
Chest pain
Abdominal pain
Fatigue
Anorexia (in older children) or poor feeding (in infants)
Circumoral cyanosis (in severe cases)

Diagnostic Tests

Chest X-ray
Gram stain and sputum culture
Complete blood count (CBC)
Pulse oximetry
Arterial blood gases
Computed tomography scan of the chest
Pleural fluid culture (pleural effusion)

Medical Management

The goals of treatment are to identify the causative microorganism, provide appropriate pharmacological therapy, and maintain adequate oxygenation to tissues until the pneumonia is resolved (Broyles, 2005). Bacterial pneumonia is treated with antibiotics prescribed based on the causative bacteria and its antibiotic sensitivity. Antimicrobials of choice include azithromycin, clarithromycin, ceftriaxone, cefotaxine, ampicillin, and cefuroxime (Broyles, Reiss, & Evans, 2007).

Antiviral agents used to treat viral pneumonia are usually reserved for moderate to severe cases. These agents include ribavirin (reconstitute 6 grams into 300 mL of sterile water to make a concentration of 20 mg/mL and administer as continuous aerosol over 12–18 hours for 24 hours for 3–7 days), oseltamivir (not indicated for infants), and zanamivir (not approved for children under the age of 7) (Broyles et al., 2007). Adjunctive supportive therapy includes oxygen administration, chest percussion, antipyretics (acetaminophen and ibuprofen), rest, and inhalation therapy (if needed). In severe cases, mechanical ventilation may be required. Refer to Chapter 90: Respiratory Distress Syndrome (RDS)/Mechanical Ventilation for discussion of mechanical ventilation.

The most effective method of preventing pneumonia is for children to be properly immunized. The pneumococcal vaccine (Pneumovax and Prevnar) prevents *S. pneumoniae*.

The flu vaccine prevents pneumonia and other infections caused by influenza viruses. The Hib vaccine prevents pneumonia in children from *Haemophilus influenzae* type b (Centers for Disease Control and Prevention, 2005).

Nursing Management

Refer to Chapter 90: Respiratory Distress Syndrome (RDS)/Mechanical Ventilation for nursing management of child receiving mechanical ventilation.

ASSESSMENT

1. Obtain client history with focus on presence of risk factors, clinical manifestations, and allergies
2. Assess oxygen saturation via pulse oximetry
3. Perform focused respiratory assessment
4. Assess vital signs
5. Obtain baseline height and weight

NURSING DIAGNOSES (INCLUDING BUT NOT LIMITED TO)

1. Impaired gas exchange R/T ineffective breathing pattern and airway clearance secondary to pneumonia and pain
2. Deficient fluid volume R/T profuse perspiration and insensible fluid loss
3. Imbalanced nutrition: less than body requirements R/T increased metabolism, anorexia, nausea, and vomiting
4. Ineffective protection R/T risk factors and presence of pneumonia
5. Activity intolerance R/T impaired gas exchange, interrupted sleep cycle, and weakness
6. Deficient knowledge R/T condition, treatment, and home care

PLANNING/GOALS

1. Client will regain and maintain adequate gas exchange as evidenced by oxygen saturation > 94%, arterial blood gases within defined limits (WDL), and improved activity tolerance and fluid and nutritional intake.
2. Client will regain and maintain fluid balance as evidenced by intake and output, serum electrolyte levels, and urine specific gravity WDL.

3. Client will regain and maintain balanced nutrition as evidenced by weight appropriate for height, consuming 80–100% of diet.
4. Client will regain and maintain vital signs WDL within 48–72 hours following initiation of treatment.
5. Client will gradually resume age-appropriate activity level and maintain at least 8 hours of undisturbed sleep each night.
6. Parents and child (if age-appropriate) will demonstrate understanding of condition, treatment, and home care.

NOC

1. Respiratory Status: Gas Exchange
2. Fluid Balance
3. Nutritional Status
4. Immune Status
5. Activity Tolerance
6. Knowledge: Illness Care, Medications, Treatment, Health Promotion

IMPLEMENTATION

1. Gas exchange
   a. Conduct respiratory assessment every 2 hours and as indicated by client condition
   b. Place on continuous cardiorespiratory monitoring
   c. Monitor continuous pulse oximetry
   d. Encourage turning, coughing, and deep breathing if age-appropriate
   e. Administer oxygen as prescribed and indicated by oxygen saturation levels and child's response
   f. Initiate and maintain patency of intravenous access, monitoring at least hourly
   g. Administer antimicrobial agents as prescribed
   h. Administer intravenous fluids as prescribed
   i. Position with head of bed elevated to facilitate breathing
   j. Provide for uninterrupted periods of rest as indicated by child's condition
   k. Encourage use of incentive spirometry as condition allows and if age-appropriate
   l. Increase oral fluid intake
   m. Perform endotracheal suctioning as prescribed and as indicated by child's condition
   n. Encourage age-appropriate activity as child's condition allows
2. Fluid volume
   a. Assess for tachypnea and diaphoresis
   b. Initiate and maintain patency of intravenous access, monitoring at least hourly
   c. Administer intravenous fluids as prescribed
   d. Monitor strict intake and output
   e. Monitor serum electrolyte levels, collaborating with health care provider when readings are abnormal
   f. Monitor urine specific gravity and notify health care provider of abnormal readings

    g. Weigh daily

    h. Encourage oral fluids when risk of aspiration is minimal

3. Nutrition

    a. Weigh daily

    b. Monitor intake and output

    c. Administer enteral feedings as prescribed if unable to take in oral nutrition

    d. Assess for gag reflex and ability to swallow when taking oral nutrition

    e. Assess child's food preferences and collaborate with dietician to provide adequate intake

    f. Assess bowel sounds every shift

    g. Encourage age-appropriate activities when condition allows

    h. Maintain adequate fluid intake orally if possible

4. Ineffective protection

    a. Instruct parents concerning recommended immunizations to prevent pneumonia

    b. Monitor vital signs every 4 hours and as needed

    c. Maintain intravenous access, monitoring at least hourly

    d. Administer antimicrobial agents as prescribed

    e. Administer antipyretics as prescribed

    f. Instruct about the importance of hand washing and demonstrate appropriate technique

5. Activity intolerance

    a. Assess for dyspnea during activity

    b. Assist as needed to complete age-appropriate activities

    c. Encourage parents to participate in care

    d. Assist with oral feedings as needed to conserve energy

    e. Maintain calm environment

    f. Provide for uninterrupted periods of rest and sleep

    g. Administer oxygen as prescribed, monitoring with pulse oximetry

6. Parent and child (if age-appropriate) teaching

    a. Assess parents' current level of understanding

    b. Provide verbal and written information regarding:

        1) Risk factors for developing pneumonia: hospitalization, immunocompromised state, and presence of chronic disease

        2) Importance of receiving pneumococcal vaccine, receiving annual influenza vaccine, and maintaining current Hib immunizations

        3) Technique for monitoring child's oral or axillary temperature

        4) Medication administration including importance of completing prescribed medication regime

        5) Manifestations of adverse effects of medications (primarily hypersensitivity reactions)

        6) Importance of adequate oral fluid intake (should not force child to eat, but should encourage child to drink fluids)

        7) Importance of avoiding cough suppressants unless under advice of health care provider

        8) Manifestations of worsening condition

        9) Contact phone numbers for reporting signs and symptoms

    10) Importance of regular hand washing and appropriate technique

    11) Importance of follow-up with health care provider

  c. Provide adequate time for teaching

  d. Document teaching and parental response

NIC

1. Oxygen Therapy, Ventilation Assistance, Respiratory Monitoring
2. Fluid Management, Fluid Monitoring
3. Nutrition Management
4. Immunization Behavior, Vital Signs Monitoring
5. Activity Therapy, Energy Management
6. Teaching: Illness Care, Medications, Treatment, Health Education

EVALUATION

1. Client regains and maintains adequate gas exchange as evidenced by oxygen saturation > 94%, arterial blood gases WDL, and improved activity tolerance and fluid and nutritional intake.

2. Client regains and maintains fluid balance as evidenced by intake and output, serum electrolyte levels, and urine specific gravity WDL.

3. Client regains and maintains balanced nutrition as evidenced by weight appropriate for height, consuming 80–100% of diet.

4. Client regains and maintains vital signs WDL within 48–72 hours following initiation of treatment.

5. Client gradually resumes age-appropriate activity level and maintains at least 8 hours of undisturbed sleep each night.

6. Parents and child (if age-appropriate) demonstrate understanding of condition, treatment, and home care.

References

American Lung Association. (2006). *Pneumonia.* Retrieved April 11, 2007, from http://www.lungusa .org/site/apps/nl/content3.asp?c=dvLUK9O0E&b=2060321&content_id={71CC3CFD-4B3E-49C8-AA88-D76EAE1FB9F5}&notoc=1

Bennett, N. J., Domachowske, J., & Verilla-Lowell, I. (2007). *Pneumonia.* Retrieved March 10, 2008, from http://www.emedicine.com/PED/topic1833.htm

Broyles, B. E. (2005). *Medical-surgical nursing clinical companion.* Durham, NC: Carolina Academic Press.

Broyles, B. E., Reiss, B. S., & Evans, M. E. (2007). *Pharmacological aspects of nursing care* (7th ed.). Clifton Park, NY: Delmar Cengage Learning.

Centers for Disease Control and Prevention. (2005). Haemophilus influenzae *serotype b (Hib) disease.* March 10, 2008, from http://www.cdc.gov/ncidod/dbmd/diseaseinfo/haeminfluserob_t.htm

Potts, N. L., & Mandleco, B. L. (2007). *Pediatric nursing: Caring for children and their families* (2nd ed.). Clifton Park, NY: Delmar Cengage Learning.

The Children's Hospital. (2006). *Pneumonia.* Retrieved April 11, 2007, from http://www .thechildrenshospital.org/wellness/info/teens/22204.aspx

84

POISONING

Definition

Poisoning is the ingestion, inhalation, or any other form of contact with a "substance that harms the body and interferes with the body's normal functioning" (Potts & Mandleco, 2007, p. 693). "Any substance can be poisonous if enough is taken" (Centers for Disease Control and Prevention, 2007, p. 1).

Pathophysiology

The exact pathophysiology of poisoning varies depending on the substance involved in the child's exposure. Neurologic, pulmonary, cardiac, hepatic, renal, and other organ/system dysfunction can result from exposure to poisons.

Complications

Organ failure
Death

Incidence

According to the latest statistics (2005) from the American Association of Poison Control Centers (AAPCC), of the 2,424,180 reports of human exposure to toxic substances made to the AAPCC in 2005, 38.1% of cases involved children under age 3 and 50.9% concerned children younger than 6 years of age. The AAPCC notes that because not all exposures are reported, these figures reflect a lower incidence than what actually occurs. Of the exposure figures, 822,536 involved males under the age of 20 and 734,531 were females in the same age bracket. The highest incidence occurred in children between the ages of 1 and 3. Poisonings accounted for 24 deaths in children in 2005 (American Association of Poison Control Centers, 2006). Poisoning is the leading cause of injury and the fourth leading cause of death in children between the ages of 1 year and 5 years. The most common medication ingested is acetaminophen. "The lowest mortality rates [for unintentional poisonings] are among children less than 15 years old" (Centers for Disease Control and Prevention, 2007, p.1).

Etiology

The primary cause of poisonings is insufficient adult supervision and reflects the normal characteristics of the age groups involved. Toddlers and preschoolers are curious, which is believed to be the primary reason for exposures in these age groups. Common agents ingested by children under 6 years of age include cosmetics, cologne, perfume, aftershave, cleaning products, plants (azalea, buttercup, English ivy, holly, mistletoe, and philodendron), foreign bodies, toys, gasoline, kerosene, lighter fluid, turpentine, and paint thinner. Adolescents' involvement may be the result of experimentation with substances with the intent of experiencing hallucinogenic effects (Potts & Mandleco, 2007).

Clinical Manifestations

Refer to Table 84-1.

Table 84-1 | Poison Agents and Clinical Manifestations of Exposure

Substance	Clinical manifestations
Acetaminophen (Tylenol)	Nausea, vomiting, malaise, right upper quadrant abdominal pain, jaundice, confusion, somnolence; coma may develop later
Salicylates	Nausea, vomiting, hyperpnea, tinnitus, fever, disorientation, lethargy, coma, seizures, diaphoresis, abdominal pain
Cyclic antidepressants	Central nervous system (CNS) excitability, confusion, blurred vision, dry mouth, fever, mydriasis, seizures, coma, arrhythmias, hypotension, tachycardia, respiratory depression; physical condition can change rapidly
Benzodiazepines	Drowsiness, lethargy, dysarthria, ataxia, hypotension, hypothermia, coma, respiratory depression with severe overdose
Cocaine	Anxiety, euphoria, nausea, headache, chest pain, fever, hypertension, tachypnea, tachycardia, vomiting, agitation, mydriasis, diaphoresis, twitching, confusion, hallucinations, abdominal cramps, seizures, hypotension, dysrhythmias, cardiopulmonary arrest
Narcotics	Drowsiness, nausea, vomiting, miosis, respiratory depression, cyanosis, coma, seizures, bradypnea, noncardiac pulmonary edema
Hydrocarbons	Coughing, gagging, and choking; altered level of consciousness; tachypnea, grunting, retractions, and cyanosis because of pulmonary aspiration; nausea and vomiting
Corrosives (toilet, drain, and oven cleaners, mildew remover, ammonia)	Severe chemical burns and burning in mouth, throat, and stomach; edema of lips, pharynx, and tongue; violent vomiting; difficulty swallowing; white, swollen mucous membranes

Adapted from Potts and Mandleco (2007). Pediatric nursing: Caring for children and their families, 2nd edition. Clifton Park, NY: Delmar Cengage Learning.

Diagnostic Tests

Identification of type and amount of substance

Laboratory evaluation of substance

Blood toxicology

Urine toxicology

Serum electrolytes

Complete blood count

Medical Management

The goals of treatment are to prevent poisonings from occurring, remove the poisonous substance, and preserve homeostasis for the child. The solution to childhood poisoning is prevention. This is a major public education initiative sponsored by the AAPCC, American Academy of Pediatrics (AAP), CDC, and National Institutes of Health.

The treatment approaches vary depending on the type of poison, the type of exposure (ingested, inhaled, etc.), the amount of exposure, and the time lapse between exposure and treatment. The first priority is assessing the child's airway, breathing, and circulation and then stabilizing the child. Regaining respiratory function may involve the placement of an endotracheal tube and mechanical ventilation. Interventions to achieve and maintain homeostasis must be the priority of health care professionals when treating any poisoning victim.

The four primary interventions for ingestion poisonings include the placement of a nasogastric tube for gastric lavage, administration of activated charcoal, administration of cathartic agents, and/or administration of antidotes specific to the poison substance. Gastric lavage is effective in diluting the poison and removing any remaining substance in the stomach, but only if treatment is performed soon after the substance is ingested. The administration of activated charcoal is useful in many oral poisonings when given alone or in conjunction with gastric lavage. The administration of cathartic agents increases gastric motility to cause more rapid expulsion of the poison.

Antidotes have been developed for several of the most common and most toxic poison agents and are administered once the child is stabilized. These include acetylcysteine for acetaminophen poisoning, deferoxamine for iron ingestion, bicarbonate for neutralizing tricyclic antidepressants, EDTA for lead, ethanol for methanol and ethylene glycol ingestion, naloxone for opiate overdose, and flumazenil for benzodiazepines (Broyles, Reiss, & Evans, 2007; Potts & Mandleco, 2007; Spratto & Woods, 2008).

Nursing Management

ASSESSMENT

1. Assess airway, breathing, and circulation
2. Obtain client history including the substance, amount of substance, and time of poisoning exposure
3. Perform rapid physical assessment
4. Assess parents' and child's (if age-appropriate) knowledge of poison prevention

NURSING DIAGNOSES (INCLUDING BUT NOT LIMITED TO)

1. Risk for injury R/T exposure to toxic substances
2. Parents' anxiety and guilt R/T child's condition
3. Deficient knowledge R/T poison prevention, growth and development, child's condition, treatment, and home care

PLANNING/GOALS

1. Client will not experience permanent injury from poisoning episode.
2. Parents will verbalize feelings and concerns and use positive coping strategies.
3. Parents and child (if age-appropriate) will demonstrate understanding of poisoning prevention, growth and development, child's condition, treatment, and home care.

NOC

1. Risk Control, Safe Home Environment
2. Anxiety, Guilt
3. Knowledge: Health Promotion, Safe Home Environment, Growth and Development: Child, Illness Care, Treatment

IMPLEMENTATION

1. Risk for injury
   a. Assess airway, breathing, and circulation
   b. Place on continuous cardiorespiratory monitoring
   c. Place on continuous pulse oximetry
   d. Administer oxygen as prescribed
   e. Insert nasogastric tube as prescribed once child is stabilized
   f. Administer gastric lavage as prescribed
   g. Administer activated charcoal as prescribed
   h. Administer antidote if available and as prescribed
   i. Monitor intake and output
   j. Monitor respiratory status
   k. Monitor cardiac status
   l. Monitor neurologic status
   m. Monitor laboratory values
   n. Monitor renal function
   o. Monitor gastrointestinal functioning
   p. Assess psychological impact of poisoning and child's condition on parents
   q. Collaborate with health care provider and social worker if concerned about parental neglect of child

2. Anxiety/guilt
   a. Encourage parents to express feelings and concerns
   b. Listen actively
   c. Provide support
   d. Assist parents in identifying positive coping strategies
   e. Encourage parents to participate in child's care when possible
   f. Keep parents informed of child's condition

3. Parent and child (if age-appropriate) teaching
   a. Assess parents' current level of understanding
   b. Provide verbal and written information regarding:
      1) Poisoning prevention using guidelines from the AAPCC:
         a) Store poisons safely
            (i) Store medicines and household products locked up where children cannot see or reach them
            (ii) Store poisons in their original containers
            (iii) Use child-resistant packaging
            (iv) Remember that nothing is child-proof, so supervision of children is necessary
         b) Use poisons safely
            (i) Read labels and follow directions for medicines and products
            (ii) Take products with you to answer the door or use the phone if children are around
            (iii) Lock up medicines and products after use
            (iv) Do not use the word *candy* when referring to medications; use the term *medicine*
            (v) Take medication out of sight of children
         c) Teach children to ask permission before eating or drinking anything

    2) Importance of keeping Poison Control Center information by the phone

    3) 10 Tips to Protect Children from Pesticide and Lead Poisoning (Environmental Protection Agency, 2007)

    4) Growth and development characteristics that place children at risk for poisonings

    5) Medication administration if applicable

    6) Referral information as needed

    7) Importance of follow-up with health care provider

  c. Provide adequate time for teaching

  d. Document teaching and parental response

NIC

1. Risk Identification
2. Coping Enhancement
3. Teaching: Health Education, Environmental Management: Safety, Developmental Enhancement: Child, Illness Care, Treatment

EVALUATION

1. Client does not experience permanent injury from poisoning episode.
2. Parents verbalize feelings and concerns and use positive coping strategies.
3. Parents and child (if age-appropriate) demonstrate understanding of poisoning prevention, growth and development, child's condition, treatment, and home care.

References

American Association of Poison Control Centers. (2006). *2005 annual report of the American Association of Poison Control Centers' national poisoning and exposure database.* Retrieved July 7, 2007, from http://www.aapcc.org/Annual%20Reports/05report/2005%20Publsihed.pdf

Broyles, B. E., Reiss, B. S., & Evans, M. E. (2007). *Pharmacological aspects of nursing care* (7th ed.). Clifton Park, NY: Delmar Cengage Learning.

Centers for Disease Control and Prevention. (2007). *Poisoning in the United States: Fact sheet.* Retrieved July 9, 2007, from http://www.cdc.gov/ncipc/factsheets/poisoning.htm

Environmental Protection Agency. (2007). *10 tips to protect children from pesticide and lead poisonings.* Retrieved July 9, 2007, from http://www.epa.gov/oppfead1/cb/10_tips

Potts, N. L., & Mandleco, B. L. (2007). *Pediatric nursing: Caring for children and their families* (2nd ed.). Clifton Park, NY: Delmar Cengage Learning.

Spratto, G. R., & Woods, A. L. (2008). *2008 Edition PDR nurse's drug handbook.* Clifton Park, NY: Delmar Cengage Learning.

PULMONARY STENOSIS (PS)

Definition

Pulmonary stenosis (PS) is the narrowing of the lumen of the major artery that exits the right ventricle in the heart and carries blood to the lungs to be oxygenated. The obstruction can be located at the valve (valvar), just before the valve (subvalve stenosis), or above the pulmonary valve (supravalve stenosis). Refer to Figure 85-1.

Pathophysiology

The thickening and fusing of the pulmonary valve leaflets or narrowing of the pulmonary artery before or above the valve causes an obstruction in the blood flow from the right ventricle into the pulmonary artery. This increases the resistance to blood flow through the artery and causes the right ventricle to work harder pumping against this resistance. This leads to right ventricular hypertrophy and resultant systemic congestion. Depending on the degree of stenosis, the neonate may be asymptomatic or may experience moderate to severe decreases in cardiac output as a result of decreased right ventricular efficiency as a pump.

Complications

Right-heart failure
Systemic congestion

Incidence

"The incidence of pulmonary stenosis is approximately 8–10% of all CHD [congenital heart disease/defects]" (Potts & Mandleco, 2007, p. 779). "Pulmonary stenosis is the second most common congenital heart defect . . . [and] is a component of half of all complex congenital heart defects" (CongenitalHeartDefects.com, 2006, p. 1).

Etiology

According to the American Heart Association, the exact cause of PS is unknown. It is presumed to be genetic, although only a few genes discovered have been linked to the presence of heart defects. Heredity may play a role in the development of PS, as well as coexisting conditions such as Down syndrome or a mother contracting rubella during the first trimester of pregnancy. The use of alcohol and illicit drugs during pregnancy increases the fetus's risk for developing PS or other congenital heart defects (American Heart Association, 2007).

Clinical Manifestations

Most are asymptomatic except for the presence of a murmur
More severe PS:
    Dyspnea on exertion
    Tachycardia
    Tachypnea
    Systemic edema

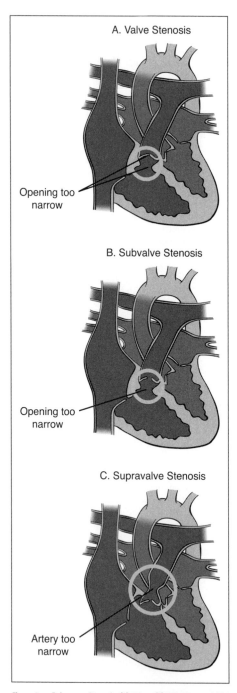

Figure 85-1: Pulmonary Stenosis: **(A)** Valvar; **(B)** Subvalvar; and **(C)** Supravalvar.

Diagnostic Tests

Chest radiography

Echocardiogram

Cardiac catheterization

Medical Management

No medical/surgical treatment is required in children with asymptomatic PS. If clinical manifestations of altered cardiac output occur, balloon valvuloplasties are used to treat small to moderate-sized PS. This procedure is performed in the cardiac catheterization lab. Severe PS or PS accompanying other defects, such as tetralogy of Fallot, requires open heart surgical repair. Refer to Medical Management in Chapter 26: Congenital Heart Disease/Open Heart Surgery.

Nursing Management

Refer to Nursing Management in Chapter 26: Congenital Heart Disease/Open Heart Surgery.

References

American Heart Association. (2007). *Congenital heart defects in children fact sheet.* Retrieved March 18, 2008, from http://americanheart.org/presenter.jhtml?identifier=12012

CongenitalHeartDefects.com. (2006). *Pulmonary stenosis (PS).* Retrieved March 18, 2008, from http://www.congenitalheartdefects.com/typesofCHD.html#PS

Potts, N. L., & Mandleco, B. L. (2007). *Pediatric nursing: Caring for children and their families* (2nd ed.). Clifton Park, NY: Delmar Cengage Learning.

86

Pyloric Stenosis/Hypertrophic Pyloric Stenosis (HPS)

Definition

Pyloric stenosis, also termed hypertrophic pyloric stenosis (HPS) or infantile hypertrophic pyloric stenosis (IHPS), is the increased size and mass of the circular layer of the lower gastric sphincter that causes gastric outlet obstruction. Refer to Figure 86-1.

Pathophysiology

Hypertrophy and hyperplasia of the circular and longitudinal muscular layers of the pylorus cause a narrowing of the gastric antrum. The pyloric canal elongates; and the entire pylorus becomes thickened, including the mucosa. If the pyloric stenosis is severe, the stomach becomes dilated in response to near-complete obstruction. As the stomach contracts to expel chyme through the pyloric stenosis, the pressure of the gastric contraction against the obstructed pyloric sphincter causes the lower esophageal sphincter (LES) to open, resulting in the classic manifestation of pyloric stenosis—projectile vomiting. This leads to a risk of aspiration, fluid and electrolyte imbalances (dehydration, hypochloremia, and hypokalemia), metabolic alkalosis (from loss of hydrogen ions in gastric secretions), and failure to thrive (from inadequate nutrient intake) (Potts & Mandleco, 2007).

Complications

- Risk of aspiration
- Dehydration
- Hypokalemia
- Hypochloremia
- Metabolic alkalosis
- Failure to thrive

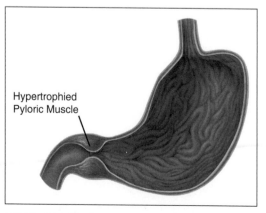

Hypertrophied
Pyloric Muscle

Figure 86-1: Pyloric Stenosis.

Incidence

Pyloric stenosis is the most common gastric outlet obstruction in infants, affecting 2–4 neonates per 1,000 live births (Kass & Sinert, 2006). Males have a higher incidence than females, with reported ratios ranging from 2:1–5:1 (Nazar & Nazar, 2006). Caucasian first-born males of European descent represent the highest incidence (Potts & Mandleco, 2007). The obstruction usually is manifested by the third week of life and is uncommon in preterm neonates.

Etiology

The exact cause of pyloric stenosis is not known; however, environmental factors and genetic factors appear to increase the risk. Other possible but still unproven causes include deficiency of nitric oxide synthase containing neurons, abnormal myenteric plexus innervation, infantile hypergastrinemia, and exposure to macrolide antibiotics (Kass & Sinert, 2006).

Clinical Manifestations

Projectile vomiting

Decreased urinary output

Depressed fontanels

Dry mucous membranes

Decreased tears

Poor skin turgor

Lethargy

Weight loss

Diagnostic Tests

Upper gastrointestinal series

Ultrasonography

Complete blood count

Serum chemistry

Medical Management

The goals of treatment are to surgically repair the stenotic sphincter, regain fluid and electrolyte and acid-base balance, and resolve the failure to thrive. Preoperatively, a nasogastric tube is inserted for gastric decompression and intravenous fluids with electrolytes are administered until the neonate is rehydrated and the serum bicarbonate is less than 30 mEq/L. The surgical procedure, termed a *pylormyotomy,* involves releasing the circular muscle fibers of the pylorus, opening the passage between the stomach and the small intestine. After surgery, the nasogastric tube is removed once bowel sounds return, and oral feedings are advanced as tolerated. This surgery is considered curative for the majority of these neonates.

Nursing Management

Refer to Chapter 100: Surgical Client.

ASSESSMENT

1. Assess airway, breathing, and circulation
2. Assess vital signs, weight, and height
3. Complete neonatal or infant physical assessment
4. Assess psychological impact of diagnosis and pending surgery on parents

Nursing Diagnoses (including but not limited to)

1. Risk for aspiration R/T projectile vomiting
2. Deficient fluid volume R/T vomiting
3. Imbalanced nutrition: less than body requirements R/T vomiting
4. Deficient knowledge (parental) R/T child's condition, treatment, and home care

Planning/Goals

1. Client will not experience aspiration as evidenced by maintaining a patent airway.
2. Client will regain and maintain hydration within defined limits (WDL) as evidenced by urinary output, fontanels, mucous membranes, and skin turgor WDL.
3. Client will regain weight lost through vomiting and meet growth guidelines (double birth weight by 6 months of age and triple birth weight by age 1 year).
4. Parents will demonstrate understanding of neonate's condition, treatment, and home care.

NOC

1. Aspiration Prevention
2. Electrolyte and Acid Base Balance, Fluid Balance
3. Nutritional Status: Nutrient Intake
4. Knowledge: Illness Care, Treatment, Health Promotion

Implementation

1. Risk for aspiration
   a. Assess airway and breathing
   b. Place on continuous cardiorespiratory monitor
   c. Place on continuous pulse oximetry
   d. Insert nasogastric tube for decompression as prescribed
   e. Maintain patency of nasogastric tube
   f. Monitor intake and output
   g. Monitor vital signs
   h. Administer oxygen as prescribed
2. Fluid and electrolyte/acid-base balance
   a. Monitor intake and output hourly
   b. Weigh wet diapers for accurate output
   c. Assess fontanels
   d. Assess skin turgor
   e. Assess mucous membranes
   f. Monitor laboratory values
   g. Maintain patency of intravenous access device, monitoring at least hourly
   h. Administer intravenous fluids and electrolytes as prescribed
3. Nutrition
   a. Weigh daily
   b. Monitor intake and output
   c. Assist breastfeeding mother with pumping of breast milk for refrigeration until neonate can resume oral intake
   d. Label stored breast milk properly

  e. Maintain patency of intravenous access device, monitoring at least hourly

  f. Administer intravenous fluids and electrolytes as prescribed

  g. Discontinue nasogastric tube after return of bowel sounds as prescribed

  h. Increase oral feedings slowly as tolerated from Infalyte to formula or breast milk

  i. Encourage parents to participate in care

 4. Parent teaching

  a. Assess current level of understanding

  b. Provide verbal and written information regarding:

   1) Postoperative care

   2) Medication administration as prescribed

   3) Infant feeding

   4) Infant care

   5) Importance of follow-up care with health care provider

   6) Contact numbers for reporting any questions or concerns to health care provider or nurse

  c. Provide adequate time for teaching

  d. Document teaching and parental response

NIC

1. Aspiration Precautions, Respiratory Management, Respiratory Monitoring

2. Fluid Management, Fluid Monitoring, Acid Base Management, Electrolyte Management

3. Nutrition Management, Nutrition Monitoring

4. Teaching: Illness Care, Treatment, Health Education

EVALUATION

1. Client does not experience aspiration as evidenced by maintaining a patent airway.

2. Client regains and maintains hydration WDL as evidenced by urinary output, fontanels, mucous membranes, and skin turgor WDL.

3. Client regains weight lost through vomiting and meets growth guidelines (double birth weight by 6 months of age and triple birth weight by age 1 year).

4. Parents demonstrate understanding of neonate's condition, treatment, and home care.

References

Kass, D. A., & Sinert, R. (2006). *Pediatrics, pyloric stenosis.* Retrieved April 13, 2007, from http://www.emedicine.com/emerg/topic397.htm

Nazar, H., & Nazar, D. (2006). *Pyloric stenosis, hypertrophied.* Retrieved April 13, 2007, from http://www.emedicine.com/ped/topic1103.htm

Potts, N. L., & Mandleco, B. L. (2007). *Pediatric nursing: Caring for children and their families* (2nd ed.). Clifton Park, NY: Delmar Cengage Learning.

87

RADIATION THERAPY

Definition

Radiation therapy is a medical treatment that uses ionizing radiation of gamma and X-rays or proton or electron beams to deliver therapeutic radiation to a tumor with minimal effects to the healthy tissue surrounding the tumor (Potts & Mandleco, 2007).

Medical Management

Radiation therapy is used in the treatment of certain pediatric malignant neoplasms, such as lymphomas, solid tumors, and brain tumors. Radiation may be employed to (1) destroy the tumor, (2) reduce the tumor's size, (3) decrease pain, or (4) relieve obstruction. Frequently, this therapy is used in combination with other cancer treatments, including chemotherapy and surgery. Ionizing radiation is believed to cause lethal injury to cellular DNA, thus resulting in cell death (Broyles, 2005).

Radiation therapy is delivered by several methods, including fractionation, hyperfractionation, stereotactic therapy, and total body irradiation. The conventional method, fractionation, uses daily doses administered in divided doses until the prescribed amount of radiation has been delivered. This produces less damage to normal cells in the path of the radiation by allowing these cells time to repair between doses (Potts & Mandleco, 2007).

Hyperfractionation is delivered as multiple doses (two or three) per day until the prescribed amount has been delivered. This method provides for higher daily radiation exposure to the tumor but uses smaller doses to preserve normal cells.

Stereotactic radiation is a successful treatment for small distinct tumors, such as brain tumors, that are not surgically accessible or otherwise cannot be surgically resected. Stereotactic radiation is administered during radiosurgery and consists of a precise delivery of a single high dose of radiation in a one-day session (IRSA, 2006).

Total body irradiation consists of external beam radiation delivered to the entire body. It is used in preparation for hematopoietic stem cell transplantation (Potts & Mandleco, 2007).

Radiation therapy can be delivered in two ways: (1) external radiation (teletherapy), which consists of applying ionizing beams to the area from a distance, and (2) internal, interstitial, or intracavity radiation (brachytherapy), where the radioactive material is placed directly into the tumor site, delivering a high dose of radiation to the tumor with the surrounding cells receiving a lower dose.

Tumor sensitivity to radiation varies; however, individuals with the highest numbers of rapidly proliferating cancer cells tend to respond more favorably to radiation. The sensitivity of the tumor types has been classified according to the radiosensitivity. Neuroblastomas, lymphomas, and chronic leukemia are very radiosensitive, whereas adenocarcinomas, fibrosarcomas, and osteogenic sarcomas have been identified as nonradiosensitive.

When administered over time, radiation therapy can destroy rapidly multiplying cancer cells. Unfortunately, it also can destroy the rapidly multiplying normal cells of the body, especially those of the mucous membranes. For instance, radiation therapy to the head and neck can cause destruction of epithelial cells of the mouth and severe pain associated with mucositis. Xerostomia, dryness of the mouth, occurs from the radiation due to decreased production or cessation of the production of salivary secretions.

Teeth sensitivity and pain can occur. This can result in an inability to intake oral fluids and nutrition. Xerostomia can cause difficulty speaking because of the dryness.

Radiation to the chest area can cause painful esophagitis from destruction of the mucous membrane lining of the esophagus. This may require hospitalization to manage the pain crisis and to provide alternative feeding techniques including insertion of tubes for enteral nutrition and fluids. Dryness, erythema, pruritis, and even burns can occur to the skin exposed to radiation therapy. In the presence of skin breakdown, further radiation therapy should be delayed until the area has healed. Alopecia results from radiation treatments to the head. Children being treated with radiation to the bones, such as for Ewing's sarcoma, or soft tissue and blood vessels may experience altered growth and development or asymmetry of bone growth (Potts & Mandleco, 2007).

Radiation pneumonitis, an acute reaction to radiation therapy, is the result of edema and sloughing of the endothelial cells of the smaller vessels of the lungs. This allows fluid to accumulate in the interstitial tissues, which can lead to respiratory compromise that may require hospitalization and mechanical ventilation (Potts & Mandleco, 2007).

Radiation therapy to the head can result in central nervous system toxicity including headache, nausea, and vomiting. Acute toxicity can lead to cerebral inflammation, edema, and increased intracranial pressure. Children with the somnolence syndrome are drowsy and may sleep up to 20 hours a day in addition to experiencing fever, dysplasia, ataxia, and transient swelling of the optic nerve called papilledema (Potts & Mandleco, 2007). Some children may exhibit fatigue, anorexia, and loss of taste (IRSA, 2006).

A recent report by a British research team that was published in the February 7, 2007, issue of the *Journal of National Cancer Institute* found that survivors of Hodgkin's lymphoma treated with radiation and certain chemotherapeutic agents are at increased risk of having a fatal heart attack for up to 25 years after undergoing treatment. The study spanned 33 years and included 7,033 clients, among whom 2,441 died during an average follow-up of 11 years. The cause of death in 166 of these clients was myocardial infarction. The researchers concluded that study participants experienced a risk of a fatal heart attack that was 2.5 times higher than that of the general population (Reuters Health Information, 2007).

Complications

Mucositis

Xerostomia

Teeth sensitivity

Esophagitis

Dryness, erythema, pruritis, burns, and breakdown of skin

Alopecia

Radiation pneumonitis

Altered bone growth

Central nervous system manifestations

Long-term higher risk of myocardial infarction

Nursing Management

ASSESSMENT

1. Obtain client history including any medications child is taking
2. Assess skin and mucous membranes for evidence of damage
3. Assess pain using age-appropriate rating scale
4. Assess current knowledge of treatment plan
5. Perform psychosocial assessment to determine impact of diagnosis and treatment

Nursing Diagnoses (including but not limited to)

1. Risk for impaired oral mucous membrane integrity R/T exposure to radioactive beams
2. Risk for impaired skin integrity R/T radiation exposure
3. Risk for injury, radiation pneumonitis, central nervous system changes, nausea, and vomiting R/T radiation toxicity
4. Imbalanced nutrition: less than body requirements R/T anorexia, nausea, and vomiting
5. Anxiety R/T radiation therapy and diagnosis of cancer
6. Deficient knowledge R/T radiation therapy, adverse effects, and importance of compliance with treatment plan

Planning/Goals

1. Client will experience minimal damage to mucous membranes; however, any damage will be treated effectively in a timely manner.
2. Client will not experience damage to skin; however, any damage will be treated effectively in a timely manner.
3. Client will not experience radiation toxicity; however, if toxicity does occur, it will be treated effectively with no residual deficits occurring.
4. Client will receive adequate nutritional intake to meet growth and development and metabolic needs.
5. Family will express feelings and concerns and use positive coping strategies.
6. Parents and child (if age-appropriate) will demonstrate understanding of treatment, adverse effects, and importance of compliance with treatment plan.

NOC

1. Tissue Integrity: Mucous Membranes
2. Tissue Integrity: Skin
3. Risk Control
4. Nutritional Status
5. Anxiety
6. Knowledge: Illness Care, Treatment, Health Promotion

Implementation

1. Mucous membranes
   a. Assess mucous membranes at least 3 times per day
   b. Monitor intake and output
   c. Initiate and maintain patency of intravenous access, monitoring at least hourly for client with esophagitis
   d. Monitor pain level hourly
   e. Collaborate with health care provider for appropriate pain management
   f. Administer analgesics as prescribed for mucositis and esophagitis
   g. Provide mouth care and teach parents/child appropriate technique
   h. Encourage fluid intake by offering favorite beverages
   i. Offer hard candy or sugarless gum to stimulate saliva production
   j. Provide enteral feedings as prescribed
   k. Teach parents/child how to administer enteral feedings
   l. Evaluate parents'/child's ability to administer enteral feedings

2. Skin integrity
    a. Assess skin at least 3 times per day
    b. Maintain radiation therapy markings on skin
    c. Provide skin care; discuss use of lotions, creams, or deodorant with radiation oncologist before using
    d. Use mild soap for hygiene
    e. Avoid friction, tight clothing, hot water, tape, and strong soaps on skin
    f. Explain importance of avoiding sun exposure
    g. Obtain culture prior to wound treatment if a wound is present
3. Risk of toxicity
    a. Monitor vital signs every 4 hours
    b. Monitor breath sounds at least 3 times per day
    c. Monitor for respiratory compromise
    d. Monitor oxygen saturation via continuous pulse oximetry
    e. Report abnormal findings to health care provider immediately
    f. Teach family importance of reporting respiratory problems to health care provider
    g. Monitor neurologic status at least 3 times per day
    h. Report changes in sensorium to health care provider immediately
    i. Protect child from falls
    j. Encourage parental presence and involvement in care
    k. Teach family importance of reporting changes in mental status to health care provider immediately
    l. Administer antiemetics proactively prior to radiation therapy
    m. Administer prednisone as prescribed prior to radiation therapy
    n. Collaborate with health care provider if medication therapy is not effective in controlling nausea and vomiting
4. Nutrition
    a. Weigh daily
    b. Monitor intake and output
    c. Provide enteral feedings as prescribed
    d. Provide parenteral feedings as prescribed
    e. Encourage intake of favorite high-protein, high-calorie fluids
    f. Collaborate with nutritionist
5. Anxiety
    a. Encourage parents/child to verbalize feelings and concerns
    b. Listen actively
    c. Encourage parents to participate in child's care
    d. Assist with identifying previously used positive coping strategies
    e. Assist with identifying support systems
    f. Provide for spiritual needs
6. Parent/child teaching
    a. Assess parents'/child's current level of understanding
    b. Provide verbal and written information regarding:
        1) Skin care including not removing skin markings identifying site of external radiation; washing skin, using water only, over markings; washing surrounding skin with mild soap; not applying deodorants, lotions, perfume, or medications

to radiation site during treatment; avoiding rubbing or scratching skin over treatment area; avoiding exposure of treatment site to heat or cold; wearing loose-fitting soft clothing over site to avoid irritation; avoiding sun exposure during treatment; using electric razor for shaving; and inspecting skin daily, noting and reporting any skin damage to health care provider

2) Medication administration

3) Signs and symptoms of adverse effects of medications

4) Signs of radiation toxicity

5) Demonstration and return demonstration of enteral feedings if applicable

6) Contact numbers for health care provider and referrals

c. Provide adequate time for teaching, demonstrations, and return demonstrations

d. Document teaching and parent/child response

NIC

1. Oral Health Restoration
2. Skin Surveillance
3. Surveillance: Safety, Risk Identification
4. Nutrition Management
5. Anxiety Reduction
6. Teaching: Illness Care, Treatment, Health Promotion

EVALUATION

1. Client experiences minimal damage to mucous membranes and receives timely and effective treatment of damage.
2. Client does not experience damage to skin.
3. Client does not experience radiation toxicity.
4. Client receives adequate nutritional intake to meet growth and development and metabolic needs.
5. Family expresses feelings and concerns and uses positive coping strategies.
6. Parents and child (if age-appropriate) demonstrate understanding of treatment, adverse effects, and importance of compliance with treatment plan.

References

Broyles, B. E. (2005). *Medical-surgical nursing clinical companion*. Durham, NC: Carolina Academic Press.

IRSA. (2006). *Stereotactic radiosurgery overview*. Retrieved July 9, 2007, from http://www.irsa.org/radiosurgery.html

Potts, N. L., & Mandleco, B. L. (2007). *Pediatric nursing: Caring for children and their families* (2nd ed.). Clifton Park, NY: Delmar Cengage Learning.

Reuters Health Information. (2007). *Hodgkin's disease therapy up heart attack risks*. Retrieved March 18, 2008, from http://www.reuters.com/article/healthNews/idUSSPI71257620070207

88

RENAL FAILURE, ACUTE (ARF)

Definition

Acute renal failure (ARF) is a severe partial or total impairment of renal function usually occurring as a result of a dramatic reduction in renal perfusion.

Pathophysiology

ARF usually is a consequence of trauma and the shock response. It has a rapid onset and is characterized by a critical reduction in renal function. Approximately 50% of the 2–3 million nephrons cease to function. The manifestations reflect the decrease in the multiple functions of the kidneys (Broyles, 2005).

ARF is comprised of three primary mechanisms according to which part of the kidney the dysfunction originates in. Prerenal ARF, also referred to as prerenal azotemia, is the most common type and is caused by hypovolemia, septic shock, cardiogenic shock, perinatal asphyxia, burns, congestive heart failure, renal artery obstruction, or severe dehydration (Potts & Mandleco, 2007). Other factors that can lead to this type of ARF are medications that block the production of prostaglandins necessary for renal function, including nonsteroidal anti-inflammatory drugs (NSAIDs), angiotensin-converting enzyme (ACE) inhibitors, and cyclooxygenase inhibitors. This leads to nephron ischemia. Intrarenal ARF results from damage to the renal parenchyma and most often results from acute tubular necrosis, but it can occur as an extension of prerenal ARF. Acute tubular necrosis is the result of ischemia secondary to renal artery stenosis or nephrotoxic substances including cyclosporine, vancomycin, aminoglycoside antimicrobials, amphotericin, and antineoplastic agents. Postrenal ARF occurs secondary to conditions that lead to blockages that cause outlet obstructions in the kidneys, including bilateral ureteral obstruction.

In 2004, the Acute Dialysis Quality Initiative (ADQI) group established a systematic method of defining ARF when it published the RIFLE classification. This method is based on changes from the child's or adult's baseline in serum creatinine level or glomerular filtration rate (GFR), urine output (UO), or both. This classification system is as follows:

Risk (R)—Increase in serum creatinine level × 1.5 or decrease in GFR by 25% or UO < 0.5 mL/kg/hr for 6 hours

Injury (I)—Increase in serum creatinine level × 2.0 or decrease in GFR by 50% or UO < 0.5 mL/kg/hr for 12 hours

Failure (F)—Increase in serum creatinine level × 3.0, decrease in GFR by 75%, or serum creatinine level ≥ 4 mg/dL; UO < 0.3 mL/kg/hr for 24 hours or anuria for 12 hours

Loss (L)—Persistent ARF, complete loss of kidney function > 4 weeks

End-stage kidney disease (E)—Loss of kidney function > 3 months (Sinert & Peacock, 2006)

The loss of renal function causes a cascade of reactions including azotemia, an accumulation of nitrogen waste products in systemic circulation, and is manifested as an increase in blood urea nitrogen (BUN) and creatinine levels. Because the kidneys are the primary route for the excretion of certain electrolytes such as potassium and sodium as well as by-products of protein metabolism, the concentrations of these substances increase in the bloodstream. Hyperkalemia can result in cardiac dysrhythmias; hypernatremia leads to fluid retention, edema, congestive heart failure, and hypertension. Fluid retention can manifest as pulmonary edema, pleural effusion, and cardiac tamponade as well as seizures and altered level of consciousness. Reduced renal perfusion activates the renin-angiotensin complex, causing an increase in aldosterone secretion that further increases the risk of hypertension. The renal system is the primary acid-base buffer reflected in the increased or decreased release of sodium bicarbonate in response to the pH level in the body. Because renal function is decreased or lost, metabolic acidosis results. Anemia occurs because of inadequate erythropoietin production, This when combined with uremia results in an increased tendency to experience gastrointestinal bleeding. As a consequence of the inverse reciprocal relationship between calcium and phosphorous in the body, hypocalcemia occurs due to the kidneys' inability to filter and excrete phosphorous, leading to elevated serum phosphorous levels (hyperphosphatemia).

ARF can lead to chronic renal failure and thus dependency on dialysis or the need for renal transplantation. Complications such as cardiac dysrhythmias, pleural effusion, pulmonary edema, and cardiac tamponade can be fatal.

Complications

Azotemia
Hyperkalemia
Cardiac dysrhythmias
Hypernatremia
Pulmonary edema
Pleural effusion
Cardiac tamponade
Metabolic acidosis
Anemia
Hypocalcemia
Hyperphosphatemia
Uremia
Chronic renal failure

Incidence

In the pediatric population, the annual rate is 1 to 2 new cases of ARF in every 100,000 children (National Kidney and Urologic Diseases Information Clearinghouse, 2006).

Etiology

The most common cause of ARF in children is prerenal etiologies. These include hypovolemia, septic shock, cardiogenic shock, perinatal asphyxia, burns, congestive heart failure, renal artery obstruction, or severe dehydration.

Clinical Manifestations

Oliguria
Anuria
Nocturia
Peripheral edema
Generalized edema
Numbness and tingling of extremities
Muscle twitching
Irritability
Decreased level of consciousness
Lethargy progressing to coma
Seizures

Nausea and vomiting

Ecchymosis

Pallor

Prolonged bleeding

Hypertension

Fatigue

Poor feeding

Tinnitus

Flank pain

Diagnostic Tests

Complete blood count

Serum electrolyte levels

Renal function tests

Urinalysis

Renal arteriography

Chest radiography

Bone scan

Renal ultrasound

Electrocardiogram

Renal biopsy

Abdominal computed tomography (CT)

Abdominal magnetic resonance imaging (MRI)

Medical Management

The goals of treatment are to identify and treat the underlying cause(s), prevent complications, and restore renal function and fluid and electrolyte balance. Intravenous fluids and pharmacological support are initiated. Medications to treat the cause are administered to stabilize the child hemodynamically and to increase renal perfusion. Antihypertensives (nifedipine) are titrated to reduce blood pressure in the presence of hypertension. However, dopamine may be required during the critical stage to increase blood pressure and renal perfusion associated with hypoperfusion secondary to shock. Diuretics such as furosemide (Lasix) may be necessary in the presence of pulmonary edema and congestive heart failure. Positive inotropic agents such as digoxin are used to increase cardiac output. Sodium bicarbonate frequently is the drug of choice for treating the metabolic acidosis (Broyles, Reiss, & Evans, 2007). Phenytoin (Dilantin) is prescribed to control seizures. To reduce potassium levels through the excretion of potassium through the large intestines, Kayexalate is the drug of choice. In addition, erythropoietin (Epogen) may be required to stimulate red blood cell production for the treatment of anemia. If the ARF persists, dialysis may be required. Refer to Chapter 89: Renal Failure, Chronic (CRF)/End-Stage Renal Disease (ESRD)/Renal Transplantation for a discussion of dialysis.

Hemodialysis or peritoneal dialysis is indicated in the presence of uremia, persistent hyperkalemia, uncompensated metabolic acidosis, persistent fluid volume excess, uremic pericarditis, and/or uremic encephalopathy. Hemodialysis is preferred because for many critically ill children, the placement of dialysate fluid in the abdominal cavity for peritoneal dialysis compromises breathing. Because dialysis removes large amounts of electrolytes, electrolyte replacement is achieved through intravenous infusion of needed electrolytes and is titrated to serum electrolyte levels. Continuous venovenous hemofiltration (CVVH) often is considered the best continuous renal replacement therapy (CRRT) approach for children who have difficulty handling large fluid and electrolyte shifts (Potts & Mandleco, 2007). CRRT requires only a double-lumen central venous catheter and is administered via a pump; it is believed to be more reliable than titrating to the mean arterial pressure. CRRT must be done in a critical care unit where the child is continuously monitored.

If dialysis needs to be continued after the child is discharged from the hospital, the current standard of care is peritoneal dialysis. This method can be performed by the parents at home and does not carry the risk of severe hypotension associated with hemodialysis.

Renal transplantation is considered if the child does not respond to dialysis. Renal transplantation is more successful in children than in adults. Refer to Chapter 89: Renal Failure, Chronic (CRF)/End-Stage Renal Disease (ESRD)/Renal Transplantation for a discussion about renal transplantation. Treatment for ARF following hospitalization varies greatly and is dependent on the level of renal function. Although complete recovery usually occurs, it can take weeks or months to fully resolve. Depending on the age of the child, dietary changes may be necessary until recovery is complete. These modifications may include sodium, potassium, and protein restrictions.

Nursing Management

Refer to Chapter 89: Renal Failure, Chronic (CRF)/End-Stage Renal Disease (ESRD)/Renal Transplantation for nursing management of children receiving renal dialysis and renal transplantation.

ASSESSMENT

1. Obtain client history with focus on risk factors for ARF
2. Assess vital signs
3. Monitor laboratory and diagnostic test results
4. Assess for presence of clinical manifestations of azotemia
5. Obtain height and weight
6. Perform pediatric assessment
7. Assess psychological impact that diagnosis has on parents and child (if age-appropriate)

NURSING DIAGNOSES (INCLUDING BUT NOT LIMITED TO)

1. Excess fluid volume R/T sodium and fluid retention
2. Deficient fluid volume R/T fluid intake restrictions, diuretic therapy, and dialysis
3. Risk for decreased cardiac output R/T dysrhythmias secondary to hyperkalemia
4. Ineffective protection R/T invasive lines, altered immune responses, and presence of uremic toxins
5. Risk for impaired skin integrity R/T edema
6. Imbalanced nutrition: less than body requirements R/T decreased intake and increased metabolic demands
7. Risk for ineffective tissue perfusion R/T decreased red blood cell production
8. Anxiety (parents and child, if age-appropriate) R/T critical care environment and uncertainty of prognosis
9. Deficient knowledge R/T child's condition, treatment, prognosis, and home care

PLANNING/GOALS

1. Client will experience fluid and electrolyte balance within 24–48 hours of onset of ARF as evidenced by intake and output, electrolyte levels, vital signs, and weight within defined limits (WDL).

2. Client will regain and maintain adequate fluid volume within 24 hours of diagnosis of ARF as evidenced by intake and output, electrolyte levels, vital signs, and weight WDL.

3. Client will not experience cardiac dysrhythmias.

4. Client will not experience infection.

5. Client's skin will remain intact.

6. Client will regain and maintain adequate nutrition within 72 hours of onset of ARF as evidenced by caloric intake and weight WDL.

7. Client will maintain adequate tissue perfusion as evidenced by capillary refill, oxygen saturation, neurologic status, and vital signs WDL.

8. Client (if age-appropriate) and parents will demonstrate use of positive coping strategies as evidenced by decreased verbal and nonverbal indicators of anxiety.

9. Parents and child (if age-appropriate) will demonstrate understanding of condition, treatment, prognosis, and home care.

NOC

1. Fluid Balance, Electrolyte and Acid/Base Balance
2. Fluid Balance, Electrolyte and Acid/Base Balance
3. Cardiac Pump Effectiveness, Vital Signs
4. Risk Control
5. Skin Integrity, Hemodialysis Access
6. Nutritional Status: Nutrient Intake
7. Risk Control, Circulation Status
8. Anxiety
9. Knowledge: Illness Care, Treatment, Health Promotion

IMPLEMENTATION

1. Excess fluid volume
   a. Monitor hourly intake and output
   b. Monitor urine specific gravity and capillary refill
   c. Weigh daily
   d. Place on continuous cardiorespiratory monitor
   e. Monitor vital signs according to child's condition
   f. Place on continuous pulse oximetry
   g. Administer oxygen titrating to maintain oxygen saturation > 94%
   h. Maintain hemodynamic monitoring
   i. Monitor central venous pressure and mean arterial pressure
   j. Auscultate lung sounds at least every 2 hours
   k. Assess for peripheral edema every 2 hours
   l. Initiate and maintain vascular access device, monitoring at least hourly
   m. Administer intravenous fluids as prescribed
   n. Restrict fluid intake as prescribed
   o. Monitor serum sodium levels
   p. Administer diuretics as prescribed
   q. Prepare for dialysis or CRRT as prescribed
   r. Turn every 2 hours

2. Deficient fluid volume
   a. Monitor hourly intake and output
   b. Monitor urine specific gravity and capillary refill
   c. Weigh daily
   d. Collaborate with health care provider to replace fluids lost through vomiting or sudden diuresis
   e. Maintain patency of vascular access device, monitoring at least hourly
   f. Administer intravenous fluids as prescribed
   g. Maintain hemodynamic monitoring
   h. Assess vital signs frequently and according to child's condition
   i. Monitor central venous pressure and mean arterial pressure
   j. Monitor hemoglobin, hematocrit, BUN, and creatinine
   k. Encourage oral fluids as prescribed and tolerated
   l. Assess mucous membranes and skin for indications of dehydration
   m. Provide oral hygiene every 2 hours and as needed
   n. Monitor fluid changes as a result of dialysis or CRRT

3. Risk for dysrhythmias
   a. Maintain continuous cardiac monitoring
   b. Auscultate heart sounds
   c. Monitor vital signs frequently according to child's condition
   d. Administer medications as prescribed
   e. Maintain safe environment with side rails up
   f. Assess neurologic status at least every 2 hours and as needed
   g. Monitor potassium, sodium, and calcium levels

4. Risk for infection
   a. Monitor continuous temperature with skin probe
   b. Assess color, odor, and appearance of all drainage
   c. Monitor white blood cell count
   d. Maintain strict surgical asepsis during dressing changes and intravenous line changes
   e. Avoid indwelling catheters if possible
   f. Provide oral hygiene every 2 hours
   g. Assess skin integrity during every 2-hour position change
   h. Encourage coughing and deep breathing and use of incentive spirometer

5. Skin integrity
   a. Assess for edema at least every 2 hours
   b. Assess skin integrity during every 2-hour position change
   c. Keep skin clean and dry
   d. Elevate extremities if edema is present
   e. Monitor invasive lines for manifestations of infection
   f. Maintain strict surgical asepsis during dressing changes
   g. Encourage age-appropriate activities as soon as condition allows
   h. Encourage ambulation as soon as condition allows

6. Nutrition
   a. Weigh daily
   b. Maintain patency of vascular device, monitoring at least hourly

    c.   Administer enteral feedings or total parenteral nutrition as prescribed

    d.   Maintain strict intake and output

    e.   Monitor BUN and creatinine levels

    f.   Maintain caloric intake between 35–45 cal/kg as prescribed

    g.   Monitor electrolyte levels

    h.   Administer medications as prescribed to treat hyperphosphatemia and hypocalcemia

    i.   Monitor for manifestations of acid-base and electrolyte imbalances

7. Tissue perfusion

    a.   Monitor vital signs frequently

    b.   Maintain hemodynamic monitoring

    c.   Monitor heart sounds

    d.   Assess capillary refill with vital signs

    e.   Monitor hemoglobin and hematocrit

    f.   Administer oxygen, titrating to maintain oxygen saturation > 94%

    g.   Monitor central venous pressure and mean arterial pressure

    h.   Maintain patency of vascular access, monitoring at least hourly

    i.   Administer intravenous fluids as prescribed

    j.   Administer medications as prescribed

    k.   Monitor neurologic status every 2 hours

8. Anxiety

    a.   Orient to environment as needed

    b.   Explain all procedures and equipment

    c.   Keep parents informed about child's condition

    d.   Encourage expression of fears and concerns

    e.   Listen actively

    f.   Encourage parental participation in care

    g.   Engage in age-appropriate activities as condition allows

    h.   Assist parents in identifying positive coping strategies and support systems

    i.   Collaborate with child /parents to determine need for referral to pastoral care

    j.   Maintain calm affect

9. Parent and child (if age-appropriate) teaching

    a.   Assess current level of understanding

    b.   Provide verbal and written information regarding:

        1) Risk factors for developing ARF

        2) Medication administration including importance of compliance with the prescribed medication regimen

        3) Manifestations of adverse effects of medications

        4) Importance of not taking over-the-counter medications without consulting health care provider

        5) Relationship between calcium and phosphorous and need to consume vitamin D with calcium

        6) Demonstration and return demonstration of procedure if being discharged on peritoneal dialysis

        7) Referral information for home health nurse

        8) Manifestations of worsening of condition

      9) Contact phone numbers for reporting manifestations

      10) Importance of regular hand washing and appropriate technique

      11) Importance of follow-up with health care provider and routine laboratory testing

   c. Provide adequate time for teaching

   d. Document teaching and parental response

NIC

1. Fluid Monitoring, Fluid/Electrolyte Management, Acid/Base Management
2. Fluid Monitoring, Fluid/Electrolyte Management, Acid/Base Management
3. Hemodynamic Regulation, Vital Signs Monitoring
4. Infection Precautions
5. Skin Surveillance, Dialysis Access Maintenance
6. Nutrition Management, Nutrition Monitoring
7. Hemodynamic Regulation
8. Anxiety Reduction, Coping Enhancement
9. Teaching: Illness Care, Treatment, Health Education

EVALUATION

1. Client experiences fluid and electrolyte balance within 24–48 hours of onset of ARF as evidenced by intake and output, electrolyte levels, vital signs, and weight WDL.
2. Client regains and maintains adequate fluid volume within 24 hours of diagnosis of ARF as evidenced by intake and output, electrolyte levels, vital signs, and weight WDL.
3. Client does not experience cardiac dysrhythmias.
4. Client does not experience infection.
5. Client's skin remains intact.
6. Client regains and maintains adequate nutrition within 72 hours of onset of ARF as evidenced by caloric intake and weight WDL.
7. Client maintains adequate tissue perfusion as evidenced by capillary refill, oxygen saturation, neurologic status, and vital signs WDL.
8. Client (if age-appropriate) and parents demonstrate use of positive coping strategies as evidenced by decreased verbal and nonverbal indicators of anxiety.
9. Parents and child (if age-appropriate) demonstrate understanding of condition, treatment, prognosis, and home care.

References

Broyles, B. E. (2005). *Medical-surgical nursing clinical companion.* Durham, NC: Carolina Academic Press.

Broyles, B. E., Reiss, B. S., & Evans, M. E. (2007). *Pharmacological aspects of nursing care* (7th ed.). Clifton Park, NY: Delmar Cengage Learning.

National Kidney and Urologic Diseases Information Clearinghouse. (2006). *Overview of kidney diseases in children.* Retrieved March 18, 2008, from http://kidney.niddk.nih.gov/kudiseases/pubs/childkidneydiseases/overview/index.htm

Potts, N. L., & Mandleco, B. L. (2007). *Pediatric nursing: Caring for children and their families* (2nd ed.). Clifton Park, NY: Delmar Cengage Learning.

Sinert, R., & Peacock, P. R. (2006). *Renal failure, acute.* Retrieved March 18, 2008, from http://www.emedicine.com/emerg/topic500.htm

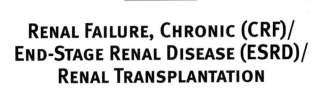

89

RENAL FAILURE, CHRONIC (CRF)/ END-STAGE RENAL DISEASE (ESRD)/ RENAL TRANSPLANTATION

Definition

Chronic renal failure (CRF) is the progressive, permanent, and irreversible damage to the nephrons, the functional cells of the kidneys. End-stage renal disease (ESRD) describes sufficient renal cell destruction that requires dialysis or renal transplantation to substitute for renal function. Renal transplantation is the placement of a functional donor kidney into a recipient with inadequate renal function.

Pathophysiology

Refer to Chapter 88: Renal Failure, Acute (ARF) for initiating factors that contribute to the development of CRF. The chronic compromise of the renal system occurs as the renal blood flow through the kidney causes loss of oxygen to the tissues and the eventual death of the nephrons. Although the pathophysiology of CRF has varying mechanisms that initiate the process (prerenal, intrarenal, or postrenal), it usually occurs as stages and reflects loss of renal regulatory functions. As renal function declines by 30–50%, a decrease in renal reserve occurs. Because serum creatinine levels usually do not begin to rise until 50% renal function is lost, this decrease in renal reserves is usually an asymptomatic stage as the remaining nephrons hypertrophy to compensate.

The next stage is renal insufficiency, which is characterized by electrolyte imbalances and an accumulation of nitrogen waste products in the bloodstream (azotemia) that manifests as an increase in blood urea nitrogen (BUN) and creatinine levels (Potts & Mandleco, 2007). Because the kidneys are the primary routes of potassium, sodium, and water excretion and this function is impaired, hyperkalemia, hypernatremia, and water retention result. Hyperkalemia places the child at risk for developing cardiac dysrhythmias. Hypernatremia and fluid retention lead to edema, congestive heart failure (CHF), and hypertension. Pulmonary edema can occur as the excess fluid third-spaces, or it can accompany the CHF. The activation of the renin-angiotensin complex causes an increase in aldosterone secretion that also increases the risk of hypertension. As a consequence of the inverse reciprocal relationship between calcium and phosphorous in the body, hypocalcemia results from hyperphosphatemia that occurs because of impairment in the kidney's inability to filter and excrete phosphorous. Normally, the renal system regulates the acid-base system by controlling the release of sodium bicarbonate. In the presence of decreased kidney function, the kidneys are unable to release sodium bicarbonate, resulting in metabolic acidosis. The kidneys also regulate erythropoietin, which is necessary for red blood cell production. The lack of erythropoietin is manifested as anemia as renal function declines. When anemia is combined with uremia, the child has an increased risk of experiencing gastrointestinal bleeding. Finally, as the nephrons continue to be destroyed, the child progresses to ESRD. At this point, manifestations are more severe, resulting in the need for dialysis or renal transplantation to sustain life. Because renal transplantation is highly successful in children, this is the ultimate goal of treatment.

Complications

Azotemia

Electrolyte imbalances (hyperkalemia, hypernatremia, hyperphosphatemia, and hypocalcemia)

Cardiac dysrhythmias

Pulmonary edema

Pleural effusion

Cardiac tamponade

Metabolic acidosis

Anemia

Uremia

ESRD

Death

Incidence

CRF in children is not as common as it is in adults. Approximately 150 cases of CRF per million people are newly diagnosed each year in the United States in the general population (Krause, 2006). In children aged 19 and under, the annual rate is only 1 or 2 new cases in every 100,000 children, with the incidence increasing with age. African Americans in their late teens are 3 times more likely than Caucasians in the same age group to develop kidney failure. CRF affects boys nearly twice as often as girls (National Kidney and Urologic Diseases Information Clearinghouse, 2006). Approximately 1 in every 65,000 children develops ESRD (Hatch & Agrawal, 2007). Renal transplantation is the treatment of choice in children. According to the Organ Procurement and Transplantation Network, as of March 14, 2008, over 15,000 pediatric kidney transplants have been performed since 1988, with the majority of recipients between the ages of 11 and 17 years of age. Over 100 kidney transplants have been performed on infants; 2,654 for children 1–5 years of age; 2,840 for children 6–10 years old; and 8,698 for individuals between 11 and 17 years of age (Organ Procurement and Transplantation Network, 2007). Eighteen and nineteen year olds are included in the data for the broader group of 18–34 year olds.

Etiology

The same conditions that cause acute renal failure (ARF) can result in CRF. Refer to Chapter 88: Renal Failure, Acute (ARF). In addition, hemolytic uremic syndrome; nephrotic syndrome; birth defects; and hereditary diseases such as polycystic kidney disease, glomerular diseases, and systemic diseases such as diabetes mellitus and lupus can result in CRF. From birth to age 14 years, birth defects and hereditary diseases are the leading causes of renal failure. Between ages 5 and 14 years, glomerular diseases become the second leading cause of CRF; and in the 15- to 19-year-old age group, glomerular diseases are the leading causes of CRF (National Kidney and Urologic Diseases Information Clearinghouse, 2006).

Clinical Manifestations

Oliguria

Anuria

Nocturia

Peripheral edema

Generalized edema

Numbness and tingling of extremities

Muscle twitching

Irritability

Decreased level of consciousness

Lethargy progressing to coma

Seizures

Nausea and vomiting

Ecchymosis

Pallor

Prolonged bleeding

Hypertension

Fatigue

Poor feeding

Tinnitus

Flank pain

Diagnostic Tests

Complete blood count

Serum electrolyte levels

Renal function tests

Urinalysis

Renal arteriography

Chest radiography

Bone scan

Renal ultrasound

Electrocardiogram

Renal biopsy

Abdominal computed tomography (CT)

Abdominal magnetic resonance imaging (MRI)

Prior to renal transplantation:

    Tissue typing

    Blood typing

    Antibody screening

    Antigen screening

Medical Management

Refer to Chapter 88: Renal Failure, Acute (ARF) for medical management of renal failure. The following discussion focuses on renal dialysis and transplantation.

Dialysis removes excess fluids and waste products and restores electrolyte and acid-base balance for the child experiencing renal failure; dialysis is necessary when the child has CRF or ESRD. Regardless of the type of dialysis, blood moves through dialysate fluid that is composed of glucose, water, sodium chloride, potassium, magnesium, calcium, and sodium bicarbonate. During the process of dialysis, the dialysate fluid draws the toxins and excess fluid out of the blood, after which the cleansed blood is returned to the body. The two types of dialysis are hemodialysis (HD) and peritoneal dialysis (PD).

For children, HD primarily is used as an emergency measure. It works by passing blood, through diffusion, through a semipermeable membrane to an external dialysis machine. An external vascular access designed specifically for HD is placed in the subclavian or internal jugular vessels for use in small children. For older children, the commonly used accesses are internally placed and are either an arteriovenous (AV) fistula or an AV graft. An AV fistula involves the surgical anastomosing of an artery and a vein under the skin. The increased blood volume enlarges the elastic vein, allowing a large volume of blood to flow through it. An AV fistula is more permanent but requires four to six weeks to engraft before it can be used for dialysis. An AV graft, created by suturing a piece of saphenous vein, bovine carotid artery, or synthetic graft to the child's own vessel, usually is used when the child's vessels are not suitable for the creation of an AV fistula.

HD is performed in a health care environment designed specifically for the treatment. Because of the risk of severe hypotension (a common complication of HD), the child's vital signs and weight are assessed and recorded prior to accessing the HD device. Once the HD device has been accessed, specimens are withdrawn for complete blood count and serum chemistry for baseline measurements. Once HD is initiated, toxins in the blood are drawn into the dialysate fluid through diffusion while water is removed from the blood by osmosis. The hydrostatic pressure that is set on the dialysis machine determines the amount of fluid drawn off the child. Potassium and sodium usually move out of the plasma into the dialysate while calcium and bicarbonate move from the dialysate into vascular plasma. The dialysate fluid is warmed as it moves through the dialyzer to facilitate diffusion and to prevent hypothermia. Hypotension occurs because of the large volume of blood moving through the dialyzer and fluid being withdrawn. Once the HD session is completed, which usually takes 2–4 hours, blood for laboratory testing is withdrawn, and the HD device is deaccessed. Although not frequently used for children because of the size of their vessels and the risk for hypotension, advantages of HD are (1) more efficient blood clearance and (2) less time needed for the procedure compared to PD. Disadvantages of HD include the fact that (1) it is a more complex procedure, (2) travel to a dialysis center is necessary for the procedure, (3) it is less convenient, and 4) vascular access care is required, including contraindications for having blood pressures and venous blood draws taken from the extremity where the access is placed (Broyles, 2005).

PD is most commonly used in children. Occurring within the peritoneal cavity, it is a process of diffusion and osmosis across a semipermeable membrane. However, with PD, the membrane is the peritoneal membrane, which is porous, large, and rich in capillaries to provide ample access to vascular supply. A silicone rubber catheter is surgically placed in the abdominal cavity through which dialysate is infused to draw out the waste products and excess fluid from the bloodstream. Dialysate fluid is infused by gravity into the abdominal cavity. The amount of each infusion depends on the size of the child and his/her tolerance. After the prescribed amount of dialysate is infused, it dwells in the peritoneal cavity for a prescribed time. Following the dwell period, the fluid, which now contains excess water, electrolytes, and nitrogen wastes, is drained by gravity out of the body into a drainage bag. This is repeated four or five times and is referred to as a PD exchange. Refer to Figure 89-1.

The amount of excess fluid removed is dependent on the concentration of the dialysate, and the number of exchanges is prescribed by the health care provider and based on laboratory values. Advantages to PD are the facts that (1) parents can perform it at home, (2) it is associated with fewer hemodynamic complications, and (3) it is a simpler process than HD. The disadvantages include that facts that it (1) is more time-consuming, (2) requires parents to learn meticulous PD catheter care, and (3) carries a high risk of infection (Broyles, 2005).

Renal transplantation is the replacing of a non-functioning kidney with a functional kidney from either a live donor or a cadaver. Transplantation is the life-sustaining therapy for children with ESRD. Although there is no age limitation for renal transplantation, most children are 2 years of age or older. Transplant donors must be free of metastatic disease. For children, most transplants are performed using live donors, usually a parent, a sibling, or another family member with immunologic similarity. The first two criteria for suitability of transplantation are that (1) blood typing must match and (2) human leukocyte antigens should match. These antigens are genetic markers located

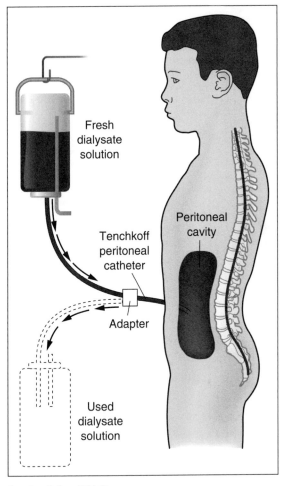

Figure 89-1: Peritoneal Dialysis.

on the surface of the leukocytes. A child inherits six antigens, a set of three from each parent. The more of these antigens that match with the donor kidney, the greater the viability of the transplanted kidney and the longer it remains viable (Broyles, 2005).

Prior to the transplant, a surgical team is organized that specializes in transplant surgery and includes circulating and scrub nurses, an anesthesiologist, clinical nurse specialists, transplant surgeons, and nephrologists. Dialysis is usually performed on the organ recipient within 24 hours prior to surgery. In addition, the child usually receives a transfusion of packed red blood cells, which, research indicates, increases the survival of the donor kidney, especially in live donor transplants. The dialysis access is maintained until sufficient renal function is established on the donor kidney postoperatively.

The donor kidney is harvested surgically, which in a live donor, can take up to 3–4 hours. A flank incision is performed to remove the donated kidney. For live donors, a new retrieval procedure involves small abdominal incisions similar to those used with laparoscopy. This allows faster donor recovery. Surgery to place the donor kidney in the recipient usually takes 4–5 hours because of the time required to anastomose the ureter and the renal artery and vein of the recipient to the donor kidney. Usually, the failed kidney is not removed because it poses no risk and allows for a smaller abdominal incision in the recipient. The donated kidney usually is situated in the right anterior iliac fossa for easier anastomosis. This positioning also facilitates assessment of tissue perfusion to the organ postoperatively. As soon as arterial access and perfusion is established to the donor kidney, evidence of renal function (urine production) becomes apparent. Following surgical closure, the child is transferred to the pediatric intensive care unit (PICU), where urine output is continuously monitored through an indwelling urinary catheter; in addition, hemodynamic stabilization can be established and maintained.

Two complications are associated with transplanting any organ. Organ rejection is prevented by postoperative administration of immunosuppressant therapy. Unfortunately, this causes the second complication, infection, which is the leading cause of death following organ transplantation. Among the common immunosuppressants are azathioprine (Imuran), prednisone, cyclosporine, monoclonal antibody (OKT-3), basiliximab (for children aged 2 and older), daclizumab (for children 11 months and older), and FK-506 (Broyles, Reiss, & Evans, 2007). Although the doses of these agents may be tapered off over time, lifelong anti-rejection drug therapy is necessary. This has dramatically reduced the incidence of rejection of donated kidneys. Cyclosporine has been the gold standard for immunosuppression therapy; however, it can be nephrotoxic. Cyclosporine stimulated the development of the other immunosuppressant agents used. Although it remains a constant agent used to prevent rejection, using combination therapy allows for a lower dosing of cyclosporine and a decrease in its nephrotoxicity (Broyles et al., 2007).

Renal graft or organ rejection, known as graft-versus-host disease (GVHD), occurs when the body's immune system attempts to destroy what it perceives as a foreign organ. This reaction can be life-threatening (Potts & Mandleco, 2007). Organ rejection is classified according to when the rejection occurs. Hyperacute rejection occurs within 24 hours following the transplant. Acute rejection usually happens within 3–14 days but may occur any time during the first year. Chronic rejection can take place many years following the transplant. Organ rejection leads to failure of the donated kidney and renewed need for dialysis. Most transplanted organs do not fail because of rejection but rather because of vascular thrombosis that interrupts tissue perfusion to the organ.

Nursing Management

Refer to Chapter 88: Renal Failure, Acute (ARF) for nursing management of renal failure and Chapter 100: Surgical Client.

ASSESSMENT

1. Obtain client history
2. Obtain vital signs, height, and weight
3. Assess for manifestations of infection related to PD
4. Assess for manifestations of decreased tissue perfusion during HD
5. Assess for manifestations of rejection
6. Assess for manifestations of infection
7. Assess renal perfusion by auscultating the renal artery through the abdomen
8. Assess wound for signs of healing or infection

NURSING DIAGNOSES (INCLUDING BUT NOT LIMITED TO)

1. Risk for infection R/T PD
2. Risk for impaired tissue perfusion R/T HD
3. Risk for injury, rejection R/T body's immune response to donor kidney

4. High risk for infection R/T immunosuppressant therapy
5. Risk for altered renal tissue perfusion R/T renal artery thrombosis or stenosis
6. Impaired skin integrity R/T surgical wound
7. Risk for injury R/T complications of immunosuppressant therapy
8. Anxiety (parental and child) R/T renal transplantation, life-long immunosuppressant therapy, and life-threatening complications of treatment
9. Deficient knowledge R/T child's condition, posttransplant care, immunosuppressant therapy, and home care.

PLANNING/GOALS

1. Client will not experience infection related to PD.
2. Client will not experience life-threatening hypotension related to HD.
3. Client will not experience rejection of transplanted kidney.
4. Client will not experience life-threatening infection secondary to immunosuppressant therapy.
5. Client will maintain adequate renal perfusion as evidenced by urine output, BUN, and creatinine within defined limits (WDL).
6. Client's wound will exhibit healing within 24 hours following surgery, with complete healing within six weeks of surgery.
7. Client will not experience complications of immunosuppressant therapy as evidenced by no manifestations of nephrotoxicity, gastrointestinal ulceration, or stomatitis.
8. Parents and client (if age-appropriate) will verbalize feelings and concerns and use positive coping strategies.
9. Parents and client (if age-appropriate) will demonstrate understanding of importance of compliance with posttransplant care, immunosuppressant therapy, and home care.

NOC

1. Infection Severity, Risk Control
2. Risk Control, Vital Signs
3. Risk Control, Renal Tissue Perfusion
4. Risk Control, Immune Status
5. Circulation Status
6. Skin Integrity
7. Risk Control
8. Anxiety
9. Knowledge: Illness Care, Treatment, Medications, Health Promotion

IMPLEMENTATION

1. Risk for infection
   a. Provide meticulous care for PD catheter
   b. Teach parents how to perform catheter care
   c. Monitor urine for cloudiness (first sign of infection)
   d. Monitor vital signs every 4 hours during hospitalization
   e. Reinforce information concerning how to perform PD at home
   f. Demonstrate procedure for PD and have parents provide return demonstrations until proficient
   g. Collaborate with health care provider to appropriate referrals

2. Risk for hypotension
   a. Obtain baseline vital signs and weight
   b. Withhold antihypertensive medication prior to HD
   c. Obtain laboratory specimens from HD device
   d. Flush HD device to determine patency
   e. Assess level of consciousness before, during, and after HD session
   f. Perform HD session, monitoring child continuously
   g. Obtain posthemodialysis laboratory specimens
   h. Flush and heparinize HD device
3. Risk for rejection
   a. Assess for signs of rejection including oliguria, edema, fever, increasing blood pressure, weight gain, swelling and tenderness over transplanted kidney, and increasing BUN and creatinine levels
   b. Monitor BUN and creatinine levels
   c. Monitor urine output and urine specific gravity hourly
   d. Monitor serum electrolyte levels
   e. Report immediately to health care provider abnormal findings indicating potential rejection
   f. Maintain patency of intravenous access, monitoring at least hourly
   g. Administer intravenous fluids as prescribed
   h. Administer immunosuppressants as prescribed
   i. Maintain patency of dialysis catheter/device
4. High risk for infection
   a. Maintain strict universal (standard) precautions
   b. Assess for signs of infection—fever
   c. Monitor vital signs at least every 4 hours
   d. Report temperature elevations immediately
   e. Monitor leukocyte/neutrophil count
   f. Administer antipyretics as prescribed, monitoring temperature 45 minutes after administration to assess effectiveness
   g. Maintain patency of intravenous access, monitoring at least hourly
   h. Administer antimicrobials as prescribed
   i. Monitor for signs of opportunistic infections (*Candida albicans,* Cytomegalovirus, and *Pneumococcus*)
   j. Monitor for manifestations of septicemia including shaking chills, fever, tachycardia, tachypnea, leukocytosis, or leukopenia
5. Renal perfusion
   a. Assess urine output hourly
   b. Monitor urine specific gravity
   c. Auscultate over renal artery every 4 hours for bruit
   d. Monitor BUN and creatinine level
   e. Monitor abdomen over transplant site for swelling and tenderness
   f. Monitor vital signs per unit protocol
   g. Monitor serum electrolyte levels
6. Skin integrity
   a. Assess wound for redness, swelling, tenderness, drainage, and incision approximation
   b. Perform wound care as prescribed

7. Complications of immunosuppressant therapy
   a. Monitor urine output hourly
   b. Monitor urine specific gravity
   c. Assess oral mucosa for evidence of candidiasis
   d. Administer nystatin "swish and swallow" or "swish and spit" as prescribed
   e. Administer prednisone and cyclosporine with food
   f. Administer proton pump inhibitors or histamine-2 antagonists as prescribed
   g. Monitor blood pressure every 4 hours
   h. Monitor cardiovascular function
8. Anxiety
   a. Encourage verbalization of feelings and concerns
   b. Listen actively
   c. Reinforce information provided by health care provider
   d. Explain all equipment and procedures
   e. Provide calm environment
   f. Assist in identifying positive coping strategies and support systems
   g. Encourage parental participation in child's care
   h. Engage child in age-appropriate activities consistent with level of stability
9. Parent/child teaching
   a. Assess current level of understanding
   b. Provide verbal and written instructions and demonstration of information regarding:
      1) PD
      2) HD
      3) Medication administration and importance of compliance with medications prescribed for CRF
      4) Importance of follow-up care with health care provider
      5) Postoperative renal transplantation instructions
      6) Immunosuppressant therapy and importance of compliance with medication
      7) Manifestations of organ rejection and infection and importance of reporting these manifestations to health care provider immediately
      8) Contact information for health care provider
      9) Referral information including local and national support groups
   c. Provide adequate time for demonstrations and return demonstration related to dialysis
   d. Provide adequate time for medication teaching
   e. Document teaching and parents'/child's response

NIC

1. Infection Precautions
2. Hemodynamic Monitoring, Vital Signs Monitoring
3. Infection Precautions
4. Risk Identification, Hemodynamic Monitoring
5. Risk Identification, Hemodynamic Monitoring

6. Wound Care
7. Risk Identification
8. Coping Enhancement
9. Teaching: Illness Care, Treatment, Medications, Health Education

EVALUATION

1. Client does not experience infection related to PD.
2. Client does not experience life-threatening hypotension related to HD.
3. Client does not experience rejection of transplanted kidney.
4. Client does not experience life-threatening infection secondary to immunosuppressant therapy.
5. Client maintains adequate renal perfusion as evidenced by urine output, BUN, and creatinine WDL.
6. Client's wound exhibits healing within 24 hours following surgery, with complete healing within six weeks of surgery.
7. Client does not experience complications of immunosuppressant therapy as evidenced by no manifestations of nephrotoxicity, gastrointestinal ulceration, or stomatitis.
8. Parents and client (if age-appropriate) verbalize feelings and concerns and use positive coping strategies.
9. Parents and client (if age-appropriate) demonstrate understanding of importance of compliance with posttransplant care, immunosuppressant therapy, and home care.

References

Broyles, B. E. (2005). *Medical-surgical nursing clinical companion.* Durham, NC: Carolina Academic Press.

Broyles, B. E., Reiss, B. S., & Evans, M. E. (2007). *Pharmacological aspects of nursing care* (7th ed.). Clifton Park, NY: Delmar Cengage Learning.

Hatch, D., & Agrawal, R. (2007). *Renal transplantation.* Retrieved March 18, 2008, from http://www.emedicine.com/ped/topic2842.htm

Krause, R. (2006). *Renal failure, chronic and dialysis complications.* Retrieved March 18, 2008, from http://www.emedicine.com/emerg/topic501.htm

National Kidney and Urologic Diseases Information Clearinghouse. (2006). *Overview of kidney diseases in children.* Retrieved July 9, 2007, from http://kidney.niddk.nih.gov/kudiseases/pubs/childkidneydiseases/overview/index.htm

Organ Procurement and Transplantation Network. (2008). *Transplants in the U.S. by recipient age.* Retrieved March 18, 2008, from http://www.optn.org/latestData/rptData.asp

Potts, N. L., & Mandleco, B. L. (2007). *Pediatric nursing: Caring for children and their families* (2nd ed.). Clifton Park, NY: Delmar Cengage Learning.

90

RESPIRATORY DISTRESS SYNDROME (RDS)/MECHANICAL VENTILATION

Definition

Respiratory distress syndrome (RDS), also known as hyaline membrane disease, is a condition common in neonates born less than 28 weeks' gestation and characterized by hypoxia. It is a medical emergency.

Pathophysiology

Hyaline membranes line the alveoli and develop within 30 minutes after birth; and by 36–72 hours following birth, surfactant begins to be synthesized (Pramanik, 2006). Surfactant, made by the cells in the airways, consists of phospholipids and protein. It begins to be produced in the fetus at about 24–28 weeks of pregnancy. Surfactant is found in amniotic fluid between 28 and 32 weeks. By about 36 weeks' gestation, most neonates have developed sufficient amounts of surfactant to maintain functional alveoli. In premature or preterm infants born prior to 36 weeks, the lungs lack enough surfactant to keep the alveoli from collapsing. Diffuse atelectasis of distal air spaces and distension of distal airways and perilymphatic areas occur in RDS, leading to impaired gas exchange, hypoxia, and cyanosis. Immediate oxygen administration and frequently the use of mechanical ventilation are required for survival (Potts & Mandleco, 2007). Metabolic acidosis results from increased levels of lactic acid, the by-product of anaerobic cellular metabolism stimulated by tissue hypoperfusion.

The treatment for RDS (oxygen administration and mechanical ventilation) can cause trauma to the pulmonary structures, leading to the inflammatory response. This leads to interstitial edema and destruction of pulmonary epithelium. "Hyperinflation, atelectasis, and tissue fibrosis result" (Potts & Mandleco, 2007, p. 743). There is an imbalance in the ventilation-perfusion ratio and a right-to-left shunt resulting in hypercapnea and hypoxemia and increased workload on the heart.

NOTE: Respiratory distress or failure can occur in children between the ages of 2 months and 21 years and is termed *acute respiratory distress syndrome,* or *ARDS*. ARDS occurs in approximately 1–4% of children admitted to pediatric intensive care units. ARDS can occur due to chronic respiratory disease such as cystic fibrosis or muscular dystrophy or as a result of chest trauma, inhalation injuries, tumor necrosis factor, sepsis, or septic shock (Feng & Steele, 2007). ARDS in the adult population is termed *adult respiratory distress syndrome.*

Complications

Impaired gas exchange
Metabolic acidosis
Hypoxemia
Respiratory failure
Hypoxemia
Death

Incidence

RDS occurs in approximately 20,000–30,000 infants each year in the United States. It is a complication in about 1% of pregnancies (Pramanik, 2006). RDS affects approximately 10% of all premature infants (MedlinePlus, 2007). The more preterm the neonate is, the more at risk the infant is for RDS. RDS occurs in over 50% of neonates born before 28 weeks' gestation but in less than 33% of those born between 32 and 36 weeks (Lucile Packard Children's Hospital at Stanford, 2008).

Etiology

For neonates born prior to 36 weeks, the most common cause of RDS is lack of sufficient surfactant to keep alveoli open to exchange gases. Infants at greatest risk include Caucasian male infants, infants born to mothers with diabetes, infants born by cesarean section, the second infant of twins, and infants with a family history of RDS (Pramanik, 2006).

Clinical Manifestations

Tachypnea
Expiratory grunting (from partial closure of glottis)
Subcostal and intercostal retractions
Cyanosis
Nasal flaring
Apnea
Hypothermia

Diagnostic Tests

Arterial blood gases
Pulse oximetry
Chest radiography
Echocardiography
Pulmonary mechanics testing (PMT)

Medical Management

The goals of treatment are to provide ventilatory support, promote tissue perfusion, and resolve the RDS with surfactant replacement. Early identification of neonates at risk for RDS and the prevention of complications are the first steps in protecting these tiny clients. Following delivery, neonates less than 28 weeks' gestation should be given immediate resuscitation provided by a neonatologist experienced in resuscitating premature neonates. An arterial line is placed in the umbilical artery (umbilical artery catheterization), and a vascular access is established to provide fluids and pharmacological agents to support the cardiopulmonary effort.

Surfactant replacement therapy should be initiated as soon as possible. Research has shown that the early provision of surfactant replacement decreases pulmonary air leaks and chronic lung disease. In addition, it allows for decreased time that these infants must be on mechanical ventilation. Prolonging mechanical ventilation increases the risk of the infant developing bronchopulmonary dysplasia (refer to Chapter 17: Bronchopulmonary Dysplasia [BPD]), risk for pulmonary infection, and oxygen dependency. Pulmonary infections can occur as soon as 24 hours following intubation and placement on mechanical ventilation. "Neonates with RDS who require assisted ventilation with a fraction of inspiratory oxygen (FIO_2) of > 0.40 should receive intratracheal surfactant as soon as possible, preferably within 2 hours after birth. . . . Recommended dosages of clinically available surfactant preparations are 50–200 mg/kg, approximately the surfactant pool of term newborn lungs" (Pramanik, 2006, p. 6).

Tracheal intubation or a tracheostomy is performed to provide an access for mechanical ventilation. The mechanical ventilation modes for neonates with RDS are positive end-expiratory pressure (PEEP) for the delivery of the surfactant therapy, synchronized intermittent mandatory ventilation (SIMV), assist-control ventilation, high-frequency ventilation (HFV), high-frequency oscillatory ventilation (HFOV), and continuous positive airway pressure (CPAP). Oxygen is administered through the mechanical ventilator. Early surfactant therapy can provide for rapid extubation and the administration of CPAP via nasal prongs or face masks after extubation.

The following is a general discussion about mechanical ventilation. The most frequently used are positive pressure ventilator settings, which apply positive pressure in the airway during inspiration to provide positive intrathoracic pressure to expand the lungs. The chest and lungs then recoil naturally, and the airway pressure returns to normal as the flow of oxygen stops. There are five types of positive pressure ventilation (PPV) systems: time-cycled, volume-cycled, pressure-cycled, HFV, and volumetric diffusion ventilation.

Time-cycled PPV delivers inspiratory flow over a specific preset time with variable airway pressures and tidal volumes. This is the most frequent type used for neonates and children. Volume-cycled PPV delivers inspiratory flow until a preset volume is established. Airway pressures vary depending on airway resistance and lung compliance. This type of ventilation can lead to barotrauma. Pressure-cycled PPV delivers inspiratory flow until a preset pressure is met. Tidal volumes vary depending on airway resistance and lung compliance. The disadvantage of this type of ventilation is that it may result in hypoventilation or hyperventilation.

A type of ventilation commonly used in neonates with RDS is HFV or jet ventilation. It delivers small tidal volumes (less than the anatomic dead space) at rapid frequencies or at high respiratory rates. It allows for lower pressures and decreases problems associated with venous return. Volumetric diffusion ventilation and HFOV deliver an inspiratory flow based on predetermined inspiratory and expiratory times with the added benefit of an oscillating action.

The settings on mechanical ventilators include the FIO_2 setting, which represents the fraction of inspired oxygen or concentration of oxygen the child is to receive. Peak inspiratory pressure, or PIP, is the maximum pressure reached at the end of the inspiratory cycle and should be less than 40. The I:E ratio, inspiratory to expiratory ratio, is a comparison of inspiratory time to expiratory time. Tidal volume is the amount of air the ventilator delivers to the child with each ventilator breath. Tidal volume is determined by multiplying the child's weight in kilograms by 10–15 mL. The respiratory rate setting is the number of positive-pressure breaths the ventilator delivers per minute (Broyles, 2005).

Mechanical ventilation can be set for a variety of modes. These are the mechanisms that end expiration and signal the beginning of inspiration. The objective is to graduate the client from the highest mode required to maintain ventilation during the acute phase of the condition to the least mechanical ventilation mode as the client's respiratory status improves.

Control mode ventilation (CMV) refers to continuous mandatory ventilation that involves a preset tidal volume and a preset rate regardless of the client's respiratory effort. The client cannot initiate a breath or change the ventilatory pattern, and CMV usually requires sedation with fentanyl to prevent the client from exerting energy "fighting the ventilator." It is used to treat chest trauma and chemical overdose and commonly is employed during anesthesia.

Assist/controlled ventilation mode (ACV) has the tidal volume and respiratory rate set in the ventilation but allows the client to trigger breathing. This mode senses the negative inspiratory force from the client and delivers the present tidal volumes. It decreases the work of breathing and respiratory muscle fatigue since the client need only initiate the breath. It is used to treat muscular dystrophy, flail chest, and other conditions in which the client has a normal respiratory drive but weak musculature. Because of the risk of hyperventilation with ACV, sedation may be required to reduce spontaneous breaths.

Intermittent mandatory ventilation (IMV) mode is set for a minimum of six-plus respirations. The client receives six (or so) breaths from the ventilator and breathes normally the rest of the time. This allows the client to breathe spontaneously between ventilator breaths; however, the ventilator delivers a predetermined number of breaths per minute regardless of the client's inspiratory effort. This mode is used with clients who have impaired ventilatory drive, such as those with apneic spells. However, it is not appropriate for neonates with RDS.

SIMV is a version of IMV that synchronizes the ventilator breath with the child's spontaneous breath. The child is able to breathe at his/her own rate and tidal volume. SIMV senses when the child does not initiate a breath and delivers one. This mode uses the child's own respiratory pattern but is preset so that the breaths are timed to pressure air into the child's lungs during inhalation. This requires the child to have spontaneous respiratory effort and is used in RDS infants after successful surfactant replacement therapy prior to weaning them from mechanical ventilation and initiating intranasal CPAP.

PPV provides positive pressure in response to the client's spontaneous inspiratory breath that augments the client's tidal volume and reduces the effort of breathing. This mode is indicated for clients with adequate respiratory drives but who become easily fatigued with the effort of breathing.

Finally, with the CPAP mode, positive airway pressure is maintained during the entire respiratory cycle, not just during expiration (as with PEEP). It is the mode used for weaning clients from other ventilatory modes, for neonates recovering from acute RDS, and for children and adults with obstructive sleep apnea.

In addition to surfactant replacement therapy and mechanical ventilation, these neonates require supportive therapy including temperature regulation, fluid therapy, return of acid-base balance, and nutritional support. Hypothermia increases oxygen consumption, causing additional compromise to the preterm neonates with RDS. Neutral thermal environment can be provided by the use of a radiant warmer or a double-walled isolette. Intravenous therapy involves the intravenous administration of 5% or 10% dextrose at a rate of 60–80 mL/kg/24 hr. These infants must be monitored carefully, including blood glucose, electrolytes, calcium, and phosphorous levels, as well as renal function and hydration. Gradually, fluid intake should be increased for adequate hydration at a rate of 120–140 mL/kg/day; however, extremely premature infants may require fluid intake of 200–300 mL/kg or more because of insensible water loss occurring from their body surfaces (Pramanik, 2006).

As soon as the neonate is stable, total parenteral nutrition (TPN) should be initiated within 24–48 hours after birth. As soon as the infant can tolerate enteral feedings, they should be resumed as frequent small feedings given per gastrostomy tube or orogastric tube (inserted through the mouth to the stomach for each feeding and then removed after each feeding) because of the energy required for sucking. A pacifier should be used to provide for the infant's sucking need. Enteral feedings are increased as tolerated; then oral feedings are initiated, providing for a given amount to be administered orally and the rest of the feeding finished through the enteral tube.

Circulation should be monitored using a cardiorespiratory monitor, vital signs, and peripheral pressure monitoring. The administration of blood products and volume-expanding intravenous fluids in addition to vasopressor agents is to treat anemia and support cardiovascular function. The immune system of a preterm infant is very immature; and with the presence of invasive lines and procedures, these infants are extremely susceptible to opportunistic pathogens. Blood cultures, a complete blood count with differential, and C-reactive protein levels are obtained; then the infant is prescribed antibiotic therapy. The antibiotics are continued until the blood cultures are negative for three consecutive days.

RDS causes stress and uncertainty for the infant's parents and family, so supportive mechanisms must be provided for these individuals. Among the techniques used are keeping the parents informed of the infant's condition, answering questions, providing referrals to community agencies, and encouraging the parents to visit the neonate as often as possible and to provide care when conditions allow.

Nursing Management

ASSESSMENT

1. Assess neonates at risk for manifestations of RDS
2. Assess airway, breathing, and circulation
3. Perform rapid physical assessment
4. Assess parents for psychosocial impact of preterm birth and presence of RDS

NURSING DIAGNOSES (INCLUDING BUT NOT LIMITED TO)

1. Impaired gas exchange and ineffective breathing pattern R/T immaturity of pulmonary system and insufficient surfactant
2. Ineffective thermoregulation R/T immaturity of regulating systems
3. Impaired tissue perfusion R/T respiratory status
4. Imbalanced nutrition: less than body requirements R/T decreased intake, fatigue
5. Risk for infection R/T invasive lines, mechanical ventilation, decreased immune status, altered nutrition
6. Deficient fluid volume R/T insensible fluid losses and decreased intake
7. Delayed growth and development R/T preterm birth
8. Anxiety (parental) R/T criticality of infant's condition, prognosis, and ability to care for ill child
9. Deficient knowledge R/T infant's condition, treatment, and home care

PLANNING/GOALS

1. Client will regain and maintain adequate gas exchange as evidenced by serum pH, $PaCO_2$, PaO_2, bicarbonate level, oxygen saturation, respiratory effort, and breathing pattern within defined limits (WDL) for age.
2. Client will regain and maintain thermoregulation as evidenced by body temperature WDL.
3. Client will regain and maintain adequate tissue perfusion as evidenced by arterial blood gases, capillary refill, skin color and hydration, and body temperature WDL.
4. Client will regain and maintain adequate nutrition as evidenced by reaching weight gain milestones.
5. Client will not experience infection.
6. Client will regain and maintain fluid, electrolyte, and acid-base balance as evidenced by urine output 1–2 mL/kg/hr and electrolyte levels and arterial blood gases WDL.
7. Child will achieve growth and development milestones.
8. Parents will verbalize feelings and concerns and use positive coping strategies.
9. Parents will demonstrate understanding of infant's condition, treatment, and home care.

NOC

1. Respiratory Status: Gas Exchange
2. Thermoregulation
3. Respiratory Status: Gas Exchange
4. Nutritional Status
5. Immune Status
6. Fluid Balance
7. Child Development
8. Anxiety
9. Knowledge: Illness Care, Treatment, Infant Care, Health Promotion

IMPLEMENTATION

1. Gas exchange and breathing pattern
   a. Assess respiratory status continuously
   b. Assist with transfer to neonatal intensive care unit (NICU)
   c. Place on continuous cardiorespiratory monitoring
   d. Place on continuous pulse oximetry
   e. Assist with insertion of arterial lines
   f. Establish and maintain intravenous access device, monitoring at least hourly
   g. Administer oxygen as prescribed
   h. Assist with establishment of artificial airway (endotracheal tube or tracheostomy)
   i. Assist with administration of surfactant replacement therapy
   j. Assist with placement on mechanical ventilation
   k. Collaborate with health care provider and respiratory therapist for ventilator settings
   l. Maintain mechanical ventilator settings
   m. Suction as needed to control secretions
   n. Monitor arterial blood gases
   o. Provide respiratory monitoring consistent with neonate's condition
2. Thermoregulation
   a. Measure continuous body temperature with use of skin probes
   b. Place on radiant warmer or in isolette
   c. Maintain neutral temperature environment
   d. Avoid drafts
   e. Wipe vernix and amniotic fluid from neonate's head and place neonatal cap on infant
   f. Wipe rest of body and wrap in warm blankets in mummy wrap after determination that body temperature is stable
3. Tissue perfusion
   a. Monitor arterial blood gases
   b. Monitor cardiopulmonary status
   c. Maintain continuous hemodynamic monitoring
   d. Maintain continuous pulse oximetry
   e. Maintain ventilator settings as prescribed and per neonate's condition
4. Nutrition
   a. Monitor strict intake and output

    b. Monitor daily weight

    c. Initiate TPN as prescribed, providing meticulous care of central venous catheter for TPN administrations, infusing intravenous fluids, and obtaining laboratory specimens

    d. Initiate enteral feedings as prescribed

    e. Increase oral intake gradually as tolerated

    f. Encourage breastfeeding

    g. Provide support for breastfeeding parent

    h. Provide pacifier to meet infant's sucking needs

5. Risk for infection

    a. Assess continuous body temperature with skin probe

    b. Provide for neutral thermal environment

    c. Assess invasive lines for indications of infection

    d. Maintain strict asepsis during care and maintain invasive lines

    e. Administer antibiotics as prescribed

    f. Monitor continuous pulse and respiratory rate via cardiorespiratory monitor

    g. Monitor continuous pulse oximetry

    h. Assist with weaning from the ventilator as soon as neonate's condition allows.

6. Fluid and electrolyte balance

    a. Monitor strict intake and output

    b. Assess skin and mucous membranes for indications of hydration

    c. Assess fontanels for manifestations of hydration

    d. Weigh diapers for accurate output

    e. Maintain intravenous access device, monitoring at least hourly

    f. Administer intravenous fluids as prescribed

    g. Maintain ventilator settings to decrease insensible fluid loss

    h. Monitor serum electrolytes

    i. Monitor arterial blood gases

7. Growth and development

    a. Assess developmental status at each clinic visit

    b. Provide information to parents about how to enhance growth and development

    c. Instruct parents about developmentally appropriate activities as child grows

    d. Support parents by providing information that most preterm infants "catch up" with their same-age full-term counterparts prior to preschool

8. Parental anxiety

    a. Encourage parents to verbalize their feelings and concerns

    b. Keep parents informed of infant's condition

    c. Assist parents in identifying positive coping strategies and support systems

    d. Collaborate with health care provider for social services referral

    e. Encourage parents to visit infant in intensive care

    f. Encourage parental participation in infant's care as condition allows

    g. Encourage parents to provide light tactile stimulation for infant and to talk to infant

9. Parent teaching
   a. Assess current level of understanding
   b. Provide verbal and written instructions and demonstration for information regarding:
      1) Infant's long-term care in hospital
      2) Infant's care and feeding at home
      3) Medication administration as needed
      4) Referral information and contact numbers
      5) Functioning of auditory infant monitor
      6) Infant cardiopulmonary resuscitation
      7) Functioning of infant's cardiorespiratory monitor if discharged with one
      8) Manifestations of respiratory compromise to report to health care provider immediately
      9) Contact numbers for health care provider and other services
      10) Importance of follow-up with health care provider
   c. Provide adequate time for teaching and demonstration of skills as well as time for return demonstrations
   d. Document teaching and parental response

NIC

1. Acid-Base Monitoring, Oxygen Therapy, Ventilatory Support, Respiratory Monitoring
2. Temperature Regulation
3. Acid-Base Monitoring, Oxygen Therapy, Ventilatory Support, Respiratory Monitoring
4. Nutritional Management
5. Infection Precautions
6. Fluid Monitoring, Fluid Management
7. Developmental Enhancement: Child, Newborn Care, Nutritional Monitoring
8. Coping Enhancement
9. Teaching: Illness Care, Treatment, Infant Care, Health Education

EVALUATION

1. Client regains and maintains adequate gas exchange as evidenced by serum pH, $PaCO_2$, PaO_2, bicarbonate level, oxygen saturation, respiratory effort, and breathing pattern WDL for age.
2. Client regains and maintains thermoregulation as evidenced by body temperature WDL.
3. Client regains and maintains adequate tissue perfusion as evidenced by arterial blood gases, capillary refill, skin color and hydration, and body temperature WDL.
4. Client regains and maintains adequate nutrition as evidenced by reaching weight gain milestones.
5. Client does not experience infection.
6. Client regains and maintains fluid, electrolyte, and acid-base balance as evidenced by urine output 1–2 mL/kg/hr and electrolyte levels and arterial blood gases WDL.
7. Child achieves growth and development milestones.

8. Parents verbalize feelings and concerns and use positive coping strategies.
9. Parents demonstrate understanding of infant's condition, treatment, and home care.

References

Broyles, B. E. (2005). *Medical-surgical nursing clinical companion.* Durham, NC: Carolina Academic Press.

Feng, A., & Steele, D. (2007). *Pediatrics, respiratory distress syndrome.* Retrieved March 18, 2008, at http://www.emedicine.com/EMERG/topic398.htm

Lucile Packard Children's Hospital at Stanford. (2008). *High-risk newborn: Hyaline membrane disease/respiratory distress syndrome.* Retrieved March 18, 2008, from http://www.lpch.org/DiseaseHealthInfo/HealthLibrary/hrnewborn/hmd.html

MedlinePlus. (2007). *Respiratory distress syndrome (RDS) in infants.* Retrieved March 18, 2008, from http://www.nlm.nih.gov/medlineplus/ency/article/001563.htm

Potts, N. L., & Mandleco, B. L. (2007). *Pediatric nursing: Caring for children and their families* (2nd ed.). Clifton Park, NY: Delmar Cengage Learning.

Pramanik, A. K. (2006). *Respiratory distress syndrome.* Retrieved March 18, 2008, from http://www.emedicine.com/ped/topic1993.htm

91

REYE SYNDROME

Definition

Reye syndrome (also termed Reye's syndrome) is a disease that affects all body systems but is most lethal to the brain and liver (National Reye's Syndrome Foundation, 2008). It involves an acute life-threatening noninflammatory encephalopathy accompanied by fatty degeneration of the liver and kidney (Potts & Mandleco, 2007).

Pathophysiology

Reye syndrome was first described by R. D. K. Reye in 1963 as an entity specific to Australia. G. M. Johnson described the same disease in the United States a few months later (Weiner, 2005). Reye syndrome is considered a two-phase process because it generally follows a viral infection most commonly associated with influenza or chickenpox. It usually occurs during the recovery phase of the viral infection, although it can develop three to five days after the onset of the viral illness (National Institute of Neurological Disorders and Stroke, 2007). Although it affects all organs of the body, the most predominant involvement is in the brain and liver, resulting in life-threatening encephalopathy and fatty metamorphosis or a more than threefold increase in alanine aminotransferase (ALT), aspartate aminotransferase (AST), and/or ammonia levels in the liver. The other organs of concern affected by the accumulation of fat deposits are the kidneys.

The encephalopathy is noninflammatory but involves a rapid increase in intracranial pressure from cerebral edema that poses a life-threatening situation. The recovery from Reye syndrome is directly related to the amount of cerebral edema and the brain damage resulting from it. If treatment is not instituted early or is unsuccessful, varying degrees of brain damage can occur, including death. Refer to Chapter 61: Increased Intracranial Pressure (ICP) and Chapter 14: Biliary Atresia/Liver Transplantation, which discusses liver failure.

Complications

Increased intracranial pressure
Cerebral tissue anoxia
Brain damage
Liver failure
Death

Incidence

With the dramatic decrease in the use of salicylates in children and the use of vaccines to prevent influenza and varicella infections, Reye syndrome has become a rare condition since its peak in 1980. The incidence in the United States currently is < 0.03–1 case per 100,000 children under the age of 18 years, although it increases to as many as 6 cases per 100,000 during regional viral epidemics (Weiner, 2005). It occurs most commonly in children between the ages of 4 and 12 years (American Liver Foundation, 2007).

Etiology

Although the exact cause of Reye syndrome shows no consensus in the literature, certain factors associated with its development have been universally identified. Among these are viral infections especially caused by influenza B, influenza A, and varicella-zoster virus; exposure to toxins such as insecticides, herbicides, aflatoxins, paint, paint thinner, hepatotoxic mushrooms, hypoglycin in ackee fruit, and margosa oil; and use of salicylates, paracetamol, outdated tetracycline, valproic acid, zidovudine, didanosine, and antiemetics in children (Weiner, 2005).

Clinical Manifestations

Previous viral infection

Previous use of salicylates during viral infection

Persistent or recurrent vomiting (although not in infants)

Listlessness

Irritability or combativeness

Seizures

Changes in level of consciousness

Coma

Diagnostic Tests

Serum electrolytes

Liver function tests

Coagulation studies

Glutamine, alanine, and lysine levels

Computed tomography of the head

Electroencephalography

Lumbar puncture with cerebrospinal fluid analysis

Medical Management

There is no cure for Reye syndrome; but the goals of treatment are to prevent irreversible neurologic damage by reducing increased intracranial pressure, reversing the metabolic injury, preventing complications in the lungs, and anticipating cardiac arrest (National Institute of Neurological Disorders and Stroke, 2007; American Liver Foundation, 2007). The neurologic recovery depends on early diagnosis and control of intracranial pressure. Refer to Chapter 61: Increased Intracranial Pressure (ICP). The Centers for Disease Control and Prevention (CDC) recommend that all children aged 6 months to 8 years receive vaccinations against influenza as the best method for preventing the development of Reye syndrome (Centers for Disease Control and Prevention, 2007).

Nursing Management

Refer to Nursing Management in Chapter 61: Increased Intracranial Pressure (ICP)

ASSESSMENT

1. Obtain client history including immunization history and use of salicylates
2. Assess parental knowledge of current immunization schedule from the CDC and use of medications by child

NURSING DIAGNOSES (INCLUDING BUT NOT LIMITED TO)

1. Deficient knowledge R/T prevention of Reye syndrome and importance of reporting neurologic changes to health care provider immediately

PLANNING/GOALS

1. Parents will demonstrate understanding of the most effective mechanisms for preventing Reye syndrome and the importance of seeking immediate medical assistance if their child experiences neurologic changes. Child does not experience Reye syndrome.

NOC

1. Knowledge: Health Promotion

IMPLEMENTATION

1. Parent teaching
   a. Assess current level of understanding
   b. Provide verbal and written information regarding:
      1) Current recommended immunization schedule from the CDC
      2) Importance of maintaining current immunizations
      3) Necessity of avoiding use of salicylates in children; acetaminophen is an excellent antipyretic and analgesic for mild pain without the risks associated with salicylates
      4) Manifestations of neurologic changes that should be reported to health care provider immediately
      5) Contact information for health care provider
      6) Importance of routine well-child visits with health care provider
   c. Provide adequate time for teaching
   d. Document teaching and parental response

NIC

1. Teaching: Health Education

EVALUATION

1. Parents demonstrate understanding of the most effective mechanisms for preventing Reye syndrome and the importance of seeking immediate medical assistance if their child experiences neurologic changes. Child does not experience Reye syndrome.

References

American Liver Foundation. (2007). *Reye syndrome.* Retrieved July 10, 2007, from http://www.liverfoundation.org/education/info/reye

Centers for Disease Control and Prevention. (2007). *Vaccines for children's program: Influenza.* Retrieved July 10, 2007, from http://www.cdc.gov/vaccines/pubs/surv-manual/downloads/chpt05_influenza.pdf

National Institute of Neurological Disorders and Stroke. (2007). *NINDS Reye's syndrome information page.* Retrieved April 17, 2007, from http://www.ninds.nih.gov/disorders/reyes_syndrome/reyes_syndrome.htm

National Reye's Syndrome Foundation, Inc. (2008). *What is Reye's syndrome?* Retrieved April 16, 2008, from http://www.reyessyndrome.org/what.htm

Potts, N. L., & Mandleco, B. L. (2007). *Pediatric nursing: Caring for children and their families* (2nd ed.). Clifton Park, NY: Delmar Cengage Learning.

Weiner, D. (2005). *Pediatrics, Reye syndrome.* Retrieved March 18, 2008, from http://www.emedicine.com/emerg/topic399.htm

92

RHABDOMYOSARCOMA

Definition

Rhabdomyosarcoma is a rapidly growing malignancy of the skeletal muscle or striated tissue that most often occurs periorbitally in the head and neck in younger children and in the trunk and extremities of older children (Potts & Mandleco, 2007).

Pathophysiology

Skeletal muscles first begin to develop during approximately the seventh week of gestation. At this time, embryonic rhabdomyoblasts (cells that eventually form voluntary and skeletal muscles) begin to form and can become malignant, eventually developing into rhabdomyosarcoma (Potts & Mandleco, 2007). As a result of its embryonic development, rhabdomyosarcoma occurs most frequently in younger children (American Cancer Society, 2007). The major sites affected by rhabdomyosarcoma are in the head and neck; around the eyes (35–40%); in the genitourinary tract (20%); in the extremities (15–20%); and in the trunk, chest, and lungs (10–15%) (National Cancer Institute, 2008).

Over 85% of rhabdomyosarcomas occur in infants, children, and teenagers (American Cancer Society, 2007). Two primary types of rhabdomyosarcomas occur in children: embryonal and alveolar. Embryonal rhabdomyosarcoma is the most common type and tends to occur in the head and neck area, bladder, and vagina and in or around the prostate and testes. It usually affects infants and young children. Cells of embryonal rhabdomyosarcomas resemble the developing muscle cells of a 6- to 8-week-old fetus. Two variants of this type, botryoid and spindle cell rhabdomyosarcomas, tend to have a better prognosis than the more common forms.

Alveolar rhabdomyosarcoma occurs more often in large muscles of the trunk, arms, and legs and most often affects older children and teenagers. It is termed *alveolar* because the malignant cells form little hollow spaces, or alveoli. Alveolar rhabdomyosarcoma cells resemble the normal muscle cells seen in a 10-week-old fetus (American Cancer Society, 2007).

As with other cancers, rhabdomyosarcoma is grouped and staged according to the extent of disease. According to the American Cancer Society, the following is a summary of this grouping:

Group I: Children with localized disease (no metastasis) that is completely removed by surgery, with no spread to nearby lymph nodes. This stage involves 10–20% of children with rhabdomyosarcoma.

Group II: Approximately 20% of the children with rhabdomyosarcoma are in Group II. This group is divided into 3 subgroups:

Group IIA: Surgery has removed all of the cancer cells visible to the surgeon. However, pathology has found a small number of cancer cells on the periphery of the removed specimen. This group has no spread to nearby lymph nodes or to any other area.

Group IIB: All of the cancer has been removed, but cancer cells have been found in nearby lymph nodes that have been removed.

Group IIC: Children in this group have had all of the cancer visible to the surgeon removed, but cancer cells have been found on the periphery of the removed specimen and in nearby lymph nodes that have been removed.

Group III: These children have tumors that cannot be completely resected, there is no evidence of metastasis, and about half of children with rhabdomyosarcoma are in this group.

Group IV: These children have evidence of distant metastasis at the time of diagnosis, and this group contains approximately 15–20% of children with rhabdomyosarcoma. Rhabdomyosarcoma can metastasize to the lungs, bones, and bone marrow.

Staging of rhabdomyosarcoma is based on the histologic type and size of the tumor, its metastasis to the lymph nodes and distant organs, and its location of origination. Staging is based on the T, N, and M characteristics, which are then combined to determine an overall stage.

Stage 1: Tumor involving the orbit (area near the eye), head, and neck area except for parameningeal sites or genitourinary tract tumors except bladder and prostate. It can be any size and may have spread to nearby lymph nodes, but not to distant sites.

Stage 2: Tumor arising in bladder/prostate, parameningeal area, and other sites not mentioned in stage 1. The tumor must be smaller than 5 cm with no evidence of metastasis.

Stage 3: Tumor arising in bladder/prostate, parameningeal area, arms or legs, and other sites not mentioned in stage 1. The tumor is smaller than 5 cm (about 2 in.) but has metastasized to nearby lymph nodes, or the tumor is larger than 5 cm and may or may not have spread to nearby lymph nodes. In either case, the cancer has not spread to distant sites.

Stage 4: The tumor has metastasized to distant sites such as the lungs, bones, or bone marrow. This can be any size or site of primary tumor.

(Adapted from American Cancer Society, 2007)

Complications

Metastasis

Tumor location not conducive to surgical resection

Complications related to chemotherapy

Complications associated with radiation therapy

Incidence

Rhabdomyosarcoma accounts for about 3% of childhood cancers, and approximately 350 new cases of rhabdomyosarcoma occur annually in the United States. This makes rhabdomyosarcoma the most common type of sarcoma occurring in the soft tissues of children. It is the sixth most common cancer in children. Over 90% of rhabdomyosarcomas are diagnosed in individuals under 25 years old, and approximately 60% are diagnosed in children under the age of 10. Overall, over 65% of children with rhabdomyosarcoma will achieve cure status with proper treatment. Younger children (excluding infants) have a better prognosis than older ones (American Cancer Society, 2007).

Etiology

Most cases of rhabdomyosarcoma occur sporadically with no recognized predisposing factor or risk factor. Recent research suggests that embryonal rhabdomyosarcoma may be caused by a lack of a piece of the DNA from chromosome 11. This piece of DNA contains two different genes that prevent overgrowth. The absence of these genes may contribute to cancer formation. In addition, heredity may play a role in the development of alveolar rhabdomyosarcoma because the incidence is higher in certain rare hereditary diseases (National Cancer Institute, 2008).

Clinical Manifestations

- Dependent on tumor location
- Palpable but painless mass
- Periorbital edema
- Ptosis
- Nasal obstruction
- Epistaxis
- Earache or sinus infection
- Genitourinary manifestations
- Vomiting
- Abdominal pain
- Constipation

Diagnostic Tests

- Chest radiography
- Computed tomography
- Magnetic resonance imaging
- Biopsy
- Positron emission tomography (PET or PET scan)

Medical Management

The goal of treatment is complete cure. Treatment involves a multifocal approach with surgical resection of the tumor and chemotherapy and radiation therapy to destroy any residual cells. Refer to Chapter 100: Surgical Client.

The primary antineoplastic agents used in the treatment of embryonal rhabdomyosarcoma that has been completely removed by surgery include vincristine and dactinomycin. Cyclophosphamide usually is included for alveolar rhabdomyosarcoma. This regimen is referred to as VAC (National Cancer Institute, 2008). Topotecan and melphalan may be added to this regimen as well (MedlinePlus, 2006). Other agents used, particularly in Europe, are ifosfamide, etoposide, and doxorubicin. Radiation therapy is used regardless of evidence of metastasis.

Current research indicates that autologous stem cell transplantation is not an effective treatment for rhabdomyosarcoma (National Cancer Institute, 2008). Refer to Chapter 22: Chemotherapy and Chapter 87: Radiation Therapy.

While aggressive treatment is usually necessary, most children with rhabdomyosarcoma achieve long-term survival. Cure depends on the specific type of tumor, its location, and the amount of metastasis (MedlinePlus, 2006). In a recent study cited on the National Cancer Institute website, children with gross residual disease after initial surgery experienced a five-year survival rate of approximately 70% compared with a greater than 90% five-year survival rate for children with no residual tumor after surgery. Approximately 80% of children with microscopic tumor residual achieved a five-year survival rate.

Nursing Management

Refer to Chapter 22: Chemotherapy, Chapter 87: Radiation Therapy, and Chapter 100: Surgical Client.

References

American Cancer Society. (2007). *What is rhabdomyosarcoma?* Retrieved March 18, 2008, from http:// www.cancer.org/docroot/CRI/content/CRI_2_4_1X_What_is_rhabdomyosarcoma_53.asp?sitearea

MedlinePlus. (2006). *Rhabdomyosarcoma*. Retrieved March 18, 2008, from http://www.nlm.nih .gov/medlineplus/ency/article/001429.htm

National Cancer Institute. (2008). *Childhood rhabdomyosarcoma treatment (PDQ)*. Retrieved
    March 18, 2008, from http://www.cancer.gov/cancertopics/pdq/treatment/childrhabdomyosarcoma/
    healthprofessional

Potts, N. L., & Mandleco, B. L. (2007). *Pediatric nursing: Caring for children and their families* (2nd ed.).
    Clifton Park, NY: Delmar Cengage Learning.

93

Rheumatic Fever

Definition

Rheumatic fever is an inflammatory autoimmune disease that follows untreated Strep throat or skin infections. It is one of the diseases responsible for acquired heart disease (Potts & Mandleco, 2007).

Pathophysiology

Although the exact pathophysiology of rheumatic fever is not completely understood, it is believed to be an autoimmune response to untreated group A beta-hemolytic streptococcal pharyngitis (Strep throat). It typically occurs two to six weeks after the initial Strep infection and appears most commonly in children with a genetic predisposition to develop the disease.

Rheumatic fever affects the connective tissue of the heart, joints, subcutaneous tissue, and vasculature of the central nervous system. Sensitized B cells produce antistreptococcal antibodies that form immune complexes that cross-react with cardiac sarcolemma. This interaction can persist for up to six months (Broyles, 2005). This interaction creates acute inflammation especially in the valves of the heart. The valves most affected are the mitral valve (the valve located between the left atrium and ventricle) and the aortic valve because of the pressure in the left side of the heart, especially the left ventricle. The valve becomes fibrosed and does not completely open and close during systole and diastole, which leads to mitral valve regurgitation. The cardiac manifestations are not initially apparent; but over time, the recurrent carditis can lead to congestive heart failure. The carditis is the major cause of morbidity and mortality associated with rheumatic fever.

Complications

- Carditis
- Mitral valve stenosis
- Aortic stenosis
- Mitral valve regurgitation
- Congestive heart failure

Incidence

The incidence of rheumatic fever is determined by the frequency of streptococcal infection and the virulence of the bacterial strain. The incidence has increased over the past two decades (Parrillo & Parrillo, 2007). An estimated 2–3% of people who have untreated group A streptococcal pharyngitis will develop acute rheumatic fever. Although anyone can develop acute rheumatic fever, its peak incidence is in children 5–15 years old (American Heart Association, 2008; Parrillo & Parrillo, 2007). The resulting rheumatic heart disease can be lifelong (American Heart Association, 2008).

Etiology

Rheumatic fever is an inflammatory autoimmune response initiated by an untreated group A beta-hemolytic streptococcal infection. There appears to be a genetic predisposition.

Clinical Manifestations

Migratory polyarthritis

Carditis

Erythema marginatum

Chorea (also referred to as Sydenham's chorea and Saint Vitus' dance)

Subcutaneous nodules (Aschoff bodies)

Jones minor criteria:

    Fever

    Elevated erythrocyte sedimentation rate

    Arthralgia

Diagnostic Tests

Throat culture

Erythrocyte sedimentation rate

C-reactive protein

Streptococcal antibody titer

Electrocardiography

Echocardiography

Medical Management

The goals of treatment are to prevent the disease and to limit the consequences of rheumatic fever. The best defense against rheumatic heart disease is to prevent rheumatic fever. This usually can be accomplished by treating streptococcal pharyngitis with penicillin. To limit the heart damage if the child develops rheumatic fever, long-term prophylactic antimicrobials are prescribed monthly (intramuscular injections) or penicillin is administered through daily oral dosing. Lifelong antimicrobial therapy may be required. Anti-inflammatory agents such as prednisone, a corticosteroid, may be prescribed during acute inflammation to limit damage. If cardiac damage has occurred from the rheumatic fever, children are given additional therapy with a different antibiotic (cephalosporin) prior to dental or surgical procedures to prevent bacterial endocarditis (American Heart Association, 2008). Most care is provided on an outpatient basis; however, if cardiac damage results in manifestations, surgery may be required to repair damaged valves.

Nursing Management

ASSESSMENT

1. Obtain client history including drug allergies
2. Assess for manifestations of Strep throat
3. Obtain throat culture
4. Perform physical assessment
5. Obtain vital signs and height and weight

NURSING DIAGNOSES (INCLUDING BUT NOT LIMITED TO)

1. Risk for decreased cardiac output R/T development of rheumatic fever secondary to untreated Strep throat
2. Deficient knowledge R/T prevention of rheumatic fever, treatment, and home care

PLANNING/GOALS

1. Client will not experience permanent heart damage.
2. Parents and child (if age-appropriate) will demonstrate understanding of prevention of rheumatic fever, treatment, and home care.

NOC

1. Cardiac Pump Effectiveness
2. Knowledge: Health Promotion, Treatment

IMPLEMENTATION

1. Risk for heart damage
   a. Assess heart sounds
   b. Assess vital signs
   c. Encourage child to rest
   d. Encourage restful age-appropriate activities
   e. Administer first dose of penicillin
   f. Monitor for hypersensitivity response to penicillin
2. Parent/child (if-age-appropriate) teaching
   a. Assess current level of understanding
   b. Provide verbal and written information regarding:
      1) Risk factors for developing streptococcal infections, including crowded living conditions, damp weather, malnutrition, immunodeficiency, and inadequate health care
      2) Ways to avoid risk factors
      3) Manifestations of streptococcal pharyngitis
      4) Importance of getting treatment for child with streptococcal pharyngitis
      5) Medication administration, including importance of completing entire antibiotic prescription and monitoring for hypersensitivity response
      6) Importance of prophylactic penicillin treatment for rheumatic fever
      7) Possibility of lifelong prophylactic antibiotic treatment
      8) Need for additional antibiotic therapy prior to dental or surgical procedures
      9) Importance of hand washing and proper technique
      10) Management of joint pain
      11) Manifestations of worsening condition
      12) Contact information for reporting manifestations
      13) Importance of lifelong follow-up care
   c. Provide adequate time for teaching
   d. Document teaching and parent/child response

NIC

1. Health Education
2. Health Education

EVALUATION

1. Client does not experience permanent heart damage.
2. Parents and child (if age-appropriate) demonstrate understanding of prevention of rheumatic fever, treatment, and home care.

References

American Heart Association. (2008). *Rheumatic heart disease/rheumatic fever*. Retrieved March 18, 2008, from http://www.americanheart.org/presenter.jhtml?identifier=4709

Broyles, B. E. (2005). *Medical-surgical nursing clinical companion.* Durham, NC: Carolina Academic Press.

Parrillo, S. J., & Parrillo, C. V. (2007). *Rheumatic fever.* Retrieved March 18, 2008, from http://www.emedicine.com/emerg/topic509.htm

Potts, N. L., & Mandleco, B. L. (2007). *Pediatric nursing: Caring for children and their families* (2nd ed.). Clifton Park, NY: Delmar Cengage Learning.

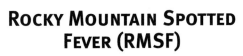
ROCKY MOUNTAIN SPOTTED FEVER (RMSF)

Definition

Rocky Mountain spotted fever (RMSF) is a rickettsial infection transmitted through the bite of a tick (Centers for Disease Control and Prevention, 2005).

Pathophysiology

Rocky Mountain spotted fever was first recognized in 1896 in the Snake River Valley of Idaho and was originally called "black measles" because of the characteristic rash (Centers for Disease Control and Prevention, 2005). RMSF is caused by the bite of a tick infected with *Rickettsia rickettsii*, a gram-negative obligate intracellular coccobacillus. These bacteria have an affinity for human endothelial cells. When the tick bites an individual, the longer the tick remains attached, the more likely it is to transmit the bacteria into the individual's vascular system. The incubation period for RMSF is from 2–14 days (Potts & Mandleco, 2007). RMSF is the most severe and most frequently reported rickettsial condition in the United States; and untreated cases can result in death, which occurs in approximately 30% of the cases.

RMSF is characterized by diffuse small-vessel vasculitis. The bacteria cause a disruption in the membranes of endothelial cells, resulting in an increased permeability. Although the exact pathophysiogenesis for cellular injury is not completely understood, "[p]ossible mechanisms for cellular injury include injury to the cell membrane, depletion of adenosine 5-triphosphate (which leads to failure of the sodium pump), and damage to the cell caused by toxic products of rickettsial metabolism" (Bennett & Domachowske, 2008, Section 2).

The vasculitis is responsible for the clinical manifestations and can be located throughout the body. It is characterized by headache, changes in level of consciousness, rash, cardiac failure, and shock. In addition, profound hyponatremia and increased intracranial pressure occur. The edema in the medulla oblongata is believed to contribute to the number of fatalities attributed to RMSF (Bennett & Domachowske, 2008).

Complications

Increased intracranial pressure
Hyponatremia
Death

Incidence

In the latest statistics from the Centers of Disease Control and Prevention (CDC), 1,936 cases of RMSF were reported in the United States in 2005 (Centers for Disease Control and Prevention, 2005). Less than 3% of ticks actually carry *Rickettsia rickettsii*, so contracting RMSF from a tick bite is not common. Approximately 500–600 cases are reported annually in the United States. Most of these cases involve children.

Although termed Rocky Mountain spotted fever, cases have been reported throughout the United States (except in the New England states, Alaska, and Hawaii), with the highest incidence in the southeastern states that border the Atlantic Ocean, including Virginia, North Carolina, South Carolina, and Georgia. It also occurs in the states west of the Atlantic states, including Tennessee, Arkansas, and Oklahoma (Centers for Disease Control and Prevention, 2005).

Etiology

RMSF is caused by *Rickettsia rickettsii*, a species of bacteria that is spread to humans by ixodid (hard) ticks (Centers for Disease Control and Prevention, 2005).

Clinical Manifestations

Usually evidence of a tick bite
Fever
Headache
Anorexia
Rash (usually on arms and ankles)
Muscle pain
Joint pain
Abdominal pain
Diarrhea

Diagnostic Tests

Serologic assays to detect anti–*R. rickettsii* immunoglobulin G (IgG) antibodies
Enzyme immunoassays (EIAs) and immunoglobulin M (IgM) antibody-capture immunoassays
Complete blood count
Serum electrolyte counts

Medical Management

The goals of treatment include prevention of tick bites, early diagnosis and treatment, and control of intracranial pressure. Prevention of tick bites can be effectively achieved by the use of insect repellents containing N, N-Diethyl-3-methylbenzamide (DEET); close inspection of the child's body after exposure to areas where ticks reside; and proper removal of an attached tick, ensuring that the head of the tick is completely removed from the skin (Bennett & Domachowske, 2008).

The best client outcomes occur when treatment for RMSF is initiated within four days of the development of clinical manifestations. A child complaining of a headache should be examined if the headache is not relieved by acetaminophen. In the presence of a history of a tick bite in someone who presents with a fever, treatment should not be withheld until laboratory confirmation. The antibiotic of choice for treating RMSF is doxycycline even in children younger than 8 years of age (Broyles, Reiss, & Evans, 2007; Bennett & Domachowske, 2008). Tetracycline has been used effectively in children who cannot tolerate doxycycline. Research shows that children "treated with chloramphenicol were more likely to die than those treated with tetracycline" (Bennett & Domachowske, 2008, Section 6).

Refer to Chapter 61: Increased Intracranial Pressure (ICP) for children admitted with evidence of RMSF that has advanced to central nervous system manifestations.

Nursing Management

Refer to Chapter 61: Increased Intracranial Pressure (ICP).

ASSESSMENT

1. Obtain client history
2. Assess for manifestations of RMSF
3. Perform neurologic assessment
4. Perform pediatric assessment
5. Assess vital signs, height, and weight

NURSING DIAGNOSES (INCLUDING BUT NOT LIMITED TO)

1. Altered protection R/T living in high-risk environment and tick bite
2. Deficient knowledge R/T prevention, child's condition, treatment, and home care

PLANNING/GOALS

1. Client will not experience a tick bite. However, if a tick bite does occur, parents will seek treatment for client early in the disease process.
2. Parents and child (if age-appropriate) will demonstrate under-standing of prevention of RMSF, child's condition, treatment, and home care.

NOC

1. Risk Control
2. Knowledge: Infection Prevention, Illness Care, Treatment, Health Promotion

IMPLEMENTATION

1. Protection
   a. Refer to "Parent/child teaching" regarding prevention techniques
   b. Begin treatment as soon as possible if child develops fever, head-ache, or neurologic changes
   c. Refer to "Parent/child teaching" regarding prevention techniques
2. Parent/child (if age-appropriate) teaching
   a. Assess parents'/child's current level of understanding
   b. Provide verbal and written information regarding:
      1) Medication administration and importance of compliance with antimicrobial therapy
      2) Importance of avoiding direct sunlight on skin because of the adverse effect of photosensitivity for child on doxycy-cline (Broyles et al., 2007)
      3) Use of protective clothing (long-sleeved shirt tucked into pants and long pants tucked into socks)
      4) Use of light-colored clothing
      5) Use of tick and insect repellents that contain DEET applied to skin or clothing. Use an insect repellent for children and check with child's health care provider before using DEET on child younger than 1 year of age.
      6) Importance of using soap and water to wash skin treated with DEET after returning indoors
      7) Necessity of checking children often for ticks, especially behind knees, between fingers and toes, under arms, in the groin, in the umbilicus, in and behind ears, on the neck and hairline, and on top of the head. In addition, check chil-dren where elastic waistband of underwear touches the skin, where bands from pants or skirts touch the skin, and any-where else clothing presses on the skin.
      8) Importance of showering or bathing children at the end of all outdoor activities
      9) Importance of walking on cleared paths and pavement through wooded areas and fields when possible.

   c. Provide adequate time for teaching
   d. Document teaching and parents' response

NIC

1. Risk Identification, Safety Surveillance
2. Teaching: Infection Precautions, Illness Care, Treatment, Health Promotion

EVALUATION

1. Client does not experience tick bite, however, if a tick bite occurs, parents will seek treatment for client early in the disease process.
2. Parents and child (if age-appropriate) demonstrate understanding of prevention of RMSF, child's condition, treatment, and home care.

References

Bennett, N. J., & Domachowske, J. (2008). *Rocky Mountain spotted fever.* Retrieved March 18, 2008, from http://www.emedicine.com/ped/topic2709.htm

Broyles, B. E., Reiss, B. S., & Evans, M. E. (2007). *Pharmacological aspects of nursing care* (7th ed.). Clifton Park, NY: Delmar Cengage Learning.

Centers for Disease Control and Prevention. (2005). *Rocky Mountain spotted fever.* Retrieved March 18, 2008, from http://www.cdc.gov/ncidod/dvrd/rmsf/Q&A.htm

Potts, N. L., & Mandleco, B. L. (2007). *Pediatric nursing: Caring for children and their families* (2nd ed.). Clifton Park, NY: Delmar Cengage Learning.

95

Scoliosis/Spinal Fusion

Definition

Scoliosis is the lateral (c-shaped or s-shaped) curvature of the vertebral spine with vertical rotation (Potts & Mandleco, 2007). Refer to Figure 95-1.

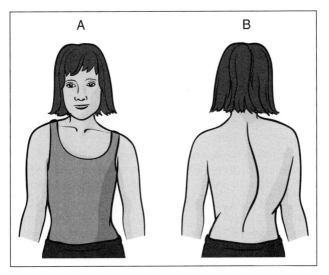

Figure 95-1: Scoliosis: **(A)** Anterior View and **(B)** Posterior View.

Pathophysiology

Scoliosis most frequently affects the thoracic and lumbar (thoracolumbar) sections of the spine. When the vertebral column curves laterally, the spine and ribs rotate toward the convex part of the curvature. The muscles and ligaments on the concave side of the curvature shorten and thicken while those on the convex side lengthen, become thin, and atrophy (Broyles, 2005; Potts & Mandleco, 2007). As this process continues, the vertebrae become deformed. The greater the initial curve of the spine, the greater the chance that scoliosis will worsen after growth is complete. Severe scoliosis (curvature > 100 degrees) can cause the rib cage to compress and compromise cardiopulmonary function (MedlinePlus, 2006). Further, compression of or damage to the spinal cord can occur in severe curvatures.

Although less life-threatening than the cardiopulmonary dysfunction, other complications can arise for the child with scoliosis. Pain frequently is a manifestation of scoliosis because of the stress on the highly innervated skeletal muscles of the trunk. The structural changes can lead to limitations in physical mobility. In addition, because most children develop scoliosis during prepubescence and early puberty, it can pose an insult to the child's body image and self-esteem.

There are three identified types of scoliosis based on etiology. Idiopathic scoliosis has no known cause. Congenital scoliosis results from malformation of the spine during vertebral development. Neuromuscular scoliosis occurs in conjunction with neuromuscular conditions that cause muscle weakness, such as cerebral palsy, muscular dystrophy, spina bifida, and polio.

Complications

PREOPERATIVE

Cardiopulmonary compromise
Spinal cord injury
Pain
Physical mobility limitations
Disturbed body image
Diminished self-esteem

POSTOPERATIVE

Pain
Neurovascular compromise
Infection
Noncompliance with postoperative instructions
Disturbed body image

Incidence

"Scoliosis affects 2–3% of the population, or an estimated 6 million people in the United States. . . . Scoliosis impacts infants, adolescents, and adults worldwide with little regard to race or socio-economic status. The primary age of onset for scoliosis is 10–15 years old, occurring equally among both genders. However, females are eight times more likely to progress to a curve magnitude that requires treatment" (National Scoliosis Foundation, 2007, p. 1).

Although the majority of scoliosis cases do not require treatment, scoliosis is responsible for more than 600,000 visits to health care provider offices annually. An estimated 30,000 children are treated medically by being placed in an orthopedic brace (Boston brace, Wilmington brace, Milwaukee brace, or Charleston brace), while 38,000 undergo spinal fusion surgery each year (National Scoliosis Foundation, 2007).

Etiology

Approximately 85% of scoliosis cases are idiopathic (National Scoliosis Foundation, 2007). Refer to the Pathophysiology section for etiology of congenital and neuromuscular scoliosis.

Clinical Manifestations

Lateral curvature of the spine
Asymmetry of the shoulders and hips
Lower back pain
Fatigue
Dyspnea
Tachypnea
Tachycardia

Diagnostic Tests

Spine radiography
Scoliometric measurements
Magnetic resonance imaging

Medical Management

The goals of treatment are to strengthen the thoracolumbar muscles if possible and to provide structural support. The type of treatment is determined by the cause and the amount and location of the curvature. Mild idiopathic scoliosis with a curvature < 20 degrees usually does not require treatment but should be monitored. Mild to moderate idiopathic scoliosis (curvatures > 25–30 degrees) usually involves placing the child in a brace. Although the Milwaukee brace is most commonly used, the Boston brace, Wilmington brace, and Charleston brace also provide pressure to help straighten the curvature and provide support to relieve asymmetrical pressure. Each brace is named for the city in which it was developed (MedlinePlus, 2006). Braces are not effective in the treatment of congenital or neuromuscular scoliosis.

Curves of 40 degrees or greater usually require surgery because curves this large pose a high risk of worsening even after bone growth stops (MedlinePlus, 2006). Surgical management involves spinal fusion using the insertion of instrumentation (Harrington rod, Dwyer cable, Luque rod, or Cotrel-Dubousset system) and bone grafts from the iliac crest. The surgical approach may be anterior or posterior depending on the degree and location of the curvature. However, for most spinal fusions, a posterior approach is taken.

A major focus postoperatively is pain management. As a result of the extent of surgical tissue trauma and required bed rest during the first 24–48 hours postoperatively, pain management frequently poses both medical and nursing challenges. Patient-controlled analgesia (PCA) with additional medication for breakthrough pain often is necessary for these children (Broyles, Reiss, & Evans, 2007). In addition, the child requires being logrolled every 2 hours for a prescribed period. Some children are fitted for a thoracic-lumbar-sacral-orthotic (TLSO) brace once ambulation begins. When this type of brace is used, the child must wear it when sitting, standing, or walking; standing for extended periods is limited at least until the follow-up visit.

Nursing Management

Refer to Nursing Management in Chapter 100: Surgical Client.

ASSESSMENT

1. Obtain client history
2. Perform physical assessment
3. Have child bend at the waist with arms pointed to the floor
4. Palpate each vertebra for position and alignment
5. Measure vital signs, height, and weight

NURSING DIAGNOSES (INCLUDING BUT NOT LIMITED TO)

PREOPERATIVE

1. Risk for impaired skin integrity R/T wearing brace
2. Disturbed body image R/T curvature of the spine, presence of brace, and postsurgical scar
3. Risk for impaired gas exchange R/T curvature of the spine compromising respiratory functioning
4. Deficient knowledge R/T child's condition, treatment, and home care

POSTOPERATIVE

5. Ineffective breathing pattern R/T anesthesia, bed rest, and supine positioning
6. Acute pain R/T surgical incision, donor site, and muscle stretching
7. Impaired physical mobility R/T postoperative restrictions
8. Risk for injury R/T altered neurovascular status secondary to surgical instrumentation placement
9. Deficient knowledge R/T postoperative care and home health promotion

PLANNING/GOALS

PREOPERATIVE

1. Client's skin will remain intact.
2. Client will verbalize feelings and concerns about how scoliosis affects his/her body image and use positive coping strategies for enhancement of body image.
3. Client will maintain adequate gas exchange as evidenced by respiratory pattern and activity level within defined limits (WDL).
4. Client/parents will demonstrate understanding about disease process, treatment, and home care as evidenced by compliance with medical regimen.

POSTOPERATIVE

5. Client will maintain effective breathing pattern as evidenced by respiratory pattern, vital signs, and oxygen saturation (per pulse oximetry) WDL.
6. Client will demonstrate effective pain management as determined by client using age-appropriate pain assessment tool.
7. Client will progress with physical activity as prescribed.
8. Client will not experience neurovascular injury as evidenced by intact sensation or movement of extremities, voluntary bladder and bowel control, warm extremities, and capillary refill < 3 seconds.
9. Client /parents will demonstrate understanding of and compliance with prescribed postoperative regimen.

NOC

PREOPERATIVE

1. Tissue Integrity: Skin
2. Body Image
3. Risk Control
4. Knowledge: Disease Process, Treatment

POSTOPERATIVE

5. Respiratory Status: Airway Patency
6. Comfort Level
7. Ambulation
8. Immobility Consequences: Physiological
9. Knowledge: Treatment, Health Promotion

IMPLEMENTATION

PREOPERATIVE

1. Skin integrity
   a. Assess brace for proper fit
   b. Assess skin for redness or pressure areas on skin
   c. Teach client/parents how to assess skin
   d. Massage pressure areas and bony prominences gently at least twice a day
   e. Collaborate with health care provider and brace shop if skin irritation is present
   f. Instruct client/parents about importance of keeping skin clean and dry

    g. Instruct client/parents that brace may be removed for bathing at least once a day during which time the skin should be assessed

    h. Instruct client/parents to avoid lotions and powders under brace

2. Body image

    a. Encourage verbalization of feelings and concerns

    b. Listen actively

    c. Maintain nonjudgmental affect

    d. Assist in identifying positive coping strategies

    e. Assist in identifying positive characteristics of self

    f. Involve in self-care and decision making about care

3. Gas exchange

    a. Assess respiratory status

    b. Assess oxygen saturation via pulse oximetry during clinic visits

    c. Collaborate with physical therapist and/or respiratory therapist for breathing exercises to assist gas exchange

4. Client/parent teaching

    a. Assess client's/parent's current level of understanding

    b. Provide verbal and written instructions and demonstration regarding:

        1) Skin surveillance

        2) Proper technique for wearing brace

        3) Importance of wearing brace a minimum of 23 hours a day and removing it only for hygiene care and skin assessment

        4) Medication administration if needed

        5) Physical exercise

        6) Referrals if needed

        7) Importance of follow-up visits with health care provider and physical therapy

        8) Contact information for reporting changes in condition

POSTOPERATIVE

5. Breathing pattern

    a. Assess respiratory status every hour during pain assessment

    b. Monitor vital signs every 4 hours until ambulatory

    c. Place on cardiopulmonary monitor

    d. Monitor continuous pulse oximetry

    e. Auscultate breath sounds every 4 hours until ambulatory

    f. Encourage use of incentive spirometer hourly while awake

6. Pain

    a. Assess pain level hourly

    b. Maintain patency of intravenous access, monitoring at least hourly

    c. Collaborate with health care provider to prescribe use of PCA

    d. Instruct client on use of PCA device

    e. Instruct client regarding importance of proactive pain management

    f. Maintain body alignment

    g. Logroll every 2 hours

    h. Maintain indwelling urinary catheter patency to prevent urinary distention

    i. Encourage early ambulation

    j. Assist client with progression to oral analgesics while continuing to ensure adequate pain management

    k. Promote climate to ensure adequate rest and sleep

7. Physical mobility

    a. Logroll every 2 hours, maintaining proper alignment

    b. Collaborate with physical therapist to measure and supply TLSO brace prior to client getting out of bed

    c. Apply TLSO brace before client sits up

    d. Assess symmetry of brace for alignment. *NOTE:* This assessment should be made with client lying supine in bed and nurse standing at foot of bed.

    e. Have client rise slowly to a sitting position following period of bed rest

    f. Assess brace for symmetry and fit while client is sitting and then again while client is standing and ambulating

    g. Collaborate with physical therapy/brace shop for adjustments to brace fit

    h. Instruct client to wear brace any time he/she is sitting, standing, or ambulating until follow-up visit with health care provider and clearance for activity without the brace. *NOTE:* The brace can be removed during times the client is lying flat in bed.

    i. Collaborate with physical therapist regarding ambulation schedule

    j. Ensure initially that client ambulates with assistance

8. Neurovascular status

    a. Assess neurovascular status every 2 hours during position change

    b. Monitor capillary refill

    c. Monitor intake and output

    d. Assess for bladder distention or bowel incontinence

    e. Provide indwelling catheter care per facility protocol and as prescribed

    f. Use fracture bedpan to meet client's elimination needs after indwelling catheter is discontinued

    g. Maintain flat position and logroll every 2 hours for prescribed postoperative period

9. Client/parent teaching

    a. Assess client's/parent's current level of understanding

    b. Provide verbal and written instructions and demonstration regarding:

        1) Importance of proactive pain management

        2) Proper technique for applying TLSO brace

        3) Need to wear brace whenever client is sitting, standing, or ambulating until health care provider has cleared client for activities without wearing the brace

        4) Skin assessment

        5) Postoperative discharge instructions

        6) Manifestations of surgical complications

        7) Contact information for reporting manifestations

        8) Importance of follow-up care with health care provider

    c. Provide adequate time for teaching

    d. Document teaching and client's/parents' response

NIC

PREOPERATIVE

1. Skin Surveillance
2. Coping Enhancement
3. Risk Identification
4. Teaching: Disease Process, Treatment

POSTOPERATIVE

5. Risk Identification
6. Pain Management
7. Exercise Therapy: Ambulation
8. Circulatory Precautions
9. Teaching: Treatment, Health Education

EVALUATION

PREOPERATIVE

1. Client's skin remains intact.
2. Client verbalizes feelings and concerns about how scoliosis affects his/her body image and uses positive coping strategies for enhancement of body image.
3. Client maintains adequate gas exchange as evidenced by respiratory pattern and activity level WDL.
4. Client/parents demonstrate understanding about disease process, treatment, and home care as evidenced by compliance with medical regimen.

POSTOPERATIVE

5. Client maintains effective breathing pattern as evidenced by respiratory pattern, vital signs, and oxygen saturation (per pulse oximetry) WDL.
6. Client demonstrates effective pain management as determined by client using age-appropriate pain assessment tool.
7. Client progresses with physical activity as prescribed.
8. Client does not experience neurovascular injury as evidenced by intact sensation or movement of extremities, voluntary bladder and bowel control, warm extremities, and capillary refill < 3 seconds.
9. Client/parents demonstrate understanding of and compliance with prescribed postoperative regimen.

References

Broyles, B. E. (2005). *Medical-surgical nursing clinical companion.* Durham, NC: Carolina Academic Press.

Broyles, B. E., Reiss, B. S., & Evans, M. E. (2007). *Pharmacological aspects of nursing care* (7th ed.). Clifton Park, NY: Delmar Cengage Learning.

MedlinePlus. (2006). *Scoliosis.* Retrieved March 18, 2008, from http://www.nlm.nih.gov/medlineplus/ency/article/001241.htm

National Scoliosis Foundation. (2007). *Information and support.* Retrieved March 18, 2008, from http://www.scoliosis.org/info.php

Potts, N. L., & Mandleco, B. L. (2007). *Pediatric nursing: Caring for children and their families* (2nd ed.). Clifton Park, NY: Delmar Cengage Learning.

96

Seizures

Definition

"Seizures are paroxysmal involuntary alterations of behavior, movement, or sensation, triggered by an abnormal or excessive electrical discharge in the brain" (Broyles, 2005, p. 745).

Pathophysiology

A seizure is an abnormal communication between neurons in the brain. Neurons communicate with each other by firing electrical impulses that travel from the neuron along the axon and then stimulating the release of neurotransmitters. These neurotransmitters flow across the synaptic cleft (the gap between the cells) to the dendrites of the receiving cell. There are excitatory transmitters, such as glutamate and acetylcholine, as well as inhibitory transmitters, such as dopamine and gamma-aminobutyric acid (GABA). If more excitatory than inhibitory transmitters are released, the cell will discharge or depolarize; if more inhibitory neurotransmitters are released, the cell will not depolarize. Because millions of these cells are involved in even simple actions, there is usually a balance in the release of neurotransmitters for control of physical and mental functioning. Each individual has a genetically determined balance between the excitatory and the inhibitory activities of the neurons, called a seizure threshold. A person with a low threshold for seizures has a higher excitatory balance, whereas an individual with a high seizure threshold has greater inhibitory balance (Epilepsy Foundation of America, 2007; Broyles, Reiss, & Evans, 2007). In children, the immaturity of the brain makes them more susceptible to seizures than adults.

In seizures, a consistently higher level of the excitatory neurotransmitters causes a decrease in inhibitory transmitters, resulting in an increased, uncontrolled continuous firing of neurons in the brain. If the neuronal firing of electrical energy has sufficient power and affects enough neurons, it will produce symptoms characteristic of the area in which the discharge took place. The result may be a sudden muscle jerk, an abrupt fall, or distorted vision. If the disturbance flashes across the whole brain at once, it may produce a convulsive seizure, temporarily disrupting multiple functions of the brain including consciousness and motor control. Most seizures last only a minute or two, although confusion afterward may last longer.

Seizures are divided into classifications, including generalized seizures (absence, atonic, tonic-clonic, and myoclonic), partial (simple and complex) seizures, nonepileptic seizures, and status epilepticus (Potts & Mandleco, 2007). Generalized tonic-clonic seizures (formerly known as grand mal seizures) are the most common type of generalized seizure. The tonic phase begins with stiffening of the limbs that is followed by jerking of the limbs and face (the clonic phase).

During the tonic phase, breathing may decrease or cease altogether, producing cyanosis of the lips, nail beds, and face. Breathing typically returns during the clonic (jerking) phase, but the breathing may be irregular. This clonic phase usually lasts less than a minute. Some individuals experience only the tonic phase of the seizure, others exhibit only the clonic phase, and still others may have a tonic-clonic-tonic pattern. Incontinence is not uncommon during tonic-clonic-tonic generalized seizure (Epilepsy Foundation of American, 2007).

Myoclonic seizures are rapid, brief contractions of bodily muscles, usually occurring at the same time on both sides of the body. Occasionally, they involve one upper extremity or a foot.

Atonic seizures, also called akinetic seizures, produce an abrupt loss of muscle tone including head flexion, loss of posture, or sudden collapse. Because they are so abrupt, without any prodromal phase, they can result in injuries to the head and face (Epilepsy Foundation of America, 2007).

Absence seizures (formerly called petit mal seizures) are lapses of awareness. The child, whether sitting or standing, simply stares vacantly, neither speaking nor apparently hearing what is said. The seizure usually lasts only a few seconds. This type is more common in children and may occur 50–100 times a day without detection. Absence seizures begin between the ages of 4 and 12 years and are sometimes misdiagnosed as a hearing impairment or behavioral problem (Lucile Packard Children's Hospital at Stanford, 2008). There is no aura, but an abrupt onset and brief duration. Some absence seizures are accompanied by brief myoclonic jerking of the eyelids or facial muscles or by variable loss of muscle tone; if the seizure is prolonged, automatisms may occur.

Infantile spasms are clusters of quick, sudden movements that start between 3 months and 2 years. If a child is sitting up, the head will fall forward and the arms will flex forward. If the child is lying down, the knees will be drawn up, with arms and head flexed forward as if the infant is reaching for support.

Simple partial seizures affect a small part of the brain and can involve movement, emotions, and sensation. These seizures do not cause loss of consciousness; however, the child frequently loses the ability to speak or move voluntarily until the seizure ends. Motor manifestations can occur in almost any part of the musculature from the eyelids to the extremities.

Usually the motor activity is accompanied by a sudden feeling of fear or a sense that something terrible is about to happen. Any of the five senses (touch, hearing, taste, smell, and vision) can be affected during the seizures, usually manifesting as abnormal sensations (tingly feelings, tinnitus, unpleasant tastes or odors, or visual distortions). Sensations such as diaphoresis, flushing, pallor, or even "out of body experiences" may occur (Epilepsy Foundation of America, 2007). Episodes of sudden diaphoresis, flushing, pallor, or having the sensation of gooseflesh (piloerections) are possible.

Complex partial seizures involve larger areas of the brain than simple partial seizures and affect consciousness, resulting in a trancelike state. Although these can affect any part of the brain, the most common are the two temporal lobes. Typically, a complex partial seizure begins with the child staring blankly and losing awareness and then making chewing movements with the mouth, picking at or fumbling with clothing, mumbling, and performing repetitive simple but unorganized movements.

Febrile seizures occur early in childhood and result from elevated temperatures associated with viral or bacterial infections common during this time of development. Characteristic of young children is a low seizure threshold. Children tend to experience higher temperatures with childhood infections, and these can cause increased neuronal excitability (Tejani & Zempsky, 2006). These seizures can manifest as generalized or absence seizures. The risk of neurologic damage and an obstructed airway (from the tongue falling back in the mouth during the seizure) is greater in young children.

Status epilepticus is a continuous state of seizure activity or seizures that are longer than 15 minutes and recurrent (Duke University Medical Center, 2007). Status epilepticus can result in neurologic damage from the death of neurons from depleted oxygen and glucose stores. In the presence of sufficient neuron death, the child can die.

Complications

Physical damage to head
Obstructed airway
Neurologic damage
Death

Incidence

Fifty percent of all seizure cases begin before the age of 25. Many start in early childhood because of the brain's immaturity, causing it to be more susceptible to seizures from any cause. Over 300,000 children and adolescents in the U.S. have seizure disorders (Epilepsy Foundation of America, 2007). In the United States, between 2% and 5% of children have experienced a febrile seizure by the time they are 5 years old. The incidence in Western Europe is similar to that in the United States; however "elsewhere in the world[, it] varies between 5% and 10% for India, 8.8% for Japan, 14% for Guam, 0.35% for Hong Kong, and 0.5–1.5% for China" (Tejani & Zempsky, 2006, Section 2). Approximately 1 in 25 children will have at least one febrile seizure (Duke University Medical Center, 2007).

Etiology

The most common causes of seizure activity in children include fever, infection such as meningitis, trauma, hemorrhage, brain malformation during gestation, anoxia during or following birth, brain immaturity, and genetic disorders (Duke University Medical Center, 2007; Epilepsy Foundation of America, 2007). For children who are being treated for a seizure disorder, the most common cause of an unexpected seizure is failure to take the medication as prescribed. There appears to be a slightly increased risk of epilepsy in close relatives of individuals with seizures compared to the risk in the general population (Epilepsy Foundation of America, 2007).

Clinical Manifestations

Trancelike staring
Jerking movements of the arms and legs
Stiffening posture
Loss of consciousness
Dyspnea
Apnea
Incontinence
Tendency to fall suddenly for no apparent reason
Tendency to be unresponsive to noise or words for brief periods
Tendency to appear confused or in a haze
Sleepiness and irritability upon waking in the morning
Nodding of the head
Periods of rapid eye blinking and staring
Refer to Pathophysiology section

Diagnostic Tests

Complete blood count
Serum chemistry
Electroencephalogram
Computed tomography
Magnetic resonance imaging
Lumbar puncture

Medical Management

The goals of treatment are to determine the cause of the child's seizure and to prevent further seizures. Monotherapy with an anticonvulsant medication is the preferred method of treatment for children with seizures.

The immediate treatment of a child during a seizure is to protect the child from injury to the head and to maintain a patent airway using the jaw thrust while noting the time the seizure began. During a seizure, nothing should be placed in the child's mouth, including a tongue blade. After the patency of the airway is assured, oxygen is administered, the child is placed on his/her side, and oral secretions should be suctioned out of the child's mouth to prevent aspiration. Because most seizures are self-limiting, lasting less than 5 minutes, usually no further management is necessary during the seizure.

In the presence of status epilepticus, the measures listed in the previous paragraph are maintained and pharmacological management is required. Intravenous administration of lorazepam or diazepam usually is performed first. If the seizure continues, phenytoin or fosphenytoin are administered. During the administration of phenytoin, a free-flowing 0.9% normal saline solution is standard and the intravenous access needs to be closely monitored for phlebitis (Broyles et al., 2007). Phenobarbital also may be used during a seizure. The child requires continuous cardiorespiratory monitoring.

After the seizure subsides, diagnostics are performed to determine the type of seizure activity and maintenance anticonvulsant therapy is initiated. For partial seizures, carbamazepine, oxycarbazepine, phenytoin, and valproic acid demonstrate similar efficacy and tolerability for both children and adults. For generalized seizures, valproic acid, felbamate, and topiramate are the drugs of choice. Infantile spasms are effectively controlled with adrenocorticotropic hormone, and valproic acid. Clonazepam is the agent of choice for treating myoclonic seizures, and phenobarbital is used to manage infantile seizures. For absence seizures, valproic acid usually is the first-line drug; however, ethosuximide (with once-daily dosing) may be used initially. Other anticonvulsant agents used as adjunctive therapy to treat partial and generalized seizures include gabapentin, lamotrigine, and topiramate (Potts & Mandleco, 2007; Broyles et al., 2007).

Other therapies include the use of a ketogenic diet. Normally, the primary source of energy is glucose; however, children usually can store only 24 hours' worth of glucose. When a child receives nothing by mouth for 24 hours (usually occurring during hospitalization for seizures), the glucose store is consumed. Fats are the secondary source of energy, and the ketogenic diet is very high in fat (about 90% of the calories come from fat) with sufficient protein to promote growth and very small amounts of carbohydrates. This diet keeps the supply of energy maintained by forcing the child's body to burn fat around the clock. It is not clear how the diet works, but some children have become seizure-free as a result of this diet (Epilepsy Foundation of America, 2007; Lucile Packard Children's Hospital at Stanford, 2008).

For some children whose seizures are not well controlled with anticonvulsant drug therapy, a procedure called vagus nerve stimulation (VNS) may be used. Currently, this procedure is approved only for children over the age of 12 who have partial seizures that are not controlled by other methods. The process involves the transmission of small pulses of energy to the brain from the vagus nerve in the neck through surgical placement of a small battery in the chest wall with wires (cutaneously placed) attached to the battery. The battery is programmed to transmit energy impulses to the brain every few minutes, and the child can activate impulses with a small magnet to help prevent the seizure from occurring (Epilepsy Foundation of America, 2007; Lucile Packard Children's Hospital at Stanford, 2008).

Brain surgery is an alternative in the treatment of seizures and may be considered in a child who "has seizures that are not controlled with medications, has seizures that always start in one specific area of the brain, or has a seizure in a part of the brain that can be removed without disrupting important behaviors such as speech, memory, or vision" (Lucile Packard Children's Hospital at Stanford, 2008, p. 1). The procedure may involve removal of a specific part of the brain where seizures are occurring or it may help interrupt the spread of negative electrical currents through the brain. This is a complex surgery that involves the child meeting specific criteria and carries risks of neurological damage as well as the other risks associated with any surgical procedure.

Nursing Management

ASSESSMENT

1. Obtain client history
2. Obtain detailed account of seizure episode
3. Perform physical assessment and detailed neurologic assessment
4. Assess vital signs, height, and weight
5. Assess diagnostic test results

NURSING DIAGNOSES (INCLUDING BUT NOT LIMITED TO)

1. Risk for ineffective airway clearance R/T airway obstruction by the tongue
2. Ineffective breathing pattern R/T dyspnea and apnea during generalized seizure activity
3. High risk for injury, physical R/T tonic-clonic movements and decreased level of consciousness
4. High risk for injury R/T adverse effects of anticonvulsant therapy, noncompliance
5. Deficient knowledge R/T child's condition, treatment, medications, and home care

PLANNING/GOALS

1. Client will maintain patent airway.
2. Client will regain and maintain effective breathing pattern.
3. Client will not experience injury during seizure activity.
4. Client will not experience adverse effects of anticonvulsant therapy and will remain compliant with therapy.
5. Parents and child (if age-appropriate) will demonstrate understanding of child's condition, treatment, medication therapy, and home care.

NOC

1. Respiratory Status: Airway Patency
2. Respiratory Status: Ventilation
3. Risk Control, Physical Injury Severity
4. Risk Control
5. Knowledge: Illness Care, Treatment, Medication, Health Promotion

IMPLEMENTATION

1. Airway patency
   a. Assess airway during seizure
   b. Use jaw thrust to maintain airway patency
   c. Place in lateral position
   d. Suction oral secretions as needed
   e. Initiate seizure precautions according to facility protocol for any child with history of seizures
   f. Assess for indicators of impending seizure activity
   g. Place padded tongue blade in mouth prior to teeth clenching, which frequently occurs during clonic phase. *NOTE:* Once teeth have clenched, *do not* attempt to insert padded tongue blade.
   h. Loosen clothing around neck
   i. Place on continuous pulse oximetry
   j. Administer oxygen as prescribed to maintain oxygen saturation > 94%

2. Breathing pattern
   a. Refer to interventions for airway patency
   b. Place on continuous cardiorespiratory monitor
   c. Position to facilitate breathing
   d. Allow child to rest/sleep immediately following seizure
   e. Monitor closely
3. Risk for physical injury
   a. Pad side rails of bed
   b. Remove all objects from bed
   c. Protect child's head from injury
   d. Gently ease child to floor if child begins to have seizure while sitting or standing and remove any furniture or objects that may cause injury
   e. Note time seizure began
   f. Document detailed description of seizure following seizure
4. Risk for medication injury
   a. Provide instructions regarding medications, including schedule, dose, route, and importance of compliance with therapy and follow-up with health care provider
   b. Monitor serum drug levels
   c. Monitor serum electrolytes
5. Parent/child teaching
   a. Assess current level of understanding
   b. Provide verbal and written information regarding:
      1) Risk factors for injuries during seizures and instructions as needed to avoid risk factors (for example, avoiding alcohol, illicit drugs, excessive fatigue, excessive caffeine, and activities that could injure the head)
      2) Assessment during seizure activity including maintenance of child's airway, protection of child, length of seizure, characteristics of child's movements during seizure, and notifying health care provider
      3) Medication administration including schedule, dose, route, and importance of compliance with prescribed medication regime
      4) Manifestations of adverse effects of medications and drug toxicity
      5) Manifestations of worsening of condition
      6) Contact numbers for reporting manifestations
      7) Importance of wearing a medical ID bracelet or necklace at all times and instructions concerning how to obtain one
      8) Importance of follow-up care with health care provider for laboratory tests
   c. Provide sufficient time for teaching
   d. Document teaching and parents'/child's response

NIC

1. Airway Management, Airway Suctioning
2. Respiratory Monitoring, Vital Signs Monitoring, Oxygen Therapy, Aspiration Precautions
3. Risk Identification, Safety Surveillance

    4. Risk Identification, Health Education

    5. Teaching: Illness Care, Treatment, Medication, Health Education

EVALUATION

    1. Client maintains patent airway.

    2. Client regains and maintains effective breathing pattern.

    3. Client does not experience injury during seizure activity.

    4. Client does not experience adverse effects of anticonvulsant therapy and remains compliant with therapy.

    5. Parents and child (if age-appropriate) demonstrate understanding of child's condition, treatment, medication therapy, and home care.

References

Broyles, B. E. (2005). *Medical-surgical nursing clinical companion.* Durham, NC: Carolina Academic Press.

Broyles, B. E., Reiss, B. S., & Evans, M. E. (2007). *Pharmacological aspects of nursing care* (7th ed.). Clifton Park, NY: Delmar Cengage Learning.

Duke University Medical Center. (2007). *Childhood seizures.* Retrieved April 30, 2007, from http://www.dukehealth.org/dr_clements/childhoodseizures

Epilepsy Foundation of America. (2007). *Living with epilepsy: Children & teens.* Retrieved March 18, 2008, from http://www.epilepsyfoundation.org/living/children/education/

Lucile Packard Children's Hospital at Stanford. (2008). *Neurological disorders: Seizures and epilepsy.* Retrieved March 18, 2008, from http://www.lpch.org/DiseaseHealthInfo/HealthLibrary/neuro/seizep.html

Potts, N. L., & Mandleco, B. L. (2007). *Pediatric nursing: Caring for children and their families* (2nd ed.). Clifton Park, NY: Delmar Cengage Learning.

Tejani, N. R., & Zempsky, W. T. (2006). *Pediatrics, febrile seizures.* Retrieved March 18, 2008, from http://www.emedicine.com/emerg/topic376.htm

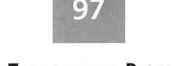

97

Sexually Transmitted Disease (STD)/ Sexually Transmitted Infection (STI)

Definition

Sexually transmitted disease (STD) is a communicable infection associated with intimate sexual activities including oral sex, sexual intercourse, and anal intercourse (Broyles, 2005; Centers for Disease Control and Prevention, 2008a). An STD also is referred to as a sexually transmitted infection (STI).

Pathophysiology

STDs are transmitted through impaired tissue integrity of the mucous membranes of the mouth, vagina, and anus. Mucous membranes are the body tissue's most sensitive to trauma. The infectious organisms enter the tissues and frequently enter the bloodstream. The exact pathophysiology of STDs depends on the type, causative organism, and invasion beyond the integrity of the tissues (Broyles, 2005). The major complication for STDs in general is transmission of these diseases.

Chlamydial infections are the most common of all bacterial STDs (Potts & Mandleco, 2007). The causative organism is *Chlamydia trachomatis*, which causes conjunctivitis, pneumonia, nongonococcal urethritis (NGU), cervicitis, and lymphogranuloma venereum. The usual incubation period is 7 days but can be as long as 5–6 weeks depending on the location of the infection. Chlamydial infection can be transmitted to the neonate during the vaginal delivery process, resulting in neonatal conjunctivitis and interstitial pneumonia.

Gonorrhea is caused by *Neisseria gonorrhoeae*, a gram-negative diplococcus; the disease has a 2–7 day incubation period. In neonates, it causes ophthalmia neonatorum, which can lead to blindness. As a result, most states in the United States require prophylactic optic medication for all neonates immediately after birth. In females, gonorrhea causes endocervicitis and pelvic inflammatory disease; in males, it causes proctitis. In both genders, it results in urethritis, pharyngitis, and conjunctivitis.

Herpes simplex type 2 virus causes herpes genitalis. In the neonate, generalized systemic infections include central nervous system (CNS) and hepatic involvement as well as infections of the eyes, mouth, and skin. There is a high mortality rate among neonates who contract herpes infections (Potts & Mandleco, 2007).

Hepatitis B is caused by the hepatitis B virus (a hepadnavirus). The incubation period averages 90 days with a range of 45–160 days (Potts & Mandleco, 2007). Hepatitis B is responsible for approximately 5,000 deaths annually in the United States (Centers for Disease Control and Prevention, 2007d).

Human papillomavirus (HPV) causes genital (venereal) and anal warts. HPV infections are the most common of all STDs. In addition, HPV has been associated with cervical, anal, and vaginal dysplasia and cervical cancer. In neonates, it is responsible for laryngeal papilloma.

Human immunodeficiency virus is caused by a retrovirus (or RNA virus). Refer to Chapter 3: Acquired Immunodeficiency Syndrome (AIDS).

Syphilis is caused by the spirocete *Treponema pallidum*. It can be contracted by the fetus transplacentally from an infected mother any time during pregnancy or at the time of delivery. It can result in stillbirth, prematurity, hydrops fetalis, hepatosplenomegaly, mucocutaneous lesions, lymphadenopathy, and thrombocytopenia. The incubation period is 3 weeks with a range of 10–90 days (Potts & Mandleco, 2007); it can lead to syphilitic heart disease in adults.

Trichomoniasis occurs as a result of infection by the single-celled protozoan parasite *Trichomonas vaginalis*. It is the most common curable STD in young sexually active females (Centers for Disease Control and Prevention, 2008b). The vagina in females and the urethra in males are the most common sites of infection. During pregnancy, trichomoniasis infection can result in prematurity or low birth weight in the neonate.

Complications

Refer to Table 97-1.

Table 97-1 | Complications of Sexually Transmitted Diseases

STD/STI	Complication
Chlamydia	Acute pelvic inflammatory disease (PID) Infertility Ectopic pregnancy
Gonorrhea	Acute epididymitis Acute PID Arthritis Dermatitis Disseminated intravascular coagulation (DIC) Infertility Ophthalmia neonatorum in newborn, which can cause blindness
Herpes Simplex Type 2	Generalized systemic (CNS, liver) infections in neonate, with high mortality rate Highly transmittable Lifelong infection Aseptic meningitis Bacterial superinfection
Hepatitis B virus (HBV)	Chronic infection Cirrhosis Liver cancer Liver failure Premature death
Human Papillomavirus (HPV)	Transmission of HPV to fetus Cancer of the cervix, vulva, vagina, anus, or penis
Syphilis	Chronic disease: Neurosyphilis Aortitis
Trichomoniasis	Increased risk of HIV infection in females

Incidence

Refer to Table 97-2.

Table 97-2 | Incidence of Sexually Transmitted Diseases

Sexually transmitted disease	Incidence	Resource
Chlamydia	976,445 in 2005; an estimated 2.8 million Americans contract this infection annually	Centers for Disease Control and Prevention (2007a)
Gonorrhea	2005 statistics: Children aged 10–14 years: 6 cases/100,000 males 35.2 cases/100,000 females Adolescents aged 15–19 years: 261.2 cases/100,000 males 624.7 cases/100,000 females	Centers for Disease Control and Prevention (2007b)
Herpes Simplex Type 2	45 million Americans aged 12 years and older	Centers for Disease Control and Prevention (2007c)
Hepatitis B virus (HBV)	In 2004, 60,000 Americans of all ages; results in 5,000 deaths annually; 90% of exposed infants will develop chronic infections.	Centers for Disease Control and Prevention (2007d) Hepatitis B Foundation (2008)
Human Papilloma-virus (HPV)	20 million Americans, with 6.2 million contracting a new HPV infection annually	Centers for Disease Control and Prevention (2007e)
Syphilis	In 2005, 8,724 cases of primary and secondary syphilis were reported in the United States, or 3 cases/100,000 people.	Centers for Disease Control and Prevention (2007f)
Trichomoniasis	7.4 million new cases annually in the United States	Centers for Disease Control and Prevention (2007g)

Etiology

Refer to Table 97-3.

Table 97-3 | Etiologies of Sexually Transmitted Diseases

Sexually transmitted disease	Etiology
Chlamydia	*Chlamydia trachomatis*
Gonorrhea	*Neisseria gonorrhoeae*
Herpes Simplex Type 2	Herpes simplex type 2 virus
Hepatitis B (HBV)	Hepadnavirus
Human Papillomavirus (HPV)	Human papillomavirus
Syphilis	*Treponema pallidum*
Trichomoniasis	*Trichomonas vaginalis*

Clinical Manifestations

Refer to Table 97-4.

Table 97-4 | Clinical Manifestations of Sexually Transmitted Diseases

Sexually transmitted disease	Clinical manifestations
Chlamydia	Nonpurulent urethritis
Gonorrhea	Purulent greenish discharge Urethritis Painful intercourse Dysuria Chronic pelvic pain (women) Pharyngitis Conjunctivitis
Herpes Simplex Type 2	Painful vesicle lesions
Hepatitis B virus (HBV)	Usually asymptomatic in young people Yellow sclera Jaundice Fatigue Anorexia Abdominal pain Dark urine and feces
Human Papillomavirus (HPV)	Genital warts (soft, moist pink or flesh-colored swellings on genitalia) Precancerous changes in the vulva, cervix, anus, and penis
Syphilis	Painless mucosal and skin lesions on genitalia Hepatosplenomegaly
Trichomoniasis	Usually no manifestations in males; however, they may experience penile irritation, mild discharge, or burn on urination or ejaculation.

Diagnostic Tests

Refer to Table 97-5.

Table 97-5 | Diagnostics for Sexually Transmitted Diseases

STD/STI	Diagnostic test
Chlamydia	Chlamydia culture enzyme immunoassay Nucleic acid amplification tests (NAAT) (American Social Health Association, 2007)
Gonorrhea	Gram stain cultures Urine for bacterial genes or DNA

(continues)

Table 97-5 | Diagnostics for Sexually Transmitted Diseases (*continued*)

STD/STI	Diagnostic test
Herpes Simplex Type 2	HSV-2 viral culture Western Blot serology
Hepatitis B virus (HBV)	Hepatitis B surface antigen (HBsAg) HBc-IgM Hbe-antigen
Human Papillomavirus (HPV)	Abnormal Pap smear HPV DNA test No diagnostic tests for men
Syphilis	Serologic VDRL
Trichomoniasis	Whiff test Wet mount Pap smear OSOM Trichomonas Rapid Test (Wilkerson & Sinert, 2006)

Medical Management
Refer to Table 97-6.

Table 97-6 | Medical Management for Sexually Transmitted Diseases

STD/STI	Medical management
Chlamydia	Azithromycin Doxycycline Erythromycin Ofloxacin

Gonorrhea	Uncomplicated infection of cervix, urethra, or rectum:
	    Ceftriaxone—new drug of choice—125 mg IM; single dose
	    Cefixime—400 mg oral; single dose
	Alternative treatment:
	    Spectinomycin—2 grams IM; single dose or single-dose cephalosporin regimens
	NOTE: Ceftriaxone is the drug of choice for uncomplicated infection of the pharynx and disseminated infection.
	NOTE: Ciprofloxacin, ofloxacin, and levofloxacin are no longer recommended because of wide-spread fluoroquinolone-resistant gonorrhea, although they may be an alternative treatment if the susceptibility of the microorganism can be documented by culture (Centers for Disease Control and Prevention, 2007b).

(*continues*)

Table 97-6 | Medical Management for Sexually Transmitted Diseases (*continued*)

STD/STI	Medical management
Herpes Simplex Type 2	No cure Acyclovir Penciclovir Famciclovir (adolescents/adults) Valacyclovir (adolescents/adults) Foscarnet (12 years old and above) Docosanol cream 10% (12 years old and above)
Hepatitis B virus (HBV)	Prevention—Hepatitis B vaccine No cure Lamividine (chronic HBV in children) Interferon-alpha Pegylated interferon (adolescents/adults) Adefovir dipivoxil (adolescents/adults) Entecavir (adolescents/adults) Telbivudine (adolescents/adults) (Broyles, Reiss, & Evans, 2007)
Human Papillomavirus (HPV)	No treatment for the virus HPV vaccine for four types (6, 11, 16, and 18) of HPV responsible for 70% of cervical cancers and 90% of cervical warts was approved in mid-2006 by the Food and Drug Administration. It is recommended for girls/women aged 9–26 years (Food and Drug Administration, 2007). Cryotherapy (genital warts) Cryosurgery Electrosurgery Laser surgery Surgical removal of genital warts Imiquimod (topical) Interferon-alfa (topical injection) Podofilox (topical) Podophyllin (applied by health care provider) 5-Fluorouracil (topical) Keratolytics (Gearhart & Randall, 2007)
Syphilis	Penicillin G benzathine (IM) Tetracycline (for penicillin-resistant syphilis) Doxycycline (for penicillin-resistant syphilis) (Broyles et al., 2007)
Trichomoniasis	Metronidazole Tinidazole (adolescents/adults) (Wilkerson & Sinert, 2006)

Nursing Management

ASSESSMENT

1. Obtain client history with focus on sexual activity
2. Perform physical assessment
3. Assess for drug allergies
4. Obtain vital signs, height, and weight
5. Assess immunization status

NURSING DIAGNOSES (INCLUDING BUT NOT LIMITED TO)

1. Risk for infection, transmission R/T contagious nature of condition
2. Risk for injury R/T complications of STD
3. Impaired skin and tissue integrity R/T inflammation and skin lesions
4. Self-esteem: situational low R/T being infected with STD
5. Deficient knowledge R/T prevention, condition, treatment, and sexual practices

PLANNING/GOALS

1. Client will be compliant with treatment protocols and will not transmit STD to others.
2. Client will be compliant with treatment protocols and refer any sexual partners for evaluation and necessary treatment.
3. Client's lesions will exhibit healing.
4. Client will demonstrate recovery of self-esteem and use positive coping strategies.
5. Client/parents will demonstrate understanding of condition, treatment, prevention, and sexual practices.

NOC

1. Risk Control: Sexually Transmitted Diseases (STDs)
2. Risk Control
3. Tissue Integrity: Skin & Mucous Membranes
4. Self-Esteem
5. Knowledge: Infection Control, Disease Process, Treatment, Sexual Functioning

IMPLEMENTATION

1. Infection
   a. Follow state and federal guidelines for reporting STDs
   b. Assess for drug allergies
   c. Administer antimicrobials as prescribed if hospitalized
   d. Monitor first dose of penicillin given in clinic or health care provider's office for 45 minutes for urticaria, itching, dyspnea, and temperature elevation
   e. Instruct about medication administration if treated as outpatient
   f. Instruct about importance of compliance with medication regimen
   g. Instruct regarding methods to prevent STDs
2. Risk for injury
   a. Be active in STD prevention programs in community and schools
   b. Stress importance of seeking medical attention if manifestations of STDs occur

    c. Stress importance of compliance with treatment

    d. Instruct about potential complications associated with untreated STDs

    e. Encourage referring sexual partners for evaluation and medical treatment if needed

    f. Instruct to abstain from sexual contact until client /contacts have completed medication regimen

    g. Stress importance of follow-up with health care provider

    h. Instruct to use condoms to prevent further infections

    i. Instruct regarding manifestations of reinfection

3. Skin/tissue integrity

    a. Assess skin lesions using standard (universal) precautions

    b. Instruct to keep lesions clean

    c. Instruct regarding use of sitz bath as prescribed

    d. Instruct concerning guidelines for use of topical agents

4. Self-esteem

    a. Provide a supportive, nonjudgmental environment for client to discuss feelings

    b. Provide privacy and confidentiality according to health care guidelines

    c. Encourage verbalization of feelings and concerns

    d. Communicate that nurse and health care provider are concerned about client

    e. Provide instructions about how to prevent reinfection

    f. Allow expressions of grief following ectopic pregnancy, referring to grief counselor as needed

    g. Collaborate with health care provider for infertility referral as needed

5. Client/parent teaching

    a. Assess client's/family's current level of knowledge

    b. Provide verbal and written information regarding:

        1) Vaccination information and schedule

        2) Risk factors for developing STDs and instructions about how to avoid risk factors; for instance, abstaining from unprotected sexual contact and individuals known to have STDs, seeking medical evaluation and treatment at first manifestations of STDs, and using barrier protection (e.g., condoms) during sexual activity

        3) Need for parents to talk to their children about STD prevention

        4) Medication administration including importance of compliance with prescribed medication regimen

        5) Manifestations of adverse effects of medications (primarily hypersensitivity reactions)

        6) Manifestations of worsening of condition

        7) Contact phone numbers for reporting manifestations

        8) Importance of regular hand washing and appropriate technique

        9) Importance of follow-up with health care provider

    c. Provide adequate time for teaching

    d. Document teaching and client's/parents' response

NIC

1. Infection Precautions, Teaching: Safe Sex
2. Risk Identification
3. Infection Protection, Medication Management, Skin Care: Topical Treatments
4. Self-Esteem Enhancement
5. Teaching: Infection Control, Disease Process, Treatment, Safe Sex

EVALUATION

1. Client is compliant with treatment protocols and does not transmit STD to others.
2. Client is compliant with treatment protocols and refers any sexual partners for evaluation and necessary treatment.
3. Client's lesions exhibit healing.
4. Client demonstrates recovery of self-esteem and uses positive coping strategies.
5. Client/parents demonstrate understanding of condition, treatment, prevention, and sexual practices.

References

American Social Health Association. (2007). *Chlamydia: Questions & answers.* Retrieved May 1, 2007, from http://www.ashastd.org/learn/learn_chlamydia.cfm#5

Broyles, B. E. (2005). *Medical-surgical nursing clinical companion.* Durham, NC: Carolina Academic Press.

Broyles, B. E., Reiss, B. S., & Evans, M. E. (2007). *Pharmacological aspects of nursing care* (7th ed.). Clifton Park, NY: Delmar Cengage Learning.

Centers for Disease Control and Prevention. (2007). *Sexually transmitted disease: Trichomoniasis—CDC fact sheet.* Retrieved March 25, 2008, from http://www.cdc.gov/std/Trichomonas/STDFact-Trichomoniasis.htm

Centers for Disease Control and Prevention. (2007a). *Sexually transmitted disease surveillance 2006 supplement: Chlamydia prevalence monitoring project annual report 2005.* Retrieved March 25, 2008, from http://www.cdc.gov/std/Chlamydia2005/CTSurvSupp2006Short.pdf

Centers for Disease Control and Prevention. (2007b). *Sexually transmitted disease surveillance 2006 supplement: Gonococcal isolate surveillance project (GISP) annual report 2006.* Retrieved March 25, 2008, from http://www.cdc.gov/std/Gisp2006/GISPSurvSupp2006short.pdf

Centers for Disease Control and Prevention. (2007c). *Sexually transmitted disease: Genital herpes—CDC fact sheet.* March 25, 2008, from http://www.cdc.gov/std/Herpes/STDFact-Herpes.htm

Centers for Disease Control and Prevention. (2007d). *Sexually transmitted disease: Hepatitis B—CDC fact sheet.* Retrieved March 25, 2008, from http://www.cdc.gov/ncidod/diseases/hepatitis/b/fact.htm

Centers for Disease Control and Prevention. (2007e). *Sexually transmitted disease: Genital HPV infection—CDC fact sheet.* Retrieved March 25, 2008, from http://www.cdc.gov/std/HPV/STDFact-HPV.htm

Centers for Disease Control and Prevention. (2007f). *STD surveillance 2006: National profile: Syphilis.* Retrieved March 25, 2008, from http://www.cdc.gov/std/stats/syphilis.htm

Centers for Disease Control and Prevention. (2008a). *Sexually transmitted diseases.* Retrieved March 25, 2008, from http://www.cdc.gov/std/default.htm

Centers for Disease Control and Prevention. (2008b). *Updated recommended treatment regimens for gonococcal infections and associated conditions—United States, April 2007.* Retrieved March 25, 2008, from http://www.cdc.gov/std/treatment/2007/updated-regimens.htm

Food and Drug Administration. (2007). *FDA licenses Gardasil.* Retrieved July 10, 2007, from http://www.fda.gov/cder/Offices/OODP/whatsnew/gardasil.htm

Gearhart, P. C., & Randall, T. C. (2007). *Human papillomavirus.* Retrieved May 1, 2007, from http://www.emedicine.com/med/topic1037.htm

Hepatitis B Foundation. (2008). *Managing HBV.* Retrieved March 25, 2008, from http://www .hepb.org/professionals/managing_hepatitis_b.htm

Potts, N. L., & Mandleco, B. L. (2007). *Pediatric nursing: Caring for children and their families* (2nd ed.). Clifton Park, NY: Delmar Cengage Learning.

Wilkerson, R. G., & Sinert, R. (2006). *Trichomoniasis.* Retrieved March 25, 2008, from http:// www.emedicine.com/emerg/topic613.htm

98

SICKLE CELL ANEMIA/
VASO-OCCLUSIVE CRISIS

Definition

Sickle cell anemia is the most common type of sickle cell disease (SCD) and is an autosomal codominant recessive genetic blood disorder characterized by the production of sickle-shaped hemoglobin, Hb S (Broyles, 2005). "Vaso-occlusive crisis refers to the aggregation of sickled cells within a vessel, causing obstruction, ischemia, and pain" (Potts & Mandleco, 2007, p. 828). The most common types of SCD in addition to sickle cell anemia are sickle-hemoglobin C disease (SC), sickle beta-plus thalassemia, and sickle beta-zero thalassemia (Sickle Cell Disease Association of America, 2005). Refer to Figure 98-1.

Pathophysiology

The genetics of SCD cause a single amino acid to change in the beta chain of hemoglobin, resulting in hemoglobin S (Hb S) molecules instead of hemoglobin A (Hb A). Inadequate oxygen causes the red blood cells (RBCs) containing Hb S to become sickle-shaped rather than the normal round shape; and because these cells cannot transport oxygen, anemia occurs. Because of their sickle shape, these RBCs clump together, or aggregate, because they are not flexible enough to flow easily through small vessels. The life span of these cells is only 10–20 days instead of the normal 120 days, so the spleen and the liver become enlarged. In addition, the splenic vessels can become occluded, resulting in the pooling of blood in the spleen. This is referred to as a sequestration crisis (Potts & Mandleco, 2007). Over time, alterations in the blood flow in the eyes can lead to blindness.

Infarctions in the lungs can produce pulmonary emboli. This impairs gas exchange and causes chest pain, cough, fever, and difficult breathing. This condition, referred to as acute chest syndrome, requires immediate medical attention, including blood transfusions, oxygen, antibiotics, and drugs to open airways in the lungs (Broyles, 2005). Pneumonia is the most common cause of death in children with sickle cell anemia (National Heart Lung and Blood Institute, 2006). Refer to Figure 98-2.

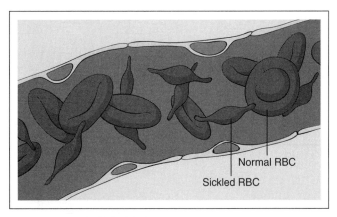

Figure 98-1: Regular and Sickled Red Blood Cells.

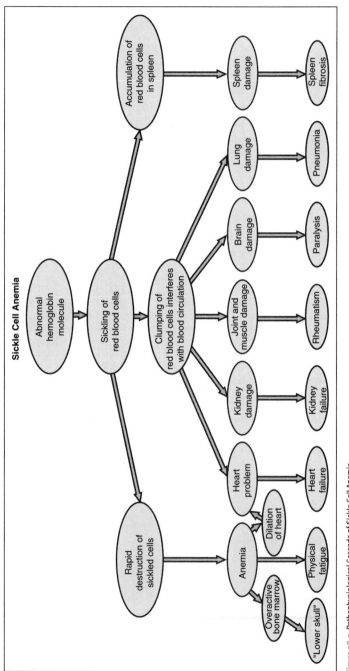

Figure 98-2: Pathophysiological Cascade of Sickle Cell Anemia.

Vaso-occlusive crisis occurs when the sickled cells aggregate, or clump together, in a blood vessel, causing obstruction. The loss of blood supply to the tissues distal to the occlusion causes the tissues to experience ischemia, resulting in damage to the tissues and severe pain. During a crisis, multiple vessels are affected, leading to severe pain throughout the body. In the event that the occlusion occurs in the small vessels of the brain, a cerebrovascular accident (CVA), or stroke, can occur. Aplastic crisis occurs when erythropoiesis decreases. In infants, hand-foot syndrome is characteristic and is so named because the hands and/or feet become tender, warm, swollen, and very painful due to microvasculature obstruction in the distal extremities (Potts & Mandleco, 2007).

Complications

Sequestration crisis causing hepatosplenomegaly
Jaundice
CVA
Vaso-occlusive crisis
Acute chest syndrome
Aplastic crisis
Blindness
Multiple organ dysfunction
Pneumonia
Bacterial septicemia, possibly leading to death

Incidence

Millions of people throughout the world are affected by sickle cell anemia. It is most common in individuals whose families come from Africa, South America, Cuba, Central American, Saudi Arabia, India, Turkey, Greece, and Italy. In the United States, sickle cell anemia affects about 72,000 people. The families of most Americans who are affected are African American. In the United States, the disease occurs in approximately 1 in every 600 African-American births and one in every 1,000–1,400 Hispanic-American births. About 1 in 12 African Americans has sickle cell trait (National Heart Lung and Blood Institute, 2006). Approximately 1 in 375 African Americans is born with SCD annually in the United States (St. Jude Children's Research Hospital, 2008). The stressors of adolescence commonly result in hospitalization of these children for vaso-occlusive crises.

Etiology

Sickle cell anemia is an autosomal codominant recessive genetic blood disease. Some individuals carry the sickle cell trait (AS) in which Hb A and Hb S are produced in the RBCs; however, more Hb A is produced than Hb S. Sickle cell trait is not a type of SCD, but rather one of the mechanisms that can result in children inheriting sickle cell anemia. If one parent has sickle cell anemia and the other does not, all of the children will have sickle cell trait. If one parent has sickle cell anemia and the other has sickle cell trait, there is a 50% chance of having a baby with either SCD or sickle cell trait with each pregnancy. When both parents have sickle cell trait, they have a 25% chance of having a baby with SCD with each pregnancy (Sickle Cell Disease Association of American, 2005).

Clinical Manifestations

Anemia:
    Fatigue
    Frequent infections
Vaso-occlusive crisis:
    Severe pain in joints
    Severe pain distal to occlusions

Fever

Decreased range of motion

Severe abdominal pain

CVA

Dyspnea

Tachycardia

Palpitations

Pallor

Weakness

Visual changes

Diagnostic Tests

Prenatal testing: chorionic villi sampling

Neonatal hemoglobinopathy screening

Sickle solubility test

Hemoglobin electrophoresis

Medical Management

The goals of treatment are early identification of neonates with SCD, prevention of infections, treatment for the anemia, and prevention and treatment of vaso-occlusive crises. Most states have adopted mandatory hemoglobinopathy screening as a part of every newborn assessment. Bone marrow transplantation is the only cure for SCD. However, its use is limited because of the difficulty in finding suitable donors (a child's parents are not suitable donors).

Hydroxyurea has been demonstrated to increase fetal hemoglobin (Hb F) and decrease the white cell count and platelet count in infants. In addition, it improves RBC hydration, decreases cytokine production, and limits RBC adhesion. Increasingly, hydroxyurea is being used throughout the world in children with SCD.

Research sponsored by the National Institutes of Health "discovered that a daily dose of penicillin could prevent fatal infections in infants with SCD. . . . Today, newborns found to have the disease are given antibiotics until age 5 when prophylaxis can be stopped safely [as demonstrated by another NIH study]. . . . [In addition,] NIH-supported researchers found ways to identify children with SCD who were likely to have strokes and established that regular blood transfusions could reduce stroke risk by 90%" (National Institutes of Health, 2007, p. 1).

Most children hospitalized with sickle cell anemia experience vaso-occlusive crisis. The standard of care for vaso-occlusive crisis is (1) pain management, (2) oxygenation, and (3) hydration. More than 20% of individuals with SCD experience as many as 40 painful episodes annually, making pain management a critical element of care. The "acute and chronic pain associated with sickle cell disease is often undertreated or otherwise inappropriately managed" (Dorman, 2005, p. 34). The standard of care for pain management "remains continuous intravenous infusion of morphine sulfate combined with patient-controlled analgesia doses of morphine for 48–72 hours (or until pain symptoms are sufficiently controlled to progress to oral opioid analgesics). Hydromorphone may be prescribed if morphine is ineffective in controlling the pain. 'As needed' dosing of these opioid analgesics is discouraged because this type of dosing does not provide continuous blood levels of the medication to achieve adequate pain management. Intramuscular dosing also is inappropriate because 1) it is a painful procedure and 2) frequent injections can lead to sclerosing of tissue that will impair absorption of the drugs" (Broyles, 2005, p. 769). Numerous studies have determined that respiratory depression is an unlikely adverse effect of opioid dosing in children and adults. However, young children should be placed on continuous cardiorespiratory monitoring as a precaution while receiving opioid analgesics (Broyles, Reiss, & Evans, 2007).

Another standard of care for vaso-occlusive crisis is the continuous administration of oxygen. It is titrated to maintain oxygen saturation > 94%. Providing oxygen to the ischemic tissues also assists in pain control.

Providing intravenous hydration also is imperative for tissue perfusion. Usually, intravenous fluids are infused at a rate of 1½ times the usual maintenance rate or at a fluid intake of 200 mL/hr according to the child's height and weight. Solutions such as 5% dextrose in water and 5% dextrose in water with 0.225% sodium chloride are used for two reasons. First, these types of intravenous fluids dilute the intracellular hemoglobin concentration, helping to prevent further crystallizing of the sickled hemoglobin. Second, because of a defect in renal concentration, dehydration is a common complication of SCD and increases pain. Providing hydration helps decrease the duration of pain. Transfusions of packed RBCs may be required to meet tissue perfusion needs to improve oxygen-carrying ability (Broyles, 2005).

During this time, physical activity is limited and determined by the child. Placing children in pain crisis on strict bed rest is not appropriate because having the child use a bedpan for elimination needs usually creates more pain than does assisting the child to the bathroom.

Following acute treatment for vaso-occlusive crisis, oxygen, intravenous hydration, and opioid analgesics are tapered according to the child's response to therapy. In some cases, removal of the spleen (splenectomy) is required. This procedure increases the risk of infection because of the immune function of the spleen, so the child requires lifelong antimicrobial prophylaxis following this surgery.

Nursing Management

ASSESSMENT

1. Perform neonatal screening
2. Obtain client history
3. Assess pain level
4. Perform physical assessment
5. Obtain vital signs, height, and weight
6. Assess psychosocial impact of disease/crisis on client/family

NURSING DIAGNOSES (INCLUDING BUT NOT LIMITED TO)

1. Acute pain R/T tissue ischemia associated with vaso-occlusive crisis
2. Ineffective tissue perfusion R/T impaired arterial blood flow
3. High risk for infection R/T splenic malfunction, splenectomy, and chronic immunosuppressed state
4. Ineffective coping R/T chronic and potentially life-threatening nature of disease
5. Deficient knowledge R/T child's condition, treatment, prevention of complications, and home care

PLANNING/GOALS

1. Client will demonstrate pain management during vaso-occlusive crisis as determined by client using an age-appropriate pain assessment scale at a level of 0 to 1 on a scale of 0 to 5 or 0 to 2 on a scale of 0 to 10 on the numeric scale. For toddlers and preschoolers a 5-point faces scale is used, with zero indicating no pain and 5 indicating the worst pain the child has ever experienced; for school-age children and adolescents, a 0–10 numerical scale is used, with zero being no pain and 10 being the worst pain the child has ever experienced.
2. Client will maintain oxygen saturation > 94%, pain management, capillary refill, and vital signs within defined limits (WDL).

3. Client will exhibit no manifestations of infection.
4. Client/family will demonstrate use of positive coping strategies.
5. Client/family will demonstrate understanding of condition, treatment, prevention of complications, and home care.

NOC

1. Pain Level, Pain Control
2. Circulation Status
3. Risk Control
4. Coping, Acceptance: Health Status, Child Adaptation to Hospitalization
5. Knowledge: Illness Care, Treatment, Medications, Health Promotion

IMPLEMENTATION

1. Pain
   a. Establish and maintain patency of intravenous access, monitoring at least hourly
   b. Assess pain hourly
   c. Instruct child about use of patient-controlled analgesia to augment continuous infusion, and importance of dosing proactively
   d. Place young child on continuous cardiorespiratory monitoring
   e. Explain purpose of cardiorespiratory monitoring and unlikelihood of respiratory depression with opioid analgesics
   f. Administer intravenous fluids as prescribed
   g. Place on continuous pulse oximetry
   h. Administer oxygen as prescribed, titrating to maintain prescribed oxygen saturation
   i. Collaborate with health care provider for increase in dosing or change of analgesic agent if pain is not managed effectively
   j. Administer bolus doses of analgesic as prescribed for breakthrough pain
   k. Position for comfort, maintaining proper alignment to avoid stress to joints and tissues
   l. Provide periods of undisturbed rest
   m. Reassure child or family that has concerns about addiction to analgesics that addiction is rare especially when used on short-term basis
   n. Collaborate with health care provider regarding use of moist heat (K-pad)
   o. Encourage child to ask for assistance to bathroom and back to bed
   p. Straighten or change bed linens while client is in bathroom to avoid discomfort of occupied bed linen change
   q. Collaborate with health care provider for alternative complementary strategies such as relaxation, hydrotherapy, massage therapy, and aroma therapy

2. Tissue perfusion
   a. Monitor continuous oxygen saturation using pulse oximetry
   b. Administer oxygen as prescribed, titrating to maintain prescribed oxygen saturation and per client response
   c. Administer intravenous fluids at prescribed rate (1½ times usual maintenance rate according to child's weight)

    d. Assess capillary refill every 8 hours and as needed

    e. Maintain quiet, restful environment to conserve energy and oxygenation

    f. Assess vital signs every 4 hours and as needed

    g. Elevate head of bed to facilitate breathing

    h. Encourage deep breathing through use of incentive spirometry

    i. Monitor laboratory test results

3. Infection

    a. Monitor vital signs during hospitalization every 4 hours and as needed

    b. Maintain strict asepsis during any invasive procedures

    c. Observe standard (universal) precautions at all times

    d. Assess breath sounds every 8 hours and as needed

    e. Administer antimicrobial agents as prescribed

    f. Administer antipyretic agents as prescribed for temperature elevation

    g. Encourage deep breathing through use of incentive spirometry

    h. Instruct about prophylaxis with penicillin and importance of immunizations

4. Coping

    a. Assess for manifestations of anxiety and caregiver stress

    b. Provide environment conducive to child's/family's expression of feelings and concerns

    c. Listen actively

    d. Assist in use of positive coping strategies

    e. Collaborate with health care provider for referrals as indicated by assessment

    f. Encourage adolescent to have contact with peers and perhaps visits depending on adolescent's needs

5. Client/family teaching

    a. Assess child's/family's current level of knowledge

    b. Provide verbal and written information regarding:

        1) Risk factors for developing infection and instructions as needed to avoid risk factors; for instance, being compliant with prophylactic antimicrobial therapy, being vaccinated against pneumonia and influenza, and avoiding people with known communicable diseases

        2) Need for lifelong antimicrobial prophylaxis, especially following splenectomy

        3) Medication administration including importance of compliance with prescribed medication regime

        4) Manifestations of adverse effects of medications (constipation with opioid analgesics and hypersensitivity response with penicillin)

        5) Manifestations of worsening condition

        6) Contact phone numbers for reporting signs and symptoms

        7) Importance of regular hand washing and appropriate technique

        8) Importance of follow-up with health care provider

    c. Provide adequate time for teaching

    d. Document teaching and client's/family's response

NIC

1. Medication Management, Pain Management, Patient-Controlled Analgesia (PCA) Assistance
2. Intravenous Therapy, Oxygen Therapy
3. Infection Precautions
4. Coping Enhancement
5. Teaching: Illness Care, Treatment, Medications, Health Education

EVALUATION

1. Client demonstrates pain management during vaso-occlusive crisis as determined by client using age-appropriate pain assessment tool at a level of 0 to 1 on a scale of 0 to 5 on the faces scale or 0 to 2 on a scale of 0 to 10 on the numeric scale.
2. Client maintains oxygen saturation > 94%, pain management, capillary refill, and vital signs WDL.
3. Client exhibits no manifestations of infection.
4. Client/family demonstrate use of positive coping strategies.
5. Client/family demonstrate understanding of condition, treatment, prevention of complications, and home care.

References

Broyles, B. E. (2005). *Medical-surgical nursing clinical companion*. Durham, NC: Carolina Academic Press.

Broyles, B. E., Reiss, B. S., & Evans, M. E. (2007). *Pharmacological aspects of nursing care* (7th ed.). Clifton Park, NY: Delmar Cengage Learning.

Dorman, K. (2005). Sickle cell crisis! Managing the pain. *RN, 68*(12).

National Heart Lung and Blood Institute. (2006). *What is sickle cell anemia?* Retrieved May 1, 2007, from http://www.nhlbi.nih.gov/health/dci/Diseases/Sca/SCA_WhatIs.html

National Institutes of Health. (2007). *Fact sheet: Sickle cell disease*. Retrieved May 2, 2007, from www.nih.gov/about/researchresultsforthepublic/SickleCellDisease.pdf

Potts, N. L., & Mandleco, B. L. (2007). *Pediatric nursing: Caring for children and their families*. (2nd ed.). Clifton Park, NY: Delmar Cengage Learning.

Sickle Cell Disease Association of America. (2005). *What is sickle cell disease?* Retrieved May 1, 2007, from http://www.sicklecelldisease.org/about_scd/index.phtml

St. Jude Children's Research Hospital. (2008). *Treating Sickle Cell Disease in children*. Retrieved March 25, 2008, from http://www.stjude.org/stjude/v/index.jsp?vgnextoid=0f3c061585f70110VgnVCM1000001e0215acRCRD&vgnextchannel=bc4fbfe82e118010VgnVCM1000000e2015acRCRD&source=overture&kw=sickle+cell+disease+in+children

99

SUDDEN INFANT DEATH SYNDROME (SIDS)

Definition

Sudden infant death syndrome (SIDS) is "the sudden, unexplained death of an infant younger than one year old" (National Institute of Child Health & Human Development, 2007, p. 1).

Pathophysiology

Because the cause of SIDS is unknown, the exact pathophysiology of the SIDS process also is not completely understood. Although theories vary concerning the mechanisms of SIDS, they seem to agree that the infant experiences hypoxia resulting in death. The mechanisms of what initiates the hypoxic process are theorized to be (1) a delay in the development of the nervous system that controls the arousal response to decreased oxygen and the cardiorespiratory center of the brain, (2) maldevelopment in the hypercapnea response system in the brain, (3) rebreathing of carbon dioxide by the infant, and (4) decreased laryngeal chemoreflex leading to apnea and bradycardia (Potts & Mandleco, 2007). Because SIDS most commonly occurs in otherwise healthy infants, the devastation to parents and family members is severe.

Complications

Death to infant
Loss and grief for family

Incidence

Annually in the United States, more than 4,500 infants die suddenly of no obvious cause. "Half of these sudden, unexplained infant deaths (SUID) are due to sudden infant death syndrome (SIDS), the leading cause of SUID and of all deaths among infants aged 1–12 months" (Centers for Disease Control and Prevention, 2007, p. 1). Boys are more likely to experience SIDS than girls, and the peak season is winter (Maindonald, 2005). SIDS is rare during the first month of life and peaks in infants aged 2–4 months, with approximately 95% of SIDS deaths occurring in infants less than 6 months of age (Potts & Mandleco, 2007). The rate declines after 6 months of age. Infants who are placed to sleep on their stomachs or sides are at higher risk for SIDS than infants who are placed on their backs to sleep. In addition, African-American infants are more than 2 times as likely to die of SIDS as Caucasian infants, and American-Indian/Alaska Native infants are nearly 3 times as likely to die of SIDS as Caucasian infants (National Institute of Child Health & Human Development, 2007).

Etiology

Currently, the cause of SIDS is unknown. However, certain risk factors have been identified, including prone positioning, soft sleep surfaces, loose bedding, use of pillows while sleeping, infant overheating, parental smoking, bed sharing, and prematurity or low birth weight (Centers for Disease Control and Prevention, 2007). Other risk factors include infants of multiple birth, infants with sibling who died of SIDS, adolescent mothers, short intervals between pregnancies, late or no prenatal care, and situations of poverty (MedlinePlus, 2007).

Clinical Manifestations

None (MedlinePlus, 2007)

Diagnostic Tests

Autopsy unable to determine cause of death

Medical Management

The goal of management of SIDS is prevention. According to the revised American Academy of Pediatrics (AAP) guidelines released in October 2005, the following recommendations should be followed by parents of infants (Colson, 2005):

1. Always put baby to sleep on his/her back, including naps.
2. Put babies to sleep in a crib only. *Never* allow a baby to sleep in bed with other children or adults and do *not* put him/her to sleep on surfaces other than cribs (e.g., a sofa).
3. Let babies sleep in the same room (*not* the same bed) as parents.
4. Avoid soft bedding materials (pillows, comforters, and quilts) and place infant on a firm, tight-fitting crib mattress. Use a light sheet to cover infant.
5. Ensure that temperature of room is not too hot. Maintain temperature so that it is comfortable for a lightly clothed adult.
6. Consider offering a pacifier at nap time and bedtime: Although the mechanism is not known, the reduced risk of SIDS associated with pacifier use during sleep is compelling, and the evidence that pacifier use inhibits breastfeeding or causes later dental complications is not. Until evidence dictates otherwise, the task force recommends use of a pacifier throughout the first year of life (American Academy of Pediatrics, 2005, p. 1)
7. Do not use breathing monitors or products marketed as ways to reduce SIDS. These are ineffective in preventing SIDS.
8. Do not expose infants to secondhand smoke.
9. Ensure that infant is placed on his/her back to sleep in day care center, in relative's home, and in all other places where infant care is provided.

Nursing Management

ASSESSMENT

1. Assess parental understanding of neonatal and infant care
2. Assess for risk factors for SIDS
3. Assess psychosocial impact of SIDS

NURSING DIAGNOSES (INCLUDING BUT NOT LIMITED TO)

1. Deficient knowledge R/T infant care and practices to prevent SIDS
2. Grieving, complicated R/T sudden death of infant

PLANNING/GOALS

1. Parents will demonstrate understanding of infant care and prevention practices for SIDS. Infant will not experience SIDS.
2. Parents (of infant who dies of SIDS) will use positive coping strategies and support systems to cope with loss of infant.

NOC

1. Knowledge: Infant Care, Health Promotion
2. Grief Resolution

IMPLEMENTATION

1. Parent teaching

   a. Assess new parents' understanding of infant care and prevention of SIDS

   b. Serve as role model by using AAP recommendations for preventing SIDS

   c. Provide verbal and written information regarding:

      1) Necessity of putting baby to sleep on his/her back, including naps

      2) Necessity of putting babies to sleep in a crib only, *never* allowing a baby to sleep in bed with other children or adults and *not* putting him/her to sleep on surfaces other than cribs (e.g., a sofa)

      3) Importance of letting babies sleep in the same room (*not* the same bed) as parents

      4) Importance of avoiding soft bedding materials (pillows, comforters, and quilts) and placing infant on a firm, tight-fitting crib mattress. A light sheet can be used to cover infant.

      5) Importance of ensuring that temperature of room is not too hot; temperature should be comfortable for a lightly clothed adult

      6) Benefit of allowing infant to sleep with a pacifier. The AAP says that one SIDS death could be prevented for every 2,733 babies who suck on a pacifier during sleep.

      7) No need to use breathing monitors or products marketed as ways to reduce SIDS. These are ineffective in preventing SIDS

      8) Benefit of not exposing infants to secondhand smoke

      9) Necessity of placing infant on his/her back to sleep in day care center, in relative's home, and in all other places where infant care is provided (Colson, 2005)

      10) Infant care and feeding (breastfeeding decreases the risk of respiratory infections that may contribute to SIDS)

      11) Importance of recommended immunizations

      12) Importance of follow-up care for infant and mother

   d. Provide adequate time for teaching

   e. Initiate referrals to Social Services for infants at risk

   f. Document teaching and parental response

2. Grief

   a. Assess for status of grief work

   b. Provide privacy for parents

   c. Encourage verbalization of feelings and concerns

   d. Assure parents (who comply with AAP guidelines) that the infant's death was not their fault

   e. Assist parents to identify positive coping strategies and support systems

   f. Provide information concerning SIDS support groups (community and national)

   g. Assist with contacting pastoral care or parents' spiritual advisor according to parents' wishes

   h. Collaborate with health care provider for continuity and follow-up care for parents

NIC

1. Teaching: Infant Care, Health Education
2. Grief Work Facilitation, Coping Enhancement

EVALUATION

1. Parents demonstrate understanding of infant care and prevention practices for SIDS. Infant does not experience SIDS.
2. Parents (of infant who dies of SIDS) use positive coping strategies and support systems to cope with loss of infant.

References

American Academy of Pediatrics. (2005). *The changing concept of Sudden Infant Death Syndrome: Diagnostic Coding Shifts, Controversies Regarding the Sleeping Environment, and New Variables to Consider in Reducing Risk.* Retrieved May 19, 2008, from http://aappolicy.aappublications.org/cgi/content/full/pediatrics;116/5/1245#SEC15

Centers for Disease Control and Prevention. (2007). *Sudden infant death syndrome (SIDS).* Retrieved March 25, 2008, from http://www.cdc.gov/SIDS/index.htm

Colson, E. R. (2005). *Revised recommendations on reducing sudden infant death syndrome.* Retrieved May 2, 2007, from http://www.ynhh.org/healthlink/pediatrics/pediatrics_12_05.html

Maindonald, E. (2005). Helping parents reduce the risk of SIDS. *Nursing, 35*(7).

MedlinePlus. (2007). *Sudden infant death syndrome.* Retrieved March 25, 2008, from http://www.nlm.nih.gov/medlineplus/ency/article/001566.htm

National Institute of Child Health & Human Development. (2007). *Sudden infant death syndrome (SIDS).* Retrieved March 25, 2008, from http://www.nichd.nih.gov/health/topics/Sudden_Infant_Death_Syndrome.cfm

Potts, N. L., & Mandleco, B. L. (2007). *Pediatric nursing: Caring for children and their families* (2nd ed.). Clifton Park, NY: Delmar Cengage Learning.

100

SURGICAL CLIENT

Definition

For this chapter, the surgical client is defined as a child who experiences a surgical procedure requiring anesthesia and preoperative, intraoperative, and postoperative nursing care. The focus is on the postoperative nursing care, remembering that adaptations need to be made for each child individually (Broyles, 2005; Smeltzer & Bare, 2008).

Nursing Management

ASSESSMENT

1. Obtain client history
2. Assess vital signs
3. Perform pediatric assessment
4. Assess preoperative diagnostic tests
5. Assess for psychosocial impact of child's surgery on child/family

NURSING DIAGNOSES (INCLUDING BUT NOT LIMITED TO)

1. Fear and anxiety R/T to diagnosis and pending surgery
2. Risk for ineffective airway clearance R/T depressed respiratory function, pain, and postoperative positioning
3. Risk for injury, bleeding R/T surgical tissue trauma
4. Acute pain R/T surgical tissue trauma
5. Ineffective thermoregulation R/T surgical environment and anesthetic agents
6. Risk for fluid volume deficit R/T surgical procedure, blood loss, presence of gastric decompression, and decreased fluid intake before and after surgery
7. Risk for infection R/T impaired tissue and skin integrity secondary to surgical procedure
8. Risk for imbalanced nutrition: less than body requirements R/T decreased oral intake
9. Risk for constipation R/T anesthetic agents, opioid analgesic medications, decreased intake, and decreased activity
10. Risk for urinary retention R/T anesthetic agents, decreased oral fluid intake
11. Deficient knowledge R/T child's condition, postoperative treatment regimen, and home care

PLANNING/GOALS

1. Client/family will verbalize concerns and demonstrate use of positive coping strategies.
2. Client will maintain a patent airway as evidenced by respiratory status within defined limits (WDL).
3. Client will not experience injury from bleeding as evidenced by hemoglobin and hematocrit and vital signs WDL.

4. Client will demonstrate pain control as determined by client as evidenced by postoperative behavioral indicators, pain level of 1 on a scale of 0 to 5 on pediatric pain scale for children under 7 years of age and 2 to 3 on a scale of 0 to 10 on numerical pain assessment scale for children over 7 years of age.

5. Client will regain and maintain body temperature WDL.

6. Client will experience fluid and electrolyte balance as evidenced by balanced intake and output and serum electrolyte levels and urine specific gravity WDL.

7. Client will not experience postoperative infection as evidenced by vital signs and white blood cell (WBC) count WDL.

8. Client will experience balanced nutrition as evidenced by consuming 90% of diet and weight gain appropriate for age.

9. Client will not experience constipation as evidenced by return of client's normal bowel pattern within 72 hours following surgery.

10. Client will not experience urinary retention as evidenced by urinary output 1–2 mL/kg/hr for young children and 30 mL/hr for older children and adolescents.

11. Parents/family and client (if age-appropriate) will demonstrate understanding of condition, treatment, and postoperative home care.

NOC

1. Fear, Anxiety
2. Respiratory Status: Airway Patency
3. Risk Control, Circulation Status
4. Pain Level
5. Thermoregulation
6. Risk Control, Fluid Balance, Electrolyte Balance
7. Risk Control, Immune Status
8. Risk Control, Nutritional Status
9. Risk Control, Bowel Elimination, Hydration
10. Risk Control, Urinary Elimination
11. Knowledge: Illness Care, Treatment, Medications, Health Promotion

IMPLEMENTATION

1. Anxiety
   a. Encourage child/family to express fears and concerns about condition and treatment
   b. Clarify and provide accurate information
   c. Allow sufficient time for questions
   d. Encourage parents to remain with child
   e. Provide preoperative instructions
   f. Encourage parents to accompany child to preoperative hold area
   g. Keep family informed of child's progress during surgery and post anesthesia care

2. Airway
   a. Monitor respiratory status continuously in post anesthesia care unit (PACU) and during immediate postoperative period on nursing unit through cardiorespiratory monitoring
   b. Monitor continuous oxygen saturation via pulse oximetry

    c. Administer oxygen to maintain prescribed oxygen saturation

    d. Position with head of bed/crib elevated

    e. Encourage turn, cough, and deep-breathing exercises

    f. Monitor vital signs according to facility postoperative protocol

    g. Auscultate breath sounds

    h. Suction respiratory secretions as needed

3. Risk for bleeding

    a. Monitor vital signs every 4 hours for 24–72 hours postoperatively according to facility protocol

    b. Assess for bleeding at incision site

    c. Monitor wound dressing (circle drainage and note time and date on dressing)

    d. Monitor hemoglobin and hematocrit and report abnormal findings to health care provider

    e. Monitor skin color and temperature

    f. Monitor oxygen saturation by pulse oximetry

    g. Administer oxygen to maintain prescribed oxygen saturation

    h. Monitor respiratory and cardiovascular status

    i. Monitor capillary refill

4. Acute pain

    a. Assess pain level hourly

    b. Maintain patency of intravenous access, monitoring at least hourly

    c. Collaborate with health care provider to prescribe use of patient-controlled analgesia (PCA) if child is old enough to press PCA button

    d. Instruct child on use of PCA device

    e. Administer opioid analgesics proactively for infant or young child

    f. Position to prevent stress on incision

    g. Turn every 2 hours

    h. Maintain indwelling urinary catheter patency to prevent urinary distention

    i. Encourage early ambulation

    j. Assist child with progression to oral analgesics while continuing to ensure adequate pain control

    k. Promote climate to ensure adequate rest and sleep

5. Thermoregulation

    a. Monitor temperature continuously with skin probe until temperature returns to WDL

    b. Place warmed blankets on child

    c. Assess for shivering, mottling, respiratory compromise, and other indicators of hypothermia

    d. Place on heating mattress if temperature does not return to normal in PACU. *NOTE: Do not use hot water bottles* as these can burn the sensitive skin of a child.

6. Fluid and electrolyte balance

    a. Maintain patency of intravenous access, monitoring at least hourly

    b. Administer intravenous fluids as prescribed

    c. Monitor intake and output

d. Maintain gastric decompression via nasogastric tube (if one is in place) by checking output every hour, maintaining prescribed suction, and irrigating tube as needed to maintain patency; administer intravenous fluid replacement for nasogastric drainage as prescribed (usually 0.5–1 mL intravenous fluids/mL of gastric drainage)

e. Maintain indwelling urinary catheter patency and assess color and amount of urine

f. Report to health care provider if urine output < 1–2 mL/kg/hr for young child and < 30 mL/hr for older child and adolescents

g. Monitor serum electrolyte levels and report abnormal values to health care provider

h. Monitor urine specific gravity

i. Assess child's favorite beverages

j. Encourage oral intake as prescribed

7. Risk for infection

a. Monitor vital signs every 4 hours

b. Monitor incision site for redness, swelling, and approximation every shift

c. Perform wound dressing changes as prescribed

d. Administer prophylactic antimicrobial agents as prescribed

e. Perform indwelling urinary catheter care per facility protocol

f. Encourage hand washing and teach appropriate technique

8. Nutrition

a. Monitor intake and output

b. Assess child's favorite foods

c. Collaborate with dietician to provide child's favorite foods as dietary restrictions, if any, allow

d. Encourage parents/family to bring child's favorite foods from home

e. Weigh daily

f. Encourage age-appropriate activities

g. Encourage parents to be present at mealtimes

9. Bowel elimination

a. Assess child's bowel patterns prior to surgery

b. Maintain intake and output

c. Monitor return of bowel sounds

d. Collaborate with health care provider for prescription for scheduled stool softener medications

e. Assist child to bathroom to defecate rather than using bedpan

f. Encourage ambulation as prescribed and tolerated

10. Urinary elimination

a. Monitor and provide catheter care per facility protocol if indwelling urinary catheter is in place

b. Monitor intake and output

c. Monitor bladder placement

d. Encourage oral intake of fluids

e. Assist child to bathroom to urinate rather than using bedpan

f. Encourage ambulation as prescribed and tolerated

11. Parent/family and child (if age-appropriate) teaching
    a. Assess parents'/family's and child's (if age-appropriate) current level of knowledge
    b. Provide verbal and written information regarding:
        1) Postoperative activity restrictions
        2) Postoperative dietary modifications as indicated
        3) Instructions about dressing changes, monitoring temperature, alternative feeding methods, etc., as appropriate
        4) Medication administration including importance of compliance with prescribed medication regimen as needed
        5) Manifestations of adverse effects of medications
        6) Manifestations of postoperative complications
        7) Importance of adequate fluid intake
        8) Instructions for providing catheter care if discharged with indwelling urinary catheter in place
        9) Contact phone numbers for reporting manifestations
        10) Importance of regular hand washing and appropriate technique
        11) Importance of follow-up with health care provider
    c. Provide adequate time for teaching, demonstrations, and return demonstrations
    d. Document teaching and parental/family response

NIC

1. Anxiety Reduction, Coping Enhancement
2. Airway Management
3. Risk Identification, Hemodynamic Regulation
4. Analgesic Administration, Pain Management
5. Temperature Regulation
6. Fluid Management, Fluid Monitoring, Electrolyte Management
7. Infection Precautions, Wound Care
8. Nutrition Management
9. Bowel Management, Fluid/Electrolyte Management
10. Urinary Elimination Management
11. Teaching: Illness Care, Treatment, Medications, Health Education

EVALUATION

1. Client/family verbalize concerns and demonstrate use of positive coping strategies.
2. Client maintains a patent airway as evidenced by respiratory status WDL.
3. Client does not experience injury from bleeding as evidenced by hemoglobin and hematocrit and vital signs WDL.
4. Client demonstrates pain control as determined by client as evidenced by postoperative behavioral indicators, pain level of 1 on a scale of 0 to 5 on pediatric pain scale for children under 7 years of age, and 2 to 3 on a scale of 0 to 10 on numerical pain assessment scale for children over 7 years of age.
5. Client regains and maintains body temperature WDL.
6. Client experiences fluid and electrolyte balance as evidenced by balanced intake and output and serum electrolyte levels and urine specific gravity WDL.

7. Client does not experience postoperative infection as evidenced by vital signs and WBC count WDL.

8. Client experiences balanced nutrition as evidenced by consuming 90% of diet and weight gain appropriate for age.

9. Client does not experience constipation as evidenced by return of normal bowel pattern within 72 hours after surgery.

10. Client does not experience urinary retention as evidenced by urinary output 1–2 mL/kg/hr for young children and 30 mL/hr for older children and adolescents.

11. Parents/family and client (if age-appropriate) demonstrate understanding of condition, treatment, and postoperative home care.

References

Broyles, B. E. (2005). *Medical-surgical nursing clinical companion*. Durham, NC: Carolina Academic Press.

Smeltzer, S. C., & Bare, B. G. (2008). *Brunner & Suddarth's textbook of medical-surgical nursing* (11th ed.). Philadelphia: Lippincott Williams & Wilkins.

101

Systemic Lupus Erythematosus (SLE)

Definition

Systemic lupus erythematosus (SLE), also referred to as lupus, is a chronic inflammatory autoimmune disorder affecting the blood vessels and connective tissues of the body (Potts & Mandleco, 2007).

Pathophysiology

The immune system normally regulates the body's defenses against invasion, specifically by developing antibodies to protect against antigens such as bacteria, viruses, and foreign bodies. In children (or adults) with SLE, the immune system is unable to distinguish between invaders and normal body cells and tissues. This results in the production of autoantibodies. These autoantibodies attack the body's own cells and, in combination with antigens, form immune complexes that develop over time. This results in a state of autoimmunity or self-immunity that deposits protein products of immunity in the vascular system, leading to inflammation, pain, and tissue damage. Although any body tissue or organ can be affected, those most commonly manifesting SLE are the blood vessels (impacting internal organs such as the lungs, heart, brain, and kidneys), skin, and joints (Potts & Mandleco, 2007). Manifestations of SLE include skin rashes, arthritis (present in 95% of clients), pleurisy, pleural effusion, hemolytic anemia, pericarditis, myocarditis, thrombocytopenia, seizures, psychosis, and nephritis. The five-year survival rate in children is approximately 90%, with most deaths attributed to infection, nephritis, renal failure, neurologic disease, or pulmonary hemorrhage (Klein-Gitelman, 2006).

One of the major hurdles for most children with SLE and for health care providers is accurately diagnosing the disease. Because three of the most common manifestations (fever, fatigue, and weight loss) are nonspecific, the organ manifestations can be confused with other disorders. In 1982, The American College of Rheumatology established 11 criteria to help assist SLE researchers and health care providers in accurately diagnosing SLE. It revised these criteria in 1996; they include (1) malar rash, (2) discoid rash, (3) photosensitivity, (4) oral ulcers, (5) arthritis, (6) serositis, (7) proteinuria, (8) seizures or psychosis, (9) hemolytic anemia, leukopenia, lymphopenia, or thrombocytopenia, (10) positive phospholipid antibody, and (11) presence of antinuclear antibody (ANA) (American College of Rheumatology, 2007). Refer to Figure 101-1. The course of SLE involves relapses and remissions and may vary from a mild episodic illness to a severe fatal disease.

"SLE is one of three primary forms of lupus. Discoid lupus erythematosus (DLE) is a form that affects only the skin and usually does not advance to SLE. Drug-induced SLE develops following the use of certain pharmacologic agents including procainamide, hydralazine hydrochloride, and chlorpromazine. This form of SLE usually completely resolves after the drug is discontinued" (Broyles, 2005, p. 811).

Complications

Arthritis

Pleurisy

Pleural effusion

Hemolytic anemia

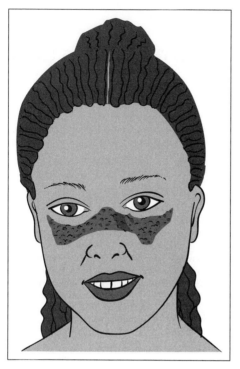

Figure 101-1: **Butterfly Rash Often Seen in SLE.**

Pericarditis
Myocarditis
Thrombocytopenia
Seizures
Psychosis
Nephritis
Infection
Renal failure
Neurologic dysfunction
Pulmonary hemorrhage
Death

Incidence

"Incidence of this disease varies by location and ethnicity. . . . Prevalence rates of 4–250 per 100,000 persons have been reported, with greater prevalence in Native Americans, Asian Americans, Latin Americans, and African Americans. . . . African American children may represent up to 60% of patients younger than 20 years" (Klein-Gitelman, 2006, Section 2). Neonatal lupus erythematosus (NLE) affects 1 in every 20,000 live births. LE of childhood occurs in 0.6 of every 100,000 children annually. NLE affects neonates and infants up to 6 months of age (Callen, 2007).

Etiology

Although the exact cause of SLE is unknown, the consensus of researchers is that SLE is an autoimmune disease with a genetic predisposition that contains environmental, hormonal, or pathogenic microorganism triggers (Potts & Mandleco, 2007; Klein-Gitelman, 2006; Callen, 2007).

Clinical Manifestations

Fever
Fatigue
Weight loss
Malar rash
Discoid rash
Photosensitivity
Oral ulcers
Arthritis
Serositis
Proteinuria
Seizures
Psychosis
Hemolytic anemia
Leukopenia
Lymphopenia
Thrombocytopenia

Diagnostic Tests

Complete blood count with platelets and reticulocyte count
Serum chemistry levels
Liver function tests
Renal function tests
Erythrocyte sedimentation rate
Urinalysis
C-reactive protein level
ANA
Anti–double-stranded DNA
Anti-Smith antibody
Lupus anticoagulant level
Antiphospholipid antibody panel
Antiribonucleoprotein (anti-RNP) antibodies
Total hemolytic complement, C3 and C4 levels
Quantitative immunoglobulins
Chest radiography
Electrocardiography
Pulmonary function tests
Magnetic resonance imaging
Ultrasonography
Skin biopsy
Liver biopsy
Renal biopsy

Medical Management

The goals of management are preventing exacerbations, effectively treating exacerbations when they do occur, and preventing organ damage and complications of the disease (Potts & Mandleco, 2007). Currently, there is no known cure for SLE. Management involves pharmacological agents including nonsteroidal anti-inflammatory drugs (NSAIDs) to manage arthritis and pleuritic pain; systemic corticosteroids (prednisone, most commonly used; hydrocortisone; methylprednisolone; and dexamethasone) used in high doses during exacerbations; corticosteroid creams to treat skin manifestations; cytotoxic drugs such as azathiaprine, cyclophosphamide, and methotrexate to help control inflammation yet are steroid-sparing; and the antimalarial agent hydroxychloroquine (Broyles, Reiss, & Evans, 2007). Other agents are used for manifestations of specific organ involvement.

Nursing Management

ASSESSMENT

1. Obtain client history
2. Perform physical assessment
3. Obtain vital signs, height, and weight
4. Assist with diagnostic testing
5. Assess psychosocial impact of disease on child/family

NURSING DIAGNOSES (INCLUDING BUT NOT LIMITED TO)

1. Chronic pain R/T disease process and inadequate pain management
2. Impaired skin integrity R/T skin rash, photosensitivity
3. Ineffective protection R/T altered immune system, immunosuppressant therapy
4. Risk for injury, falls, or bleeding R/T anemia, thrombocytopenia
5. Activity intolerance R/T arthralgia, arthritis, fatigue, and weakness secondary to pain, anemia, and weight loss
6. Ineffective coping R/T chronic nature of condition and disease manifestations
7. Deficient knowledge R/T condition, management of symptoms, treatment, and home care

PLANNING/GOALS

1. Client will verbalize adequate pain management as determined by client (using age-appropriate pain assessment tool) and participate in age-appropriate activities.
2. Client will regain and maintain skin integrity.
3. Client will remain free of infection.
4. Client will not experience injury related to disease process.
5. Client will demonstrate increased energy level by participating in age-appropriate activities.
6. Client/family will demonstrate use of positive coping strategies.
7. Client/family will demonstrate understanding of condition, symptom management, treatment, and home care.

NOC

1. Pain Control
2. Tissue Integrity: Skin & Mucous Membranes
3. Immune Status

4. Risk Control
5. Activity Intolerance
6. Coping
7. Knowledge: Illness Care, Medications, Treatment, Health Promotion

IMPLEMENTATION

1. Chronic pain
   a. Assess pain using age-appropriate pain assessment tool at each clinic/health care provider visit
   b. Ask family about child's pain behavior
   c. Instruct about use of anti-inflammatory agents
   d. Instruct to administer corticosteroids with food to decrease gastric upset
   e. Instruct regarding how to position for comfort
   f. Monitor for effectiveness of pain management
   g. Collaborate with health care provider if pain is not effectively managed
   h. Assess vital signs
   i. Monitor laboratory values
2. Skin integrity
   a. Assess skin with each clinic/health care provider office visit
   b. Instruct regarding medication administration for skin lesions
   c. Instruct to wear sunscreen when outdoors
   d. Instruct to avoid direct sunlight when possible as child's skin will burn easily
3. Immune status
   a. Instruct about how to avoid infections
   b. Monitor vital signs every 4 hours if hospitalized with infection
   c. Monitor breath sounds
   d. Monitor leukocyte values
   e. Institute protective precautions
4. Risk for injury
   a. Instruct about how to prevent injury while allowing child to participate in age-appropriate activities
   b. Monitor platelet count
   c. Establish intravenous access, maintaining patency and monitoring at least hourly
   d. Administer platelets as prescribed
   e. Reevaluate platelet count following platelet administration
5. Activity intolerance
   a. Assess child's energy and pain level
   b. Instruct about energy conservation while providing for growth and development needs
   c. Encourage rest periods when child exhibits fatigue
   d. Encourage dietary intake
   e. Instruct to gradually increase activities as fatigue and arthralgia decrease
   f. Collaborate with health care provider for child life therapy referral if hospitalized

6. Coping
   a. Assess for manifestations of ineffective coping
   b. Encourage verbalization of feelings and concerns
   c. Listen actively
   d. Assist in identifying positive coping strategies
   e. Collaborate with health care provider for necessary referrals
7. Client/family teaching
   a. Assess client's/family's current level of understanding
   b. Provide verbal and written information regarding:
      1) Disease process
      2) Medication administration including action, use, dose, schedule, and adverse effects of each medication
      3) Pain management
      4) Infection precautions
      5) Skin protection from sunlight in presence of photosensitivity
      6) Injury prevention
      7) Age-appropriate activities and growth and development needs
      8) Referrals and community and national support groups
      9) Manifestations of worsening condition
      10) Manifestations of adverse effects of medications
      11) Contact phone numbers for reporting manifestations
      12) Importance of lifelong follow-up care for monitoring and laboratory testing
   c. Provide adequate time for teaching
   d. Document teaching and child's/family's response

NIC

1. Medication Management, Pain Management
2. Skin Surveillance, Medication Management
3. Infection Protection
4. Risk Identification
5. Energy Conservation
6. Coping Enhancement
7. Teaching: Illness Care, Medications, Treatment, Health Education

EVALUATION

1. Client verbalizes adequate pain management as determined by client (using age-appropriate pain assessment tool) and participates in age-appropriate activities.
2. Client regains and maintains skin integrity.
3. Client remains free of infection.
4. Client does not experience injury related to disease process.
5. Client demonstrates increased energy level by participating in age-appropriate activities.
6. Client/family demonstrate use of positive coping strategies.
7. Client/family demonstrate understanding of condition, symptom management, treatment, and home care.

References

American Academy of Rheumatology. (2007). *Classification criteria for rheumatic diseases.* Retrieved May 2, 2007, from http://www.rheumatology.org/publications/classification/index .asp?aud=mem

Broyles, B. E. (2005). *Medical-surgical nursing clinical companion.* Durham, NC: Carolina Academic Press.

Broyles, B. E., Reiss, B. S., & Evans, M. E. (2007). *Pharmacological aspects of nursing care* (7th ed.). Clifton Park, NY: Delmar Cengage Learning.

Callen, J. P. (2007). *Neonatal lupus and cutaneous lupus erythematosus in children.* Retrieved May 2, 2007, from http://www.emedicine.com/ped/topic602.htm

Klein-Gitelman, M. S. (2006). *Systemic lupus erythematosus.* Retrieved May 2, 2007, from http://www.emedicine.com/PED/topic2199.htm

Potts, N. L., & Mandleco, B. L. (2007). *Pediatric nursing: Caring for children and their families* (2nd ed.). Clifton Park, NY: Delmar Cengage Learning.

TETHERED SPINAL CORD SYNDROME (TSCS)

Definition

Tethered spinal cord syndrome (TSCS), also termed tethered cord syndrome (TCS), is a congenital neural tube defect characterized by tissue attachments that limit the movement of the spinal cord within the spinal column (Children's Hospital of Boston, 2006, National Organization for Rare Disorders, 2007).

Pathophysiology

As the embryo develops in its cephalocaudal direction, the spinal cord begins as a flat plate of cells on the surface of the embryo. This flat plate of cells later rolls into a tube (neural tube) and becomes surrounded by a tough covering called the dura, then by muscle and bone that form later in the process. During fetal development, the spine lengthens faster than the spinal cord so that the lower tip of the spinal cord is located opposite the spinal disc between the first and second lumbar vertebrae. Normally, the spinal cord grows so that it can move up and down freely in the spinal column.

Dermal sinus tracts are small dimplelike openings in the midline of the spine; the majority of these sinus tracts are located at the lumbar-sacral level of the spine. A dermal sinus tract may connect deep into the spinal cord and attach to the end of the spinal cord. This causes tethering of the cord. The tissue attachments prevent the cord from moving freely. As a result, the cord becomes tight and stretched as the child grows, causing symptoms of nerve hypoxia and damage such as weakness or numbness of the legs, back pain, and neurologic bladder and bowel. Depending on the severity of the tethered cord, these symptoms may be present at birth or develop anytime during childhood and adulthood (National Institute of Neurological Disorders and Stroke, 2007). Refer to Figure 102-1.

The spinal cord may be connected to the skin through an opening in the bone. In some cases, the spinal cord may have fat at the end of it (spinal lipoma) that overlies the thecal sac. It may be associated with myelodysplasia (spina bifida), tumor, or injury. The most common cause is the presence of a fatty or tight filament of tissue that extends from the distal end of the spinal cord (filum) (Bui, Tubbs, & Oakes, 2007).

Complications

Impaired mobility
Pain
Neurogenic bladder
Neurogenic bowel
Scoliosis
Lordosis

Incidence

Tethered spinal cord syndrome affects from 2–24% of the population and occurs in varying degrees in the U.S. population (Khan, et al. 2007). In the embryo, this syndrome occurs beginning the 27th day of gestation during the caudal closure of the spine. The lesions predominantly are restricted to the lumbosacral cord (Bui et al., 2007).

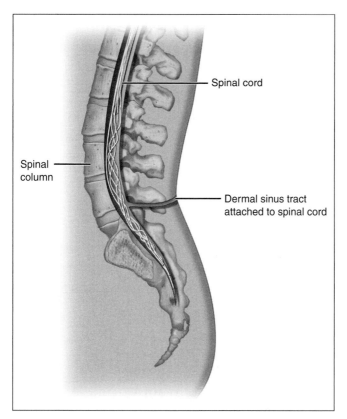

Spinal cord

Spinal column

Dermal sinus tract attached to spinal cord

Figure 102-1: Tethered Cord.

Etiology

TSCS is most commonly found in children with myelomeningocele and lipomyelo-meningocele. TSCS may result from the thickening of the terminal filum attached to the elongated spinal cord or from any nonelastic tissue such as fibromas or fibroadipose filum, tumors, lipoma, or epidermoid tumor. Other causes of tethered cord include dermal sinus tract, diastematomyelia (split cord malformation), myelomyeloceles, lipomylomyncelos, and scar formation following surgical repair for spina bifida including intrauterine surgery (Tethered Spinal Cord Syndrome Association, 2006; Lucile Packard Children's Hospital at Stanford, 2007). Because of the increased incidence of tethered cord in children with spina bifida, surgery to untether the cord may be required even in children with spina bifida occulta (Spina Bifida Association, 2007).

Clinical Manifestations

Skin on infant's/child's back:

Fatty mass
Hairy patch
Discoloration patch
Skin tags
Dimples

Bowel or bladder signs:

   Diaper being constantly wet between changing

   Frequent urinary tract infections (secondary to bladder not emptying)

   Difficulty in toilet training in younger children

   Changes in bowel control patterns

Orthopedic signs:

   Persistent crying in infant resulting from constant back pain

   Unequal changes in size of legs or feet

   Weakness of legs or feet

   Stumbling or walking changes

Diagnostic Tests

Presence of clinical manifestations

Magnetic resonance imaging (MRI)

Bladder and bowel function evaluation

Manual muscle test

Medical Management

The goal of management is to reverse or minimize manifestations of nerve injury. If clinical manifestations are present, which may not occur until the child experiences a growth spurt, surgical untethering of the spinal cord should be performed. If not treated, 90% of these children will develop irreversible neurologic damage. The procedure involves careful dissecting of the spinal cord and nerve roots from the attaching tissues. If a lipoma is involved and its growth is inside the dura of the spinal cord (the cover of the spinal cord), the dura needs to be ligated and as much of the lipoma removed without the healthy nerve roots being damaged. This usually involves the placement of an external drain so that the drainage will not apply internal pressure to the wound and so the wound can heal in a dry environment (Children's Hospital of Boston, 2006).

If the syndrome is associated with myelomeningocele, it usually will be repaired at the same time as the neural tube defect. In cases of fatty or tight filum, this surgery is relatively quick and straightforward. In the presence of ambulation difficulties, physical therapy will be an integral part of the management team. Monitoring is a very important element of the management of tethered cord because of the potential for the spinal cord to retether as the child grows.

Nursing Management

Refer to Chapter 100: Surgical Client.

ASSESSMENT

1. Verify presence of clinical manifestations
2. Assess pain level using age-appropriate pain evaluation tool
3. Assess neurologic function
4. Assess bowel and bladder function including changes
5. Assess diagnostic findings

NURSING DIAGNOSES (INCLUDING BUT NOT LIMITED TO)

1. Acute and chronic pain R/T nerve tightening and infringement
2. Risk for disturbed sensory perception R/T nerve damage
3. Impaired urinary and bowel elimination R/T damage to nerve supply
4. Risk for latex allergy response R/T urinary catheterization for neurogenic bladder

5. Deficient knowledge (child/parent) R/T condition, treatment, and home care

PLANNING/GOALS

1. Client will demonstrate effective pain management as evidenced by nonverbal (infant) or verbal manifestations of pain level 1 on a scale of 0–5 or 0–10.
2. Client will not experience permanent mobility deficits as evidenced by physical development within defined limits (WDL) for age.
3. Client will maintain bladder and bowel function WDL if no permanent damage has occurred and will not experience further damage if damage already has occurred.
4. Client will not develop latex allergy; but if this occurs, latex precautions will be consistently maintained for child.
5. Client/parent will demonstrate understanding of child's condition, treatment, and home care.

NOC

1. Comfort Level, Pain Control, Pain Level
2. Mobility Level
3. Bladder Elimination, Bowel Elimination
4. Allergy Response: Localized/Allergy Manifestations, Latex Precautions
5. Knowledge: Treatment Regimen, Health Promotion

IMPLEMENTATION

1. Pain
   a. Assess pain level hourly using age-appropriate pain assessment tool
   b. Position for comfort with back support
   c. Administer analgesics as prescribed
   d. Evaluate effectiveness of interventions
   e. Collaborate with health care provider if analgesia prescribed is not effective in managing child's pain level
   f. Provide age-appropriate diversionary activities
2. Mobility
   a. Assess for mobility deficits including neurosensory assessment
   b. Collaborate with health care provider for physical therapy consult
   c. Assist with movement as indicated by pain level and mobility
3. Bladder and bowel elimination
   a. Assess child's bowel and bladder habits at home
   b. Monitor intake and output
   c. Scan bladder at time intervals appropriate for child's level of development
   d. Catheterize as prescribed and indicated
   e. Administer medications as prescribed for bladder and bowel training
   f. Teach parents how to catheterize child using clean technique at home
4. Latex allergy
   a. Collaborate with health care provider for presence of latex allergy
   b. Place child on latex precautions if necessary according to facility protocol
   c. Communicate precautions to all staff, family, and visitors and to child

5. Client/parent teaching
   a. Assess current level of knowledge regarding child's condition
   b. Provide verbal and written information regarding:
      1) Reinforcement of health care provider information regarding surgical repair of tethered cord
      2) Clean catheterization technique including return demonstration from caregiver
      3) Medication administration if prescribed
      4) Clinical manifestations indicating worsening of condition
      5) Phone numbers for reporting clinical manifestations
      6) Importance of follow-up with health care provider
   c. Provide sufficient time for child's/parents' questions, providing answers or referring as needed
   d. Document teaching and child's/parents' response

NIC

1. Positioning, Analgesic Administration, Pain Management
2. Exercise Therapy
3. Bladder Management, Bowel Management
4. Allergy Manifestations, Latex Precautions
5. Teaching: Treatment, Health Education

EVALUATION

1. Client demonstrates effective pain management as evidenced by nonverbal (infant) or verbal manifestations of pain level of 1 on a scale of 0–5 or 0–10.
2. Client does not experience permanent mobility deficits as evidenced by physical development WDL for age.
3. Client maintains bladder and bowel function WDL if no permanent damage has occurred and does not experience further damage if damage already has occurred.
4. Client does not develop latex allergy; but if this occurs, latex precautions are consistently maintained for child.
5. Client/parent demonstrate understanding of child's condition, treatment, and home care.

References

Bui, C. J., Tubbs, R. S., & Oakes, W. J. (2007). *Tethered cord syndrome in children: A review.* Retrieved March 25, 2008, from http://www.aans.org/education/journal/neurosurgical/Aug07/23-2-2-1206.pdf

Children's Hospital Boston. (2006). *Tethered cord.* Retrieved March 25, 2008, from http://www.childrenshospital.org/clinicalservices/Site2163/mainpageS2163P4.html

Khan, A. N., Turnbull, I., MacDonald, S., Sabih, D., & Al-Okaili, R. (2007). *Spinal Dysraphism/Myelomeningocele.* Retrieved March 25, 2008, from http://www.emedicine.com/radio/TOPIC643.HTM

Lucile Packard Children's Hospital at Stanford. (2007). *Tethered cord syndrome.* Retrieved April 24, 2007, from http://www.lpch.org/clinicalSpecialtiesServices/COE/BrainBehavior/Neurosurgery/tetheredCord.html

National Institute of Neurological Disorders and Stroke. (2007). *NINDS tethered spinal cord syndrome information page.* Retrieved April 24, 2007, from http://www.ninds.nih.gov/disorders/tethered_cord/tethered_cord.htm

National Organization for Rare Disorders. (2007). *Tethered spinal cord syndrome.* Retrieved March 25, 2008, from http://www.rarediseases.org/search/rdbdetail_abstract.html?disname=Tethered%20Spinal%20Cord%20Syndrome

Spina Bifida Association. (2007). *Spotlight on spina bifida.* Retrieved March 25, 2008, from http://www.spinabifidaassociation.org/site/c.liKWL7PLLrF/b.2725873/

Tethered Spinal Cord Syndrome Association. (2006). *Tethered cord.* Retrieved March 25, 2008, from http://www.tscsa.org/id2.html

TETRALOGY OF FALLOT (TOF)

Definition

Tetralogy of Fallot (TOF) is a complex congenital heart defect (CHD) with four components: (1) ventricular septal defect, (2) pulmonary stenosis, (3) overriding aorta, and (4) right ventricular hypertrophy. Refer to Figure 103-1.

Pathophysiology

In TOF, the presence of an overriding aorta over a ventricular septal defect and pulmonary stenosis allows deoxygenated blood (that the pulmonary artery is attempting to carry into the lungs for oxygenation) to be shunted into the aorta because the pulmonary stenosis creates higher pressure at the opening of the pulmonary artery. Due to the increased pressure that the smaller lumen of the pulmonary artery creates, the aorta becomes the vessel of lesser pressure and the point of least resistance. Then through the

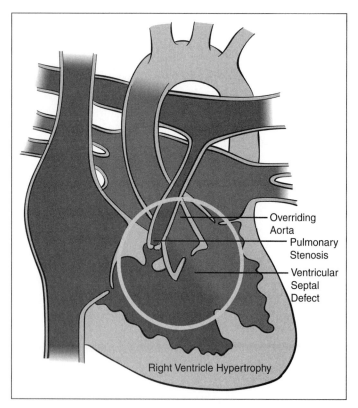

Figure 103-1: Tetralogy of Fallot.

usually large ventricular septal defect (that provides equal pressure between the right and left ventricles), the deoxygenated blood is shunted into the aorta and pumped into systemic circulation. The extent of the pulmonary stenosis determines the severity of cyanotic manifestations. The child with mild TOF may delay surgical repair until the age of 2–3 years; however, the child's survival with moderate to severe TOF depends on immediate medical/surgical attention.

Complications

Hypoxemia
Ineffective tissue perfusion
Delayed growth and development
Cardiovascular collapse
Death

Incidence

"TOF is the most common cyanotic heart defect accounting for approximately 10% of all CHD" (Potts & Mandleco, 2007. p. 780). "Tetralogy of Fallot occurs in about two out of every 10,000 live births. Tetralogy of Fallot occurs equally in boys and in girls" (CongenitalHeartDefects.com, 2006, p. 1).

Etiology

According to the American Heart Association, most of the time the cause of CHDs is unknown. Although the reason defects occur is presumed to be genetic, only a few genes have been discovered that have been linked to the presence of heart defects.

Heredity may play a role in CHD as well as coexisting conditions such as Down syndrome or a mother contracting rubella during the first trimester of pregnancy. The use of alcohol and illicit drugs during pregnancy increases the fetus's risk for developing CHD (American Heart Association, 2007).

Clinical Manifestations

Cyanosis
Hypercyanotic episodes or "tet spells" (Potts & Mandleco, 2007, p. 780)
Polycythemia
Tachypnea
Respiratory distress
Clubbing of digits
Squatting episodes
Delayed growth and development

Diagnostic Tests

Chest radiography
Echocardiogram
Cardiac catheterization

Medical Management

The definitive treatment for the infant/child with TOF is open-heart surgery to repair the ventricular septal defect and pulmonary stenosis. Preoperative medical management includes the treatment of hypercyanotic spells by placing the infant/child in a knee/chest position to decrease systemic venous return of unoxygenated blood as an attempt to decrease the pressure of the right-to-left shunt in the heart. Maintaining the patency of the ductus arteriosus with prostaglandin shunts some of the deoxygenated blood in the aorta to the pulmonary artery and into the lungs for oxygenation. The placement of a Blalock-Taussig (BT) shunt often is performed to "assure pulmonary blood flow until complete surgical repair is performed." (Potts & Mandleco, 2007, p. 781). Complete repair performed during open-heart surgery usually is performed by the time the infant is 3–12 months of age. Refer to Chapter 26: Congenital Heart Disease/Open Heart Surgery for medical management of TOF.

Nursing Management

Refer to Nursing Management in Chapter 26: Congenital Heart Disease/Open Heart Surgery.

References

American Heart Association. (2007). *Tetralogy of Fallot.* Retrieved March 26, 2008, from http://www.americanheart.org/presenter.jhtml?identifier=11071

CongenitalHeartDefects.com. (2006). *Descriptions of congenital heart defects.* Retrieved March 26, 2008, from http://www.congenitalheartdefects.com/typesofCHD.html#TOF

Potts, N. L., & Mandleco, B. L. (2007). *Pediatric nursing: Caring for children and their families* (2nd ed.). Clifton Park, NY: Delmar Cengage Learning.

104

THYROID DYSFUNCTION
(HYPERTHYROIDISM/HYPOTHYROIDISM)

Definition

Hyperthyroidism is the overproduction of hormones by the endocrine gland that controls metabolism in every body cell—the thyroid gland. Hypothyroidism is the underproduction of hormones by the thyroid gland. Congenital hypothyroidism is sometimes termed *cretinism* (Broyles, 2005; Potts & Mandleco, 2007).

Pathophysiology

The thyroid glands, located in the lower anterior neck between the larynx and the clavicles, secrete the hormones thyroxine, triiodothyronine, and thyrocalcitonin. The functioning of the thyroid glands plays a vital role in normal growth and development in children. Thyroxine and triiodothyronine are essential for cellular metabolism; thyrocalcitonin is secreted in response to calcium levels to maintain this electrolyte balance. An overproduction of these hormones by the thyroid glands increases the rate of body metabolism, and an underproduction decreases the metabolic rate. Thyroid dysfunction affects all systems, especially the cardiovascular, gastrointestinal, integumentary, and central nervous systems.

The body's metabolic rate can be compared to the speed of an automobile engine. If the speed of activity in the body normally is 55 mph, hypothyroidism would represent the body processes occurring at a speed of 35 mph and hyperthyroidism would represent the body processes speeding at 75 mph.

The hypometabolic state occurring with hypothyroidism decreases sympathetic nervous system activity and is reflected in the cardiovascular system by bradycardia, hypotension, and bradypnea; the gastrointestinal system, by poor feeding, weight gain, and constipation. Cold intolerance occurs in response to decreased heat production; the skin is dry, coarse, scaly, and edematous (periorbital edema, facial puffiness, non-pitting edema of the extremities, and thickened tongue). The central nervous system responds with lethargy, somnolence, and lack of responsiveness expected in a neonate/infant. Cognitive impairment can result due to internal sensory deprivation.

Hyperthyroidism is characterized by increases in sympathetic nervous system activity and is reflected in the cardiovascular system by tachycardia, hypertension, and tachypnea. The effects on the gastrointestinal system include polyphagia with weight loss, nausea, vomiting, and diarrhea. Diaphoresis and heat intolerance occur; and the central nervous system responds with agitation, irritability, and tremors. The skin is moist, thin, and flushed; if not treated, exophthalmos (bulging of the eyes) can develop due to elevation of the upper eyelids. In addition, cognitive impairment can result due to internal sensory overstimulation.

Complications

Cognitive impairment
Potentially fatal cardiac dysrhythmias
Constipation/diarrhea
Hyperstimulatory state
Hypostimulatory state

Incidence

Congenital hyperthyroidism is rare, and the incidence rate is not available; however, congenital hypothyroidism occurs in approximately 1 per 4,000 live births in the United

States (The Magic Foundation, 2007). Although childhood hyperthyroidism is uncommon, the predominance of cases occurs between the ages of 11 and 14 and is 5 times more common in girls than boys.

Etiology

When a pregnant woman is hyperthyroid, thyroid-stimulating immunoglobulin can cross the placental barrier and stimulate the fetal thyroid gland, causing neonatal hyperthyroidism (Shomon, 2007). The most common cause of congenital hypothyroidism is the failure of the thyroid gland to develop in the embryo. Sometimes the thyroid gland is absent, or ectopic (The Magic Foundation, 2007).

Causes of childhood hypothyroidism include treatment with irradiation for another condition, such as head or neck cancer, which can lead to hypothyroidism because the thyroid glands of children are especially sensitive to radiation (American Thyroid Association, 2005). An adverse effect of the drug amiodarone used to treat tachydysrhythmias in infants and children is hypothyroidism. Although childhood hyperthyroidism is uncommon, the predominance of cases results from a genetic marker common in this disease. In addition, approximately 60% of children with childhood hyperthyroidism have a family history of autoimmune thyroid disease.

Clinical Manifestations

CONGENITAL HYPERTHYROIDISM

Tachycardia (neonatal heart rate > 160 bpm)

Small for gestational age

Warm, moist skin

Irritability

Fatigue

Diarrhea

Decreased urinary output

Little or no growth

Muscle tremors

Good appetite but loss of weight

Exophthalmos

CONGENITAL HYPOTHYROIDISM

Bradycardia (neonatal heart rate < 100 bpm)

Large despite poor feeding habits and increased birth weight

Puffy face and swollen tongue

Hoarse cry

Floppy muscle tone

Cold extremities and mottled skin

Persistent constipation

Abdominal distention

Lethargy (lacks energy, sleeps most of the time, appears tired even
    when awake)

Little to no growth

Poor feeding

Thick, coarse hair that goes low on the forehead

Large fontanel

Prolonged jaundice

Herniated umbilicus

Diagnostic Tests

Serum thyroid hormone (T4) level

Serum thyroid-stimulating hormone (TSH) level

Thyroid scan (for children)

Medical Management

The goals of treatment are early detection of thyroid dysfunction and establishment of a euthyroid state. Congenital hypothyroidism is treated medically with lifelong thyroid replacement therapy. The usual agents are levothyroxine sodium, a synthetic form of thyroxine, or L-thyroxine. The usual starting dose for levothyroxine in a neonate is between 25 and 50 mcg per day or 8–10 mcg/kg of body weight/day. The dose increases dependent upon the individual needs of the child. The dosage form (a tablet) can be crushed and administered in a small amount of water/formula during infancy. Parents must be cautioned not to mix L-thyroxine with soy-based formula because the formula interferes in absorption (Broyles, Reiss, & Evans, 2007). The goal is to maintain the concentration of T4 in the middle to upper half of the normal range (10–16 mcg/dL) for the first years of life. The TSH level should be maintained within the normal reference range for infants (The Magic Foundation, 2007).

The treatment of hyperthyroidism in children may be medical or surgical. Most children respond to antithyroid therapy with propylthiouracil (PTU) or methimazole (MTZ). If antithyroid drug therapy is not successful or if the parents/child want to avoid long-term drug therapy, radioactive iodine (RAI) therapy is used. Oral RAI is administered, resulting in destruction of the thyroid gland in approximately 6–18 weeks (Potts & Mandleco, 2007).

The surgical option for the treatment of hyperthyroidism is a subtotal thyroidectomy during which the overactive thyroid tissue is surgically excised. Risks involved with this surgery include airway obstruction secondary to tissue trauma, hypoparathyroidism, laryngeal nerve damage, hemorrhage, and thyroid storm. Thyroid storm occurs as a result of the manipulation and resulting hypersecretion of the gland as it is being excised. This can lead to a severe calcium imbalance and result in life-threatening cardiac dysrhythmias.

Nursing Management

ASSESSMENT

1. Perform newborn/child assessment
2. Assess for manifestations of thyroid dysfunction including vital signs
3. Assess psychosocial impact of thyroid therapy or surgery

NURSING DIAGNOSES (INCLUDING BUT NOT LIMITED TO)

HYPOTHYROIDISM

1. Decreased cardiac output R/T bradycardia
2. Risk for delayed growth and development R/T internal sensory deprivation
3. Deficient knowledge R/T infant's/child's condition, drug therapy, and home care

HYPERTHYROIDISM

4. Risk for delayed growth and development R/T internal sensory overload and glucose deficiency
5. Risk for disturbed visual sensory perception R/T presence of exophthalmos
6. Deficient knowledge R/T infant's/child's condition, drug therapy, RAI treatment, and home care

7. Risk for ineffective tissue perfusion R/T postoperative hemorrhage
8. Risk for decreased cardiac output R/T intraoperative/postoperative thyroid storm
9. Risk for injury, laryngeal nerve damage R/T surgical removal of thyroid gland
10. Deficient knowledge R/T postoperative hospital and home care

PLANNING/GOALS

HYPOTHYROIDISM

1. Client will not experience decreased cardiac output as evidenced by hemodynamic stability.
2. Client will not experience developmental delays.
3. Parents will demonstrate understanding of infant's/child's condition, medication treatment, and home care.

HYPERTHYROIDISM

4. Client will not experience developmental delays.
5. Client will not develop exophthalmos.
6. Parents will demonstrate understanding of infant's/child's condition, drug therapy, RAI treatment, and home care.
7. Client will not experience postoperative hemorrhage as evidenced by dry and intact dressing and vital sign stability.
8. Client will not experience thyroid storm as evidenced by cardiac rate and rhythm within defined limits (WDL).
9. Client will not experience laryngeal nerve damage during surgery.
10. Parents will demonstrate understanding of postoperative hospital and home care.

NOC

HYPOTHYROIDISM

1. Circulation Status
2. Child Development
3. Knowledge: Illness Care, Medication, Health Promotion

HYPERTHYROIDISM

4. Child Development
5. Neurologic Status
6. Knowledge: Illness Care, Treatment, Health Promotion
7. Circulation Status
8. Circulation Status
9. Risk Control
10. Knowledge: Illness Care, Health Promotion

IMPLEMENTATION

HYPOTHYROIDISM

1. Decreased cardiac output
   a. Monitor neonates pulse rate and rhythm
   b. Monitor respiratory rate and effort
   c. Monitor continuous pulse oximetry
   d. Administer oxygen to maintain saturation within prescribed parameters
   e. Initiate thyroid replacement drug therapy as prescribed
   f. Teach parents how to prepare and administer medications

2. Growth and development
    a. Assess for developmental milestones during follow-up office visits
    b. Teach parents about age-appropriate activities to encourage meeting appropriate growth and developmental milestones
    c. Monitor parental compliance with medication therapy
3. Parent teaching
    a. Assess parents' current level of understanding
    b. Provide verbal and written instructions regarding:
        1) Infant care and feeding
        2) Administration of thyroid replacement medication
        3) Importance of compliance with medication therapy
        4) Manifestations of adverse effects of medications (hyperthyroidism)
        5) Contact information for reporting manifestations to health care provider
        6) Referral information if needed
        7) Importance of life-long follow-up care
    c. Provide adequate time for teaching
    d. Document teaching and parental response

HYPERTHYROIDISM

4. Growth and development
    a. Assess for developmental milestones during follow-up office visits
    b. Teach parents about age-appropriate activities to encourage meeting appropriate growth and developmental milestones
    c. Monitor parental compliance with medication therapy
5. Parent teaching
    a. Assess parents' current level of understanding
    b. Provide verbal and written instructions regarding:
        1) Infant care and feeding
        2) Antithyroid medication administration
        3) Importance of compliance with medication therapy
        4) Manifestations of adverse effects of medications (hypothyroidism)
        5) RAI information
        6) Contact information for reporting manifestations to health care provider
        7) Referral information if needed
        8) Importance of follow-up with health care provider
    c. Provide adequate time for teaching
    d. Document teaching and parental response
6. Visual impairment
    a. Monitor for presence of exophthalmos
    b. Encourage parents to provide for optical assessment and care for child
    c. Administer medications if prescribed
7. Tissue perfusion
    a. Assess for postoperative bleeding by placing gloved fingers behind child's neck
    b. Monitor vital signs hourly during first 4 hours

    c. Assess for swelling in neck and respiratory compromise

    d. Maintain tracheostomy insertion equipment at bedside

    e. Monitor continuous pulse oximetry

    f. Administer oxygen titrating of prescribed oxygen saturation parameters

    g. Position head of crib/bed elevated 30–45 degrees

8. Cardiac output

    a. Assess for manifestations of thyroid storm (tachydysrhythmias, fever, and systolic hypertension)

    b. Maintain patent airway

    c. Collaborate immediately with health care provider if thyroid storm is suspected

    d. Transfer to pediatric intensive care unit for hemodynamic monitoring if manifestations occur

9. Laryngeal nerve damage

    a. Assess infant's/child's voice for hoarseness every 2 hours

    b. Instruct parents to notify health care provider if hoarseness persists following discharge

10. Parent teaching

    a. Assess parents' current level of understanding

    b. Provide verbal and written instructions regarding:

       1) Manifestations of postoperative complications

       2) Pain management

       3) Importance of compliance with medication therapy

       4) Manifestations of adverse effects of medications

       5) Contact information for reporting manifestations to health care provider

       6) Referral information if needed

       7) Importance of follow-up with health care provider

    c. Provide adequate time for teaching

    d. Document teaching and parental response

NIC

HYPOTHYROIDISM

1. Hemodynamic Monitoring
2. Developmental Enhancement
3. Teaching: Illness Care, Medication, Health Promotion

HYPERTHYROIDISM

4. Developmental Enhancement
5. Teaching: Illness Care, Treatment, Health Promotion
6. Neurologic Monitoring
7. Vital Signs Monitoring
8. Hemodynamic Monitoring
9. Surveillance: Safety
10. Teaching: Illness Care, Health Promotion

EVALUATION

HYPOTHYROIDISM

1. Client does not experience decreased cardiac output as evidenced by hemodynamic stability.

2. Client does not experience developmental delays.

3. Parents demonstrate understanding of infant's/child's condition, medication treatment, and home care.

HYPERTHYROIDISM

4. Client does not experience developmental delays.

5. Client does not develop exophthalmos.

6. Parents demonstrate understanding of infant's/child's condition, drug therapy, RAI treatment, and home care.

7. Client does not experience postoperative hemorrhage as evidenced by dry and intact dressing and vital sign stability.

8. Client does not experience thyroid storm as evidenced by cardiac rate and rhythm WDL.

9. Client does not experience laryngeal nerve damage during surgery.

10. Parents demonstrate understanding of postoperative hospital and home care.

References

American Thyroid Association. (2005). *Childhood head and neck irradiation.* Retrieved March 12, 2007, from http://www.thyroid.org/patients/brochures/Head_Neck_IrradiationFAQ.pdf

Broyles, B. E. (2005). *Medical-surgical nursing clinical companion.* Durham, NC: Carolina Academic Press.

Broyles, B. E., Reiss, B. S., & Evans, M. E. (2007). *Pharmacological aspects of nursing care* (7th ed.). Clifton Park, NY: Delmar Cengage Learning.

Potts, N. L., & Mandleco, B. L. (2007). *Pediatric nursing: Caring for children and their families* (2nd ed.). Clifton Park, NY: Delmar Cengage Learning.

Shomon, M. (2007). *Congenital heart disease/thyroid disease connection.* Retrieved March 12, 2007, from http://thyroid.about.com/cs/symptomsproblems/a/congenital.htm

The Magic Foundation. (2007). *Congenital hypothyroidism—general information.* Retrieved March 12, 2007, from http://www.magicfoundation.org/www/docs/114.125/congenital_hypothyroidism_hypothyroid.html

105

TONSILLITIS/TONSILLECTOMY AND ADENOIDECTOMY

Definition

Tonsillitis is the inflammation of the masses of lymphatic tissue located in the oropharynx called the palatine and pharyngeal tonsils (Broyles, 2005). A tonsillectomy and adenoidectomy is the surgical removal of the palatine tonsils and the hypertrophied pharyngeal tonsils (adenoids). Refer to Figure 105-1.

Pathophysiology

The tonsils normally provide protection from invading microorganisms that enter the body through the nose or mouth. Usually, tonsillitis is of viral origin. However, bacterial tonsillitis caused by *Streptococcus pyogenes* can lead to serious health problems such as rheumatic fever, acute glomerulonephritis, and meningitis (Potts & Mandleco, 2007). Episodes of tonsillitis usually occur as a result of upper respiratory infection causing inflammation and infection of the tonsils. The tonsils become edematous and enlarged, causing pain and difficulty swallowing.

The lymph nodes of the jaw and neck also may be enlarged and tender (MedlinePlus, 2007). Normally, the course of the disease is 7–10 days; however, the infection can spread to the pharynx and abscess or can spread to the middle ear resulting in otitis media. Especially in children, difficulty swallowing can lead to dehydration. In severe cases, airway obstruction can occur from enlargement that encroaches on the airway. Repeated episodes of tonsillitis cause the pharyngeal tonsils to hypertrophy, and surgical removal of the tonsils usually is required.

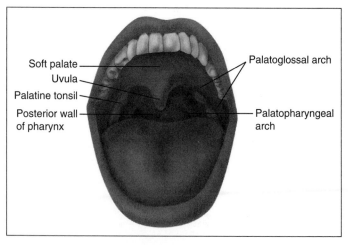

Figure 105-1: Tonsils and the Pharyngeal Cavity.

Complications

Bacterial pharyngitis
Viral pharyngitis
Pharyngeal abscess
Otitis media
Dehydration
Rheumatic fever
Acute glomerulonephritis
Meningitis

Incidence

Almost all children in the United States experience at least one episode of tonsillitis (Shah, 2008). Tonsillitis and pharyngitis most often affect children between the ages of 6 and 8 years and rarely occur in children less than 2 years of age. Children 2 years of age rarely develop group A β-hemolytic streptococcus (GABHS), or Strep throat which most commonly occurs in children 5–15 years of age. (Lucile Packard Children's Hospital at Stanford, 2007).

Etiology

Five major viruses cause tonsillitis: (1) adenovirus, (2) influenza virus, (3) Epstein-Barr virus, (4) herpes simplex virus, and (5) cytomegalovirus. The influenza virus is most common. The primary bacterial etiology is GABHS; however, *Neisseria gonorrhoeae*, *Haemophilus influenzae* type B, and mycoplasma also can cause tonsillitis. Cigarette smoking and secondhand smoke dry and atrophy the cilia in the respiratory system, making children more susceptible to upper respiratory infections, tonsillitis, and otitis media. In children who are immunosuppressed, fungal infections and parasitic infections can be causes of tonsillitis (Lucile Packard Children's Hospital at Stanford, 2007).

Clinical Manifestations

Sore throat persisting longer than 48 hours
Severe sore throat
Fever
Dysphagia
Malaise
Erythema of posterior tonsils
Dyspnea
Laryngitis

Diagnostic Tests

Throat culture
Rapid antigen detection test (RADT), also known as rapid strep test
Complete blood count
Monospot serum test

Medical Management

The goals of treatment are to cure the infection and remove the tonsils if they remain enlarged following conservative treatment or if the child experiences recurrent episodes of tonsillitis. To treat bacterial infections, prescribing penicillins, cephalosporins, or erythromycins for 7–10 days is the standard of care. Viral infections are treated symptomatically with antipyretics (acetaminophen and ibuprofen), analgesics, and saline gargles. Children should not be given aspirin for fever or pain because of the risk of

Reye syndrome. Surgical removal of the palatine tonsils is a tonsillectomy, and removal of hypertrophied pharyngeal tonsils is an adenoidectomy. Frequently, getting the child to consume oral fluids following surgery is a challenge, resulting in dehydration being the most common cause of readmission following surgery.

Nursing Management

Refer to Chapter 100: Surgical Client.

ASSESSMENT

1. Obtain client history
2. Inspect tonsils for erythema and enlargement
3. Obtain vital signs, height, and weight

NURSING DIAGNOSES (INCLUDING BUT NOT LIMITED TO)

PREOPERATIVE

1. Ineffective protection R/T pathogen invasion and risk for spread
2. Acute pain R/T inflammation
3. Risk for ineffective airway clearance R/T encroachment on the airway by enlarged tonsils
4. Risk for deficient fluid volume R/T decreased intake secondary to pain

POSTOPERATIVE

5. Risk for injury, hemorrhage R/T vessel and tissue trauma secondary to surgery
6. Acute pain R/T tissue trauma secondary to surgery
7. Risk for deficient fluid volume R/T difficulty swallowing secondary to pain of surgical incision
8. Deficient knowledge R/T postoperative hospital care and home care

PLANNING/GOALS

PREOPERATIVE

1. Client will not experience complications related to tonsillitis.
2. Client will demonstrate effective pain management as determined by client using age-appropriate pain assessment tool at a level of 0 to 1 on a scale of 0 to 5 on the faces scale (for toddlers and preschoolers) or 0 to 2 on a scale of 0 to 10 (for school-age children and adolescents) with 0 being no pain and 10 being the worst pain the client has ever experienced.
3. Client will maintain patent airway.
4. Client will maintain fluid balance as evidenced by urine output and status of mucous membranes within defined limits (WDL).

POSTOPERATIVE

5. Client will not experience postoperative hemorrhage.
6. Client will demonstrate effective pain management as determined by client using age-appropriate pain assessment tool at a level of 0 to 1 on a scale of 0 to 5 on the faces scale (for toddlers and preschoolers) or at a level of 0 to 2 on a scale of 0 to 10 (for school-age children and adolescents) with 0 being no pain and 10 being the worst pain the client has ever experienced as evidenced by verbalization and intake of oral fluids.
7. Client will maintain fluid balance as evidenced by urine output and status of mucous membranes WDL.
8. Parents/child will demonstrate understanding of postoperative care and home care.

NOC

PREOPERATIVE

1. Immune Status
2. Pain Level
3. Risk Control, Respiratory Status: Airway Patency
4. Risk Control, Fluid Balance

POSTOPERATIVE

5. Circulatory Status
6. Pain Control
7. Fluid Balance
8. Knowledge: Illness Care, Medications, Treatment, Health Promotion

IMPLEMENTATION

PREOPERATIVE

1. Infection
   a. Assess pharyngeal area of child's throat
   b. Obtain throat culture
   c. Monitor culture results
   d. Instruct parents regarding medication administration and importance of completing entire antibiotic prescription
2. Pain
   a. Assess child's pain level using age-appropriate pain assessment tool
   b. Instruct about use of acetaminophen or ibuprofen for pain
   c. Instruct not to administer aspirin to children
   d. Instruct concerning saline gargles
   e. Instruct to notify health care provider if pain is not effectively managed
3. Airway patency
   a. Assess child's airway
   b. Ask parents if child has had any difficulty breathing
   c. Instruct to notify health care provider immediately if child exhibits any respiratory difficulty
4. Fluid balance
   a. Instruct about importance of fluid intake in children
   b. Ask child about favorite fluids
   c. Encourage use of cool, nonacid fluids that child likes
   d. Instruct parents to monitor child's urinary output
   e. Instruct to notify health care provider if urine output decreases

POSTOPERATIVE

5. Bleeding
   a. Assess for airway patency
   b. Place in prone or side-lying position during postoperative period with head of bed (HOB) elevated 15–30 degrees
   c. Assess for continuous drooling of bright red secretions from mouth
   d. Assess for frequent swallowing or throat clearing
   e. Assess vital signs per postoperative protocol and as needed
   f. Notify health care provider immediately if bleeding occurs

      g.   Offer cool, clear liquids (avoid red liquids) when child is responsive from anesthesia

      h.   Monitor closely for nausea and vomiting, medicating as prescribed

      i.   Do not discharge from health care facility until client is taking adequate fluids

6. Pain
   a. Assess pain level hourly
   b. Administer oral liquid opioid analgesics proactively and as prescribed
   c. Maintain intravenous fluids until taking adequate amounts of oral fluids
   d. Assess child's fluid likes and dislikes
   e. Offer cool nonacidic, nonred fluids hourly

7. Fluid balance
   a. Monitor intake and output
   b. Maintain intravenous fluids until taking adequate amounts of oral fluids
   c. Assess child's fluid likes and dislikes
   d. Offer cool nonacidic, nonred fluids hourly
   e. Monitor urinary output, skin turgor, and oral mucous membranes

8. Parent/child teaching
   a. Assess parents'/child's (if age-appropriate) current level of knowledge
   b. Provide verbal and written information regarding:
      1) Postoperative activity restrictions
      2) Postoperative dietary modifications as indicated
      3) Medication administration including importance of compliance with prescribed medication regime as needed
      4) Manifestations of adverse effects of medications
      5) Manifestations of postoperative complications
      6) Importance of adequate fluid intake
      7) Contact phone numbers for reporting manifestations
      8) Importance of regular hand washing and appropriate technique
      9) Importance of follow-up with health care provider
   c. Provide adequate time for teaching
   d. Document teaching and parents'/child's response

NIC

PREOPERATIVE

1. Infection Protections
2. Pain Management
3. Respiratory Management
4. Fluid Management, Fluid Monitoring

POSTOPERATIVE

5. Bleeding Precautions
6. Analgesic Administration, Pain Management
7. Fluid Management, Fluid Monitoring
8. Teaching: Illness Care, Medications, Treatment, Health Education

Evaluation

Preoperative

1. Client does not experience complications related to tonsillitis.
2. Client demonstrates effective pain management as determined by client using age-appropriate pain assessment tool at a level of 0 to 1 on a scale of 0 to 5 on the faces scale (for toddlers and preschoolers) or 0 to 2 on a scale of 0 to 10 (for school-age children and adolescents) with 0 being no pain and 10 being the worst pain the client has ever experienced.
3. Client maintains patent airway.
4. Client maintains fluid balance as evidenced by urine output and status of mucous membranes WDL.

Postoperative

5. Client does not experience postoperative hemorrhage.
6. Client demonstrates effective pain management as determined by client using age-appropriate pain assessment tool at a level of 0 to 1 on a scale of 0 to 5 on the faces scale (for toddlers and preschoolers) or at a level of 0 to 2 on a scale of 0 to 10 (for school-age children and adolescents) with 0 being no pain and 10 being the worst pain the client has ever experienced as evidenced by verbalization and intake of oral fluids.
7. Client maintains fluid balance as evidenced by urine output and status of mucous membranes WDL.
8. Parents/child demonstrate understanding of postoperative care and home care.

References

Broyles, B. E. (2005). *Medical-surgical nursing clinical companion.* Durham, NC: Carolina Academic Press.

Lucile Packard Children's Hospital at Stanford. (2007). *Pharyngitis and tonsillitis.* Retrieved May 4, 2007, from http://www.lpch.org/DiseaseHealthInfo/HealthLibrary/ent/tonphar.html

MedlinePlus. (2007). *Tonsillitis.* Retrieved May 4, 2007, from http://www.nlm.nih.gov/medlineplus/ency/article/001043.htm

Potts, N. L., & Mandleco, B. L. (2007). *Pediatric nursing: Caring for children and their families* (2nd ed.). Clifton Park, NY: Delmar Cengage Learning.

Shah, U. K. (2008). *Tonsillitis and peritonsillar abscess.* Retrieved March 26, 2008, from http://www.emedicine.com/ent/topic314.htm

106

TOTAL PARENTERAL NUTRITION (TPN)

Definition

Total parenteral nutrition (TPN) "is nutritional support supplying glucose, protein, vitamins, electrolytes, trace elements, and . . . fats to maintain the body's growth, development, and tissue repair" (Daniels, Nosek, & Nicoll, 2007, p. 360). Peripheral parenteral nutrition (PPN) is not used in young children because of the fragility and size of their peripheral vessels.

Medical Management

"When adequate nutrition cannot be provided through the gastrointestinal system, parenteral nutrition is required to maintain homeostasis" (Broyles, Reiss, & Evans, 2007, p. 552). The highly concentrated TPN solution is administered through a central venous access device (CVAD) because of the need for vessels with sufficient diameter, blood volume, and turbulence for rapid dilution. CVADs are placed in vessels that empty into the subclavian vein (femoral vein or external or internal jugular veins) leading to the superior vena cava (Hockenberry, 2005). The highly irritating nature of high glucose concentrations (50–70% for neonates and infants) is too irritating to infuse in the small peripheral veins of children. For older children who require short-term parenteral nutrition, a large peripheral vein may be used; however, the primary source of energy calories for these children becomes lipids (fats) rather than glucose. PPN cannot contain a glucose concentration greater than 10% or an osmolality greater than 900 mmol. (As previously noted, PPN is rarely used in children.) Typically, TPN is infused through tunneled central venous catheters because of the potential for long-term TPN therapy. Tunneled CVADs have an antimicrobial filter on the part of the catheter that is tunneled under the skin to help prevent pathogens from entering the vascular system. Tunneled catheters include Hickmans, Broviacs, and implanted ports. Refer to Figures 22-1 and 22-2 in Chapter 22: Chemotherapy. CVADs are inserted as a surgical procedure in children.

TPN supplies nutrients in their most elemental forms so that they are immediately available for cellular metabolism (Broyles, 2005). TPN is infused using regular intravenous tubing with a special filter attached to remove particulate matter that may be in the TPN solution. The 70% glucose solutions are needed in infants to manage the growth spurt of infancy and to meet the metabolic needs placed on the infant by the pathophysiologic condition. Added to these base solutions are proteins in the form of amino acids, vitamins, minerals, and trace elements. In pediatrics, the intralipids (fats) are administered concurrently with the TPN solution but are packaged in separate containers.

High dextrose contents of TPN can lead to hyperglycemia The hyperosmolarity of the solution due to the amino acids and the dextrose content can result in fluid and electrolyte imbalances. Hyperglycemia and hyperosmolarity can cause fluid to shift from the interstitial and intracellular spaces to the plasma. This causes the plasma to expand; and with hyperglycemia, it can trigger osmotic diuresis resulting in losses of fluid, sodium, and potassium. This can lead to dehydration and hypovolemia, especially in children.

The goals of management are to provide complete nutrition, to prevent negative energy and nitrogen balance, to prevent complications associated with TPN and the presence of a CVAD, and to wean the child from TPN to enteral feedings as soon as medically feasible. The anatomy and physiology of the gastrointestinal tract is best suited for nutritional digestion and absorption when it is functioning sufficiently to provide adequate nutrition.

The indication for prescribing TPN for children is any condition that renders the gastrointestinal tract unable to absorb adequate nutrition and fluid to meet the body's metabolic needs to maintain homeostasis. These conditions include all of the following:

Severe gastrointestinal damage as occurs with Crohn's disease

Congenital gastrointestinal anomalies that increase metabolic needs and short bowel syndrome

Abdominal gunshot wounds that result in removal of all or a significant part of the small intestines

Gastrointestinal surgery

Complete blockage of the intestines

Severe vomiting or diarrhea

Complications from cancer or treatment that prevents eating or using a feeding tube (American Cancer Society, 2007)

Major burns

Trauma

Protein wasting associated with acquired immunodeficiency syndrome (AIDS)

There are advantages and disadvantages to prescribing TPN. Among the advantages are that (1) dextrose solutions come in a variety of concentrations to provide a caloric source, (2) TPN can be used long-term, (3) TPN is nutritionally complete, (4) TPN promotes tissue synthesis and normal metabolic function, and (5) TPN provides calories, protein, vitamins, minerals, trace elements, and lipid solutions in elemental forms easily used by the cells. Disadvantages of TPN include (1) a high risk of infection because of the CVAD and the high glucose content of TPN solutions, (2) metabolic complications, (3) hyperglycemia and glucose intolerance, (4) electrolyte imbalances secondary to hyperosmolarity of TPN, (5) risk of fat embolism with some lipid emulsions, and (6) risk for liver dysfunction.

The exact solution is the result of a collaborative effort by health care providers, dieticians, and pharmacists and is based on child's height, weight, and metabolic needs. TPN solutions also are available in alternative formulas suitable to children in liver failure and renal failure and those in metabolic stress, such as children with major burns. The TPN prescription must be renewed every 24 hours for hospitalized children to ensure that their metabolic needs are being met. Each day's prescription follows the obtaining of daily TPN panel blood work (Broyles, 2005). The National Institutes of Health provide clinical guidelines for prescribing components of TPN for children based the child's weight (National Institutes of Health, 2005). Medications such as insulin, heparin, and ranitidine can be added to the TPN solutions if needed. Each prescription for TPN must be individually determined for each child requiring TPN.

Prior to the discharge of an infant or a child who is receiving TPN and intralipids, the parents/caregivers must demonstrate an understanding of the infusion device (pump), the administration procedure, care of the child's CVAD, and indications for notifying the health care provider. Members of the nursing staff usually are responsible for demonstrating these skills to parents/caregivers and evaluating their understanding and skill proficiency.

Complications

Pneumothorax or hemothorax during central venous access insertion

Sepsis (related to central venous access and high glucose content of TPN solutions)

Hyperglycemia

Hyperosmolarity

Fluid and electrolyte imbalances

Fat embolism

Nursing Management

ASSESSMENT

1. Obtain client history
2. Assess CVAD at least hourly
3. Compare TPN solution contents on label with prescribed solution guidelines
4. Monitor temperature every 4 hours
5. Monitor capillary glucose levels every 6 hours

NURSING DIAGNOSES (INCLUDING BUT NOT LIMITED TO)

1. Imbalanced nutrition: less than body requirements R/T inadequate nutritional intake to maintain homeostasis
2. High risk for infection R/T central venous access and dextrose concentration of TPN solutions
3. Risk for injury, fat embolism R/T improper administration of TPN and intralipids
4. Risk for imbalanced fluid volume R/T osmolarity of TPN solutions
5. Deficient knowledge R/T CVAD care, administration of TPN, care and use of volumetric intravenous infusion pump, prevention of complications, and signs and symptoms to report immediately

PLANNING/GOALS

1. Client will regain and maintain adequate nutrition to meet body's metabolic needs and progress to enteral feedings when medically feasible.
2. Client will not experience infection; however, if infection does occur, it will be treated immediately.
3. Client will not experience fat embolism.
4. Client will maintain fluid and electrolyte balance as evidenced by electrolyte levels and intake and output within defined limits (WDL).
5. Parents/caregivers will demonstrate ability to provide home TPN without complications as evidenced by verbalizations and return demonstrations exhibiting understanding of and compliance with instructions. Client will not experience hyperglycemia.

NOC

1. Nutritional Status
2. Immune Status, Risk Control
3. Risk Control
4. Risk Control, Fluid Balance
5. Knowledge, Illness Care, Medications, Procedures, Infection Control, Health Promotion

IMPLEMENTATION

1. Nutrition
   a. Assess daily weight
   b. Monitor strict intake and output
   c. Confirm TPN solution with written prescription

    d. Maintain a dedicated line for TPN and intralipids administration

    e. Obtain lab specimens, including TPN panel from CVAD port other than the one infusing the TPN and intralipids. *NOTE:* If TPN/intralipids line is used, these solutions are difficult to flush from the line; consequently, lab specimens may produce inaccurate readings.

    f. Monitor lab results

    g. Monitor capillary blood glucose every 6 hours

    h. Administer insulin when indicated using prescribed sliding scale

    i. Remove TPN solution from refrigerator 1 hour prior to administration so it can warm to room temperature

    j. Administer TPN as prescribed using 1.2 micron filter

    k. Administer intralipids as prescribed

    l. If the next TPN solution is not available, infuse 10% dextrose infusion until TPN is available

    m. Never abruptly discontinue TPN

    n. Offer pacifier for short periods during the day for non-nutritive sucking to prevent infant from losing sucking ability (necessary when infant progresses to oral feedings)

2. Risk for infection

    a. Monitor vital signs every 4 hours

    b. Monitor CVAD site hourly for redness and/or discharge

    c. Perform CVAD care per facility protocol (at least every 48–72 hours) using aseptic technique including wearing mask

    d. Obtain lab specimens from CVAD using strict asepsis including wearing mask

    e. Ensure that dressing on CVAD is occlusive

    f. Change TPN intravenous lines completely each time a new TPN solution is hung (every 24 hours) using aseptic technique including wearing mask and sterile gloves and, in many facilities, a sterile gown per facility protocol

    g. Change TPN and intralipid solution containers and filter every 24 hours per facility protocol

    h. Demonstrate procedures to parents/caregivers

    i. Ensure that parents/caregivers can perform return demonstrations using appropriate technique

    j. Stress to parents/caregivers importance of preventing infection (which has the potential for being life-threatening)

3. Risk for fat embolism

    a. Ensure that TPN and intralipids are infused using volumetric infusion device

    b. Administer TPN and intralipids as prescribed, ensuring that intralipids infuse concurrently with TPN. *NOTE:* TPN can be infused without intralipids, but intralipids should not be administered without TPN. Lipoproteins in the TPN solution are necessary for intralipids to move safely through the vascular system; without these lipoproteins, intralipids will develop fat embolism that can lead to death.

    c. Avoid too rapid infusion on intralipids

    d. Monitor closely for manifestations of fat embolism including respiratory distress, chest pain, and vascular collapse

4. Fluid imbalance risk
   a. Weigh daily
   b. Monitor strict intake and output
   c. Monitor daily electrolyte values including blood urea nitrogen (BUN) and creatinine
   d. Monitor capillary blood glucose every 6 hours
   e. Administer insulin when indicated using prescribed sliding scale
   f. Report abnormal laboratory values to health care provider
   g. Assess mucous membranes every shift
   h. Monitor for manifestations of hypovolemia
   i. Maintain intravenous access, monitoring at least hourly
5. Parent/caregiver teaching
   a. Assess parents'/caregivers' current level of understanding
   b. Provide demonstration and adequate opportunities for return demonstrations regarding:
      1) Care of central venous access using aseptic technique
      2) Use of volumetric intravenous infusion pump
      3) Confirmation that TPN solution is the one prescribed
      4) Importance of accurately programming infusion pump if TPN and intralipids are administered in separate solution containers to ensure that intralipids are infused concurrently with TPN (to prevent fat embolism)
      5) Monitoring of urine and/or capillary glucose levels
      6) Monitoring of temperature and parameters prescribed
   c. Provide verbal and written information regarding:
      1) Daily weight
      2) Medication administration including importance of compliance with prescribed medication regime
      3) Manifestations of adverse effects of TPN
      4) Manifestations of adverse effects of medications
      5) Manifestations of worsening of condition
      6) Contact information for reporting signs and symptoms
      7) Importance of regular hand washing and appropriate technique
      8) Home health and nutrition referrals and contact people and phone numbers
      9) Importance of follow-up with health care provider
   d. Provide adequate time for teaching. *NOTE:* In many acute care facilities, parents/caregivers must remain at the child's bedside overnight as a part of the learning experience for caring for a child with TPN. This gives parents/caregivers experience with dealing with a volumetric infusion pump and alarms and ways to address them.
   e. Document teaching and parents'/caregivers' response

NIC

1. Nutrition Management, Nutritional Monitoring
2. Infection Control, Infection Protection, Infection Precautions
3. Surveillance: Safety
4. Fluid Management, Fluid Monitoring
5. Teaching: Illness Care, Medications, Procedures, Infection Control, Health Education

EVALUATION

1. Client regains and maintains adequate nutrition to meet body's metabolic needs and progresses to enteral feedings when medically feasible.
2. Client does not experience infection; however if infection does occur, it will be treated immediately.
3. Client does not experience fat embolism.
4. Client maintains fluid and electrolyte balance as evidenced by electrolyte levels and intake and output WDL.
5. Parents/caregivers demonstrate ability to provide home TPN without complications as evidenced by verbalizations and return demonstrations exhibiting understanding of and compliance with instructions. Client does not experience hyperglycemia.

References

American Cancer Society. (2007). *Ways to provide nutrition.* Retrieved May 4, 2007, from http://www.cancer.org/docroot/MBC/content/MBC_6_2X_Ways_to_provide_nutrition_7.asp?sitearea=MBC

Broyles, B. E. (2005). *Medical-surgical nursing clinical companion.* Durham, NC: Carolina Academic Press.

Broyles, B. E., Reiss, B. S., & Evans, M. E. (2007). *Pharmacological aspects of nursing care* (7th ed.). Clifton Park, NY: Delmar Cengage Learning.

Daniels, R., Nosek, L. J., & Nicoll, L. H. (2007). *Contemporary medical-surgical nursing.* Clifton Park, NY: Delmar Cengage Learning.

Hockenberry, M. J. (2005). *Wong's essentials of pediatric nursing* (7th ed.). St. Louis, MO: Elsevier Mosby.

National Institutes of Health. (2005). *Total parenteral nutrition (TPN).* Retrieved May 4, 2007, from http://www.cc.nih.gov/ccc/pedweb/pedsstaff/tpn.html

Urinary Tract Infection (UTI)

Definition

"[A] urinary tract infection (UTI) is an infection of one or more structures in the urinary tract and can be classified as lower urinary tract (urethritis, cystitis) or upper urinary tract (ureteritis, pyelonephritis)" (Potts & Mandleco, 2007, p. 625).

Pathophysiology

Urethritis is an inflammation or infection of the urethra (the tube leading to the urinary bladder from the outside), and cystitis is an infection of the urinary bladder. Ureteritis is an infection in the ureters (the tubes leading from the urinary bladder to the kidneys), and pyelonephritis is an infection in the kidneys. Most infections in the body descend through gravity, but UTIs ascend through the urinary system with increasing severity. The focus of this chapter is infection in the lower urinary tract.

UTIs occur when bacteria enter the urinary system by ascending up the urethra. Girls are especially prone to these infections because of their short urethra, whereas boys have a longer urethra and the secretions from the prostate gland have antibacterial properties (Potts & Mandleco, 2007). The short urethra in females is susceptible to pathogen microorganism invasion because of its close proximity to the anus. If girls are not taught to wipe from front to back after defecating, microorganisms from the feces can enter through the urinary meatus. In addition, underwear worn by little girls tends to be tighter, allowing residual fecal material in the anal area to attach to the underwear and come in contact with the meatus. Finally, because most infants and small girls take tub baths, the warmth of the water causes the meatus to dilate, allowing microorganisms in the bathtub and water to enter the meatus. A characteristic of many young children is urinary stasis from infrequent voiding because they do not want to stop playing long enough to regularly and completely empty the urinary bladder.

Boys can contract UTIs; however, the infections are not as common as they are in girls. In boys under the age of 5 years, structural abnormalities should be investigated in the presence of UTIs.

Microorganisms can flourish in the alkaline environment of the urinary structures, causing irritation and tissue damage. As previously noted, lower UTIs can lead to more serious upper UTIs. Because of the high vascular volume that flows through the kidneys, bacteremia or sepsis can result in children who are immune-compromised.

Complications

Chronic or recurrent UTI
Complicated UTI
Pyelonephritis
Bacteremia
Sepsis

Incidence

UTIs affect approximately 3% of children in the United States annually. Throughout the course of childhood, the risk of a UTI in boys is 2% and in girls it is 8%. UTIs are responsible for more than 1 million visits to pediatricians' offices annually in the United States (National Kidney and Urologic Diseases Information Clearinghouse (NKUDIC),

2005; Cleveland Clinic, 2007). "Approximately 5–10% of children with symptomatic UTI and fever develop renal scarring" (Egland & Egland, 2006, Section 2).

Etiology

The three primary causes of UTIs in children are classified as urinary abnormalities, immune dysfunction, or dysfunctional voiding. Urinary abnormalities include vesicoureteral reflux or neurogenic bladder from conditions such as spina bifida. Some children are more susceptible to developing UTIs because of their immune system. Dysfunctional voiding actions include not voiding regularly, not completely emptying the bladder when voiding, practicing improper hygiene, wearing tight underclothing, and bathing in a tub. Urethral irritation in females is common as sexual activity is initiated or is frequent. This irritation increases the urethra's susceptibility to infection. Constipation and localized infections also can cause UTIs.

Clinical Manifestations

Urgency
Frequency
Pain on urination
Pain from bladder spasms
Burning on urination
Incontinence
Fever

Diagnostic Tests

Urinalysis
Urine culture and sensitivity

Medical Management

The goals of treatment are to cure the infection and prevent further UTIs. The standard of care for UTIs in children is oral medication therapy with sulfamethoxazole with trimethoprim (8–10 mg/kg/24 hr for children and infants over 2 months of age) for 7–10 days. This is the most commonly used urinary anti-infective agent (Broyles, Reiss, & Evans, 2007). Other agents that may be prescribed include ciprofloxacin (4 mg/kg/dose not to exceed 500 mg/dose or 8 mg/kg/day), amoxicillin (500 mg every 8 hours or every 12 hours in children weighing more than 40 kg and 8 mg/kg/day in divided doses for children over 3 months and weighing less than 40 kg), or nitrofurantoin (5–7 mg/kg/day in four divided doses) (Spratto & Woods, 2008; Broyles et al., 2007).

Nursing Management

Assessment

1. Obtain client history
2. Obtain urine for culture and sensitivity prior to beginning of anti-infective therapy
3. Assess current voiding and hygiene habits
4. Obtain vital signs, height, and weight

Nursing Diagnoses (including but not limited to)

1. Risk for injury R/T complications of infectious process
2. Risk for deficient fluid volume R/T nausea, decreased intake, and fever
3. Acute pain R/T nerve irritation secondary to inflammation
4. Deficient knowledge R/T condition, predisposing factors, treatment, and home care

PLANNING/GOALS

1. Client will not experience complications of cystitis or recurrence of infection, and the infection will be successfully treated.
2. Client will maintain fluid balance.
3. Client will demonstrate pain control as determined by client and as evidenced by verbalizations using age-appropriate pain assessment tool and will experience decrease/absence of bladder spasms.
4. Parents and client (if age-appropriate) will demonstrate understanding of condition, predisposing factors, treatment, and home care.

NOC

1. Infection Severity
2. Fluid Balance
3. Pain Control
4. Knowledge: Disease Process, Diagnostic Procedures, Medications, Health Promotion

IMPLEMENTATION

1. Risk for injury
   a. Assess child's normal urinary pattern
   b. Assess urine for clarity, sediment, and gross blood, including lab stick urine
   c. Monitor intake and output
   d. Obtain urine for urinalysis and culture and sensitivity
   e. Instruct child/parent regarding hygiene practices that will help prevent UTIs
   f. Instruct regarding manifestations of pyelonephritis
   g. Instruct about importance of follow-up care and repeat urine for culture to evaluate success of treatment
   h. Monitor vital signs
2. Fluid balance
   a. Monitor intake and output
   b. Instruct parents regarding medication administration
   c. Monitor vital signs
   d. Instruct parents and client (if age-appropriate) to complete prescribed medications to fully treat infection and to prevent development of antibiotic-resistant microorganisms
   e. Encourage favorite fluids by mouth in small amounts frequently
   f. Instruct to monitor temperature
   g. Instruct parents/child how to monitor fluid intake
   h. Encourage intake of cranberry juice (to decrease microorganisms from adhering to bladder wall) and/or orange juice to acidify urine
   i. Monitor urine specific gravity
3. Pain
   a. Assess pain level hourly using age-appropriate pain assessment tool
   b. Administer analgesics as prescribed
   c. Instruct on use of analgesics at home
   d. Apply warm, moist heat to abdomen to decrease bladder spasms
4. Parent/child teaching
   a. Assess parents'/child's current level of understanding
   b. Provide verbal and written instructions regarding:

1) Risk factors for developing UTI

2) Appropriate technique for perineal care

3) Need to avoid tub baths

4) Importance of wearing cotton rather than nylon underwear

5) Importance of drinking adequate fluids (preferably water and juice) frequently during the day

6) Necessity of voiding frequently and completely

7) Medication administration and importance of completing prescribed medication therapy

8) Manifestations of adverse effects of medications

9) Manifestations of worsening condition

10) Contact phone numbers for reporting signs and symptoms

11) Importance of regular hand washing and appropriate technique

12) Importance of follow-up with health care provider to reculture urine

c. Provide adequate time for teaching

d. Document teaching and parents'/client's response

NIC

1. Infection Control

2. Fluid Management, Fluid Monitoring

3. Analgesic Administration

4. Teaching: Disease Process, Diagnostic Procedures, Medications, Health Education

EVALUATION

1. Client does not experience complications of cystitis or recurrence of infection, and the infection is successfully treated.

2. Client maintains fluid balance.

3. Client demonstrates pain control as determined by client and as evidenced by verbalizations using age-appropriate pain assessment tool and experiences decrease/absence of bladder spasms.

4. Parents and client (if age-appropriate) demonstrate understanding of condition, predisposing factors, treatment, and home care.

References

Broyles, B. E., Reiss, B. S., & Evans, M. E. (2007). *Pharmacological aspects of nursing care* (7th ed.). Clifton Park, NY: Delmar Cengage Learning.

Cleveland Clinic. (2007). *Urinary tract infections in children.* Retrieved May 5, 2007, from http://www.clevelandclinic.org/health/health-info/docs/0800/0867.asp?index=5472

Egland, A. G., & Egland, T. K. (2006). *Pediatrics, urinary tract infections and pyelonephritis.* Retrieved March 25, 2008, from http://www.emedicine.com/emerg/topic769.htm

National Kidney and Urologic Diseases Information Clearinghouse (NKUDIC). (2005). *Urinary tract infections in children.* Retrieved March 25, 2008, from http://kidney.niddk.nih.gov/kudiseases/pubs/utichildren

Potts, N. L., & Mandleco, B. L. (2007). *Pediatric nursing: Caring for children and their families* (2nd ed.). Clifton Park, NY: Delmar Cengage Learning.

Spratto, G. R., & Woods, A. L. (2008). *2008 edition: PDR nurse's drug handbook.* Clifton Park, NY: Delmar Cengage Learning.

108

Ventricular Septal Defect (VSD)

Definition

A ventricular septal defect (VSD) is an abnormal connection between the two larger lower chambers of the heart (American Heart Association, 2008) that occurs during fetal development, resulting in a left-to-right shunt. Refer to Figure 108-1.

Pathophysiology

The VSD can vary in size from a small hole that is 1 mm in diameter to as large as the complete absence of the septum. Small defects usually produce no symptoms beyond a vague murmur, whereas larger defects can produce symptoms of decreased cardiac output requiring open-heart surgery to close the connection between the two ventricles. Normally, blood (deoxygenated for systemic circulation) entering the right chambers of the heart remains in the right side until pumped into the lungs from the right ventricle,

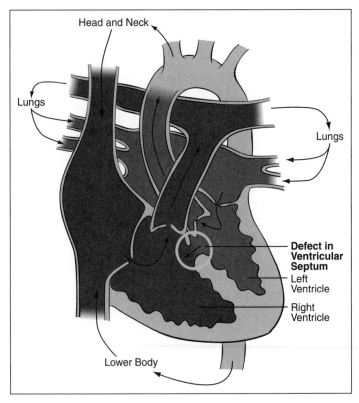

Figure 108-1: Ventricular Septal Defect.

and oxygenated blood in the left chambers stays on the left side until pumped from the left ventricle into systemic circulation. In the presence of a VSD, blood in the left ventricle is forced through the opening to the right side each time the ventricle contracts because of higher pressure in the left ventricle than in the right ventricle. This oxygenated blood is recirculated to the lungs; consequently, deoxygenated blood is unable to reach the lungs. This causes an increased workload on the right ventricle and eventually permanent damage to the walls of the blood vessels in the lungs. Right ventricular hypertrophy is more likely to occur in the presence of a large VSD. Most infants/children with small VSD are asymptomatic, requiring neither medical nor surgical interventions (CongenitalHeartDefects.com, 2006).

Complications

Right ventricular hypertrophy
Decreased cardiac output
Failure to thrive
Altered gas exchange

Incidence

"A ventricular septal defect, or VSD, is the most common kind of congenital heart defect" (CongenitalHeartDefects.com, 2006, p. 1). "Isolated VSDs and those VSDs associated with other congenital anomalies account for approximately 50% of infants with congenital heart disease" (Potts & Mandleco, 2007, p. 774).

Etiology

Most of the time the cause of congenital heart defects is unknown. Although the reason defects occur is presumed to be genetic, only a few genes have been discovered that have been linked to the presence of heart defects. Heredity may play a role in CHD, as well as coexisting conditions such as Down syndrome or a mother contracting rubella during the first trimester of pregnancy. The use of alcohol and illicit drugs during pregnancy increases the fetus's risk for developing CHD (American Heart Association, 2008).

Clinical Manifestations

Most VSDs produce no symptoms except a murmur. Severe defects can
produce:
Murmur
Dyspnea on exertion
Feeding difficulties
Fatigue
Growth retardation
Failure to thrive
Right ventricular hypertrophy
Right-sided heart failure

Diagnostic Tests

Auscultation of a murmur
Pulse oximetry
Electrocardiogram
Chest radiography
Echocardiogram
Cardiac catheterization

Medical Management

Most infants/children with VSDs are asymptomatic and require no medical intervention; and many, if not most, VSDs close due to the increased pressure the excess blood creates in the right ventricle. These VSDs usually are small, and closure occurs within the first year of life. However, a complex VSD requires medical/surgical management, which is discussed in Chapter 26: Congenital Heart Disease/Open Heart Surgery.

Nursing Management

Refer to Nursing Management in Chapter 26: Congenital Heart Disease/Open Heart Surgery.

References

American Heart Association. (2008). *Ventricular septal defect.* Retrieved March 26, 2008, from http://www.americanheart.org/presenter.jhtml?identifier=11066

CongenitalHeartDefects.com. (2006). *Ventricular septal defect (VSD).* Retrieved April 24, 2007, from http://www.congenitalheartdefects.com/typesofCHD.html#VSD

Potts, N. L., & Mandleco, B. L. (2007). *Pediatric nursing: Caring for children and their families* (2nd ed.). Clifton Park, NY: Delmar Cengage Learning.

109

VISUAL IMPAIRMENT

Definition

Visual impairment is a decrease in the ability to see (Broyles, 2005).

Pathophysiology

Visual impairments include a variety of conditions and are classified according to the type of impairment. Refractive errors are alterations in the pathway of light rays through the eyes. Myopia, also called nearsightedness, is characterized by the inability to see objects at a distance. It results from light focusing on an object in front of the retina rather than at the rear of the retina. Hyperopia, or farsightedness, is the inability to see objects close. It is caused by light focusing on an object beyond the retina. Astigmatism "occurs when there is an uneven curvature of the cornea or lens, preventing light rays from focusing correctly on the retina" (Potts & Mandleco, 2007, p. 1035). Refer to Figure 109-1.

Strabismus, or cross-eyed appearance, is a condition of lack of coordination in the musculature of the eye. It occurs when both eyes do not simultaneously focus on the same object, resulting in double images. Amblyopia, also called lazy eye, results most often from the brain's response to suppress the vision in the deviated eye of strabismus to compensate and avoid the diplopia. Eventually, if not treated, sight will be lost in the deviated eye (Potts & Mandleco, 2007).

Some visual impairments result from lack of integrity of eye structures. Congenital cataract is the presence of an opaque lens. Congenital glaucoma occurs when there is increased intraocular pressure.

Infections also can impair vision. Acute conjunctivitis is inflammation of the conjunctiva usually caused by infection and referred to as pink eye. Neonatal conjunctivitis results from an infection caused by *Haemophilus influenzae* or *Streptococcus pneumoniae* or by chemical irritants such as the medications administered into the eyes of neonates to prevent ophthalmia neonatorum. "Trachoma is a chronic form of conjunctivitis caused by *Chlamydia trachomatis* that results in scarring of the conjunctiva and eyelids and is the leading cause of blindness worldwide" (Broyles, 2005, p. 868).

Blindness has a number of definitions. Legal blindness is defined as visual acuity of 20/200. A child also is considered blind if he/she uses the other senses (hearing, touch, and smell) as the primary means of perceiving, learning, and performing tasks. Blindness also is the complete lack of ability to see. This can result from damage to the optic nerve during gestational development or from damage due to trauma, untreated infections, cataracts, or glaucoma.

Complications

Inability to see clearly
Risk for physical injuries
Blindness

Incidence

In the United States, blindness and serious visual impairment occur in 30–64 children/100,000 population. Less serious visual impairment occurs in an additional

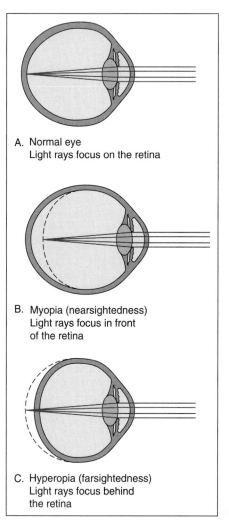

A. Normal eye
   Light rays focus on the retina

B. Myopia (nearsightedness)
   Light rays focus in front
   of the retina

C. Hyperopia (farsightedness)
   Light rays focus behind
   the retina

Figure 109-1: Refractory Errors.

100 children/100,000 population (Hockenberry, 2005). Refractory errors are the most common type of conditions resulting in visual impairment in children. Approximately 2–3% of the pediatric population experiences amblyopia during preschool years; cataracts affect 1 in 250 neonates; and congenital glaucoma occurs in 1 out of 10,000 live births (Potts & Mandleco, 2007).

Etiology

The cause of refractory errors is believed to be heredity. Approximately 50% of children with strabismus have a family history of the condition (Potts & Mandleco, 2007). Amblyopia is believed to be most often the result of strabismus. Congenital cataracts and glaucoma are present at birth as gestational anomalies.

Clinical Manifestations

Redness

Itching

Purulent drainage

Squinting

Sitting close to television to see

Headache

Irritability

Complaints of difficulty seeing when reading or watching television

Difficulty with motor skills because of inability to see

Photophobia

Inability to see oncoming traffic or other types of danger

Diagnostic Tests

Acuity testing with Snellen "E" or "Big E" chart

Hirschberg corneal reflex test (strabismus)

Corneal red reflex (cataract)

Intraocular pressure tonometry (glaucoma)

Visual fields assessment

Ophthalmic examination to visualize eye structures

Medical Management

The goals of treatment are early detection of the child's visual impairment, treatment of the condition, prevention of blindness, and rehabilitation for serious visual impairments or blindness. Refractory errors are treated with corrective lens. Glasses are recommended for young children and contact lens for children mature enough to care for contacts responsibly. Strabismus is treated medically with eye patching; however, if this does not correct the impairment, surgery is required. The definitive treatment for congenital cataracts is surgical removal of the opaque lens. Surgical opening of the outflow of aqueous humor from the anterior chamber of the eye is the definitive treatment for congenital glaucoma. Infections are treated with antimicrobials including gentamicin 3% ophthalmic ointment for trachoma; erythromycin ophthalmic ointment or ciprofloxacin ophthalmic ointment for conjunctivitis caused by *C. trachomatis, H. influenzae,* or *S. pneumoniae*; and silver nitrate to prevent ophthalmia neonatorum (Broyles, Reiss, & Evans, 2007; Spratto & Woods, 2008).

Nursing Management

Assessment

1. Obtain client history
2. Examine visual acuity
3. Assess level of growth and development

Nursing Diagnoses (including but not limited to)

1. Disturbed visual sensory perception R/T visual impairment
2. Risk for injury R/T visual impairment
3. Deficient knowledge R/T child's condition, treatment, and home care

Planning/Goals

1. Client will regain and maintain highest level of visual acuity through compliance with treatment regimen.

2. Client will not experience injury.

3. Parents and client (if age-appropriate) will demonstrate understanding of child's condition, treatment, and home care

NOC

1. Sensory Function: Vision
2. Risk Control
3. Knowledge: Disease Process, Procedures, Treatment, Medication, Health Promotion

IMPLEMENTATION

1. Vision
   a. Assess child's vision
   b. Assess for manifestations of eye infection
   c. Encourage parents to verbalize feelings and concerns
   d. Listen actively
   e. Explain procedures
   f. Discuss care of corrective lenses
2. Risk for injury
   a. Assess child's level of growth and development
   b. Discuss with parents behaviors that would place child at risk for injury
   c. Explain to parents and child (if age-appropriate) importance of compliance with treatment plan
3. Parent/child teaching
   a. Assess parents' and child's (if age-appropriate) level of understanding
   b. Demonstrate use of ophthalmic medications and provide for return demonstration
   c. Provide verbal and written information regarding:
      1) Importance of visual screening
      2) Growth and development behaviors
      3) Avoidance of behaviors that may result in eye injury
      4) Medication administration including importance of administering ophthalmic medications only in the eye, applying medication to conjunctival sac (not directly on cornea or retina), keeping eye medication sterile, not touching the eye with the medication applicator, and never using ophthalmic medications that have been contaminated or solutions that are cloudy
      5) Hand washing and proper technique
      6) Importance of follow-up care with health care provider
   d. Provide adequate time for teaching
   e. Document teaching and parents'/child's response

NIC

1. Visual Enhancement
2. Risk Identification
3. Teaching: Disease Process, Procedures, Treatment, Medication, Health Education

EVALUATION

1. Client regains and maintains highest level of visual acuity through compliance with treatment regimen.

2. Client does not experience injury.
3. Parents and client (if age-appropriate) demonstrate understanding of child's condition, treatment, and home care

References

Broyles, B. E. (2005). *Medical-surgical nursing clinical companion.* Durham, NC: Carolina Academic Press.

Broyles, B. E., Reiss, B. S., & Evans, M. E. (2007). *Pharmacological aspects of nursing care* (7th ed.). Clifton Park, NY: Delmar Cengage Learning.

Hockenberry, M. J. (2005). *Wong's essentials of pediatric nursing* (7th ed.). St. Louis, MO: Elsevier Mosby.

Potts, N. L., & Mandleco, B. L. (2007). *Pediatric nursing: Caring for children and their families* (2nd ed.). Clifton Park, NY: Delmar Cengage Learning.

Spratto, G. R., & Woods, A. L. (2008). *2008 edition: PDR nurse's drug handbook.* Clifton Park, NY: Delmar Cengage Learning.

WILMS' TUMOR

Definition

Wilms' tumor, also called nephroblastoma, is a rare type of renal cancer that affects children (MedlinePlus, 2007). Wilms' tumor is the most common renal cancer in children, making up 95% of all pediatric renal cancers (American Cancer Society, 2008).

Pathophysiology

Wilms' tumor was named after Max Wilms, a German physician who wrote about the tumor in 1899. It is a rapidly growing tumor on the kidney (usually the left kidney) encapsulated in a thin, fragile capsule that can be easily torn, providing a mechanism for seeding of the cancer cells. Usually, it forms unilaterally, but a small percentage of children develop the tumor on both kidneys (American Cancer Society, 2008).

Two categories describe the histology of Wilms' tumor: favorable and unfavorable according to how it appears microscopically. Favorable histology tumors are more responsive to treatment and provide a more favorable prognosis (Potts & Mandleco, 2007).

"A tumor has an unfavorable appearance [unfavorable histology] when the nuclei (the central part of the cell that contains the DNA) of the cancer cells are very large and distorted. In addition, the cells are not uniform and their appearance varies widely. This is called anaplasia. The more anaplasia that is found, the poorer the chance is for a cure. Favorable appearance [favorable histology] means there is no anaplasia and the chance of cure is very good. About 95% of Wilms' tumors have a favorable histology" (American Cancer Society, 2008, p. 1).

In addition to histologic classifications, Wilms' tumor is staged according to the National Wilms' Tumor Study Group (NWTSG) staging system. A Stage I tumor involves only one kidney and is completely removed by surgery; approximately 42% of all Wilms' tumors are stage I. The four-year survival rate in stage I is 96% for favorable tumors and 93% for unfavorable (anaplastic) tumors. Stage II tumors extend beyond the kidney but are completely removed surgically. Approximately 22% of all Wilms' tumors are stage II, and the four-year survival rate is 91% for favorable tumors and 70% for unfavorable tumors. Stage III Wilms' tumors cannot be completely removed, but the remaining cancer cells are limited to the abdominal cavity. The remaining cancer cells may be in the abdominal or pelvic lymph nodes, may be present at the edge of the tissue removed by surgery, may be the result of seeding before or during surgery, or may be present in structures near the kidney involved. Approximately 22% of all Wilms' tumors are stage III with a four-year survival rate of 91% for favorable tumors and 56% for unfavorable tumors. In Stage IV tumors, the cancer cells have disseminated through the vascular system to the lungs, liver, bone, or lymph nodes distant from the kidneys. These tumors make up about 9% of all Wilms' tumors with a four-year survival rate of 81% for favorable tumors and 17% for unfavorable tumors. Finally, Stage V tumors are in both kidneys at the time of diagnosis and constitute approximately 5% of all Wilms' tumors. The four-year survival rate is 82% for favorable tumors with no available figures for unfavorable tumors at this time (American Cancer Society, 2008).

Complications

Metastasis

Death with unfavorable histology and staging

Incidence

Approximately 500 new cases of Wilms' tumors are diagnosed annually in the United States. These tumors constitute about 5.6% of all pediatric cancers. They usually occur in children under the age of 6 years and are uncommon after this age. Wilms' tumor is more common in girls than boys and is slightly more prevalent among African-American children. The overall five-year survival rate for children with Wilms' tumor is more than 92% (American Cancer Society, 2008).

Etiology

As with most cancers, the exact cause of Wilms' tumor is unknown. Identified risk factors include genetics, heredity, race, gender, and the presence of certain birth defects including WAGR syndrome, Beckwith-Wiedemann syndrome, Denys-Drash syndrome, Perlman syndrome, Sotos syndrome, Simpson-Golabi-Behmel syndrome, and Bloom syndrome (American Cancer Society, 2008).

Clinical Manifestations

Abdominal mass

Flank mass

Abdominal pain

Fever

Hematuria

Diagnostic Tests

Ultrasonography

Computed tomography

Magnetic resonance imaging

Angiography of the renal veins or inferior vena cava

Chest radiography

Bone scan

Medical Management

The goal of treatment is to remove the tumor surgically and provide chemotherapy to destroy any remaining tumor cells. It is extremely important to avoid vigorous abdominal palpation in a child expected of having Wilms' tumor; this can cause the thin capsule around the tumor to tear, allowing the tumor to seed to adjacent areas. The standard of care for children with Wilms' tumor is surgery to resect the tumor followed by chemotherapy. For stage III, IV, and V tumors, radiation therapy also is used. Antineoplastic agents most often used to treat Wilms' tumor are actinomycin D and vincristine for stages I, II, and III with favorable histology. For advanced stages and those with unfavorable histology, doxorubicin, cyclophosphamide, and/or etoposide are used (Broyles, Reiss, & Evans, 2007; American Cancer Society, 2008).

Nursing Management

Refer to Chapter 22: Chemotherapy, Chapter 87: Radiation Therapy, and Chapter 100: Surgical Client.

References

American Cancer Society. (2008). *Detailed guide: Wilms tumor.* Retrieved March 26, 2008, from http://www.cancer.org/docroot/CRI/content/CRI_2_4_1x_What_is_wilms_tumor_46.asp?sitearea

Broyles, B. E., Reiss, B. S., & Evans, M. E. (2007). *Pharmacological aspects of nursing care* (7th ed.). Clifton Park, NY: Delmar Cengage Learning.

MedlinePlus. (2007). *Wilms' tumor.* Retrieved March 26, 2008, from http://www.nlm.nih.gov/medlineplus/wilmstumor.html

Potts, N. L., & Mandleco, B. L. (2007). *Pediatric nursing: Caring for children and their families* (2nd ed.). Clifton Park, NY: Delmar Cengage Learning.

DIAGNOSTIC TESTS

> *NOTE:* In large acute care facilities, child life therapists who may be on staff should be incorporated in the care of children undergoing diagnostic studies.

Angiography

DEFINITION AND USE

Angiography is used to visualize the structure and circulation through the blood vessels and lymphatics. It also can be helpful in evaluating the vascularity of tumors (Potts & Mandleco, 2007). Radiopaque contrast medium is injected into the circulation so that the vessels can be visualized.

PROCEDURE AND NURSING CARE

The procedure should be explained to the parents and child in developmentally appropriate terminology, and they should be provided adequate time to ask questions. Angiography is performed in the radiology department or vascular laboratory in an acute care facility, so the child will be transported to the appropriate department. The site of the injection should be prepped with EMLA cream 1 hour prior to or LMX4 applied 30 minutes prior to the injection of the dye to prevent pain from the injection. The older child should be reassured that EMLA will help prevent the procedure from being painful. In infants and younger children, conscious sedation or general anesthesia may be used. If sedation or general anesthesia is used, the child must have nothing by mouth for a prescribed period based on the child's age.

Prior to the procedure, the nurse performs an assessment including vital signs, height, and weight, and assesses the child for allergies to iodine, contrast media, or shellfish. The child should have nothing by mouth for a prescribed period (depending on the age of the child) prior to the procedure. Following the procedure, the child must be closely monitored until fully recovered from sedation/anesthesia. If the procedure is performed in an outpatient setting, the child is released following a 1–2 hour recovery period. Parents are instructed to monitor the injection site for bleeding, which should be reported immediately to the child's health care provider. The nurse should instruct the parents about the importance of returning for the scheduled health care provider appointment.

Bone Marrow Aspiration and Biopsy

DEFINITION AND USE

Bone marrow aspiration and biopsy is performed to obtain specimens of the soft jellylike substance (marrow) that fills the inner cavity of large bones (Beattie, 2007). This procedure is used to diagnose and manage diseases such as leukemia, aplastic anemia, and polycythemia, and exposure to certain chemicals; the procedure also is used to diagnose whether some cancers have metastasized to the bone.

PROCEDURE AND NURSING CARE

The procedure should be explained to the parents and child in developmentally appropriate terminology, and they should be provided adequate time to ask questions. Prior to the procedure, the nurse performs an assessment including vital signs, height, and weight; coagulation studies are also performed due to the risk of bleeding with this procedure. The results of the complete blood count and coagulation studies should be available for review by the pathologist.

The procedure lasts approximately 20 minutes and involves the use of a 14- to 18-gauge needle inserted in the iliac crest (site of choice). The area should be prepped with EMLA at least 1 hour before the procedure or LMX4 at least 30 minutes prior to the procedure, and the health care provider performing the procedure administers a local injection of 1% lidocaine immediately prior to the aspiration. This procedure is performed under conscious sedation for young children and general anesthesia for infants. If sedation or general anesthesia is used, the child must have nothing by mouth for a prescribed period based on the child's age.

The child and parents should be instructed that the child experiences a great deal of pressure throughout the procedure. The child should be reassured that a nurse will be in attendance during the entire procedure. If the procedure is performed in a treatment area, parents may be permitted to remain with the child if they feel comfortable being present. They should not be asked to restrain the child, but they can offer comfort.

The child is positioned on the side not being accessed for the aspiration with the upper leg flexed. If the child is conscious, the nurse should talk softly to him/her throughout the procedure, keeping the child's leg flexed and observing the sterile field. Immediately following the procedure, firm pressure should be applied to the site for several minutes to prevent bleeding. A sterile pressure dressing is applied.

Extra-strength acetaminophen is the drug of choice for any discomfort the child may experience following the procedure. The parents and child are instructed to leave the pressure dressing on and intact for 24 hours. Parents should report any bleeding through the dressing or a temperature elevation to 38°C (100.4°F) to the health care provider immediately. The nurse should instruct the parents about the importance of returning for the scheduled health care provider appointment.

Bronchoscopy

DEFINITION AND USE

Bronchoscopy is performed to visualize the anatomical structures of the trachea and bronchial tree. During the procedures, lesions can be biopsied, cultures can be obtained, and foreign objects can be removed.

PROCEDURE AND NURSING CARE

Bronchoscopies are performed in the operating room. Rigid bronchoscopy requires general anesthesia, and flexible bronchoscopy can be done under conscious sedation. Prior to the procedure, the nurse performs an assessment including vital signs, height, and weight. The parents and child should be instructed about the procedure and given specific instructions regarding conscious sedation if it is to be used. The child should have nothing by mouth for a prescribed period (depending on the age of the child) prior to the procedure.

During and after the procedure, the child should be continuously monitored because of the risk of trauma to the upper airway during the bronchoscopy. Humidified air may be administered after the procedure to reduce swelling and edema. If the bronchoscopy is performed in an outpatient facility, the child must be fully recovered from general anesthesia or conscious sedation prior to discharge. Parents should be instructed regarding manifestations of airway obstruction, which should be reported immediately to the health care provider if they occur. The nurse should instruct the parents about the importance of returning for the scheduled health care provider appointment and given the approximate time that test results will be available.

Cardiac Catheterization

DEFINITION AND USE

Cardiac catheterization is an invasive procedure involving the introduction of a catheter into the femoral artery or vein. Dye is injected through the catheter to allow the visualization of the structures of the heart. This procedure is performed to identify specific cardiac defects and usually is performed in the cardiac catheterization laboratory, which is situated in close proximity to the surgical area.

PROCEDURE AND NURSING CARE

Prior to the procedure, pretesting, including electrocardiography, echocardiography, complete blood count, and coagulation studies, usually is performed. The nurse should review the results and collaborate with the health care provider regarding the results. The nurse performs an assessment including vital signs, height, and weight, and assesses the child for allergies to iodine, contrast media, or shellfish. The child should have nothing by mouth for a prescribed period (usually 4–6 hours depending on the age of the child) prior to the procedure. Both groin areas should be prepped with EMLA or LMX4 to prevent the pain of inserting the catheter through the skin. Although the left groin vessel is preferred, prepping both groins allows for use of either one. The child and parents should be provided with verbal and written information regarding the procedure and allowed time to verbalize any concerns or questions they may have. The primary complication during the cardiac catheterization is the initiation of cardiac dysrhythmias.

Following the procedure, the child is closely monitored for the primary complications that can occur after a cardiac catheterization: (1) bleeding at the catheter insertion site, (2) hematoma formation at the insertion site, and (3) infection (manifestations usually are not apparent for 12–24 hours). The affected leg must remain extended for a prescribed period (usually 4–8 hours) following the procedure. At prescribed intervals (initially 15–30 minutes for an hour then 30 minutes to every hour for 4 hours then every 4 hours for 24 hours), vital signs, groin dressing, peripheral pulses (femoral, posttibial, and pedal), and temperature and sensation of both extremities are assessed. Both extremities should be assessed concurrently for comparison of pulses, skin temperature, and color, and the results documented. The child should be offered oral fluids as soon as fully recovered from anesthesia, and intake and output should be monitored. The pressure dressing can be removed after 24 hours (Potts & Mandleco, 2007).

The parents should be instructed regarding how to care for the pressure dressing. The child should not bathe in a tub for 48–72 hours, and oral fluids should be encouraged. Parents should report any bleeding through the dressing or a temperature elevation to 38°C (100.4°F) to the health care provider immediately. The nurse should instruct the parents about the importance of returning for the scheduled health care provider appointment.

Computed Tomography (CT) Scan

DEFINITION AND USE

A computed tomography (CT) scan involves the use of narrow beam X-rays combined with a computer and allows the visualization of any body structure in successive layers. Each beam or pulse of the X-ray lasts less than a second and provides data via the computer of thin slices of body tissue. A CT scan can provide a 360-degree view of the brain in small increments. Contrast media may be used for CT scans.

PROCEDURE AND NURSING CARE

The nurse should provide developmentally appropriate information to the child and parents about the CT scan. A CT scan usually is quite lengthy, and the child is required to remain still during the procedure. As a result, conscious sedation is used for young children, and they must have nothing by mouth for a prescribed period prior to sedation. The parents and child should be reassured that the procedure is not painful.

No special precautions are necessary before or after a CT scan unless conscious sedation is used. Following conscious sedation, the child must be closely monitored for respiratory compromise and must remain in the outpatient or same-day surgery facility until fully responsive from the sedation. The parents should be instructed to report any worsening of the child's condition to the health care provider immediately and to return for the scheduled health care provider appointment.

Echocardiography

DEFINITION AND USE

An echocardiogram uses sound waves emitted from a transducer to produce a two-dimensional and Doppler evaluation of cardiac structures, size, and function (Potts & Mandleco, 2007). It is a noninvasive procedure that can detect cardiac anomalies, ejection fraction of the heart, and valve leakages even in the fetus. If abnormalities that require surgery are noted, a cardiac catheterization frequently is performed prior to surgery for confirmation of the need for surgery and for more exact measurements of anatomical anomalies. There are different types of echocardiograms, including transthoracic, transesophageal, and fetal.

PROCEDURE AND NURSING CARE

For an echocardiogram to be performed accurately, the child must cooperate; so young children usually require conscious sedation. If sedation is to be used, the child must have nothing by mouth for a prescribed period based on the child's age.

As with any procedure for which conscious sedation is used, the child must be monitored with continuous pulse oximetry and cardiorespiratory monitoring. The procedure should be explained to the parents and child in developmentally appropriate language with sufficient time for their questions. No specific precautions are needed except those noted for conscious sedation. Following the procedure, the child can be discharged with parental instructions regarding the importance of returning for the scheduled follow-up visit with the health care provider. Children who have received conscious sedation cannot be discharged until fully responsive from sedation.

Electrocardiography (ECG)

DEFINITION AND USE

An electrocardiogram (ECG) is the recording of the electrical activity of the heart (Daniels, Nosek, & Nicoll, 2007). The electrical waveforms are produced through leads placed on the skin of the child's chest and extremities. The ECG machine prints the cardiac rhythm on paper specifically designed for recording cardiac electrical activity. This is a noninvasive procedure.

PROCEDURE AND NURSING CARE

The procedure should be explained to the parents and child in developmentally appropriate terminology, and they should have adequate time to ask questions. For best results, the child should lie still in a supine position during this short procedure. Holding the child or providing distraction may be needed.

No specific precautions or diagnostic studies are required prior to the ECG. Any lotion or powders need to be removed from the skin, and the specific skin sites for electrode placement should be cleansed with alcohol. Electrode pads containing transponder gel covered with a foam pad are applied to the chest and extremities, and the electrode leads then are attached to the pads. Usually, 12 leads are used; however, as many as 15 may be required. Because the electrode pads have an adhesive backing that sticks to the skin, they should be removed carefully after the recording has been completed. Children may remove these pads themselves as long as the nurse supervises the activity.

No special instructions for home care are needed. The parents should be instructed to report any worsening of the child's condition to the health care provider immediately and to return for the scheduled health care provider appointment.

Electroencephalography (EEG)

DEFINITION AND USE

An electroencephalogram (EEG) is a recording of the electrical activity of the brain. It is used to diagnose specific seizure activity. This is achieved through electrodes placed on the scalp that conduct and amplify the brain's electrical activity.

PROCEDURE AND NURSING CARE

An EEG is a noninvasive procedure that does not involve special precautions. The procedure should be explained to the parents and child in developmentally appropriate terminology, and they should be provided adequate time to ask questions. The hair and scalp are cleansed to remove any hair care products. The electrodes are placed directly on the scalp and remain in place due to the adhesive backing on the electrode pads or the use of electrode gel. The child is instructed to remain still and not to touch the electrodes. Frequently, the EEG is performed while the child sleeps to prevent movement or dislodging of the electrodes. Sedation is contraindicated because it alters brain activity.

No special home care instructions are required following an EEG. The parents should be instructed to report any worsening of the child's condition to the health care provider immediately and to return for the scheduled health care provider appointment.

Endoscopy

DEFINITION AND USE

An endoscopy is the visualization through a scope of the gastric structures for the diagnosing of gastrointestinal abnormalities. Fiber-optic gastrointestinal endoscopy or esophagogastroduodenoscopy (EGD) is the visualization of the esophagus, stomach, and duodenum. It is used to diagnose gastroesophageal reflux, esophageal atresia, pyloric stenosis, duodenal atresia, and the presence of lesions or ulcerations.

PROCEDURE AND NURSING CARE

The procedure should be explained to the parents and child in developmentally appropriate terminology, and they should be provided adequate time to ask questions. This is considered an invasive procedure, and the child must have nothing by mouth for 4–6 hours prior to the procedure. For infants and young children, endoscopy may be performed under general anesthesia. For older children, conscious sedation is used. The child should be continuously monitored using pulse oximetry and a cardiorespiratory monitor throughout the procedure and at its conclusion until the child is fully responsive.

A lighted scope is passed down the esophagus into the stomach and then advanced to the duodenum. During the procedure, the structures are displayed on a visual monitor and as still photographs.

This procedure can be performed in an acute care facility or in an outpatient facility. The child cannot be discharged until fully responsive from anesthesia or sedation. The parents should be instructed to report any worsening of the child's condition to the health care provider immediately and to return for the scheduled health care provider appointment.

Kidney, Ureter, and Bladder (KUB) Radiography

DEFINITION AND USE

A kidney, ureter, and bladder (KUB) radiography is a flat-plate abdominal X-ray used to diagnose the presence of renal calculi or size changes in the structures. This noninvasive procedure is performed prior to renal studies.

PROCEDURE AND NURSING CARE

No special precautions are required for this procedure. The procedure should be explained to the parents and child in developmentally appropriate terminology, and they should be provided adequate time to ask questions. They should be assured that the procedure does not cause discomfort to the child. The child is transported to the radiology department and may be discharged as soon as the radiologist is sure the X-rays are complete.

The procedure can be performed in an inpatient or outpatient facility. The parents should be instructed to report any worsening of the child's condition to the health care provider immediately and to return for the scheduled health care provider appointment.

Laryngoscopy

DEFINITION AND USE

Laryngoscopy is the direct visualization of the larynx with a scope to diagnose structural reasons for stridor and local abnormalities (Daniels, 2003). This procedure is performed in the operating room.

PROCEDURE AND NURSING CARE

The procedure should be explained to the parents and child in developmentally appropriate terminology, and they should be provided adequate time to ask questions. General anesthesia or conscious sedation is required, and the child must have nothing by mouth for a prescribed period based on the child's age. During and following the procedure, the child must be continuously monitored for cardiopulmonary status.

The child is positioned supine with the head tilted back. The laryngoscope is inserted, and the structures are examined. A tissue specimen can be obtained for laboratory analysis. Following the procedure, the child is transported to a recovery area to be continuously monitored until responsive from anesthesia/sedation. The child cannot be discharged until the nurse is sure the child's gag reflex has returned and the child can take oral fluids. The parents should be instructed to report any symptoms of respiratory compromise or any worsening of the child's condition to the health care provider immediately and to return for the scheduled health care provider appointment.

Liver Biopsy

DEFINITION AND USE

A liver biopsy is the removal of hepatic tissue for laboratory analysis. It is an invasive procedure used to detect hepatic disease.

PROCEDURE AND NURSING CARE

The procedure should be explained to the parents and child in developmentally appropriate terminology, and they should be provided adequate time to ask questions. Because of the vascular nature of the liver and the risk of bleeding, preprocedural coagulation studies are performed. The procedure can be performed in a treatment room on the pediatric nursing care unit or in an operating room setting. Very young children and infants require sedation for the procedure and must be monitored continuously throughout the procedure with pulse oximetry and cardiorespiratory monitoring. If sedation is used, the child must have nothing by mouth for a prescribed period of time based on the child's age. If the biopsy is performed in a treatment area, parents may be permitted to remain with the child (if the child is not sedated) if they feel comfortable being present. They should not be asked to restrain the child, but they can offer comfort. The child's right side over the site of the liver may have EMLA applied at least 1 hour before the procedure or LMX4 applied 30 minutes prior to the procedure.

The child is positioned in a supine or left lateral position with the right arm over the head. This is a sterile procedure, and the sterile field must remain intact. The skin over the liver is prepped, and a local anesthetic is injected (if the child is awake). The EMLA or LMX4 should ensure that the child is not hurt by the anesthetic injection. To avoid a pneumothorax, the child must hold his/her breath for approximately 10 seconds as the needle for the biopsy is being inserted. After the needle is inserted into the liver tissue, a tissue sample is withdrawn. After the needle is removed, pressure must be applied to the site for several minutes; then a pressure dressing is applied.

Following the procedure, the child is positioned on his/her right side with a pillow under the right side to apply further pressure to the biopsy site. The child remains on strict bed rest for up to 4 hours with frequent monitoring of vital signs and the pressure dressing.

This procedure can be performed in an acute care facility or in an outpatient facility; however, inpatient is preferred. The child cannot be discharged until fully responsive from anesthesia or sedation and after the prescribed assessment of his/her vital signs and biopsy pressure dressing. The pressure dressing should remain for 24 hours. The parents should be instructed to report any bleeding from the dressing or worsening of the child's condition to the health care provider immediately and to return for the scheduled health care provider appointment.

Lumbar Puncture (LP)

DEFINITION AND USE

A lumbar puncture (LP), also referred to as a spinal tap, is an invasive procedure involving the insertion of a needle into the subarachnoid space at the level of the lumbar spine for the purpose of aspirating cerebrospinal fluid (CSF) for analysis. It also is performed to instill medications such as anesthesia and intrathecal antimicrobials and antineoplastic agents (DeLaune & Ladner, 2006). This is the procedure of choice for diagnosing meningitis.

PROCEDURE AND NURSING CARE

The procedure should be explained to the parents and child in developmentally appropriate terminology, and they should be provided adequate time to ask questions. Prior to the procedure, the nurse assesses the child for allergies to iodine. EMLA should be applied at least 1 hour before the procedure or LMX4 applied 30 minutes prior to the procedure to the site of the puncture.

The child must lie still; so for very young children, some level of sedation usually is required. The child is placed in a lateral recumbent position "with the craniospinal axis parallel to the floor and the flat of the back perpendicular to the procedure table" (DeLaune & Ladner, 2006, p. 651) with the knees flexed against the chest so the back is bowed to separate the vertebrae. The nurse must hold the child in position for the procedure.

This is a sterile procedure, so the sterile field must remain intact. The site of the puncture is prepped, and a local anesthetic agent is injected. The needle and stylet are inserted into the midsagittal space and advanced into the subarachnoid space. The stylet is removed, and the needle remains in place. A pressure reading is obtained, and the CSF specimen is removed. The needle is removed at the end of the procedure, and pressure is applied to the site to prevent the leakage of CSF. Then a sterile bandage is applied.

The procedure can be performed in an inpatient or outpatient facility. The child is monitored for CSF leakage and neurologic status until stable. The bandage should remain on the site for 24 hours. The parents should be instructed to report any worsening of the child's condition to the health care provider immediately and to return for the scheduled health care provider appointment.

Magnetic Resonance Imaging (MRI)

DEFINITION AND USE

Magnetic resonance imaging (MRI) "is an imaging technique that uses radiowaves and a strong magnetic field to make continuous cross-sectional images of the body" (DeLaune & Ladner, 2006, p. 646). The client is supplied with headphones to muffle the clanging sound the machine makes.

PROCEDURE AND NURSING CARE

The procedure should be explained to the parents and child in developmentally appropriate terminology, and they should be provided adequate time to ask questions. The child is instructed to remain still during the procedure. For infants and young children, conscious sedation may be required. All metal objects and jewelry must be removed so the magnet is not attracted to them.

The procedure is lengthy, requiring up to an hour to perform depending on the part(s) of the body being scanned. If sedation is used, the child must have nothing by mouth for a prescribed period based on the child's age. For children under conscious sedation, continuous monitoring of respiratory status must be performed. During and following the procedure, the child should be continuously monitored using pulse oximetry and a cardiorespiratory monitor until the child is fully responsive.

This procedure can be performed in an acute care facility or in an outpatient facility. The child cannot be discharged until fully responsive from anesthesia or sedation. The parents should be instructed to report any worsening of the child's condition to the health care provider immediately and to return for the scheduled health care provider appointment.

Renal Biopsy

DEFINITION AND USE

Renal biopsy is an invasive procedure performed to remove renal tissue for laboratory analysis. This procedure is used to detect the presence of cancer cells and to evaluate renal cellular function.

PROCEDURE AND NURSING CARE

The procedure should be explained to the parents and child in developmentally appropriate terminology, and they should be provided adequate time to ask questions. Because of the vascular nature of the kidney and the risk of bleeding, preprocedural coagulation studies may be performed. The procedure can be performed in a treatment room on the pediatric nursing care unit or in an operating room setting. Very young children and infants require sedation for the procedure and must be monitored continuously throughout the procedure with pulse oximetry and cardiorespiratory monitoring. If sedation is used, the child must have nothing by mouth for a prescribed period based on the child's age. If the biopsy is performed in a treatment area, parents may be permitted to remain with the child (if the child is not sedated) if they feel comfortable being present. They should not be asked to restrain the child, but they can offer comfort. EMLA can be applied at least 1 hour before the procedure or LMX4 30 minutes prior to the procedure to the area where the biopsy will be performed.

The child is positioned prone and instructed to lie very still. For postrenal transplant children, the supine position is used. This is a sterile procedure, and the sterile field must be maintained. If EMLA or LMX4 has not been used, a local anesthetic is injected into the skin over the proposed biopsy site. Then the site is prepped, and the needle is inserted into the kidney. Tissue is withdrawn and sent to the laboratory for analysis. Pressure is applied for several minutes over the biopsy site, and a pressure dressing is applied.

This procedure can be performed in an acute care facility or in an outpatient facility; however, inpatient is preferred. The child cannot be discharged until fully responsive from sedation and after the prescribed assessment of his/her vital signs and biopsy pressure dressing. The pressure dressing should remain for 24 hours. The parents should be instructed to report any bleeding from the dressing or worsening of the child's condition to the health care provider immediately and to return for the scheduled health care provider appointment.

Sweat Test (Pilocarpine Iontophoresis)

Definition and Use

The sweat test, also called a chloride sweat test, measures sweat electrolyte concentrations on the skin and is used to confirm a diagnosis of cystic fibrosis.

Procedure and Nursing Care

The procedure should be explained to the parents and child in developmentally appropriate terminology, and they should be provided adequate time to ask questions. No special precautions or preparation is needed. Sweating is stimulated on the child's forearm with pilocarpine, and a sweat specimen is collected on absorbent material. At least a 50 mL sample is needed for accuracy in measuring the amount of sodium and chloride in the sample. Because of the quantity of specimen needed for this test, it is not used on neonates.

This procedure can be performed in an acute care facility if the child is hospitalized or on an outpatient basis. The nurse should provide support to the parents as they face the implications of a positive result. The parents should be instructed about the importance of returning for the scheduled health care provider appointment.

Ultrasonography

Definition and Use

Ultrasound "is a non-invasive study that uses high-frequency sound waves to visualize deep body structures" (DeLaune & Ladner, 2006, p. 644). It does not require contrast media, so it should be scheduled before other diagnostic tests that do require contrast. It is used to evaluate the brain, thyroid gland, heart, abdominal organs, and kidneys.

Procedure and Nursing Care

The procedure should be explained to the parents and child in developmentally appropriate terminology, and they should be provided adequate time to ask questions. The child is instructed to remain still during the procedure. For infants and young children, conscious sedation may be required.

No special precautions are needed for this procedure. A coupling gel that increases the contact between the transducer and the skin is placed on the surface of the body area to be studied. The transducer converts electrical energy to sound waves that are reflected off soft tissue structures. The density of the structures deflects the waves to form varying images on an oscilloscope. The images are individually recorded as photographs.

This procedure can be performed in an acute care facility or in an outpatient facility. The child cannot be discharged until fully responsive from anesthesia or sedation. The parents should be instructed to report any worsening of the child's condition to the health care provider immediately and to return for the scheduled health care provider appointment.

References

Beattie, S. (2007). Hands-on help: Bone marrow aspiration and biopsy. *RN 70*(2).

Daniels, R. (2003). *Delmar's manual of laboratory and diagnostic tests.* Clifton Park, NY: Delmar Cengage Learning.

Daniels, R., Nosek, L. J., & Nicoll, L. H. (2007). *Contemporary medical-surgical nursing.* Clifton Park, NY: Delmar Cengage Learning.

DeLaune, S. C., & Ladner, P. K. (2006). *Fundamentals of nursing: Standards and practice* (4th ed.). Clifton Park, NY: Delmar Cengage Learning.

Potts, N. L., & Mandleco, B. L. (2007). *Pediatric nursing: Caring for children and their families* (2nd ed.). Clifton Park, NY: Delmar Cengage Learning.

COMMON LABORATORY TESTS AND NORMAL VALUES

Acetaminophen (serum or plasma)

Therapeutic concentration	10–30 µg/mL
Toxic concentration	> 200 µg/mL

Albumin (plasma)

Newborn	2.5–3.4 grams/dL
< 5 yr	3.4–5.0 grams/dL
5–19 yr	4.0–5.6 grams/dL

Alkaline phosphatase (ALP) (serum)

1–9 yr	145–420 units/L
2–10 yr	100–320 units/L
11–18 yr male	100–390 units/L
11–18 yr female	100–320 units/L

Ammonia nitrogen (serum or plasma)

Newborn	90–150 mg/dL
Child	40–80 mg/dL

Amylase (serum)

1–19 yr	35–127 units/L

Antistreptolysin O titer (ASO titer) (serum)

2–4 yr	< 166 Todd units
School-age	170–330 Todd units

Bicarbonate (HCO_3) (serum)

Infant (venous)	20–24 mEq/L
> 2 years (venous)	22–29 mEq/L
> 2 years (arterial)	21–28 mEq/L

Bilirubin (conjugated) (serum) 0.0–0.2 mg/dL

Bilirubin (total) (serum)

Premature infant

Cord blood	< 2 mg/dL
0–1 day	< 8 mg/dL
1–2 days	< 12 mg/dL
2–5 days	< 16 mg/dL
> 5 days	< 20 mg/dL

Full-term infant

Cord blood	< 2.8 mg/dL
0–1 day	< 2–6 mg/dL
1–2 days	< 6–8 mg/dL
2–5 days	< 4–6 mg/dL
> 5 days	< 10 mg/dL

Blood volume (whole blood)

Male	52–83 mL/kg
Female	50–75 mL/kg

C-reactive protein (CRP) (serum)

2–12 yr	67–1800 ng/mL

Calcium (Ca)—Total (serum)

Newborn	9.0–10.6 mg/dL
Child	8.8–10.8 mg/dL

Carbon dioxide

   Partial pressure (PCO$_2$) (whole blood, arterial)

Newborn	27–40 mm Hg
Infant	27–41 mm Hg
Thereafter: Male	35–48 mm Hg
Female	35–45 mm Hg

   Total (tCO$_2$) (serum or plasma)

Newborn	13–22 mmol/L
Infant	20–28 mmol/L
Child	20–28 mmol/L
Thereafter	23–30 mmol/L

Chloride (Cl) (serum)

Newborn	97–110 mmol/L
Thereafter	98–106 mmol/L

Chloride (sweat)

Normal	< 40 mmol/L
Borderline	45–60 mmol/L
Cystic fibrosis	> 60 mmol/L

Cholesterol (total)

Newborn	53–135 mg/dL
Infant	70–175 mg/dL
Child	120–200 mg/dL
Adolescent	< 200 mg/dL

Creatinine (serum)

Newborn	0.3–1.0 mg/dL
Infant	0.2–0.4 mg/dL
Child	0.3–0.7 mg/dL
Adolescent	0.5–1.0 mg/dL

Creatine kinase (CK, CPK) (serum)

Newborn	87–725 units/L

Digoxin (serum or plasma)

Therapeutic concentration

Congestive heart failure (CHF)	0.8–1.5 ng/mL
Arrhythmias	1.5–2.0 ng/mL
Toxic concentration	> 2.5 ng/mL

Erythrocyte (RBC) count (whole blood)

Newborn	4.8–7.1 million/mm^3
3–6 mo	3.1–4.5 million/mm^3
0.5–2 yr	3.7–5.3 million/mm^3
2–6 yr	3.9–5.3 million/mm^3
6–12 yr	4.0–5.2 million/mm^3
12–18 yr: Male	4.5–5.3 million/mm^3
Female	4.1–5.1 million/mm^3

Erythrocyte sedimentation rate (ESR) (whole blood)

Westergren (modified)	0–10 mm/hr
Wintrobe	0–13 mm/hr

Fibrinogen (plasma)

Newborn	125–300 mg/dL
Thereafter	200–400 mg/dL

Glucose (serum)

Newborn	50–90 mg/dL
Child	60–100 mg/dL
Thereafter	70–105 mg/dL

Glycosylated hemoglobin

Nondiabetic child	1.8–4%
Good diabetic control	2.5–5.9%
Fair diabetic control	6–8%
Poor diabetic control	> 8%

Growth hormone (hGH, somatotropin) (plasma, fasting)

Newborn	15–40 ng/mL
Child	0–10 ng/mL

Hematocrit (HCT, Hct) (whole blood)

Newborn	44–72%
2 mo	28–42%
6–12 yr	35–45%
12–18 yr: Male	37–49%
Female	36–46%

Hemoglobin (Hb) (whole blood)

Newborn	14–27 grams/dL
2 mo	9–14 grams/dL
6–12 yr	11.5–15.5 grams/dL
12–18 yr: Male	13–16 grams/dL
Female	12–16 grams/dL

Iron (serum)

Newborn	100–250 µg/dL
Infant	40–100 µg/dL
Child	50–120 µg/dL
Thereafter: Male	50–160 µg/dL
Female	40–150 µg/dL

Lead (whole blood)

Child	< 10 µg/dL

Leukocyte (WBC) count (whole blood)

Newborn	9–30 × 1000 cells/mm³
1–3 yr	6.0–17.5 × 1000 cells/mm³
4–7 yr	5.5–15.5 × 1000 cells/mm³
8–13 yr	4.5–13.5 × 1000 cells/mm³
Adult	4.5–11.0 × 1000 cells/mm³

Leukocyte differential count (whole blood)

Myelocytes	0%
Neutrophils—"bands"	3–5%
Neutrophils—"segs"	54–62%
Lymphocytes	25–33%
Monocytes	3–7%
Eosinophils	1–3%
Basophils	0–0.75%

Osmolality (serum)

Child, adult	275–295 mOsmol/kg H_2O

Oxygen, partial pressure (PO_2) (whole blood, arterial)

Birth	8–24 mm Hg
1 day	54–95 mm Hg
Thereafter (decreased with age)	83–108 mm Hg

Oxygen saturation (SaO_2) (whole blood, arterial)

Newborn	85–90%
Thereafter	95–99%

Partial thromboplastin time (PTT) (whole blood) (Na citrate)

Nonactivated	60–85 seconds (Platelin)
Activated	25–35 seconds (differs with methods)

Phenylalanine (serum)

Premature	2.0–7.5 mg/dL
Newborn	1.2–3.4 mg/dL
Thereafter	0.8–1.8 mg/dL

Plasma volume (plasma)

Male	25–43 mL/kg
Female	28–45 mL/kg

Platelet count (thrombocyte count) (whole blood)

Newborn (after 1 wk same as adult)	84–478 × 1000/mm³ (µL)
Adult	150–400 × 1000/mm³ (µL)

Potassium (serum)

< 2 yr	3.0–6.0 mmol/L
2–12 yr	3.5–7.0 mmol/L
> 12 yr	3.5–5.0 mmol/L

Protein (serum, total)

Premature	4.3–7.5 grams/dL
Newborn	4.6–7.4 grams/dL
1–7 yr	6.1–7.9 grams/dL
8–12 yr	6.4–8.1 grams/dL
13–19 yr	6.6–8.2 grams/dL

Prothrombin time (PT)

One-stage (Quick) (whole blood)

In general	11–15 seconds (varies with type of thromboplastin)
Newborn	Prolonged by 2–3 sec

Sodium (serum or plasma)

Newborn	136–146 mmol/L
Infant	139–146 mmol/L
Child	138–145 mmol/L
Thereafter	136–146 mmol/L

Specific gravity (urine)

Newborn	1.016–1.030
Infant	1.002–1.006
Thereafter	1.016–1.030

Thyrotropin (thyroid stimulating hormone [TSH])

Newborn	3–18 μ International Units/L by day 3 of life
Thereafter	2–10 m International Units/L

Thyroxine (T$_4$, T$_4$ total, T$_4$ RIA) (serum)

Newborn	9–18 μg/dL
Infant	7–15 μg/dL
1–5 yr	7.3–15 μg/dL
5–10 yr	6.4–13.3 μg/dL
Thereafter	5–12 μg/dL

Triglycerides (TG) (serum) (after ≥ 12-hr fast)

	Male	Female
0–5 yr	30–86 mg/dL	32–99 mg/dL
6–11 yr	31–108 mg/dL	35–114 mg/dL
12–15 yr	36–138 mg/dL	41–138 mg/dL
16–19 yr	40–163 mg/dL	40–128 mg/dL

Triiodothyronine (T$_3$, T$_3$ total, T$_3$ RIA) (serum)

Newborn	72–260 ng/dL
1–5 yr	100–260 ng/dL
5–10 yr	90–240 ng/dL
10–15 yr	80–210 ng/dL
Thereafter	115–190 ng/dL

Urea nitrogen (serum or plasma)

Newborn	3–12 mg/dL
Infant or child	5–18 mg/dL
Thereafter	7–18 mg/dL

Urine volume (urine, 24-hr)

Newborn	50–300 mL/day
Infant	350–550 mL/day
Child	500–1000 mL/day
Adolescent	700–1400 mL/day
Thereafter: Male	800–1800 mL/day
Female	600–1600 mL/day (varies with intake and other factors)

NOTE: Normal laboratory values differ depending on laboratories and methods used to determine values. Verify your facility's normal values.

Modified from *Delmar's Manual of Laboratory and Diagnostic Tests* by R. Daniels. (2003). Clifton Park, NY: Delmar Cengage Learning; *Nelson Textbook of Pediatrics* (18th ed.) by R. Behrman, R. Kliegman, H. Jenson, & B. Stanton (2007). Philadelphia: W. B. Saunders; *A Manual of Laboratory and Diagnostic Tests* (8th ed.) by F. Fischbach. (2009). Philadelphia: Lippincott Williams & Wilkins.

Pediatric Physical Assessment, Growth Charts, BMI Charts, Pain Scales

Biographical Data

1. Child's name
2. Address and phone number
3. Sources of information
4. Parent/legal guardian

Health History

1. Birth history
   a. Prenatal
   b. Labor and delivery
   c. Postnatal
2. Client profile
   a. Age
   b. Eating habits
   c. Sleeping habits
   d. Developmental level
   e. Education levels (school, day care, etc.)
   f. Behavior
   g. Person/people with whom client lives
   h. Work environment (school-age and adolescence)
   i. Current medications
3. Past health history
   a. Immunizations
   b. Childhood illnesses
   c. Previous hospitalizations
   d. Accidents or injuries
   e. Allergies
   f. Medications

Nutritional Assessment

1. Dietary intake
2. Dietary history
3. Assessment of obesity
4. Laboratory evaluation
5. Anthropometric data
   a. Weight
   b. Height
   c. Size of component parts
   d. Skinfolds
   e. Plot on growth charts and BMI charts. Refer to Figure C-1 A-H.

6. Physical examination data
7. Evaluation of data including laboratory values

Developmental Assessment
Refer to Appendix E: Pediatric Growth and Development.

Physical Assessment

VITAL SIGNS
Refer to Appendix D: Pediatric Vital Signs.

1. Temperature
   a. Axillary in neonates, infants, and children less than 5 years old
   b. Tympanic can be quick and noninvasive

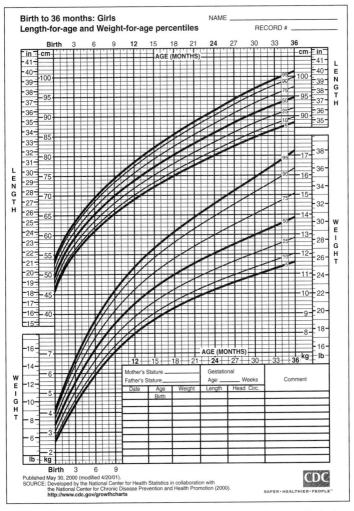

Figure C-1A: Physical Growth Chart: Girls: Birth to 36 Months (Length and Weight). Courtesy of National Center for Health Statistics, U.S. Centers for Disease Control and Prevention, 2001.

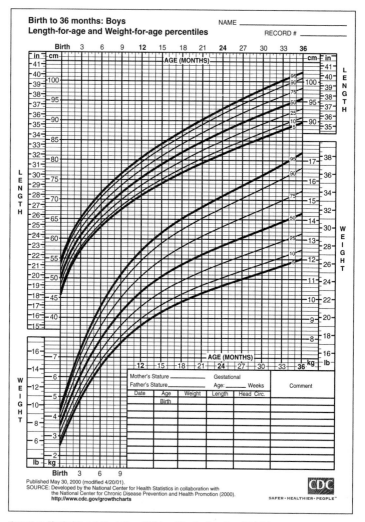

Figure C-1B: Physical Growth Chart: Boys: Birth to 36 Months (Length and Weight). Courtesy of National Center for Health Statistics, U.S. Centers for Disease Control and Prevention, 2001.

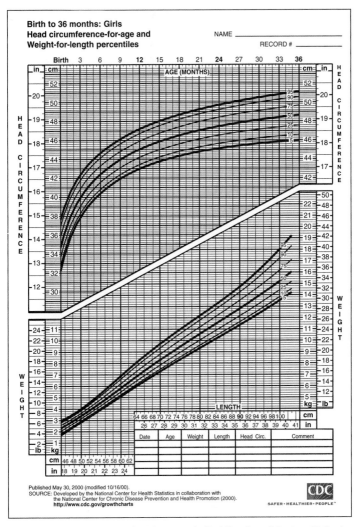

Figure C-1C: Physical Growth Chart: Girls: Birth to 36 Months (Head Circumference). Courtesy of National Center for Health Statistics, U.S. Centers for Disease Control and Prevention, 2001.

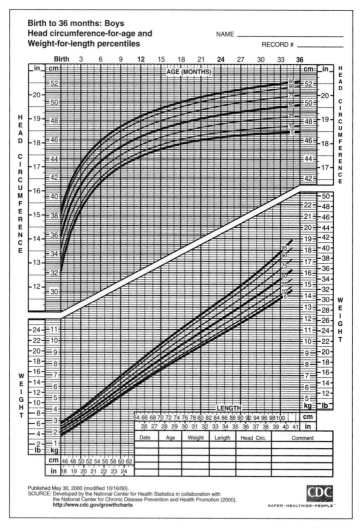

Figure C-1D: Physical Growth Chart: Boys: Birth to 36 Months (Head Circumference). Courtesy of National Center for Health Statistics, U.S. Centers for Disease Control and Prevention, 2001.

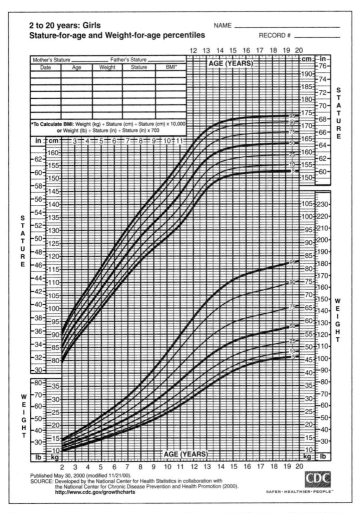

Figure C-1E: Physical Growth Chart: Girls: 2 to 20 Years (Stature and Weight). Courtesy of National Center for Health Statistics, U.S. Centers for Disease Control and Prevention, 2001.

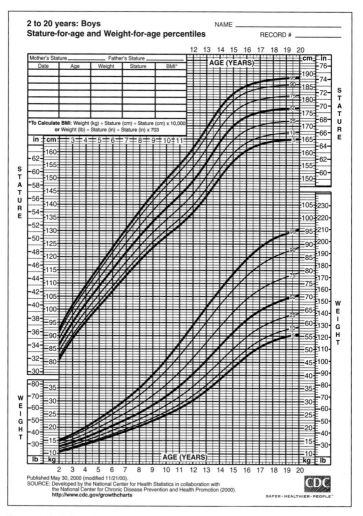

Figure C-1F: Physical Growth Chart: Boys: 2 to 20 Years (Stature and Weight). Courtesy of National Center for Health Statistics, U.S. Centers for Disease Control and Prevention, 2001.

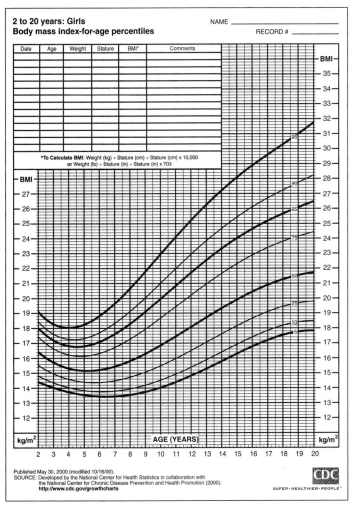

Figure C-1G: Physical Growth Chart: Girls: 2 to 20 Years (Body Mass Index for Age). Courtesy of National Center for Health Statistics, U.S. Centers for Disease Control and Prevention, 2001.

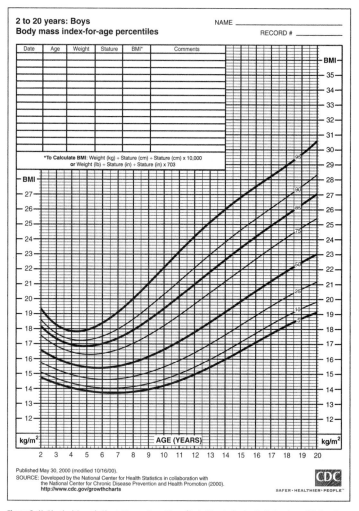

Figure C-1H: Physical Growth Chart: Boys: 2 to 20 Years (Body Mass Index for Age). Courtesy of National Center for Health Statistics, U.S. Centers for Disease Control and Prevention, 2001.

    c. Oral in children over 5 years of age

    d. Rectal only when no other feasible route is available

2. Pulse

    a. Apical pulse for neonates, infants, and toddlers

    b. Apical pulse for children on digoxin

    c. Radial pulse in children over 3 years of age

    d. Presence or absence, rate, rhythm, and quality

3. Respirations

    a. Monitor rate, depth, effort, and symmetry

    b. Monitor expansion of abdomen in infants and toddlers (abdominal breathers)

    c. Position for comfort

    d. Note presence of retractions, nasal flaring (infants), or use of accessory muscles

4. Blood pressure

    a. Use correct cuff size (width of bladder cuff should be 40% of arm's circumference and should cover 80–100% of arm's circumference) (Potts & Mandleco, 2007; DeLaune & Ladner, 2007; Hockenberry, 2005)

    b. Monitor systolic–diastolic pressures and quality

    c. Start monitoring blood pressure in children 3 years and older (National High Blood Pressure Education Program Working Group on High Blood Pressure in Children and Adolescents, 2004)

PHYSICAL GROWTH

Refer to Figures C-1A–H

1. Weight

    a. Place infants in supine position on balanced scales with all clothing removed

    b. Measure child who can cooperate and stand without support, using vertical balanced scales

    c. Plot measurements on standardized physical growth chart for appropriate age and gender

2. Length and height

    a. Measure neonates and infants by linear length

    b. Measure child who can cooperate and stand without support, using vertical height bar or measuring tape

    c. Plot measurements on standardized physical growth chart for appropriate age and gender

3. Head circumference

    a. Measure on all children less than 2 years of age or children suspected of brain injury

    b. Compare with previous serial measurements

    c. Measure with tape measure anteriorly from just above eyebrows posteriorly to occipital protuberance

    d. Note that normal head growth is 1.0–1.5 cm per month for first 6 months of life then slow to 0.5 cm for second 6 months

    e. Note that head circumference is greater than chest circumference up to 1 year of age

    f. Plot measurements on standardized physical growth chart for appropriate age and gender

4. Chest circumference
   a. Measure in infants
   b. Measure across nipple line
   c. Compare to head circumference
   d. Plot measurements on standardized physical growth chart for appropriate age and gender
   e. Note that chest circumference exceeds head circumference after 1 year of age

5. Skin
   a. Color and pigmentation
   b. Moisture
   c. Turgor
   d. Presence of lesions

6. Hair
   a. Texture
   b. Dryness and moisture
   c. Color
   d. Distribution
   e. Cleanliness
   f. Presence of lesions, infestation, scales, or crusts on scalp

7. Nails
   a. Color
   b. Capillary refill
   c. Presence of cyanosis or cracking of nails

CARDIOVASCULAR ASSESSMENT

1. Apical pulse—rate, rhythm, and quality
2. Heart sounds
   a. S_1 is best heard at apex of the heart
   b. S_2 is best heard at heart base
   c. Auscultation for sinus rhythm
   d. Auscultation of murmurs
      1) Approximately half of all children develop a murmur without pathology during childhood
      2) Murmur is audible until ductus arteriosus closes (as late as 3 months)

3. Peripheral pulses
   a. Rate, rhythm, presence, or absence
   b. Differences between upper and lower extremity pulses
   c. Radial, brachial, carotid, femoral, popliteal, posttibial, and pedal

4. Activity level
5. Skin color
6. Extremities—clubbing of toes or fingers
7. Abdominal auscultation for bruits over aortic, renal, iliac, and femoral arteries

RESPIRATORY ASSESSMENT

1. Behavior
2. Activity level

3. Chest examination
   a. Inspection of chest shape and symmetry
   b. Palpation for tactile fremitus
   c. Percussion
   d. Respirations
      1) Rate, depth, effort, rhythm, symmetry, and pattern
      2) Position of comfort
      3) Presence of retractions or use of accessory muscles
      4) Presence of nasal flaring
   e. Auscultation of lung sounds
      1) Listen over all five lobes (two on the left; three on the right)
      2) Listen anteriorly and posteriorly
      3) Note characteristic sounds
         a) Tracheal—very loud, very high, and harsh; heard over extrathoracic trachea (Daniels, Nosek, & Nicoll, 2007)
         b) Bronchial—loud, high, and tubular; heard over malubrium
         c) Bronchovesicular—moderate loudness and pitch, rustling; heard over bronchial mainstem
         d) Vesicular—soft, low, gentle rustling; heard over most of peripheral lung
      4) Listen for adventitious breath sounds (stridor, rales, rhonchi, or wheeze)

NEUROLOGIC ASSESSMENT

1. Level of consciousness
   a. Alertness appropriate for developmental level
   b. Orientation appropriate for developmental level
2. Behavior
   a. Appropriate for developmental level
   b. Affect
   c. Cognition
   d. Thought processes
   e. Presence of irritability
   f. Glasgow coma scale for pediatrics (modified Glasgow coma scale)
3. Vital signs
   a. Respirations—erratic in presence of increased intracranial pressure (ICP)
   b. Pulse—bradycardic in presence of increased ICP
   c. Blood pressure—elevated in presence of increased ICP
   d. Temperature—altered if hypothalamus is dysfunctional or if there is presence of infection
4. Motor function
   a. Appropriate for developmental level
   b. Strength
   c. Coordination
   d. Movement of all extremities
   e. Gait
5. Sensory function (Refer to Figures C-2, C-3, C-4)
   a. Reflex status
      1) In neonates (Refer to Appendix E: Pediatric Growth and Development)

Facial expression	0– relaxed	1–grimace	2–vigorous
Cry	0– no cry	1– whimper	
Breathing pattern	0– relaxed	1– change in breathing	
Arms	0– relaxed or restrained	1–flexed or extended	
Legs	0– relaxed or restrained	1–flexed or extended	
State of arousal	0–sleeping or awake	1–fussy	

Figure C-2: Neonatal Infant Pain Scale (NIPS). Source: Lawrence, J., and others (1993). The development of a tool to assess neonatal pain. *Neonatal Network, 12*(6), 59–66.

    2) Other reflexes for infants and children over 6 months of age
      a) Deep tendon
      b) Biceps
      c) Triceps
      d) Brachioradial
      e) Patellar
      f) Achilles
  b. Cranial nerves (modified for age)
  c. Proprioception (modified for age)
  d. Response to pain and temperature
  e. Visual function
    1) Visual acuity (use of age-appropriate Snellen chart)
    2) Color vision (Ishihara chart)
    3) Epicanthal folds
    4) Eyebrows, eyelashes, and eyelids
    5) Symmetry of iris and pupils
    6) Lacrimal function
    7) Conjunctiva
    8) Corneal light reflex
    9) Retinal red reflex
  f. Auditory function
    1) Testing of 8th cranial nerve
    2) Quantitative assessment with audiometer
    3) External ear
      a) Placement and position
      b) Discharge
      c) Palpation of mastoid bone prominences
      d) Auricles
      e) Otoscopic exam to visualize tympanic membrane, ear canal, and cerumen
    4) Balance and gait
  g. Olfactory function
    1) Visualization of nares
    2) Familiar odors offered for identification

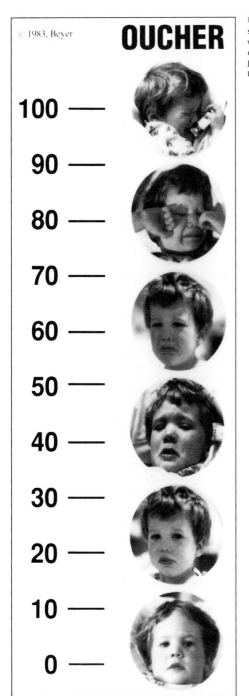

Figure C-3: The Oucher Pain Assessment Tool. The Caucasian version of the Oucher, further developed and copyrighted by Judith E. Beyer, RN, PhD, 1983. Used with permission.

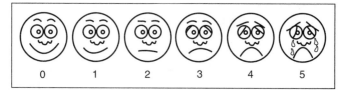

Figure C-4: Wong-Baker FACES Pain Rating Scale. From Hockenberry, M. J., Wilson, D., & Winkelstein, M. L. (2005). *Wong's essentials of pediatric nursing* (7th ed., p. 1259). St. Louis: Mosby. Copyright Mosby. Used with permission.

      h. Head assessment

         1) Symmetry

         2) Circumference in neonates and infants

         3) Fontanels

            a) Anterior—diamond shape on top of head; soft and flat

            b) Posterior—triangular located on occiput, soft, and flat

            c) Assessment for depression or bulging

6. Pupillary action

    a. Dilate and constrict to light equally

    b. Size

    c. Shape

MUSCULOSKELETAL ASSESSMENT

1. General appearance
2. Muscle mass
3. Muscle tone
4. Muscle strength
5. Gross and fine motor skills appropriate for developmental level
6. Joints

    a. Symmetry

    b. Range of motion

    c. Flexibility

    d. Hips—legs equal in length and gluteal folds equal

7. Spine

    a. Curvature (vertical and horizontal)

    b. Assessment of shoes for abnormal wear

    c. Gait

8. Symmetry of muscles, bones, and spine
9. Ability to participate in developmentally appropriate activities

GASTROINTESTINAL ASSESSMENT

1. Bowel function

    a. Bowel sounds over all four abdominal quadrants

    b. Bowel habits including toilet training experience

    c. Presence of constipation or diarrhea

2. Food and fluid intake

    a. Changes in eating or drinking habits

    b. Complaints of abdominal pain, nausea, or vomiting

3. Abdomen

    a. Inspection of contour, symmetry, and characteristics of umbilicus

    b. Skin color and turgor

    c. Presence of lesions

    d. Gentle palpation for tenderness, guarding, rigidity, masses, and distention

4. Rectal exam only if dysfunction is suspected

Lymphatic Assessment

1. Inspection of lymph nodes—presence of enlargement
2. Palpation (Potts & Mandleco, 2007) Refer to Figure C-5.

    a. Submental—under chin

    b. Submandibular—under mandible

    c. Tonsillar—behind temporomandibular joint, under angle of jaw

    d. Superficial cervical—superficial to sternomastoid muscle

    e. Deep cervical—from sternomastoid muscle down to clavicle

    f. Posterior cervical—along anterior edge of trapezius muscle

    g. Preauricular—in front of auricle of the ear

    h. Parotid—along upper jaw line

    i. Postauricular—behind auricle of the ear

    j. Axillary (pectoral)—along lower border of pectoralis major muscle

    k. Axillary (subscapular)—along border of the scapula bone

    l. Axillary (lateral)—along upper humerus and midaxillary line

    m. Epitrochlear—medial aspect of upper arm

    n. Infraclavicular—behind clavicle

    o. Supraclavicular—above clavicle

    p. Subclavicular—below the clavicle

    q. Horizontal inguinal—high in anterior thigh below inguinal ligament

    r. Vertical inguinal—clustered near upper edge of saphenous vein

Endocrine Assessment

1. Most assessments obtained through laboratory values drawn when suspicion of endocrine dysfunction exists
2. Palpation of thyroid gland for presence of masses or enlargement

Genitourinary

1. Urinary function

    a. Fluid intake

    b. Bladder habits including bladder training

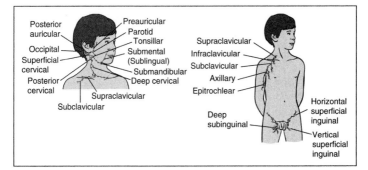

Figure C-5: Location of Lymph Nodes

    c. Urinary pattern
    d. Urinalysis evaluation
    e. Palpation of bladder
  2. Female reproductive
    a. Breasts
      1) Inspection performed throughout childhood for symmetry and enlargement
      2) Examinations begin with puberty
    b. Genitalia
      1) Inspection performed throughout childhood
      2) Examination prior to menarche only if abuse is suspected
      3) Sexual activity status
      4) Annual pelvic examinations should begin at onset of menarche
  3. Male reproductive
    a. General appearance
    b. Genitalia
      1) Penis
        a) Circumcision status
        b) Position of urinary meatus
        c) Hygiene habits
        d) Sexual activity status
        e) Presence of discharge
      2) Scrotum
        a) Cremasteric reflex—retraction of testes from scrotum in cross-legged position
        b) Presence of both testes
        c) Presence of inguinal hernia

REFERENCES

Centers for Disease Control and Prevention. (2007). *2000 CDC growth charts: United States.* Retrieved April 14, 2008, from http://www.cdc.gov/growthcharts

Centers for Disease Control and Prevention. (2007). *BMI-Body mass index.* Retrieved April 14, 2008, from http://www.cdc.gov/nccdphp/dnpa/bmi

Daniels, R., Nosek, L. J., & Nicoll, L. H. (2007). *Contemporary medical-surgical nursing.* Clifton Park, NY: Delmar Cengage Learning.

DeLaune, S. C., & Ladner, P. K. (2007). *Fundamentals of nursing: Standards and practice* (4th ed.). Clifton Park, NY: Delmar Cengage Learning.

Hockenberry, M. J. (2005). *Wong's essentials of pediatric nursing* (7th ed.). St. Louis, MO: Elsevier Mosby.

National High Blood Pressure Education Program Working Group on High Blood Pressure in Children and Adolescents. (2004). The fourth report on the diagnosis, evaluation, and treatment of high blood pressure in children and adolescents. *Pediatrics, 114*(2). Retrieved May 9, 2007, from http://pediatrics.aappublications.org/cgi/content/full/114/2/S2/555#SEC4

Potts, N. L., & Mandleco, B. L. (2007). *Pediatric nursing: Caring for children and their families* (2nd ed.). Clifton Park, NY: Delmar Cengage Learning.

PEDIATRIC VITAL SIGNS

Body Temperature

AGE	CENTIGRADE	FAHRENHEIT	METHOD
Neonate to 1 year	35.5°–37.7°	95.9°–99.7°	Axillary
3 to 5 years	37.0°–37.2°	98.6°–99.0°	Axillary
7 to 9 years	36.7°–36.8°	98°–98.2°	Oral
10 years old and older	36.6°	97.8°	Oral

Pulse/Respirations

AGE	PULSE (BEATS/MINUTE)	RESPIRATIONS (BREATHS/MINUTE)
Newborn	100–170	30–50
1 year	80–170	20–40
3 years	80–130	20–30
6 years	70–115	16–22
10 years	70–110	16–20
14 years	60–110	14–20
18 years	60–100	16–20

Courtesy of Potts, N. L., & Mandleco, B. L. (2007). Pediatric nursing: Caring for children and their families *(2nd ed.). Clifton Park, NY: Delmar Cengage Learning.*

Blood Pressure

Age	Systolic	Diastolic
Newborn	46–92	38–71
3 years	72–110	40–73
10 years	83–121	45–79
16 years	93–131	49–85

PEDIATRIC GROWTH AND DEVELOPMENT

Neonate/Newborn (Birth–4 Weeks)

See Figure E-1.

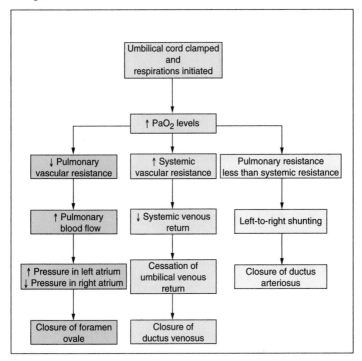

Figure E-1: Neonate's Transition to Extrauterine Life.

PHYSICAL DEVELOPMENT

1. Weight
   a. 2812–4173 grams (6 lb. 2 oz.–9 lb. 2 oz.) (KidsHealth, 2007)
   b. < 10th percentile—SGA (small for gestational age)
   c. > 90th percentile—LGA (large for gestational age)
2. Length (height)
   a. Measured from crown to heel
   b. 48–53 cm (19–21 in.) (KidsHealth, 2007)
3. Head circumference
   a. 32–38 cm with average of 34 cm (approximately 13.4 in.)
   b. Approximately 2 cm larger than chest circumference
4. Fontanels (See Figure E-2)
   a. Anterior fontanel

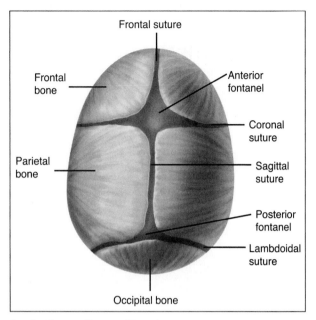

Figure E-2: Placement of Sutures and Fontanels.

        1) Diamond-shaped, soft, and flat
        2) Located on top of the head
        3) Up to 4–5 cm in diameter
        4) Typically closed by 12–18 months of age
    b. Posterior fontanel
        1) Triangular-shaped, soft, and flat
        2) Located at midline occipital region
        3) Smaller than anterior fontanel
        4) Typically closed by 3 months of age if open at birth
  5. Chest circumference
    a. Measured at nipple line
    b. 30–37.5 cm (12–15 in.)
    c. Approximately 2 cm smaller than head circumference
  6. Reflexes (all are present at birth but the noted point that some of them disappear are averages not absolutes)
    a. Blink (ciliary)
        1) Eyes blink at sudden appearance of light or object
        2) Persists throughout life
    b. Doll's eye
        1) Eyes lag behind and do not immediately adjust to change in head position
        2) Diminishes as ability to focus develops
    c. Pupillary
        1) Pupils constrict when bright light is shone toward pupil
        2) Persists throughout life

   d. Sneeze
      1) Sneezes with irritation or nasal obstruction
      2) Persists throughout life
   e. Cough
      1) Coughs with laryngeal irritation
      2) Persists throughout life
   f. Extrusion of tongue
      1) Occurs when tongue is depressed or touched
      2) Absent by 4 months
   g. Gag
      1) Occurs with stimulation of pharynx
      2) Persists throughout life
   h. Rooting
      1) Head turns toward stimulus when cheek is stroked or touched
      2) Absent by approximately 4 months
   i. Sucking
      1) Occurs when object touches lips or is placed in mouth
      2) Absent by 7 months
   j. Yawn
      1) Occurs with decreased oxygen
      2) Persists throughout life
   k. Babinski
      1) Hyperextension of toes when lateral aspect of the sole is touched
      2) Absent by 1 year
   l. Grasp
      1) Flexion of hands and toes when palms of hands or soles of feet are stroked
      2) Absent by 8 months
   m. Crawl
      1) Crawling motion when placed on abdomen
      2) Absent by approximately 6 weeks
   n. Dance or step
      1) Alternating stepping motion when neonate is held upright and one foot is allowed to touch a surface
      2) Absent by 4 months
   o. Moro
      1) Arms extend, head moves back, fingers spread and then arms flex, fist clenches, and spine and lower extremities extend
      2) Occurs with sudden change of position
      3) Absent by 3–4 months
   p. Placing
      1) When held upright and dorsal surface of feet touch the edge of a table, flexion of the knees and hips occur and the legs move up the table surface (Potts & Mandleco, 2007)
      2) Absent by 4 months
   q. Tonic neck
      1) Arm and leg extend in a fencing pose when neonate turns head to one side while lying supine
      2) Absent by 3–4 months

7. Nutrition
   a. Has stomach capacity of approximately 90 mL (3 oz.)
   b. Prefers sweet to salty taste
   c. Needs 120 kcal/kg of body weight per day
   d. Fluid requirements for 1–10 kg weight neonates: 100 mL/kg
   e. Needs nonnutritive sucking also (pacifier) but is unable to hold pacifier in mouth without adult holding it in place because of tongue extrusion reflex
   f. Breastfeeding
      1) Colostrum (foremilk)—present for first 3 days after delivery and serves as excellent source of protein and immunity
      2) Breast milk begins secreting approximately 3 days after neonate begins suckling
      3) Both breasts should be suckled at each feeding, beginning with alternating breast (to promote emptying of each breast and to help decrease nipple tenderness)
      4) Feeding time can be gradually increased from 3 minutes to 10 minutes for first breast and 6 minutes for second breast
      5) Neonate needs to feed every 2–3 hours
      6) 6–10 wet diapers a day indicates adequate hydration
8. Formula feeding (using prepared formula)
   a. Pediatrician provides guidance for which formula to use
   b. Neonate should drink 60–90 mL/feeding every 3–4 hours
   c. Neonate's intake is better on demand feedings
   d. Prepared formulas are designed to simulate human milk
   e. Neonates and infants should never be fed cow's milk
   f. Concentrated or ready-to-feed formulas should be used
9. Teeth
   a. Teething is very individual
   b. Usually, first deciduous teeth (lower central incisors) erupt between 3–4 months of age followed by upper central incisors by 5–6 months
   c. Dental care should begin with gentle washing with soft cloth
10. Elimination needs
   a. Urine output
      1) First urine output should be within 24 hours after birth
      2) Neonate voids 1–3 mL/kg/hr, or approximately 250 mL/day
      3) Usually voids 6–10 times/day
      4) Bladder capacity is approximately 15 mL
   b. Bowel output
      1) Meconium is first stool; sticky, dark green in color, odorless
      2) First stool should occur within 36 hours after birth
      3) After 2–3 days, stools gain consistency and change to soft, yellow-brown if infant is formula-fed, yellow and seedy appearance if infant is breastfed

PSYCHOSOCIAL DEVELOPMENT

1. Erikson—trust versus mistrust
2. Piaget—sensorineural period
3. Freud—oral stage

4. Born with distinctive behavioral styles; however, easily affected by family and social environment
5. Fascinated by movement, adults, and colors although sees figures as black and white contrasts
6. Responsive to auditory stimuli
7. "Learning occurs through imitation and habituation" (Potts & Mandleco, 2007, p. 185)
8. Learns from operant conditioning
9. Cries when has needs—hunger, discomfort, need to be held and cuddled, and overstimulation
10. Play consists of being held, talked to, sung to, and tickled

SAFETY ISSUES

1. Choking
2. Thermoregulation

Infant (1–12 Months)

PHYSICAL DEVELOPMENT

1. Weight
   a. Doubles birth weight in first 6 months, gaining approximately 1.5 lb. per month or 5–7 oz. per week
   b. Triples birth weight by 12 months
   c. Gains approximately 2–3 oz. per week or less than 1 lb. per month during second six months
2. Height
   a. Increases approximately 1 in. per month during first 6 months
   b. Increases approximately ½ in. per month during second 6 months
3. Head circumference/brain growth
   a. Head circumference increases by ½ in. per month during first 6 months
   b. Head circumference increases by ¼ in. per month during second 6 months
   c. Posterior fontanel closes by 3 months of age
   d. Infant's brain grows to 2/3 the size of an adult's brain by 12 months
4. Motor development. *NOTE:* These are approximations, not absolutes.
   a. 1–3 months
      1) Can turn head to side when prone (at 1 month)
      2) Can put hand in mouth
      3) Can lift head from prone position
      4) Displays head lag when pulled up from lying to sitting position
      5) Can hold hand open, look at fingers, and place fingers in mouth (by 3 months)
      6) Can hold pacifier in mouth but still requires assistance if pacifier falls out of mouth (by 3 months)
   b. 4–5 months
      1) Plays with own feet
      2) Puts foot in mouth
      3) Turns from abdomen to back
      4) Begins reaching to grasp items with palm of hand

    c. 5–6 months
1) Is able to hold head, chest, and abdomen up by bearing weight with hands
2) Turns from supine to prone

    d. 6–7 months
1) Sits, leaning forward on both hands—3-point stance or tri-pod stance
2) Transfers objects from one hand to the other
3) Is able to place pacifier in mouth without assistance

    e. 7–8 months
1) Is able to sit alone without support
2) Attempts to propel self by kicking feet when prone
3) Bears weight with some support

    f. 8–10 months
1) Moves from prone to sitting without assistance
2) Is able to crawl (moving on hands and knees with abdomen on floor)
3) Creeps (moving forward on hands and knees with abdomen off floor) after learning to crawl
4) Pulls self up to standing position
5) Uses pincer grasp (8–9 months)

    g. 10–12 months
1) Is able to cruise by holding onto a stationary object, but prefers to creep most of the time
2) Stands alone
3) Attempts to walk
4) Drops items purposefully
5) Can hold and mark paper with large crayon
6) Can feed self finger foods
7) Can turn multiple pages of a book

5. Nutrition
    a. Infancy is the first of two major growth spurts during life
    b. Eating progresses from reflex → dependent on assistance → attempts to feeds self
    c. Nutrition needs are based on activity and growth; however, caloric intake is generally as follows:
1) 650 kcal per day for months 1–6
2) 850 kcal per day for months 6–12
    d. Fluid requirements for infants are based on weight: 1–10 kg: 100 mL/kg
    e. By 12 months, weaning from bottle and pacifier should begin so that at 1 year, when child no longer needs formula, bottle and pacifier can be removed
    f. Semisolid foods can be started when infant is able to sit well with support
    g. Foods should be introduced gradually with intervals between each food to detect possible food allergies and to allow infant to adjust to new taste; usually, a new food can be introduced every 3–7 days
    h. First semisolid food introduced should be iron-fortified rice cereal liquefied with breast milk or formula

      i.   Vegetables usually are introduced next, then fruits

      j.   Fruit juice can be offered at the same time fruits are begun; citrus fruit juices (rich in vitamin C, which helps with iron absorption) can be introduced by 6 months

      k.   Finger foods can be introduced by 8–10 months

      l.   Infants generally eat every 2–4 hours during first 6 months

      m.   After introduction of solid foods, infant gradually advances to three meals and two or three nutritious snacks per day

      n.   Formula remains primary source of nutrition through infancy

Psychosocial Development

1. Erikson—trust versus mistrust
2. Piaget—sensorimotor period
3. Freud—oral stage
4. Infancy is foundation for future development
5. Infant should learn that needs will be met, the environment is a good place, and self is "good"
6. Infant is entirely dependent on having needs met by someone else
7. Stimulation of other senses is very important, especially touch
8. Infant explores world orally
9. Stranger anxiety begins at approximately 8–12 months of age
10. Language and communication
    a. 1–3 months
       1) Smiles—reflective action at first, then more voluntary and reciprocal
       2) Coos
    b. 3–6 months
       1) Babbles
       2) Makes repetitive sounds
       3) Identifies primary caregiver's voice
       4) Enjoys hearing own voice
       5) Squeals
       6) Laughs aloud
       7) Uses single vowel and consonant combinations—ba, ga, ah, and da
    c. 7–9 months
       1) Strings vowels and consonants together—baba, dada, and gaga
       2) Responds gradually to own name
    d. 9–12 months
       1) Uses gestures to communicate
       2) Says "mama" and "dada" to identify caregivers
       3) Learns three to five words
11. Play is narcissistic in nature
12. Short attention span gradually increasing to 5 minutes
13. Refer to Appendix F: Pediatric Play

Safety Issues

1. Motor vehicle accidents
2. SIDS risk
3. Choking
4. Falls

Toddler (12–36 Months, 1–3 Years)

PHYSICAL DEVELOPMENT

1. Weight
   a. Weight gain slows with focus on gross motor and language skills
   b. Average weight gain is approximately 5 lb. per year
   c. Birth weight quadruples by 2–3 years of age
   d. Brain growth by 3 years is 80–90% of that of adult
2. Height
   a. Toddler grows approximately 3 in. per year
   b. Height is about one third of adult height by 3 years
3. Potbellied appearance is due to immature abdominal muscles
4. Adipose tissue is gradually replaced by muscle as gross motor skills develop
5. Anterior fontanel closes by 12–18 months
6. Gross motor skills
   a. Focus is on locomotion
   b. Is always on the move
   c. Is able to explore environment beyond same room as parent, but periodically "takes attendance" to make sure parent is still there
   d. Is able to walk independently by 15 months
   e. Is able to push or pull toys
   f. Attempts to run by 18 months with frequent falls
   g. Begins climbing stairs by 12–15 months (non-alternating feet); by 3 years of age can alternate feet when climbing
   h. Shows improved hand-eye coordination
   i. Enjoys removing shoes and socks and clothes, but not selective as to where these are removed
   j. Can zip zippers by 18 months
   k. Can dress self by 24 months in easy-to-put-on clothing
   l. Is able to wash and dry hands
   m. Is able to control urinary bladder (by 2–3 years)
7. Teeth
   a. First and second molars and cuspids erupt
   b. Can brush teeth, but needs assistance for plaque removal
8. Nutrition
   a. Gains proficiency with use of cup and spoon
   b. Likes feeding self; likes finger foods
   c. Sees growth rate slow
   d. Has decreased appetite, called "physiologic anorexia"
   e. May be picky about food choices
   f. Does not like to stop playing to eat
   g. Is influenced by family and cultural eating habits
   h. Can be impacted by mealtime environment
   i. Fluid requirements: 10–20 kg in weight should have 1000 mL plus 50 mL/kg for over 10 kg
   j. Nutrient requirements
      1) 1300 kcal/kg of body weight/day
      2) No offering of bottle as substitute for solid foods

3) 500 mg of calcium per day

4) 7 mg of iron per day

Psychosocial Development

1. Erikson—autonomy versus shame and doubt
2. Piaget—preoperational period (2–7 years); sensorimotor (2 years)
3. Freud—anal stage
4. Negativism can dominate but subsides as child approaches 3 years of age
   a. Common expressions of independence: "No!"
   b. Need for autonomy apparent in "Me do" or "Me have" or "Me go"
   c. At the same time, fear of being abandoned
   d. Sometimes resistant to bedtime, bath, and dental care
   e. Possessive of toys
   f. Temper tantrums are common because of inability to verbalize frustration especially at limit setting
5. Ritualistic behavior
   a. Finds comfort in scheduled routines
   b. Has difficulty with any flexibility
   c. Routines offer security and allow toddler to venture out of direct sight of parent
6. Separation anxiety
   a. Peaks during toddler years
   b. Major stressor of hospitalization
   c. Needs transitional object (blanket, stuffed animal, or toy) when away from parents (day care, or babysitter, hospital)
7. Play—Refer to Appendix F: Pediatric Play
8. Sexual identity
   a. Recognizes gender and sex differences, but does not understand the differences
   b. Focuses attention on bowel and bladder training and independence
   c. Focuses on genital area and structures
9. Discipline
   a. Is necessary to maintain safety and safe behaviors (toddlers are very curious)
   b. Use of time-out for discipline (time frame of 1–2 minutes per year of age)
10. Language and communication
    a. 12–15 months old
       1) Speaks three or four words easily understood by others
       2) Develops own language
    b. 18 months old
       1) Speaks at least ten words
       2) Speaks language and terms heard at home
       3) Uses gestures well
    c. 24 months old
       1) Uses spoken language that is largely understandable
       2) Displays rapid growth in language
       3) Uses pronouns
       4) Speaks in two- to three-words sentences

    d. 36 months old
      1) Speaks in three- to five-word sentences
      2) Has a vocabulary of approximately 900 words
      3) Has a concept of time based on events—after lunch, after dinner, when a particular television program is on, in the morning)

SAFETY ISSUES

1. Motor vehicle accidents
2. Poisoning
3. Burns
4. Drowning

Preschooler (3–6 Years)

PHYSICAL DEVELOPMENT

1. Weight
    a. Shows gradual growth
    b. Gains approximately 2.3 kg (5 lb.) per year
2. Height
    a. Gains 7.5 cm (5 in.) per year
    b. Achieves approximately half of adult height by age 5
3. Body shape
    a. Loses potbellied appearance
    b. Becomes slimmer and more agile and graceful
    c. Is more posturally erect
4. Teeth
    a. Usually has all 20 deciduous teeth by age 5
    b. Deciduous teeth may begin to be replaced by permanent teeth
5. Coordination and muscle strength rapidly increase
6. Visual acuity is 20/20; color vision is fully developed
7. Gross motor skills
    a. Achieves bowel and bladder control during this period; because of anatomical differences, boys achieve toilet training later than girls
    b. 3 years old
      1) Walks, runs, and jumps
      2) Pedals tricycle
      3) Balances on one foot for a few seconds
      4) Can walk a straight line and can walk backwards
      5) Throws ball with one hand
      6) Jumps off bottom step
      7) Alternates feet going up stairs
    c. 4 years old
      1) Skips and hops on one foot
      2) Alternates feet going up and down stairs holding onto stair rail
      3) Climbs jungle gym
      4) Catches ball with both hands
      5) Runs well
      6) Walks heel to toe
    d. 5 years old
      1) Runs with more control and power; shows coordination of arm and leg movements when running

        2) Skips on alternating feet

        3) Jumps from height of 12 in., landing on toes

        4) Begins to skate and swim

        5) Rides bicycle with training wheels

        6) Throws and catches ball well

        7) Proficient climber

        8) Can play in competitive exercise sports (T-ball, soccer) for the exercise and fun of socializing with other children of same age

8. Fine motor skills

   a. 3 years old

      1) Builds towers of 9–10 blocks

      2) Copies circle and cross

      3) Draws circle and adds face

      4) Can cut on straight line; needs safety scissors

      5) Strings large beads

      6) Can build a bridge with blocks

      7) Dresses and undresses self

   b. 4 years old

      1) Uses scissors well

      2) Draws stick figure with three parts

      3) Can lace shoes but is unable to tie shoes

      4) Can cut on curved line

      5) Has established hand dominance

      6) Tries to print letters

   c. 5 years old

      1) Begins to tie shoes

      2) Uses pencil well

      3) Draws person figure with six parts

      4) Prints first name and some letters

      5) Cuts out simple shapes

      6) Copies square and triangle

      7) Hits nail on head with hammer

9. Nutrition

   a. Needs serving size of 1 tablespoon of each solid food per meal per year of age

   b. Feeds self proficiently

   c. Begins using fork by 3–4 years

   d. Should continue to try new foods

   e. Likes to eat at table and chairs consistent with child's height

   f. Should sit at table with family for meals to help with communication and socialization skills

   g. Prefers single foods rather than combinations

   h. Will eat vegetables that were properly introduced earlier

   i. Prefers finger foods

   j. Needs 1800 kcal or 90 kcal/kg body weight per day

   k. Requires 1500 mL of fluids (children over 20 kg) plus 20 mL/kg for over 20 kg

   l. Must have adequate vitamin, mineral, and fluid intake

Psychosocial Development

1. Erikson—initiative versus guilt
2. Piaget—preoperational period
3. Freud—phallic or Oedipal stage
4. Displays imagination and socialization as driving forces
5. Uses imaginary friends when social relationships are absent
6. Imitates behaviors of family members
7. Feels responsible when "bad" things happen
8. Understands right and wrong
9. Learns spiritual behavior and practices by imitating parents and family
10. Develops fears of dark (related to vivid imagination) at 3 years of age
11. Displays magical thinking during third and fourth year, which decreases beginning at age 5
12. Begins daydreaming by age 5
13. Likes to please family members and to help with household tasks
14. Shows increase in attention span (approximately 1–5 minutes per year)
15. Is very energetic and active; enjoys socializing with other children and exploring
16. Shows increasing independence in activities of daily living (dresses self, brushes teeth, and washes and dries hands by 3 years of age; completes toilet training during third year)
17. Sexual development
    a. Is curious; may masturbate
    b. Knows sexual differences and own sex by age 3
18. Understands past and future but not yesterday or tomorrow by 3 years of age; understands yesterday and tomorrow and next week by age 4
19. Becomes less argumentative and rebellious and gets along well with parents by age 5
20. Continues to require limit setting to learn safe, acceptable behaviors
21. Refer to Appendix F: Pediatric Play
22. Language development
    a. 3 years old
        1) Knows name and age
        2) Forms sentences of three or four words
        3) Is very inquisitive; wants to know "why"
        4) Uses plurals and pronouns correctly
        5) May use made-up words due to influence of imagination
        6) Is perpetually talkative, including having conversations with self if no one else is around to listen
        7) Has a vocabulary of approximately 900 words
        8) Correct use of plurals and pronouns
    b. 4 years old
        1) Uses four- or five-word sentences
        2) Tells imaginative and exaggerated stories
        3) Uses prepositions correctly
        4) Names one or more colors
        5) Has a vocabulary of approximately 1,500 words
        6) Counts to 4
        7) Questioning is constant

   c. 5 years old
1) Uses six- to eight-word sentences
2) Uses past tense verbs, prepositions, and adjectives correctly
3) Names four or more colors
4) Knows days of week and other time-related words
5) Follows three commands in succession
6) Has a vocabulary of approximately 2100 words

SAFETY ISSUES

1. Motor vehicle accidents
2. Pedestrian versus motor vehicle accidents
3. Burns
4. Drowning

School-Age Child (6–12 Years)

PHYSICAL DEVELOPMENT

1. Weight
   a. Child gains approximately 5–6 lb. per year
   b. Average 6-year-old weighs 45 lb.
   c. Average male at 12 years old weighs 88 lb.; average female at 12 years weighs 91 lb.
   d. Focus is on prevention of childhood obesity
2. Height
   a. Child gains approximately 2 in. per year
   b. Average 6-year-old is 46 in. tall
   c. Average male at 12 years old is 59 in. tall; average female at 12 years is 60 in. tall
3. Physical coordination reaches its peak during this stage of pediatric development
4. Lymphatic tissues continue to grow until age 9
5. Frontal sinuses develop at age 7
6. Gross motor skills
   a. 6–7 years
   1) Rides two-wheel bicycle
   2) Completes mastery of gross motor skills
   3) Is active in cooperative games and some sports
   4) Throws ball overhand
   5) Walks a straight line
   b. 8–9 years
   1) Develops hand-eye coordination
   2) Displays increasing motor coordination
   3) Plays team sports
   4) Shows increased body flexibility
   c. 10–12 years
   1) Displays well-developed hand-eye coordination
   2) May become awkward at gross motor skills with beginning of second growth spurt and puberty
   3) Balances on one foot for 15 seconds
   4) Catches a fly ball
   5) Cooks and sews

7. Fine motor skills
   a. 6–7 years
      1) Prints letters legibly
      2) Uses eating utensils well
      3) Displays improved dexterity
      4) Cuts, pastes, and folds paper
      5) Copies diamond
      6) Is able to fix hair
      7) Ties shoelaces
   b. 8–9 years
      1) Is able to use household tools
      2) Dresses self completely
      3) Has dexterity to use cursive writing
      4) Draws three-dimensional figures
   c. 10–12 years—displays well-developed fine motor skills
8. Nutrition
   a. Growth continues to slow but at a steady rate
   b. Caloric intake should match energy and growth expenditure
   c. Child needs approximately 2000 kcal/day
   d. Fluid requirements are 2000 mL/day
   e. Child has adult meal behavior
   f. Child may rush through meals to resume play activities with friends
   g. Child should be limited to how much junk food he/she eats
9. Focus is on dental health with replacement of deciduous teeth with permanent teeth

Psychosocial Development

1. Erikson—industry versus inferiority
2. Piaget—concrete operations (7–12 year); preoperational (6–7 years)
3. Freud—latency stage
4. Interacts well with others
5. Has friends who are same age and same gender; period of "best friends"
6. Becomes sensitive to norms and values of peer groups
7. Shows an increase in belonging to clubs and organizations
8. Develops a conscience
9. Develops strong religious feelings and can describe God abstractly
10. Understands the rules of games and is willing to adhere to them
11. Focuses on a sense of accomplishment in school and social settings
12. Is still dependent on adults to meet needs of love and security, but self-esteem and belonging gradually become more established in school and with friends
13. Needs praise and recognition
14. Cognitive development
    a. 6–7 years
       1) Learns to tell time
       2) Learns to read; can read from memory
       3) Knows right from wrong
       4) Understands the value of currency
       5) Continues to have an active imagination

      6) Understands concept of numbers

      7) Enjoys word and spelling games

      8) Attends first and second grade in school

      9) Enjoys learning

      10) Shares and cooperates

      11) Is an attentive listener within attention span

      12) Has a vocabulary of approximately 8,000–14,000 words

      13) Demonstrates increasing independence

      14) Is able to play quietly by self

  b. 8–9 years

      1) Understands concept of time; is punctual

      2) Knows date and month

      3) Collects and classifies objects

      4) Shows increased reading comprehension

      5) Knows space, cause, effect, and conservation

      6) Learns fractions, multiplication, and division

      7) Counts backward from 20

      8) Shows appreciation for art and music

      9) Learns from experiences

      10) Continues to be idealistic in thinking

      11) Can make change with small currency

      12) Improvises simple activities

      13) Knows similarities and differences

      14) Attends third and fourth grades

  c. 10–12 years

      1) Develops ability to think abstractly

      2) Is able to write stories

      3) Is easily distracted

      4) Knows death is irreversible

      5) Is more realistic than idealistic

      6) Is truthful

      7) Reads well and enjoys reading

      8) Likes to memorize and enjoys facts

      9) Likes to discuss and debate

      10) Begins formal operations

      11) Rules are important

      12) Begins to show interest in the opposite sex

      13) Easy to please

      14) Obedient

      15) Affectionate, sensitive, respectful to parents

      16) Can stay at home alone for short periods of time

      17) Attends fifth to seventh grades

15. Attention span lengthens to 50 minutes

SAFETY ISSUES

1. Motor vehicle accidents
2. Pedestrian versus motor vehicle accidents
3. Drowning
4. Accidents with firearms and violent crime

Adolescent (12–21 Years)

PHYSICAL DEVELOPMENT

1. Weight
   a. Males gain 12–14 lb. (skeletal growth ends between 18–21 years of age)
   b. Females gain 8–10 lb. (skeletal growth ends between 15–17 years of age)
2. Height
   a. Males gain 3–6 in./yr
   b. Females gain 2.5–5 in./yr
3. Second and final physiological growth spurt
4. Gross motor skills
   a. Gangly and awkward early in adolescence
   b. More adept at sports later
   c. Greater physical endurance
5. Fine motor skills—greater skill at drawing, writing, and playing musical instruments
6. Physiological milestones
   a. 11–14 years
      1) Males
         a) Growth of testes, scrotum, and penis
         b) Development of pubic hair (curly)
         c) Fine and downy facial hair
         d) Axillary hair growth
         e) Gynecomastia
      2) Females
         a) Breast development
         b) Onset of menarche
         c) Initiation of ovulation
         d) Development of pubic hair (curly with triangular distribution)
         e) Heavier than males
   b. 15–17 years
      1) Males
         a) Adult genitalia
         b) Mature sperm production
         c) Presence of facial and body hair
         d) Muscle mass and strength greater than females
         e) Increased appetite
         f) Voice change
         g) Disappearance of gynecomastia
         h) Presence of acne
      2) Females
         a) End of skeletal growth; sexually mature
         b) Decrease in percentage of body fat but fat stores are maintained for childbearing
         c) Decreased appetite
         d) Presence of acne

      c.   18–21 years—End of skeletal growth

  7. Nutrition

      a.   Has a busy schedule—school, sports, dating, and peer activities

      b.   Is concerned about body image

      c.   Eats away from home often

      d.   Appears to be constantly hungry and eating

      e.   May acquire eating disorders

      f.   Caloric intake

          1) Males—2500 to 3000 kcal/day and 52 grams of protein

          2) Females—2000 kcal/day and 46 grams of protein

  8. Teeth

      a.   All permanent teeth present

      b.   Dental care becomes as much appearance-driven as dental health-focused

PSYCHOSOCIAL DEVELOPMENT

1. Erikson—identity versus role confusion
2. Piaget—formal operations
3. Freud—genital stage
4. Struggles for independence
5. Exhibits period of internal confusion with hormonal and growth pressures
6. Rebels against parents, often exhibiting intense child-parent conflict especially with same-gender parent
7. Sees peers as central figures who provide primary sense of belonging
8. Displays risk-taking behavior and sense of own immortality; short-term oriented
9. Finds difficulty coping with death of a peer of the same age because of immortality thinking
10. Is impulsive, impatient, narcissistic, and intensely private
11. Is self-conscious about appearance
12. Displays intense relationships with members of the opposite sex; may experiment with sex
13. May experiment with drugs and alcohol
14. Begins thinking of future (college, work plans, and permanent intimate relationship) during middle adolescence
15. Understands ethical and moral boundaries, but short-term thinking can result in opposition of own responsibilities

SAFETY ISSUES

1. Motor vehicle accidents
2. Substance abuse
3. Accidental and non-accidental trauma including suicide and homicide

REFERENCES

KidsHealth. (2007). *Growth and your newborn.* Retrieved May 9, 2007, from http://www.kidshealth.org/parent/growth/growth/grownewborn.html

Potts, N. L., & Mandleco, B. L. (2007). *Pediatric nursing: Caring for children and their families* (2nd ed.). Clifton Park, NY: Delmar Cengage Learning.

PEDIATRIC PLAY

Functions of Play (Play Is the Work of Children)

1. Physical development
    a.   Exploration
    b.   Joint and muscle development
    c.   Muscle coordination
    d.   Gross and fine motor skill development
    e.   Kinesthetic stimulation
2. Cognitive development
    a.   Use of senses—tactile, vision, auditory, olfactory, and taste
    b.   Numbers, colors, sizes, shapes, and textures
    c.   Importance of objects
    d.   Problem solving
    e.   Critical thinking
    f.   Hand-eye coordination
    g.   Creativity
3. Social development
    a.   Social skills
    b.   Right from wrong
    c.   Different roles
4. Emotional development
    a.   Sense of belonging
    b.   Coping strategies
    c.   Self-awareness
    d.   Sense of security
    e.   Sense of self-worth
5. Moral development
    a.   Ethical behavior
    b.   Sharing
    c.   Awareness of feelings of others
    d.   Self-awareness and who they are in perspective of the world

Types of Play

1. Solitary
    a.   Begins in infancy and is common in toddlers
    b.   Is necessary for all age groups to develop independent play
2. Parallel
    a.   Involves child playing next to another child but not with that child
    b.   Is characteristic of toddlers
    c.   Is not characteristic of sharing
3. Associative
    a.   Involves interaction with other children
    b.   Although rules are present, imaginative play results in frequent rule changes

    c. Begins in late toddlerhood and extends through preschool years

    d. Helps develop ability to share

4. Cooperative

    a. Involves organized play of groups

    b. Usually involves a leader

    c. Follows standardized rules of games

    d. Begins in late preschool and extends throughout life

5. Onlooker

    a. Child is a bystander

    b. Child observes the play of others but does not join in

    c. Method of learning rules and players

    d. Common in toddlers, but occurs at older levels

6. Therapeutic

    a. Is guided by members of health care team to assist child in coping with hospitalization

    b. Involves supervised play with medical equipment to be used with child

    c. Enhances compliance with therapy and nursing care

    d. Provides emotional outlet during stressful periods

7. Dramatic

    a. Is an emotional outlet

    b. Provides child with opportunity to act out stressful events

    c. Is used by psychologists as a means of child communicating traumatic events

Play Characteristic of Each Level of Growth and Development

Level of Growth and Development	Characteristics	Play Items
Infant	Is narcissistic in nature Enjoys watching others Is aware of little beyond boundaries of own body Human interaction is very important Needs activities to develop senses Puts most toys in mouth so they must not have small parts	Colorful crib mobile Peek-a-boo Rattles Busy boxes Mirrors Musical toys Water toys during bath Colorful blocks Safe kitchen utensils Picture books Items large enough for infant to pick up
Toddler	Focus is on gross motor skills Is beginning to use fine motor skills Focus is on developing autonomy Is very curious	Push-pull toys Containers to empty and fill Books to be read to Blocks, trucks, dolls Coloring or creating with large crayons

(continues)

Play Characteristic of Each Level of Growth and Development *(continued)*

LEVEL OF GROWTH AND DEVELOPMENT	CHARACTERISTICS	PLAY ITEMS
Toddler	Begins exploration of home environment Is very active Begins associating things Does not like to be told "no"	Nesting toys Clay, finger paints, sand, bubbles Increase in language development
Preschooler	Is driven by imagination and socialization Focus is on fine motor skills Has imaginary playmates Likes to run, hop, jump Likes to build, draw, create Begins simple collections Is very active Is very verbal	Riding toys Building materials Coloring books and crayons Cars, dolls, stuffed animals Cutting and pasting Puzzles Books Beginning to read but tends to make up stories Dress-up Singing games, tapes Nonsense rhymes Games, but changes rules at will Age-appropriate video games Age-appropriate television programs, videos, DVDs Play that mimics same-gender parent
School-age child	Time of greatest coordination Play is more organized with rules and leaders Is aware of rules and wants to accomplish tasks Employs higher-level thinking skills Begins competitive sports Has same-gender playmates	Riddles Board games with friends and family members Age-appropriate video games Collections Dolls Reading Bicycle riding Hobbies Continues same-gender parent activities (cooking, fishing, sewing) Competitive games/sports Drawing

(continues)

Play Characteristic of Each Level of Growth and
Development *(continued)*

LEVEL OF GROWTH AND DEVELOPMENT	CHARACTERISTICS	PLAY ITEMS
Adolescent	Activities with peers Strict rules Competitiveness Risk-taking behavior Games Athletics Music	Playing sports Playing video games Listening to music Experimenting with appearance Reading teen magazines Talking on telephone Texting on cell phone Being active with peers

PEDIATRIC IMMUNIZATION SCHEDULE

Recommended Immunization
Schedule for Persons Aged 0 to 6 Years

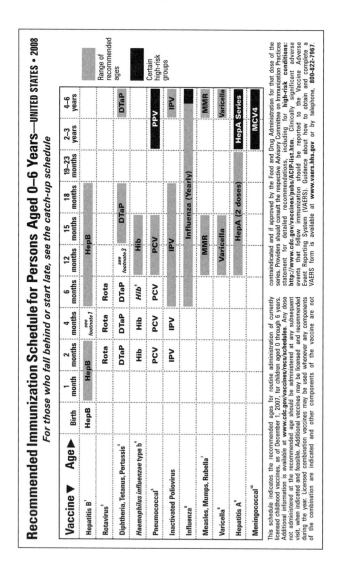

Recommended Immunization Schedule for Persons Aged 0–6 Years—UNITED STATES • 2008

For those who fall behind or start late, see the catch-up schedule

Vaccine ▼ Age ▶	Birth	1 month	2 months	4 months	6 months	12 months	15 months	18 months	19–23 months	2–3 years	4–6 years
Hepatitis B[1]	HepB	HepB		see footnote 1		HepB					
Rotavirus[2]			Rota	Rota	Rota						
Diphtheria, Tetanus, Pertussis[3]			DTaP	DTaP	DTaP		DTaP				DTaP
Haemophilus influenzae type b[4]			Hib	Hib	Hib[4]	Hib					
Pneumococcal[5]			PCV	PCV	PCV	PCV				PPV	
Inactivated Poliovirus			IPV	IPV		IPV					IPV
Influenza[6]						Influenza (Yearly)					
Measles, Mumps, Rubella[7]						MMR					MMR
Varicella[8]						Varicella					Varicella
Hepatitis A[9]						HepA (2 doses)				HepA Series	
Meningococcal[10]										MCV4	

Range of recommended ages

Certain high-risk groups

This schedule indicates the recommended ages for routine administration of currently licensed childhood vaccines, as of December 1, 2007, for children aged 0 through 6 years. Additional information is available at www.cdc.gov/vaccines/recs/schedules. Any dose not administered at the recommended age should be administered at any subsequent visit, when indicated and feasible. Additional vaccines may be licensed and recommended during the year. Licensed combination vaccines may be used whenever any components of the combination are indicated and other components of the vaccine are not contraindicated and if approved by the Food and Drug Administration for that dose of the series. Providers should consult the respective Advisory Committee on Immunization Practices statement for detailed recommendations, including for **high-risk conditions: http://www.cdc.gov/vaccines/pubs/ACIP-list.htm.** Clinically significant adverse events that follow immunization should be reported to the Vaccine Adverse Event Reporting System (VAERS). Guidance about how to obtain and complete a VAERS form is available at **www.vaers.hhs.gov** or by telephone, **800-822-7967.**

CS103164

1. Hepatitis B vaccine (HepB). *(Minimum age: birth)*

At birth:

- Administer monovalent HepB to all newborns prior to hospital discharge.
- If mother is hepatitis B surface antigen (HBsAg) positive, administer HepB and 0.5 mL of hepatitis B immune globulin (HBIG) within 12 hours of birth.
- If mother's HBsAg status is unknown, administer HepB within 12 hours of birth. Determine the HBsAg status as soon as possible and if HBsAg positive, administer HBIG (no later than age 1 week).
- If mother is HBsAg negative, the birth dose can be delayed, in rare cases, with a provider's order and a copy of the mother's negative HBsAg laboratory report in the infant's medical record.

4-month dose:

- The HepB series should be completed with either monovalent HepB or a combination vaccine containing HepB. The second dose should be administered at age 1–2 months. The final dose should be administered no earlier than age 24 weeks. Infants born to HBsAg-positive mothers should be tested for HBsAg and antibody to HBsAg after completion of at least 3 doses of a licensed HepB series, at age 9–18 months (generally at the next well-child visit).
- It is permissible to administer 4 doses of HepB when combination vaccines are administered after the birth dose. If monovalent HepB is used for doses after the birth dose, a dose at age 4 months is not needed.

2. Rotavirus vaccine (Rota). *(Minimum age: 6 weeks)*

- Administer the first dose at age 6–12 weeks.
- Do not start the series later than age 12 weeks.
- Administer the final dose in the series by age 32 weeks. Do not administer any dose later than age 32 weeks.
- Data on safety and efficacy outside of these age ranges are insufficient.

3. Diphtheria and tetanus toxoids and acellular pertussis vaccine (DTaP). *(Minimum age: 6 weeks)*

- The fourth dose of DTaP may be administered as early as age 12 months, provided 6 months have elapsed since the third dose.
- Administer the final dose in the series at age 4–6 years.

4. Haemophilus influenzae type b conjugate vaccine (Hib). *(Minimum age: 6 weeks)*

- If PRP-OMP (PedvaxHIB® or ComVax® [Merck]) is administered at ages 2 and 4 months, a dose at age 6 months is not required.
- TriHiB® (DTaP/Hib) combination products should not be used for primary immunization but can be used as boosters following any Hib vaccine in children age 12 months or older.

5. Pneumococcal vaccine. *(Minimum age: 6 weeks for pneumococcal conjugate vaccine [PCV]; 2 years for pneumococcal polysaccharide vaccine [PPV])*

- Administer one dose of PCV to all healthy children aged 24–59 months having any incomplete schedule.
- Administer PPV to children aged 2 years and older with underlying medical conditions.

6. Influenza vaccine. *(Minimum age: 6 months for trivalent inactivated influenza vaccine [TIV]; 2 years for live, attenuated influenza vaccine [LAIV])*

- Administer annually to children aged 6–59 months and to all eligible close contacts of children aged 0–59 months.
- Administer annually to children 5 years of age and older with certain risk factors, to other persons (including household members) in close contact with persons in groups at higher risk, and to any child whose parents request vaccination.
- For healthy persons (those who do not have underlying medical conditions that predispose them to influenza complications) aged 2–49 years, either LAIV or TIV may be used.
- Children receiving TIV should receive 0.25 mL if age 6–35 months or 0.5 mL if age 3 years or older.
- Administer 2 doses (separated by 4 weeks or longer) to children younger than 9 years who are receiving influenza vaccine for the first time or who were vaccinated for the first time last season but only received one dose.

7. Measles, mumps, and rubella vaccine (MMR). *(Minimum age: 12 months)*

- Administer the second dose of MMR at age 4–6 years. MMR may be administered before age 4–6 years, provided 4 weeks or more have elapsed since the first dose.

8. Varicella vaccine. *(Minimum age: 12 months)*

- Administer second dose at age 4–6 years; may be administered 3 months or more after first dose.
- Do not repeat second dose if administered 28 days or more after first dose.

9. Hepatitis A vaccine (HepA). *(Minimum age: 12 months)*

- Administer to all children aged 1 year (i.e., aged 12–23 months). Administer the 2 doses in the series at least 6 months apart.
- Children not fully vaccinated by age 2 years can be vaccinated at subsequent visits.
- HepA is recommended for certain other groups of children, including in areas where vaccination programs target older children.

10. Meningococcal vaccine. *(Minimum age: 2 years for meningococcal conjugate vaccine [MCV4] and for meningococcal polysaccharide vaccine [MPSV4])*

- Administer MCV4 to children aged 2–10 years with terminal complement deficiencies or anatomic or functional asplenia and certain other high-risk groups. MPSV4 is also acceptable.
- Administer MCV4 to persons who received MPSV4 3 or more years previously and remain at increased risk for meningococcal disease.

The Recommended Immunization Schedules for Persons Aged 0–18 Years are approved by the Advisory Committee on Immunization Practices (www.cdc.gov/vaccines/recs/acip), the American Academy of Pediatrics (http://www.aap.org), and the American Academy of Family Physicians (http://www.aafp.org).

DEPARTMENT OF HEALTH AND HUMAN SERVICES • CENTERS FOR DISEASE CONTROL AND PREVENTION • SAFER • HEATHIER • PEOPLE™

Courtesy of the Centers for Disease Control and Prevention, 2008.

Recommended Immunization Schedule for Persons Aged 7 to 18 Years

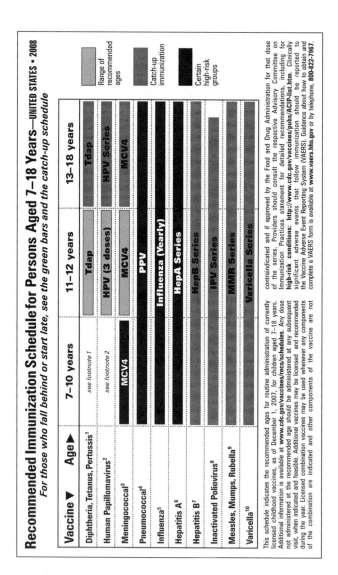

Recommended Immunization Schedule for Persons Aged 7–18 Years—UNITED STATES • 2008

For those who fall behind or start late, see the green bars and the catch-up schedule

Vaccine ▼ Age ►	7–10 years	11–12 years	13–18 years
Diphtheria, Tetanus, Pertussis[1]	see footnote 1	Tdap	Tdap
Human Papillomavirus[2]	see footnote 2	HPV (3 doses)	HPV Series
Meningococcal[3]	MCV4	MCV4	MCV4
Pneumococcal[4]	PPV	PPV	
Influenza[5]	Influenza (Yearly)		
Hepatitis A[6]	HepA Series		
Hepatitis B[7]	HepB Series		
Inactivated Poliovirus[8]	IPV Series		
Measles, Mumps, Rubella[9]	MMR Series		
Varicella[10]	Varicella Series		

Legend:
- Range of recommended ages
- Catch-up immunization
- Certain high-risk groups

This schedule indicates the recommended ages for routine administration of currently licensed childhood vaccines, as of December 1, 2007, for children aged 7–18 years. Additional information is available at **www.cdc.gov/vaccines/recs/schedules**. Any dose not administered at the recommended age should be administered at any subsequent visit, when indicated and feasible. Additional vaccines may be licensed and recommended during the year. Licensed combination vaccines may be used whenever any components of the combination are indicated and other components of the vaccine are not contraindicated and if approved by the Food and Drug Administration for that dose of the series. Providers should consult the respective Advisory Committee on Immunization Practices statement for detailed recommendations, including for **high-risk conditions: http://www.cdc.gov/vaccines/pubs/ACIP-list.htm**. Clinically significant adverse events that follow immunization should be reported to the Vaccine Adverse Event Reporting System (VAERS). Guidance about how to obtain and complete a VAERS form is available at **www.vaers.hhs.gov** or by telephone, **800-822-7967**.

CS103164

1. Tetanus and diphtheria toxoids and acellular pertussis vaccine (Tdap). *(Minimum age: 10 years for BOOSTRIX® and 11 years for ADACEL™)*

- Administer at age 11–12 years for those who have completed the recommended childhood DTP/DTaP vaccination series and have not received a tetanus and diphtheria toxoids (Td) booster dose.
- 13–18-year-olds who missed the 11–12 year Tdap or received Td only are encouraged to receive one dose of Tdap 5 years after the last Td/DTaP dose.

2. Human papillomavirus vaccine (HPV). *(Minimum age: 9 years)*

- Administer the first dose of the HPV vaccine series to females at age 11–12 years.
- Administer the second dose 2 months after the first dose and the third dose 6 months after the first dose.
- Administer the HPV vaccine series to females at age 13–18 years if not previously vaccinated.

3. Meningococcal vaccine.

- Administer MCV4 at age 11–12 years and at age 13–18 years if not previously vaccinated. MPSV4 is an acceptable alternative.
- Administer MCV4 to previously unvaccinated college freshmen living in dormitories.
- MCV4 is recommended for children aged 2–10 years with terminal complement deficiencies or anatomic or functional asplenia and certain other high-risk groups.
- Persons who received MPSV4 3 or more years previously and remain at increased risk for meningococcal disease should be vaccinated with MCV4.

4. Pneumococcal polysaccharide vaccine (PPV).

- Administer PPV to certain high-risk groups.

5. Influenza vaccine.

- Administer annually to all close contacts of children aged 0–59 months.
- Administer annually to persons with certain risk factors, health-care workers, and other persons (including household members) in close contact with persons in groups at higher risk.

- Administer 2 doses (separated by 4 weeks or longer) to children younger than 9 years who are receiving influenza vaccine for the first time or who were vaccinated for the first time last season but only received one dose.
- For healthy nonpregnant persons (those who do not have underlying medical conditions that predispose them to influenza complications) ages 2–49 years, either LAIV or TIV may be used.

6. Hepatitis A vaccine (HepA).

- Administer the 2 doses in the series at least 6 months apart.
- HepA is recommended for certain other groups of children, including in areas where vaccination programs target older children.

7. Hepatitis B vaccine (HepB).

- Administer the 3-dose series to those who were not previously vaccinated.
- A 2-dose series of Recombivax HB® is licensed for children aged 11–15 years.

8. Inactivated poliovirus vaccine (IPV).

- For children who received an all-IPV or all-oral poliovirus (OPV) series, a fourth dose is not necessary if the third dose was administered at age 4 years or older.
- If both OPV and IPV were administered as part of a series, a total of 4 doses should be administered, regardless of the child's current age.

9. Measles, mumps, and rubella vaccine (MMR).

- If not previously vaccinated, administer 2 doses of MMR during any visit, with 4 or more weeks between the doses.

10. Varicella vaccine.

- Administer 2 doses of varicella vaccine to persons younger than 13 years of age at least 3 months apart. Do not repeat the second dose if administered 28 or more days following the first dose.
- Administer 2 doses of varicella vaccine to persons aged 13 years or older at least 4 weeks apart.

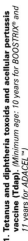

The Recommended Immunization Schedules for Persons Aged 0–18 Years are approved by the Advisory Committee on Immunization Practices (www.cdc.gov/vaccines/recs/acip), the American Academy of Pediatrics (http://www.aap.org), and the American Academy of Family Physicians (http://www.aafp.org).

DEPARTMENT OF HEALTH AND HUMAN SERVICES • CENTERS FOR DISEASE CONTROL AND PREVENTION
SAFER • HEALTHIER • PEOPLE™

Courtesy of the Centers for Disease Control and Prevention, 2008.

Catch Up Immunization Schedule

Catch-up Immunization Schedule
UNITED STATES • 2008

for Persons Aged 4 Months–18 Years Who Start Late or Who Are More Than 1 Month Behind

The table below provides catch-up schedules and minimum intervals between doses for children whose vaccinations have been delayed. A vaccine series does not need to be restarted, regardless of the time that has elapsed between doses. Use the section appropriate for the child's age.

CATCH-UP SCHEDULE FOR PERSONS AGED 4 MONTHS–6 YEARS

Vaccine	Minimum Age for Dose 1	Minimum Interval Between Doses			
		Dose 1 to Dose 2	Dose 2 to Dose 3	Dose 3 to Dose 4	Dose 4 to Dose 5
Hepatitis B[1]	Birth	4 weeks	8 weeks (and 16 weeks after first dose)		
Rotavirus[2]	6 wks	4 weeks	4 weeks		
Diphtheria, Tetanus, Pertussis[3]	6 wks	4 weeks	4 weeks	6 months	6 months[3]
Haemophilus influenzae type b[4]	6 wks	4 weeks if first dose administered at younger than 12 months of age **8 weeks (as final dose)** if first dose administered at age 12-14 months **No further doses needed** if first dose administered at 15 months of age or older	4 weeks[4] if current age is younger than 12 months **8 weeks (as final dose)**[4] if current age is 12 months or older and second dose administered at younger than 15 months of age **No further doses needed** if previous dose administered at age 15 months or older	**8 weeks (as final dose)** This dose only necessary for children aged 12 months–5 years who received 3 doses before age 12 months	
Pneumococcal[5]	6 wks	4 weeks if first dose administered at younger than 12 months of age **8 weeks (as final dose)** if first dose administered at age 12 months or older or current age 24-59 months **No further doses needed** for healthy children if first dose administered at age 24 months or older	4 weeks if current age is younger than 12 months **8 weeks (as final dose)** if current age is 12 months or older **No further doses needed** for healthy children if previous dose administered at age 24 months or older	**8 weeks (as final dose)** This dose only necessary for children aged 12 months–5 years who received 3 doses before age 12 months	
Inactivated Poliovirus[6]	6 wks	4 weeks	4 weeks	4 weeks[6]	
Measles, Mumps, Rubella[7]	12 mos	4 weeks			
Varicella[8]	12 mos	3 months			
Hepatitis A[9]	12 mos	6 months			

CS113897

CATCH-UP SCHEDULE FOR PERSONS AGED 7–18 YEARS

Vaccine	Minimum Age for Dose 1	Dose 1 to Dose 2	Dose 2 to Dose 3	Dose 3 to Booster Dose
Tetanus, Diphtheria/ Tetanus, Diphtheria, Pertussis[10]	7 yrs[10]	4 weeks	4 weeks if first dose administered at younger than 12 months of age / 6 months if first dose administered at age 12 months or older (and 24 weeks after the first dose)	6 months if first dose administered at younger than 12 months of age
Human Papillomavirus[11]	9 yrs	4 weeks	12 weeks	
Hepatitis A[9]	12 mos	6 months		
Hepatitis B[1]	Birth	4 weeks	8 weeks (and 16 weeks after first dose)	
Inactivated Poliovirus[6]	6 wks	4 weeks	4 weeks	4 weeks[6]
Measles, Mumps, Rubella[7]	12 mos	4 weeks		
Varicella[8]	12 mos	3 months if first dose administered at younger than 13 years of age / 4 weeks if first dose administered at age 13 years or older		

1. Hepatitis B vaccine (HepB).
- Administer the 3-dose series to those who were not previously vaccinated.
- A 2-dose series of Recombivax HB® is licensed for children aged 11–15 years.

2. Rotavirus vaccine (Rota).
- Do not start the series later than age 12 weeks.
- Administer the final dose in the series by age 32 weeks.
- Do not administer a dose later than age 32 weeks.
- Data on safety and efficacy outside of these age ranges are insufficient.

3. Diphtheria and tetanus toxoids and acellular pertussis vaccine (DTaP).
- The fifth dose is not necessary if the fourth dose was administered at age 4 years or older.
- DTaP is not indicated for persons aged 7 years or older.

4. Haemophilus influenzae type b conjugate vaccine (Hib).
- Vaccine is not generally recommended for children aged 5 years or older.
- If current age is younger than 12 months and the first 2 doses were PRP-OMP (PedvaxHIB® or ComVax® [Merck]), the third (and final) dose should be administered at age 12–15 months and at least 8 weeks after the second dose.
- If first dose was administered at age 7–11 months, administer 2 doses separated by 4 weeks plus a booster at age 12–15 months.

5. Pneumococcal conjugate vaccine (PCV).
- Administer one dose of PCV to all healthy children aged 24–59 months having any incomplete schedule.
- For children with underlying medical conditions, administer 2 doses of PCV at least 8 weeks apart if previously received less than 3 doses, or 1 dose of PCV if previously received 3 doses.

6. Inactivated poliovirus vaccine (IPV).
- For children who received an all-IPV or all-oral poliovirus (OPV) series, a fourth dose is not necessary if third dose was administered at age 4 years or older.

- If both OPV and IPV were administered as part of a series, a total of 4 doses should be administered, regardless of the child's current age.
- IPV is not routinely recommended for persons aged 18 years and older.

7. Measles, mumps, and rubella vaccine (MMR).
- The second dose of MMR is recommended routinely at age 4–6 years but may be administered earlier if desired.
- If not previously vaccinated, administer 2 doses of MMR during any visit with 4 or more weeks between the doses.

8. Varicella vaccine.
- The second dose of varicella vaccine is recommended routinely at age 4–6 years but may be administered earlier if desired.
- Do not repeat the second dose in persons younger than 13 years of age if administered 28 or more days after the first dose.

9. Hepatitis A vaccine (HepA).
- HepA is recommended for certain groups of children, including in areas where vaccination programs target older children. See MMWR 2006;55(No. RR-7);1–23.

10. Tetanus and diphtheria toxoids vaccine (Td) and tetanus and diphtheria toxoids and acellular pertussis vaccine (Tdap).
- Tdap should be substituted for a single dose of Td in the primary catch-up series or as a booster if age appropriate; use Td for other doses.
- A 5-year interval from the last Td dose is encouraged when Tdap is used as a booster dose. A booster (fourth) dose is needed if any of the previous doses were administered at younger than 12 months of age. Refer to ACIP recommendations for further information. See MMWR 2006;55(No. RR-3).

11. Human papillomavirus vaccine (HPV).
- Administer the HPV vaccine series to females at age 13–18 years if not previously vaccinated.

Information about reporting reactions after immunization is available online at http://www.vaers.hhs.gov or by telephone via the 24-hour national toll-free information line 800-822-7967. Suspected cases of vaccine-preventable diseases should be reported to the state or local health department. Additional information, including precautions and contraindications for immunization, is available from the National Center for Immunization and Respiratory Diseases at http://www.cdc.gov/vaccines or telephone, 800-CDC-INFO (800-232-4636).

DEPARTMENT OF HEALTH AND HUMAN SERVICES • CENTERS FOR DISEASE CONTROL AND PREVENTION • SAFER • HEALTHIER • PEOPLE

Courtesy of the Centers for Disease Control and Prevention, 2008.

COMMON CONVERSIONS

Weight/Volume

1 kg = 1000 grams
1 gram = 1000 mg
1 mg = 1000 mcg
1 mcg = 0.001 mg
1 liter = 1000 mL

Weight

1 gram = 15 gr
1 gr = 60 mg
0.6 mg = 1/100 gr
0.4 mg = 1/150 gr
0.3 mg = 1/200 gr
1 kg = 2.2 lb.

Volume

1 qt. = 960 mL
4 fl. oz. = 120 mL
1 fl. oz. = 30 mL
1 tsp. = 5 mL (approximate)
1 tbs. = 15 mL (approximate)
2 tbs. = 30 mL (approximate)

Body Temperature Conversions (Celsius to Fahrenheit)

CELSIUS	FAHRENHEIT	CELSIUS	FAHRENHEIT
34.0	93.2	38.4	101.1
34.2	93.6	38.6	101.4
34.4	93.9	38.8	101.8
34.6	94.3	39.0	102.2
34.8	94.6	39.2	102.5
35.0	95.0	39.4	102.9
35.2	95.4	39.6	103.2
35.4	95.7	39.8	103.6
35.6	96.1	40.0	104.0
35.8	96.4	40.2	104.3
36.0	96.8	40.4	104.7
36.2	97.1	40.6	105.1
36.4	97.5	40.8	105.4
36.6	97.8	41.0	105.8
36.8	98.2	41.2	106.1
		41.4	106.5
37.0	98.6	41.6	106.8
37.2	98.9	41.8	107.2
37.4	99.3	42.0	107.6
37.6	99.6	42.2	108.0
37.8	100.0	42.4	108.3
38.0	100.4	42.6	108.7
38.2	100.7	42.8	109.0

Conversion formulas:

Fahrenheit to Celsius $(°F - 32) \times (5/9) = °C$

Celsius to Fahrenheit $(°C) \times (9/5) + 32 = °F$

Pediatric Weight Conversion (Pounds to Kilograms)

POUNDS	0	1	2	3	4	5	6	7	8	9
0	0.00	0.45	0.90	1.36	1.81	2.26	2.72	3.17	3.62	4.08
10	4.53	4.98	5.44	5.89	6.35	6.80	7.35	7.71	8.16	8.61
20	9.07	9.52	9.97	10.43	10.88	11.34	11.79	12.24	12.70	13.15
30	13.60	14.06	14.51	14.96	15.42	15.87	16.32	16.78	17.23	17.69
40	18.14	18.59	19.05	19.50	19.95	20.41	20.86	21.31	21.77	22.22
50	22.68	23.13	23.58	24.04	24.49	24.94	25.40	25.85	26.30	26.76
60	27.21	27.66	28.22	28.57	29.03	29.48	29.93	30.39	30.84	31.29
70	31.75	32.20	32.65	33.11	33.56	34.02	34.47	34.92	35.38	35.83
80	36.28	36.74	37.19	37.64	38.10	38.55	39.00	39.46	39.93	40.37
90	40.82	41.27	41.73	42.18	42.63	43.09	43.54	43.99	44.45	44.90
100	45.36	45.81	46.26	46.72	47.17	47.62	48.08	48.53	48.98	49.44
110	49.89	50.34	50.80	51.25	51.71	52.16	52.61	53.07	53.52	53.97
120	54.43	54.88	55.33	55.79	56.24	56.70	57.15	57.60	58.06	58.51
130	58.96	59.42	59.87	60.32	60.78	61.23	61.68	62.14	62.59	63.05
140	63.50	63.95	64.41	64.86	65.31	65.77	66.22	66.67	67.13	67.58
150	68.04	68.49	68.94	69.40	69.85	70.30	70.76	71.21	71.66	72.12
160	72.57	73.02	73.48	73.93	74.39	74.84	75.29	75.75	76.20	76.62
170	77.11	77.56	78.01	78.47	78.92	79.38	79.83	80.28	80.74	81.19
180	81.64	82.10	82.55	83.00	83.46	83.91	84.36	84.82	85.27	85.73
190	86.18	86.68	87.09	87.54	87.99	88.45	88.90	89.35	89.81	90.26
200	90.72	91.17	91.62	92.08	92.53	92.98	93.44	93.89	94.34	94.80

Example: To determine the kilogram equivalent of 43 pounds, read 40 pounds on the vertical scale, read 3 pounds on the horizontal scale, then add. 43 pounds equals 19.5 kilograms.

ABBREVIATIONS

ABG	Arterial blood gas
ADHD	Attention deficit hyperactivity disorder
ADL	Activities of daily living
AHA	American Heart Association
AIDS	Acquired immunodeficiency syndrome
ALL	Acute lymphocytic (lymphoblastic) leukemia
AML	Acute myelocytic (myeloblastic) leukemia
AOM	Acute otitis media
AOME	Acute otitis media with effusion
ARF	Acute renal failure
AS	Aortic stenosis
ASD	Atrial septal defect
ATV	All-terrain vehicle
AZT	Zidovudine
BMT	Bone marrow transplant
BN	Bulimia nervosa
BP	Blood pressure
BPD	Bronchopulmonary dysplasia
BT shunt	Blalock-Taussig shunt
BUN	Blood urea nitrogen
CBC	Complete blood count
CD	Crohn's disease
CDC	Centers for Disease Control and Prevention
CF	Cystic fibrosis
CHAAD	Children and adults with attention deficit/hyperactivity disorder
CHD	Congenital heart defect
CHF	Congestive heart failure
CL	Cleft lip
CL/CP	Cleft lip/cleft palate
cm	Centimeter
CMV	Cytomegalovirus
CNS	Central nervous system
CP	Cerebral palsy
CPT	Chest physiotherapy
CRF	Chronic renal failure
CRRT	Continuous renal replacement therapy
CSF	Cerebrospinal fluid
CT	Computed tomography
CVA	Cerebral vascular accident
CVAD	Central venous access device
CVVH	Continuous veno-venous hemofiltration
dB	Decibel

DD ....Developmentally delayed
DDAVP ....Desmopressin acetate
DDH ....Developmental dysplasia of the hip
DEET ....N-N-diethyl-M-toluamide
DI ....Diabetes insipidus
DIC ....Disseminated intravascular coagulation
dL ....Deciliter
DM ....Diabetes mellitus
DNA ....Deoxyribonucleic acid
DS ....Down syndrome
DtaP ....Diphtheria toxoid, tetanus toxoid, acellular pertussis vaccine
EA..Esophageal atresia
EBV ....Epstein-Barr virus
ECF ....Extracellular fluid
ECG..Electrocardiogram
ECHO ....Echocardiogram
ED ....Emergency department
EDH ....Epidural hematoma
EEG ....Electroencephalogram
ELISA...Enzyme-linked immunosorbent assay
EMLA..Eutectic mixture of local anesthetics
ES ....Ewing's sarcoma
ESR ....Erythrocyte sedimentation rate
ESRD ....End-stage renal disease
FA...Fanconi's anemia
FBA ....Foreign body aspiration
FDA...Food and Drug Administration
FTT ....Failure to thrive
GCS...Glasgow Coma Scale
G&D ....Growth and development
GER...Gastroesophageal reflux
GFR...Glomerular filtration rate
GI ....Gastrointestinal
GN...Glomerulonephritis
gr ....Grain
HAART ....Highly active antiretroviral therapy
HAV...Hepatitis A
Hb S ....Hemoglobin S
HBV ....Hepatitis B
Hct ....Hematocrit
HCV ....Hepatitis C
HD ....Hemodialysis
HD ....Hirschsprung's disease
Hep B ....Hepatitis B vaccine
HIB ....*Haemophilus influenzae* Type B
HIV ....Human immunodeficiency virus
HLHS...Hypoplastic left heart syndrome
HPV ....Human papilloma virus

HR..Heart rate
HUS ....Hemolytic uremic syndrome
HSV-1...Herpex simplex type 1
HSV-2...Herpex simplex type 2
IBD ....Inflammatory bowel disease
ICF ....Intracellular fluid
ICH ....Intracranial hemorrhage
ICHF...International Children's Heart
                                                       Foundation
ICP ....Intracranial pressure
IDA ....Iron deficiency anemia
IgA..Immunoglobulin A
IgD ....Immunoglobulin D
IgE..Immunoglobulin E
IgG ....Immunoglobulin G
IgM...Immunoglobulin M
IM ....Intramuscular
INR ....International normalized ratio
IPV ....Inactivated polio vaccine
ISHLT ....International Society for Heart & Lung
                                                       Transplantation
ITP ....Idiopathic thrombocytopenia purpura; immune
                                                       thrombocytopenia purpura
IV ....Intravenous
IVIG ....Intravenous immunoglobulin
IVP ....Intravenous pyelogram
JA..Juvenile arthritis
JRA..Juvenile rheumatoid arthritis
KD...Kawasaki disease
kg...Kilogram
LA...Left atrium
LES...Lower esophageal sphincter
LV ....Left ventricle
mcg...Microgram
MD...Muscular dystrophy
MDI ....Metered dose inhaler
mg ....Milligram
mL...Milliliter
MMR..Measles-mumps-rubella (vaccine)
MR ....Mental retardation
MRA...Magnetic resonance angiography
MRI..Magnetic resonance imaging
MVA..Motor vehicle accident
MVC...Motor vehicle crash
NAMI ....National Alliance on Mental Illness
ND ....Nasoduodenal
NEC ....Necrotizing enterocolitis
NG..Nasogastric
NHL..Non-Hodgkin's lymphoma

NHLBI	National Heart Lung and Blood Institute (of the National Institutes of Health)
NICHCY	National Dissemination Center for Children with Disabilities
NICU	Neonatal intensive care unit
NIGMS	National Institute of General Medical Sciences (of the National Institutes of Health)
NIH	National Institutes of Health
NINDS	National Institute of Neurological Disorders and Stroke
NLM	National Library of Medicine (of National Institutes of Health)
NOFTT	Non-organic failure to thrive
NPO	Nothing by mouth/nothing per OS
NS	Nephrotic syndrome
NS	Normal saline
NSAID	Nonsteroidal anti-inflammatory drug
OFTT	Organic failure to thrive
OI	Osteogenesis imperfecta
OM	Otitis media
OME	Otitis media with effusion
OPV	Oral polio vaccine
ORS	Oral rehydration solution
ORT	Oral rehydration therapy
OS	Osteogenic sarcoma
PA	Pulmonary artery
PCA	Patient-controlled analgesia
PCC	Poison Control Center
PD	Peritoneal dialysis
PDA	Patent ductus arteriosus
PICU	Pediatric intensive care unit
PPD	Purified protein derivative
PPN	Peripheral parenteral nutrition
PS	Pulmonary stenosis
PT	Prothrombin time
PTT	Partial thromboplastin time
RA	Right atrium
RAD	Reactive airway disease
RBC	Red blood cell; red blood count
RDS	Respiratory distress syndrome
RMSF	Rocky Mountain spotted fever
RR	Respiratory rate
RSV	Respiratory syncytial virus
R/T	Related to
RV	Right ventricle
SA	Sinoatrial
SAH	Subarachnoid hemorrhage
SaO_2	Oxygen saturation
SBS	Shaken-baby syndrome

SC...Subcutaneous
SCA ....Sickle cell anemia
SCD..Sickle cell disease
SDH ....Subdural hematoma
SIDS..Sudden infant death syndrome
SLE..Systemic lupus erythematosus
SSRI ....Selective serotonin reuptake inhibitor
STD...Sexually transmitted disease
TBI ....Traumatic brain injury
TBSA..Total body surface area
TCDB..Traumatic Coma Data Bank
Td..Tetanus toxoid
TEACCH.......................................Treatment and Education of Autistic and Related
                                                           Communication-Handicapped Children
TEF ....Tracheoesophageal fistula
TIBC ....Total iron binding capacity
TM ....Tympanic membrane
TOF...Tetralogy of Fallot
TPN...Total parenteral nutrition
UA ....Urinalysis
UC..Ulcerative colitis
UNOS ....United Network for Organ Sharing
URI ....Upper respiratory infection
Urine C&S ....Urine culture and sensitivity
UTI..Urinary tract infection
VA Shunt.......................................Ventriculoatrial shunt
VP Shunt.......................................Ventriculoperitoneal shunt
VSD...Ventricular septal defect
VUR ....Vesicoureteral reflux
WBC ....White blood cell; white blood count
WNL ....Within normal limits
WDL ....Within defined limits
WHO ....World Health Organization

Suggested Readings

Autism Speaks. (2007). Retrieved April 14, 2008, from http://www.autismspeaks.org

Avery, R. A., Frank, G., Glutting, J. J., & Eppes, S. C. (2006). Prediction of Lyme meningitis in children from Lyme disease-endemic regions: A logistic-regression model using history, physical and laboratory findings. *Pediatrics, 117*(1).

Baumann, B. M., Welsh, B. E., Rogers, C. J., & Newbury, K. (2008). Nursing using volumetric bladder ultrasound in the pediatric ED. *American Journal of Nursing, 108*(4).

Beard-Pfeuffer, M. (2008). Understanding the world of children with autism. *RN, 71*(2).

Beattie, S. (2007). Hands-on help: Bone marrow aspiration and biopsy. *RN, 70*(2).

Briguglio, A. (2007). Should the family stay? *RN, 70*(5).

Broyles, B. E., Reiss, B. S., & Evans, M. E. (2007). *Pharmacological aspects of nursing care* (7th ed.). Clifton Park, NY: Delmar Cengage Learning.

Chiafery, M. (2006). Care and management of the child with shunted hydrocephalus. *Pediatric Nursing, 32*(3).

Chiocca, E. M. (2006). Action stat: Pertussis. *Nursing, 36*(7).

Clinical rounds: News, updates, research. (2007). *Nursing, 37*(6).

Colby-Graham, M. F., & Chordas, C. (2003). The childhood leukemias. *Journal of Pediatric Nursing, 18*(2).

Delahanty, K. M., & Myer, F. E. (2007). Nursing 2007 infection control survey report. *Nursing, 37*(6).

Dest, V. (2006). Drug watch '06: Cancer therapies. *RN, 69*(6).

Down Syndrome Information Network. (2007). Retrieved February 16, 2007 from http://www.down-syndrome.org

Dunne, E. F., Unger, E. R., Sternberg, M., McQuillan, G., Swan, D. C., Patel, S. S., & Markowitz, L. E. (2007). Prevalence of HPV infection among females in the United States. *JAMA, 297*(8).

Fagley, M. U. (2007). Taking charge of a seizure. *Nursing, 37*(9).

Fink, J. L. (2007). Pacifiers help prevent SIDS. *RN, 70*(11).

Gallon, H. J., Armstrong, B. G., & Fiese, M. A. (2006). Before you give that vaccination . . . . *Nursing, 36*(11).

Gardner, J. (2007). What you need to know about cystic fibrosis. *Nursing, 37*(7).

Gardner, J. (2008). Combating infection: Viral croup in children. *Nursing, 38*(4).

Hydrocephalus Association (2007). Retrieved April 14, 2008, from http://www.hydroassoc.org/

Hydrocephalus Foundation, Inc. (2007) Retrieved April 15, 2008, from http://www.hydrocephalus.org/

Johnson, M., Bulechek, G., Burcher, H., Dochterman, J. M., Maas, M., Moorhead, S., & Swanson, E. (2006). *NANDA, NOC, and NIC linkages: Nursing diagnoses, outcomes, & interventions*. St. Louis, MO: Elsevier Mosby.

Kawasaki Disease Foundation. (2004). Retrieved March 17, 2007, from http://www.kdfoundation.org

King, J. E. (2007). Does my patient have ulcerative colitis or Crohn's disease? *Nursing, 37*(3).

Krueger, A. (2007). Need help finding a vein? *Nursing, 37*(6).

Kyles, D. (2007). Is your patient having a transfusion reaction? *Nursing, 37*(4).

Laskowski-Jones, L. (2006). First aid for burns. *Nursing, 36*(1).

Laskowski-Jones, L. (2006). First aid for sprains. *Nursing, 36*(8).

Laskowski-Jones, L. (2007). Should families be present during resuscitation? *Nursing, 37*(5).

Lauts, N. M. (2005). RSV: Protecting the littlest patients. *RN, 68*(12).

Leung-Chen, P. (2008). Emerging infections: Syphilis makes another comeback. *American Journal of Nursing, 108*(2).

March of Dimes. (2007). *Down syndrome*. Retrieved April 15, 2008, from http://www.marchofdimes.com/pnhec/4439_1214.asp

Matthews, C., Miller, L., & Mott, M. (2007). Getting ahead of acute meningitis & encephalitis. *Nursing, 37*(11).

Mennick, F. (2008). Adolescent depression: Recipe for success. *American Journal of Nursing, 108*(2).

Miller, E. R., Iskander, J., Pickering, S., & Varricchio, F. (2007). How can you promote vaccine safety? *Nursing, 37*(4).

NANDA International. (2007). NANDA Nursing diagnoses: Definitions & classifications 2007–2008. Author.

National Dissemination Center for Children with Disabilities. (2004). *Spina bifida fact sheet*. Retrieved April 15, 2008, from http://www.nichcy.org/pubs/factshe/fs12txt.htm

Nowlin, A. (2006). The delicate business of burn care. *RN, 69*(1).

Nunnelee, J. D. (2007). Snakebite! How do you know then it's poisonous. *RN, 70*(9).

Pediatric Fractures. (2006). *Fractures in children: Broken bones*. Retrieved February 27, 2007, from http://www.fracturesinchildren.org/index.htm

Pittman, H. J. (2008). Action stat: Rattlesnake bite. *Nursing, 38*(4).

Prevent Child Abuse America. (2008). Retrieved April 15, 2008, from http://www.preventchildabuse.org/index.shtml

Rice, D. (2008). Lullaby for Ferd. *Nursing, 38*(2).

Sakakeeny-Zaal, K. (2007). Emergency: Pediatric orthopnea and total airway obstruction. *American Journal of Nursing, 107*(4).

Salati, D. S. (2006). Responding to foreign-body airway obstruction. *Nursing, 36*(12).

Spina Bifida Association. (2008). *Fact sheets*. Retrieved April 15, 2008, from http://www.spinabifidaassociation.org/site/c.liKWL7PLLrF/b.2642343/k.8D2D/Fact_Sheets.htm

Stocker, P. K. (2005). Touched by an angel. *Nursing, 35*(5).

Thomas, D. O. (2007). Let the family in. *RN, 70*(5).

Thorne, A. (2007). Are you ready to give care to a child with autism? *Nursing, 37*(5).

UNICEF. (2007). *Children with HIV and AIDS.* Retrieved April 15, 2008, from http://www.unicef.org/aids/index.php

Zeigler, S. A. (2007). Prevent dangerous hemodialysis catheter disconnections. *Nursing, 37*(3).

INDEX

Page numbers followed by a "t" or "f" indicate that the entry is included in a table or figure.

DATE DUE | DATE DUE